PULMONARY EDEMA

LUNG BIOLOGY IN HEALTH AND DISEASE

Executive Editor

Claude Lenfant
Director, National Heart, Lung and Blood Institute
National Institutes of Health
Bethesda, Maryland

1. Immunologic and Infectious Reactions in the Lung, *edited by Charles H. Kirkpatrick and Herbert Y. Reynolds*
2. The Biochemical Basis of Pulmonary Function, *edited by Ronald G. Crystal*
3. Bioengineering Aspects of the Lung, *edited by John B. West*
4. Metabolic Functions of the Lung, *edited by Y. S. Bakhle and John R. Vane*
5. Respiratory Defense Mechanisms (in two parts), *edited by Joseph D. Brain, Donald F. Proctor, and Lynne M. Reid*
6. Development of the Lung, *edited by W. Alan Hodson*
7. Lung Water and Solute Exchange, *edited by Norman C. Staub*
8. Extrapulmonary Manifestations of Respiratory Disease, *edited by Eugene Debs Robin*
9. Chronic Obstructive Pulmonary Disease, *edited by Thomas L. Petty*
10. Pathogenesis and Therapy of Lung Cancer, *edited by Curtis C. Harris*
11. Genetic Determinants of Pulmonary Disease, *edited by Stephen D. Litwin*
12. The Lung in the Transition Between Health and Disease, *edited by Peter T. Macklem and Solbert Permutt*
13. Evolution of Respiratory Processes: A Comparative Approach, *edited by Stephen C. Wood and Claude Lenfant*
14. Pulmonary Vascular Diseases, *edited by Kenneth M. Moser*
15. Physiology and Pharmacology of the Airways, *edited by Jay A. Nadel*
16. Diagnostic Techniques in Pulmonary Disease (in two parts), *edited by Marvin A. Sackner*
17. Regulation of Breathing (in two parts), *edited by Thomas F. Hornbein*
18. Occupational Lung Diseases: Research Approaches and Methods, *edited by Hans Weill and Margaret Turner-Warwick*
19. Immunopharmacology of the Lung, *edited by Harold H. Newball*
20. Sarcoidosis and Other Granulomatous Diseases of the Lung, *edited by Barry L. Fanburg*

21. Sleep and Breathing, *edited by Nicholas A. Saunders and Colin E. Sullivan*
22. *Pneumocystis carinii* Pneumonia: Pathogenesis, Diagnosis, and Treatment, *edited by Lowell S. Young*
23. Pulmonary Nuclear Medicine: Techniques in Diagnosis of Lung Disease, *edited by Harold L. Atkins*
24. Acute Respiratory Failure, *edited by Warren M. Zapol and Konrad J. Falke*
25. Gas Mixing and Distribution in the Lung, *edited by Ludwig A. Engel and Manuel Paiva*
26. High-Frequency Ventilation in Intensive Care and During Surgery, *edited by Graziano Carlon and William S. Howland*
27. Pulmonary Development: Transition from Intrauterine to Extrauterine Life, *edited by George H. Nelson*
28. Chronic Obstructive Pulmonary Disease: Second Edition, Revised and Expanded, *edited by Thomas L. Petty*
29. The Thorax (in two parts), *edited by Charis Roussos and Peter T. Macklem*
30. The Pleura in Health and Disease, *edited by Jacques Chrétien, Jean Bignon, and Albert Hirsch*
31. Drug Therapy for Asthma: Research and Clinical Practice, *edited by John W. Jenne and Shirley Murphy*
32. Pulmonary Endothelium in Health and Disease, *edited by Una S. Ryan*
33. The Airways: Neural Control in Health and Disease, *edited by Michael A. Kaliner and Peter J. Barnes*
34. Pathophysiology and Treatment of Inhalation Injuries, *edited by Jacob Loke*
35. Respiratory Function of the Upper Airway, *edited by Oommen P. Mathew and Giuseppe Sant'Ambrogio*
36. Chronic Obstructive Pulmonary Disease: A Behavioral Perspective, *edited by A. John McSweeny and Igor Grant*
37. Biology of Lung Cancer: Diagnosis and Treatment, *edited by Steven T. Rosen, James L. Mulshine, Frank Cuttitta, and Paul G. Abrams*
38. Pulmonary Vascular Physiology and Pathophysiology, *edited by E. Kenneth Weir and John T. Reeves*
39. Comparative Pulmonary Physiology: Current Concepts, *edited by Stephen C. Wood*
40. Respiratory Physiology: An Analytical Approach, *edited by H. K. Chang and Manuel Paiva*
41. Lung Cell Biology, *edited by Donald Massaro*
42. Heart–Lung Interactions in Health and Disease, *edited by Steven M. Scharf and Sharon S. Cassidy*
43. Clinical Epidemiology of Chronic Obstructive Pulmonary Disease, *edited by Michael J. Hensley and Nicholas A. Saunders*
44. Surgical Pathology of Lung Neoplasms, *edited by Alberto M. Marchevsky*
45. The Lung in Rheumatic Diseases, *edited by Grant W. Cannon and Guy A. Zimmerman*

46. Diagnostic Imaging of the Lung, *edited by Charles E. Putman*
47. Models of Lung Disease: Microscopy and Structural Methods, *edited by Joan Gil*
48. Electron Microscopy of the Lung, *edited by Dean E. Schraufnagel*
49. Asthma: Its Pathology and Treatment, *edited by Michael A. Kaliner, Peter J. Barnes, and Carl G. A. Persson*
50. Acute Respiratory Failure: Second Edition, *edited by Warren M. Zapol and Francois Lemaire*
51. Lung Disease in the Tropics, *edited by Om P. Sharma*
52. Exercise: Pulmonary Physiology and Pathophysiology, *edited by Brian J. Whipp and Karlman Wasserman*
53. Developmental Neurobiology of Breathing, *edited by Gabriel G. Haddad and Jay P. Farber*
54. Mediators of Pulmonary Inflammation, *edited by Michael A. Bray and Wayne H. Anderson*
55. The Airway Epithelium, *edited by Stephen G. Farmer and Douglas Hay*
56. Physiological Adaptations in Vertebrates: Respiration, Circulation, and Metabolism, *edited by Stephen C. Wood, Roy E. Weber, Alan R. Hargens, and Ronald W. Millard*
57. The Bronchial Circulation, *edited by John Butler*
58. Lung Cancer Differentiation: Implications for Diagnosis and Treatment, *edited by Samuel D. Bernal and Paul J. Hesketh*
59. Pulmonary Complications of Systemic Disease, *edited by John F. Murray*
60. Lung Vascular Injury: Molecular and Cellular Response, *edited by Arnold Johnson and Thomas J. Ferro*
61. Cytokines of the Lung, *edited by Jason Kelley*
62. The Mast Cell in Health and Disease, *edited by Michael A. Kaliner and Dean D. Metcalfe*
63. Pulmonary Disease in the Elderly Patient, *edited by Donald A. Mahler*
64. Cystic Fibrosis, *edited by Pamela B. Davis*
65. Signal Transduction in Lung Cells, *edited by Jerome S. Brody, David M. Center, and Vsevolod A. Tkachuk*
66. Tuberculosis: A Comprehensive International Approach, *edited by Lee B. Reichman and Earl S. Hershfield*
67. Pharmacology of the Respiratory Tract: Experimental and Clinical Research, *edited by K. Fan Chung and Peter J. Barnes*
68. Prevention of Respiratory Diseases, *edited by Albert Hirsch, Marcel Goldberg, Jean-Pierre Martin, and Roland Masse*
69. *Pneumocystis carinii* Pneumonia: Second Edition, Revised and Expanded, *edited by Peter D. Walzer*
70. Fluid and Solute Transport in the Airspaces of the Lungs, *edited by Richard M. Effros and H. K. Chang*
71. Sleep and Breathing: Second Edition, Revised and Expanded, *edited by Nicholas A. Saunders and Colin E. Sullivan*
72. Airway Secretion: Physiological Bases for the Control of Mucous Hypersecretion, *edited by Tamotsu Takishima and Sanae Shimura*

73. Sarcoidosis and Other Granulomatous Disorders, *edited by D. Geraint James*
74. Epidemiology of Lung Cancer, *edited by Jonathan M. Samet*
75. Pulmonary Embolism, *edited by Mario Morpurgo*
76. Sports and Exercise Medicine, *edited by Stephen C. Wood and Robert C. Roach*
77. Endotoxin and the Lungs, *edited by Kenneth L. Brigham*
78. The Mesothelial Cell and Mesothelioma, *edited by Marie-Claude Jaurand and Jean Bignon*
79. Regulation of Breathing: Second Edition, Revised and Expanded, *edited by Jerome A. Dempsey and Allan I. Pack*
80. Pulmonary Fibrosis, *edited by Sem Hin Phan and Roger S. Thrall*
81. Long-Term Oxygen Therapy: Scientific Basis and Clinical Application, *edited by Walter J. O'Donohue, Jr.*
82. Ventral Brainstem Mechanisms and Control of Respiration and Blood Pressure, *edited by C. Ovid Trouth, Richard M. Millis, Heidrun F. Kiwull-Schöne, and Marianne E. Schläfke*
83. A History of Breathing Physiology, *edited by Donald F. Proctor*
84. Surfactant Therapy for Lung Disease, *edited by Bengt Robertson and H. William Taeusch*
85. The Thorax: Second Edition, Revised and Expanded (in three parts), *edited by Charis Roussos*
86. Severe Asthma: Pathogenesis and Clinical Management, *edited by Stanley J. Szefler and Donald Y. M. Leung*
87. *Mycobacterium avium*–Complex Infection: Progress in Research and Treatment, *edited by Joyce A. Korvick and Constance A. Benson*
88. Alpha 1–Antitrypsin Deficiency: Biology • Pathogenesis • Clinical Manifestations • Therapy, *edited by Ronald G. Crystal*
89. Adhesion Molecules and the Lung, *edited by Peter A. Ward and Joseph C. Fantone*
90. Respiratory Sensation, *edited by Lewis Adams and Abraham Guz*
91. Pulmonary Rehabilitation, *edited by Alfred P. Fishman*
92. Acute Respiratory Failure in Chronic Obstructive Pulmonary Disease, *edited by Jean-Philippe Derenne, William A. Whitelaw, and Thomas Similowski*
93. Environmental Impact on the Airways: From Injury to Repair, *edited by Jacques Chrétien and Daniel Dusser*
94. Inhalation Aerosols: Physical and Biological Basis for Therapy, *edited by Anthony J. Hickey*
95. Tissue Oxygen Deprivation: From Molecular to Integrated Function, *edited by Gabriel G. Haddad and George Lister*
96. The Genetics of Asthma, *edited by Stephen B. Liggett and Deborah A. Meyers*
97. Inhaled Glucocorticoids in Asthma: Mechanisms and Clinical Actions, *edited by Robert P. Schleimer, William W. Busse, and Paul M. O'Byrne*
98. Nitric Oxide and the Lung, *edited by Warren M. Zapol and Kenneth D. Bloch*

99. Primary Pulmonary Hypertension, *edited by Lewis J. Rubin and Stuart Rich*
100. Lung Growth and Development, *edited by John A. McDonald*
101. Parasitic Lung Diseases, *edited by Adel A. F. Mahmoud*
102. Lung Macrophages and Dendritic Cells in Health and Disease, *edited by Mary F. Lipscomb and Stephen W. Russell*
103. Pulmonary and Cardiac Imaging, *edited by Caroline Chiles and Charles E. Putman*
104. Gene Therapy for Diseases of the Lung, *edited by Kenneth L. Brigham*
105. Oxygen, Gene Expression, and Cellular Function, *edited by Linda Biadasz Clerch and Donald J. Massaro*
106. $Beta_2$-Agonists in Asthma Treatment, *edited by Romain Pauwels and Paul M. O'Byrne*
107. Inhalation Delivery of Therapeutic Peptides and Proteins, *edited by Akwete Lex Adjei and Pramod K. Gupta*
108. Asthma in the Elderly, *edited by Robert A. Barbee and John W. Bloom*
109. Treatment of the Hospitalized Cystic Fibrosis Patient, *edited by David M. Orenstein and Robert C. Stern*
110. Asthma and Immunological Diseases in Pregnancy and Early Infancy, *edited by Michael Schatz, Robert S. Zeiger, and Henry N. Claman*
111. Dyspnea, *edited by Donald A. Mahler*
112. Proinflammatory and Antiinflammatory Peptides, *edited by Sami I. Said*
113. Self-Management of Asthma, *edited by Harry Kotses and Andrew Harver*
114. Eicosanoids, Aspirin, and Asthma, *edited by Andrew Szczeklik, Ryszard J. Gryglewski, and John R. Vane*
115. Fatal Asthma, *edited by Albert L. Sheffer*
116. Pulmonary Edema, *edited by Michael A. Matthay and David H. Ingbar*
117. Inflammatory Mechanisms in Asthma, *edited by Stephen T. Holgate and William W. Busse*

ADDITIONAL VOLUMES IN PREPARATION

Biology of Lung Cancer, *edited by Madeleine A. Kane and Paul A. Bunn, Jr.*

The Lung at Depth, *edited by Claes Lundgren and John N. Miller*

Lung Tumors, *edited by Christian Brambilla and Elizabeth Brambilla*

Five-Lypoxygenase Products in Asthma, *edited by Jeffrey M. Drazen, Sven-Erik Dahlén, and Tak H. Lee*

Diagnostic Pulmonary Pathology, *edited by Philip Cagle*

Immunotherapy of Asthma, *edited by Jean Bousquet and Hans Yssel*

Rhinitis, *edited by Robert M. Naclerio, Stephen R. Durham, and Niels Mygind*

Interleukin-5: From Molecule to Drug Target for Asthma, *edited by Colin Sanderson*

Viral Infections of the Lung, *edited by Raphael Dolin and Peter F. Wright*

Pediatric Asthma, *edited by Shirley J. Murphy, H. William Kelly, and Bennie C. McWilliams*

LAM and Other Diseases Characterized by Smooth Muscle Proliferation, *edited by Joel Moss*

Control of Breathing in Health and Disease, *edited by Murray D. Altose and Yoshikazu Kawakami*

Physiological Basis of Ventilatory Support, *edited by John J. Marini and Arthur S. Slutsky*

Complexity in Structure and Function of the Lung, *edited by Michael P. Hlastala and H. Thomas Robertson*

Human Immunodeficiency Virus and the Lung, *edited by Mark J. Rosen and James M. Beck*

Neurobiology of Sleep and Circadian Rhythms, *edited by Fred Turek and Phyllis Zee*

PULMONARY EDEMA

Edited by

Michael A. Matthay

University of California at San Francisco
San Francisco, California

David H. Ingbar

University of Minnesota School of Medicine
Minneapolis, Minnesota

MARCEL DEKKER, INC. NEW YORK • BASEL • HONG KONG

Library of Congress Cataloging-in-Publication Data

Pulmonary edema / edited by Michael A. Matthay, David H. Ingbar.
p. cm. — (Lung biology in health and disease; v. 116)
Includes bibliographical references and index.
ISBN 0-8247-0150-X (alk. paper)
1. Pulmonary edema. I. Matthay, Michael A. II. Ingbar, David H. III. Series
[DNLM: 1. Pulmonary Edema. W1 LU62 v.116 1998 / WF 600
P98343029 1998]
RC776. P8P843 1998
616.2' 4—dc21
DNLM/DLC
for Library of Congress 98-3647
CIP

The publisher offers discounts on this book when ordered in bulk quantities. For more information, write to Special Sales/Professional Marketing at the address below.

This book is printed on acid-free paper.

MARCEL DEKKER, INC.
270 Madison Avenue, New York, New York 10016
http://www.dekker.com

Current printing (last digit):
10 9 8 7 6 5 4 3 2 1

PRINTED IN THE UNITED STATES OF AMERICA

INTRODUCTION

Heart–lung interactions have been the subject of intense research for a long time, in great part because a disruption of the normal interactions often results in life-threatening situations. The Lung Biology in Health and Disease series of monographs has acknowledged the importance of this area of investigation by including several volumes on either basic research studies or the clinical disorders resulting from disrupted heart–lung interactions.

The first volume addressing this topic appeared twenty years ago. It was titled *Lung Water and Solute Exchange* and was edited by Norman C. Staub, a giant in the field, whose important contributions paved the way for years of basic and clinical investigations in which his disciples have played a major role. In Dr. Staub's volume, the chapter "Lung Edema Due to Increased Vascular Permeability" by Kenneth Brigham discusses the foundation of pulmonary capillary permeability in health and disease.

Since then, enormous progress in understanding the mechanisms leading to pulmonary edema has been achieved. The new tools of molecular and cellular approaches have been used with talent and with success. Perhaps few fields of basic and clinical investigation illustrate as well that acquisition of new knowledge is a dynamic process in perpetual movement. From this, the beneficiaries are the patients. Indeed, today many patients with acute lung injury in which pulmonary edema is one of the manifestations survive, whereas twenty years ago they would have died. This success is a tribute to the research investigators in this field. However, much remains to be done if we are eventually to eliminate the toll of pulmonary edema and it consequences.

When Michael Matthay and David Ingbar decided to undertake the editing of this volume, they set out on a difficult and tortuous road, but they also knew that at the end of it was the potential for a major contribution to contemporary biomedical literature. There is no doubt that the potential has been fully realized . . . and more!

This monograph blends together fundamental and clinical research into a perfect state of the art! However, it does more, as it both implies and states important new questions that require attention and investigation. The editors have drawn on the expertise of leaders in the field. In a way, this volume is the "Who's Who" of pulmonary edema science.

The Lung Biology in Health and Disease series and its readership are privileged by the inclusion of this volume.

Claude Lenfant, M.D.
Bethesda, Maryland

PREFACE

Pulmonary edema is a major, life-threatening cause of acute respiratory failure in patients with acute and chronic cardiac failure as well as in patients with acute lung injury and the acute respiratory distress syndrome from sepsis, pneumonia, shock and trauma, aspiration syndromes, as well as several other clinical disorders. Between 1959 and 1985, several classical studies by Guyton, Staub, Fishman, Taylor and other investigors established the physiological basis for hydrostatic versus increased-permeability edema, thereby providing rational guidelines for the diagnosis and treatment of patients with pulmonary edema. In the last ten years there has been remarkable progress in understanding the molecular and cellular mechanisms responsible for the formation and resolution of pulmonary edema. Therefore, a comprehensive update on *Pulmonary Edema* is warranted to integrate these new insights into the classical understanding of the physiological basis for pulmonary edema.

This volume in the Lung Biology in Health and Disease series is designed to integrate progress in both basic science and clinical research and is organized into three sections: (1) general pathophysiology and clinical assessment, (2) specific etiologic syndromes, and (3) mechanisms of resolution and treatment. Most of the chapters consider pulmonary edema with some reference to selected aspects of the clinical problems posed by pulmonary edema, although the primary objective is to highlight new information regarding mechanisms that relate to the formation or resolution of pulmonary edema. Some of the chapters focus more on pathogenesis than treatment, while the final chapter is organized to integrate the new information on therapy, including possible new strategies to hasten the resolution of pulmonary edema.

In the first part, Chapters 1 and 2 provide a detailed update of the physiological and morphological basis for pulmonary edema. Chapters 3 and 4 present the radiographic, clinical, and laboratory features of pulmonary edema as they occur in critically ill patients.

In the second part on specific etiologies and syndromes, Chapter 5 discusses hydrostatic pulmonary edema, taking advantage of new information from novel animal modes. Chapter 6 provides an update on the mechanisms responsible for increased-permeability pulmonary edema from endotoxemia and septicemia, the most lethal cause of ARDS. Chapter 7 discusses how pneumonia, the second most important clinical cause of ARDS, leads to injury of both the endothelial and epithelial barriers of the lung. Chapter 8 reviews exciting new insights into the mechanisms that account for pulmonary edema following aspiration of low pH gastric contents, salt water, or fresh water. Chapter 9 provides integrated information on the mechanisms responsible for the development and clearance of pulmonary edema following hemorrhagic shock, a common cause of ARDS following major trauma. Chapter 10 discusses new insights into the mechanisms that lead to the formation and resolution of pulmonary edema in the setting of neurologic injury. Chapter 11 reviews the new information on the pathogenesis, prevention, and treatment of high-altitude pulmonary edema. Chapter 12 considers how ischemia and reperfusion can lead to increased-permeability pulmonary edema, a mechanism that is relevant for lung transplantation and probably other causes of pulmonary edema, including shock. Chapter 13 discusses new theories regarding how positive pressure ventilation, under some conditions, may amplify the degree of lung injury and pulmonary edema.

In the third part, on resolution and treatment, Chapters 14–17 provide a detailed discussion of the exciting new information on the mechanisms that regulate reabsorption of alveolar edema fluid in the adult lung, under both normal and pathological conditions. Chapter 18 discusses the potential role of aquaporins, the recently discovered transcellular water channels, in the formation and resolution of pulmonary edema. Although resolution of pulmonary edema fluid is sometimes considered simply to be a problem of fluid transport, the complete resolution requires removal of both the soluble and insoluble protein that has extravasated into the interstitium and distal airspaces of the lung. Therefore, Chapter 19 provides the latest information on the mechanisms responsible for removal of excess protein from the airspaces and interstitium of the lung. Finally, Chapter 20 discusses both current and future strategies for treatment of hydrostatic and increased-permeability pulmonary edema (ARDS) with an emphasis on the results of clinically relevant experimental work as well as phase II and III clinical studies.

We very much appreciate the hard work of each of the contributors to this edition, as well as the excellent editoral work provided by Moraima Suarez, Sandra Beberman, and Dr. Lenfant.

Michael A. Matthay
David H. Ingbar

CONTRIBUTORS

Denise R. Aberle, M.D. Professor and Chief of Thoracic Imaging, Department of Radiological Sciences, University of California at Los Angeles School of Medicine, Los Angeles, California

Kurt H. Albertine, Ph.D. Professor, Departments of Pediatrics, Medicine, and Neurobiology and Anatomy, University of Utah Health Sciences Center, Salt Lake City, Utah

Yves Berthiaume, M.D., M.Sc. Associate Professor, Department of Medicine, University of Montreal, Montreal, Quebec, Canada

Jahar Bhattacharya, M.D., D.Phil. Associate Professor, Department of Medicine, St. Luke's—Roosevelt Hospital Center, and Columbia College of Physicians and Surgeons, New York, New York

Kenneth L. Brigham, M.D. Professor, Department of Medicine, Vanderbilt University Medical Center, Nashville, Tennessee

Andre R. Campbell, M.D. Assistant Professor, Department of Surgery, University of California at San Francisco, San Francisco, California

Ethan P. Carter, Ph.D.* Research Physiologist, Cardiovascular Research Institute, University of California at San Francisco, San Francisco, California

Edward D. Crandall, Ph.D., M.D. Hastings Professor of Medicine and Norris Chair of Medicine, Will Rogers Institute Pulmonary Research Center, University of Southern California, Los Angeles, California

---

Current affiliation: Research Physiologist, Pulmonary Laboratory, Colorado Health Sciences Center, Denver, Colorado

Didier Dreyfuss, M.D. Professor of Medicine and Critical Care, Faculté Xavier Bichat, and Hôpital Louis Mourier, Paris, France

Michael D. DuVall, D.V.M., Ph.D. Postdoctoral Fellow, Department of Anesthesiology, University of Alabama at Birmingham, Birmingham, Alabama

Richard M. Effros, M.D. Professor and Division Chief, Pulmonary and Critical Care Medicine, Medical College of Wisconsin, Milwaukee, Wisconsin

Hans G. Folkesson, Ph.D. Associate Professor, Department of Animal Physiology, Lund University, Lund, Sweden

Chrystelle Garat, Ph.D. Postdoctoral Fellow, Department of Medicine, National Jewish Center for Immunology and Respiratory Medicine, Denver, Colorado

Michael A. Gropper, M.D., Ph.D. Assistant Professor, Department of Anesthesia, University of California at San Francisco, San Francisco, California

Yi Guo, Ph.D. Postdoctoral Fellow, Department of Anesthesiology, University of Alabama at Birmingham, Birmingham, Alabama

Randolph H. Hastings, M.D., Ph.D. Staff Physician, Department of Anesthesiology, San Diego VA Medical Center, San Diego, California

John E. Heffner, M.D., F.A.C.P., F.C.C.P. Professor of Clinical Medicine, Department of Medicine, University of Arizona Health Sciences Center, and St. Joseph's Hospital and Medical Center, Phoenix, Arizona

Herbert N. Hultgren, M.D.† Professor Emeritus, Division of Cardiology, Department of Medicine, Stanford University School of Medicine, Stanford, California

David H. Ingbar, M.D. Associate Professor, Departments of Medicine and Pediatrics, University of Minnesota School of Medicine, Minneapolis, Minnesota

Kwang-Jin Kim, Ph.D. Associate Professor, Department of Medicine, University of Southern California, Los Angeles, California

† Deceased

Kiyoyasu Kurahashi, M.D. Postdoctoral Fellow, Department of Anesthesia, University of California at San Francisco, San Francisco, California

Michael B. Maron, Ph.D. Professor and Chairperson, Department of Physiology, Northeastern Ohio Universities College of Medicine, Rootstown, Ohio

Sadis Matalon, Ph.D. Professor of Anesthesiology, Physiology and Biophysics, and Pediatrics, Department of Anesthesiology, University of Alabama at Birmingham, Birmingham, Alabama

Michael A. Matthay, M.D. Professor, Cardiovascular Research Institute, Departments of Medicine and Anesthesia, University of California at San Francisco, San Francisco, California

Katharina Modelska, M.D. Senior Research Fellow, Department of Anesthesia, University of California at San Francisco, San Francisco, California

John H. Newman, M.D. Chief, Medical Service, Nashville Veterans Administration Hospital, Interim Chairman, Department of Medicine, Vanderbilt University School of Medicine, Nashville, Tennessee

Maria Ohara, M.D. Postdoctoral Fellow, Department of Anesthesia, University of California at San Francisco, San Francisco, California

Charles F. Pilati, Ph.D. Associate Professor, Department of Physiology, Northeastern Ohio Universities College of Medicine, Rootstown, Ohio

Jean-François Pittet, M.D. Assistant Professor in Residence, Department of Anesthesia, University of California at San Francisco, San Francisco, California

Karen M. Ridge, Ph.D. Department of Medicine, Pulmonary and Critical Care, Michael Reese Hospital and University of Illinois, Chicago, Illinois

Ivan M. Robbins, M.D. Instructor, Department of Medicine, Vanderbilt University Medical Center, Nashville, Tennessee

Tsutomu Sakuma, M.D., Ph.D. Assistant Professor, Department of Respiratory Medicine, Kanazawa Medical University, Ishikawa, Japan

Georges Saumon, M.D. Career Researcher, Unité 82, Institut National de la Santé et de la Recherche Médicale, Paris, France

Teiji Sawa, M.D., Ph.D. Assistant Research Anesthesiologist, Department of Anesthesia, University of California at San Francisco, San Francisco, California

Daniel P. Schuster, M.D. Professor of Medicine and Radiology, Department of Internal Medicine, Washington University School of Medicine, St. Louis, Missouri

Robert D. Suh, M.D. Director of Thoracic Imaging and Intervention, Department of Radiology, Loma Linda University Medical Center, Loma Linda, California

Jacob Iasha Sznajder, M.D. Professor, Departments of Medicine and Pulmonary and Critical Care, Michael Reese Hospital, and University of Illinois, Chicago, Illinois

Mary I. Townsley, Ph.D. Professor, Department of Physiology, University of South Alabama, Mobile, Alabama

Alan S. Verkman, M.D., Ph.D. Professor of Medicine and Physiology, Cardiovascular Research Institute, University of California at San Francisco, San Francisco, California

Yibing Wang, M.D. Visiting Scientist, Cardiovascular Research Institute, University of California at San Francisco, San Francisco, California

Lorraine B. Ware, M.D. Postdoctoral Fellow, Department of Pulmonary and Critical Care, Cardiovascular Research Institute, University of California at San Francisco, San Francisco, California

Christine H. Wendt, M.D. Assistant Professor, Department of Medicine, University of Minnesota School of Medicine, Minneapolis, Minnesota

Jeanine P. Wiener-Kronish, M.D. Professor of Anesthesia and Medicine and Vice-Chairman, Department of Anesthesia, University of California at San Francisco, San Francisco, California

CONTENTS

Part III: RESOLUTION AND TREATMENT

1

Physiological Basis of Pulmonary Edema

JAHAR BHATTACHARYA

St. Luke's–Roosevelt Hospital Center and
Columbia College of Physicians and Surgeons
New York, New York

I. Introduction

The lung has long puzzled microvascular physiologists because of its tendency to develop edema under differing pathophysiological conditions. For example, pulmonary edema is associated with conditions as diverse as left ventricular failure (Chap. 5), liquid aspiration (Chap. 8), sepsis (Chap. 6), trauma (Chap. 9), high altitude sickness (Chap. 11) and mismatched blood transfusions, to name a few (1). Hence, the basic mechanisms by which the lung produces and transports liquid in both normal and pathophysiological conditions have elicited longstanding interest.

The modern understanding of pulmonary edema arises out of extensive experimental data that address the formation, interstitial drainage, and lymphatic removal of the lung microvascular filtrate. The landmark paper by Guyton and Lindsey (2) established the importance of lung vascular pressures in edema formation and intitiated the modern inquiry of pulmonary edema. In classical studies that followed, development of the lymph fistula, the gravimetry and the indicator dilution techniques, as well as new morphological methods, led to pioneering advances in the understanding of lung liquid transport. The consensus reached by the end of the 1970s was, first, that lung liquid production is attributable to passive microvascular filtration across endothelial junctions, and second, that pulmonary edema results from the imbalance between excess liquid formation by microvascular filtration and inadequate removal of the liquid by lung lymphatics (3).

Although the underpinnings of this classical theory remain unchallenged, major questions remain concerning the predominant sites of microvascular filtration, mechanisms of alveolar flooding, and the role of the interstitial matrix in liquid exchange. Advances in endothelial biology challenge the classical view that the microvascular wall plays a passive role in liquid formation and raise an entirely new set of questions concerning the endothelial role in lung microvascular barrier regulation.

A detailed consideration of all of these issues is outside the scope of this chapter. Much of the classical material has been reviewed several times (1,4,5) and will be discussed here only in brief. The aim of this review is to consider the processes of lung liquid balance through the microphysiological perspective that is emerging from the application of intravital microscopy and micropuncture to the lung microvascular bed. Other recent reviews may be consulted for more detailed discussions on pulmonary hemodynamics (6) and lung interstitial mechanics (7). Chapter 4 provides a discussion of methods to measure transvascular fluid and protein flux in patients with pulmonary edema.

II. Determination of Lung Microvascular Transport

A. Lung Microvascular Bed

Lung microvessels subsume 90% of the lung's vast vascular surface area (90 m^2 in man) and comprise a dense network of alveolar septal capillaries and the first two or three generations of arterioles and venules respectively, up- and downstream of the septum. The vastness of the microvascular bed predicates nonuniformity of regional filtration (see Sec. IV.B) and other heterogeneities that complicate understanding of lung liquid production.

An example of the microvascular heterogeneity is the nonuniformity of vascular diameter responses during lung expansion. Increased alveolar pressure (positive-pressure inflation) decreases diameter in septal vessels, increases diameter in extraseptal vessels of diameter >100 μm, but causes no diameter changes in vessels of the first two vascular generations both proximal and distal to the septal capillary bed (8). The decrease of diameter in septal vessels is attributable to the compressive effect of alveolar pressure, while the increase of diameter in extraseptal vessels occurs in response to tissue stretch caused by the lung expansion that accompanies increased alveolar pressure.

These effects of increased alveolar pressure are potentially important from the standpoint of liquid exchange. The alveolar pressure-induced septal compression may increase microvascular flow resistance which, by increasing pressures, increases filtration in the proximal microvascular bed. On the other hand, obstruction of blood flow by septal compression results in decreased perfused surface area, hence decreased surface area of filtration. The net effect may be an increase or no change in filtration rate, depending on the relative extents of these two hemodynamic effects.

B. Theory of Transport Quantification

Major Transport Equations

Lung microvascular liquid transport is described by the Starling and the Kedem-Katchalsky equations, which are respectively,

$$Jv = Lp \cdot S\ (\Delta P - \sigma\ \Delta\pi) \tag{1}$$

and

$$Jp = PS\Delta C + (1 - \sigma)\overline{C} \cdot Jv \tag{2}$$

where Jv is filtration rate, Lp the microvascular hydraulic conductivity, S the surface area of filtration, ΔP and $\Delta\pi$ respectively, the transmembrane hydrostatic and colloid osmotic pressure differences, σ the osmotic reflection coefficient, Jp the transmicrovascular protein flux, P the microvascular permeability coefficient, and $\overline{C}$ the mean protein concentration in the transendothelial transport pathway (Table 1).

In Equation 1, the product LpS equals the filtration coefficient, K*f*; ΔP equals (Pc − Pi) and $\Delta\pi$ equals ($\pi c - \pi i$), where Pc and Pi are, respectively, the microvascular and interstitial hydrostatic pressures, and πc and πi are the corresponding colloid osmotic pressures.

The Starling equation provides the basis for classifying pulmonary edemas into the "hydrostatic" and the "permeability" types (1). "Hydrostatic" edema results from increased filtration attributable to the force differences ΔP and $\Delta\pi$, when the barrier constants Lp and σ are unchanged. "Permeability" edema results when, despite unaltered forces, filtration is increased by increase of Lp or decrease of σ. Such changes in the barrier constants signify loss of barrier properties, so the filtrate is relatively more protein-rich in the permeability than in the hydrostatic form of edema.

As discussed in Section IV.B, the bulk of the lung's filtration may normally occur in the proximal half of the lung microvascular bed. A pathogenic increase of microvascular pressure that elevates ΔP in all regions may recruit the distal half for filtration, thereby increasing S. According to Equation 1, S and ΔP each relate directly to filtration rate. Hence, hydrostatic edema may be attributable to the additive effects of increases in S and ΔP.

Table 1 Glossary of Terms

Term	Definition
Convection	Water flow driven by pressure difference
Diffusion	Solute flow driven by concentration difference of solute
Jv	Microvascular filtration rate
ΔC	Transmembrane difference of protein concentration
$\overline{C}$	Mean protein concentration of the transmicrovascular transport pathway
C_L	Protein concentration of lung lymph
C_P	Plasma protein concentration
$C_{P_{avg}}$	The average **plasma** protein concentration
Jp	Transmicrovascular protein flux
K*f*	Microvascular filtration coefficient
Lp	Hydraulic conductivity
P	Microvascular permeability coefficient
Pc	Microvascular pressure
πc	Plasma colloid osmotic pressure
Pi	Interstitial pressure
$\pi\iota$	Interstitial colloid osmotic pressure
Q_L	Lung lymph flow
S	Surface area of filtration
σd	Microvascular osmotic reflection coefficient
σf	Microvascular filtration reflection coefficient
Padv	Interstitial pressure in microvessel adventitia
Pjct	Interstitial pressure at alveolar junctions

The Starling equation also indicates that the transmicrovascular convective flux (Jv) depends on the transmicrovascular *differences* of, respectively, the hydrostatic and the osmotic pressure pairs, rather than on single pressures of either kind. A second important consideration is that osmotic pressures of small solutes (<10 kD) do not determine the transmicrovascular flux. The plasma (πc) and and interstitial (πi) colloid osmotic pressures are determined, respectively, by the plasma and interstitial protein concentrations alone. It should be pointed out, however, that increased small solute concentration deteriorates the barrier as indicated by increase of the hydraulic conductivity (Lp) (9). This effect is probably attributable to hyperosmolarity-induced osmotic endothelial shrinkage, and could be relevant in diseases associated with serum hyperosmolarity (e.g., renal failure).

Inclusion of the convective flux term, Jv, in the Kedem-Katchalsky equation indicates that transmicrovascular protein transport is filtration-dependent. Thus, vascular pressure determines not only filtration rate but also protein transport. However, the ΔC term in Equation 2 indicates that the transmembrane gradient of protein concentration may also drive diffusive protein transport. Under baseline conditions, however, most authorities attribute greater than 80% of the total protein flux to convection (10), which ascribes a relatively minor role in the transport for diffusive or other concentration dependent processes.

Although πc and πi are indicated as independent variables in the Starling equation, they are in fact coupled. This is because the plasma protein concentration not only determines πc, but it also uniquely defines the interstitial protein concentration relevant to πi. When a decrease in πc is maintained for several hours, πi ultimately decreases by a similar extent. Hence, the baseline $\Delta\pi$ is reestablished. However, when πc is decreased rapidly, a similar πi does not occur in the short term. Hence $\Delta\pi$ increases transiently. Because of these effects, a decrease of C_P is followed by transient increase of filtration rate which soon returns to baseline (11–13).

Decrease of πc does not affect membrane barrier properties. Thus, reduction of plasma protein concentration by 50% of normal has no effect on the baseline lung microvascular hydraulic conductivity, Lp (14). By contrast, when πc is increased by increasing plasma albumin concentration, Lp increases (15). This barrier deteriorating effect is consistent with clinical findings that hyperoncotic albumin therapy fails to reduce pulmonary edema and may in fact increase lung water (16,17). By contrast, no barrier deterioration occurs when πc is increased using macromolecules such as neutral dextran or IgG (15). Therefore, the hyperoncotic barrier deterioration may be albumin-specific and the relevant mechanisms may be attributable to albumin-endothelial interactions (see discussion on albumin-binding poteins in Sec. III.D).

Microvascular Protein Restriction

As envisaged by Starling in 1896, plasma proteins exert absorptive osmotic pressure across the microvascular membrane. This is attributable to the membrane's protein-restrictive property that establishes higher protein concentration, hence higher colloid osmotic pressure in plasma than in interstitial fluid. As indicated in the Starling equation, the $\Delta\pi$ that drives osmotic flow is itself modified by intrinsic membrane properties that are described by the osmotic reflection coefficient σ, which varies from 0 to 1. Thus the change in osmotic flow following a given change of $\Delta\pi$, is greater when $\sigma = 1$ than when $\sigma < 1$. No osmotic flow occurs when $\sigma = 0$. Decrease of σ following experimental intervention signifies loss of the membrane's ability to generate osmotic flow and thereby reports deterioration of a fundamental barrier property.

The fact that a transmicrovascular osmotic gradient should contribute to bulk flow at all, is counterintuitive and is attributable to the thermodynamic properties of water as explained in Figure 1. This figure also illustrates the pore model of the lung microvascular membrane (18), which exists in several cognate versions and is presented here in simplified form. According to this model, protein transport is restricted by small but not large pores. Therefore small pores

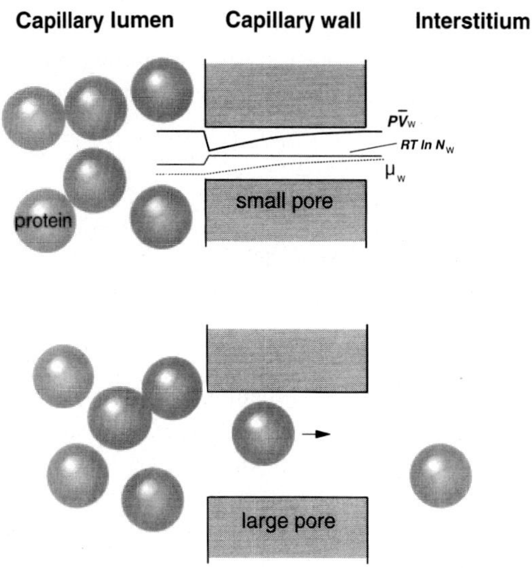

Figure 1 The pore model of transmicrovascular transport. Transport of proteins (spheres) occurs from capillary lumen on left, across the capillary wall to the interstitial space. *Upper panel.* Proteins are excluded from a small pore. Protein concentration is higher in capillary lumen than in the interstitium. μ_w is the chemical potential of water, P is hydrostatic pressure, V_w is the partial molal volume of water, and N_w is the mole fraction of water (≈ number of water molecules). $\mu_w = PV_w + RT \ln N_w$. As proposed by Dainty (92), osmotic water flow occurs from right to left across the pore because of the thermodynamic difference in the chemical potential of water on the two sides of the membrane. The explanation is as follows: Assume (1) that the capillary lumen contains water and proteins, while the pore and the interstitium contain pure water. Assume (2) that P is constant on both sides of the capillary wall. Since the pore is protein-free, the mole fraction of water is higher in the pore. Hence a step increase occurs in RT ln N_w at the pore entrance. Since μ_w is constant throughout the capillary lumen, PV_w must fall at the pore entrance to maintain the sum (PV_w + RT ln N_w) constant. However, by Assumption 1, water activity is higher within the pore and in the interstitium. Hence, μ_w increases along the pore from left to right. Since the pore contains pure water, RT ln N_w remains constant from left to right along the pore. Therefore, to account for the increase of μ_w, PV_w must increase along the pore from left to right as shown. Therefore P is higher at the exit end than at the entrance end of the pore. This P difference provides the hydrostatic pressure gradient required for driving bulk flow across the pore from right to left. *Lower panel.* A large pore accommodates protein flow in the direction of the arrow. Some restriction to protein flow occurs because the pore diameter is not much larger than the protein diameter.

Other methods for σ determination include the single-microvessel approach based on the zero-filtration pressure, discussed in Section II.C, and one introduced by Wolf et al. (22) using the relation:

$$\sigma = 1 - (M[T]/G \cdot C_{P_{avg}}) \quad (5)$$

where M[T] and G are, respectively, total macromolecular mass and volume transported from blood to tissue in a given filtration period and $C_{P_{avg}}$ is the average plasma protein concentration.

Besides these approaches, barrier quantification through estimation of the PS product has been widely used on the basis of the extraction equation:

$$E = 1 - e^{-PS/F} \quad (6)$$

where E is the extraction from blood to tissue of a diffusible tracer such as urea or inulin, and F is blood flow. The assumptions, limitations, and applications of the method, as applied to the lung vascular bed, have been reviewed (5).

C. Methods for Quantifying Lung Microvascular Flux

Lung Lymph Flow

Pure lung lymph as obtained by the lymph-fistula technique reflects the quantity and composition of filtrate that reaches the lymphatics. To the extent that the microvascular filtrate bypasses the lymphatics, the lung lymph flow underestimates microvascular filtration. The filtrate may bypass lymphatics if it enters the alveolar space either under normal conditions to form the liquid that underlies alveolar surfactant, or under abnormal conditons as edema liquid. Nevertheless, the existence of lung lymph flow which varies from 4 to 12 mL/h in unanesthetized sheep (1) and is probably double that in man, confirms the existence of net filtration in lung. Since lung vascular pressures are less than πc,* a substantial πi must oppose πc in order to support filtration (see Eq. 1). πi has not been directly determined. However, based on the direct relation between π and protein concentration and the CL/CP ratio of ~0.7 for sheep lung, $\Delta\pi$ is estimated to be ~10 cm H_2O.

The CL/CP ratio may be interpreted as a marker of microvascular barrier properties when data are obtained in the filtration-independent condition (see Sec. II.B) (1). An increase of vascular pressure causes greater water than protein flow across the microvascular membrane. This dilutes the lymph and decreases CL. Since CP remains constant, the ratio decreases for the normal barrier. Barrier deterioration is interpreted when decrease of the ratio is absent or blunted. The

---

*The mean pulmonary artery pressure in man is 25 to 30 cm H_2O, whereas πc is 30 cm H_2O.

alone support osmotic flow. Large pores permit protein transport by sol\ (the convective flow literally drags along the proteins); however, the t is restricted by size-dependent solute-pore interactions.*

By pore theory postulates, the interstitial protein concentration, hen is determined by (1) the protein-poor small-pore flow that tends to dilu protein concentration hence decrease πi, and (2) the protein-containing la pore flow that tends to add to the interstitial protein content and increase π complexity is that large-pore transport includes convective and diffusive co ponents. At low vascular pressure, convection is low and diffusion is hig Hence, protein concentration in the large pore tends to increase as protein diffuse in from the plasma. At high vascular pressure, convection dominates the diffusive effect is less, and the large pore flow is more dilute. In other words, πi is filtration-dependent and it varies inversely with transmicrovascular flux.

The uncertainty of the aggregate protein concentration of the filtered liquid contributes to the difficulty of σ quantification. This problem was addressed by Patlak and Rappoport (19), who integrated Equation 2 for solute concentration along the length of the transport pathway. Their formulation, called the Patlak equation, has been rearranged by Granger and Taylor (20) in a form that is applicable to lung lymph data (see Sec. II.C) as:

$$C_L/C_P = (1 - \sigma)/(1 - \sigma_f \cdot e^{-x}) \tag{3}$$

where $x = (1 - \sigma)\, Q_L/PS$. Q_L the lymph flow, is an indirect estimate of J_v, and PS is the permeability-surface area product for the microvascular bed.

As Q_L increases by ~4 times the baseline value, $(1 - \sigma e^{-x})$ term in Equation 4 approaches 1. Hence, under such high filtration conditions

$$C_L/C_P = 1 - \sigma \tag{4}$$

Hence, the asymptotic, or the filtration-independent C_L/C_P ratio obtained during high filtration conditions provides a method for quantifying σ. The limitations of this method are that lymph determinations are applicable only to a single animal model, the sheep, and that sustained increases of lung vascular pressure may change Pi (21) and induce undetermined endothelial responses that independently affect barrier properties.

---

*I have not considered here the solvent drag reflection coefficient (σf), which has been extensively discussed in the literature. The similarity of terminology to the osmotic reflection coefficient is confusing, because σf quantifies the large-pore restriction to protein transport and bears no direct relation to small-pore osmotic flow. However, the solvent drag consideration is important in the theoretical understanding of σ quantification by lymph methods, and is discussed in several reviews (18,39,91).

advantages are that the CL/CP ratio is surface area-independent and yet provides a quantification of barrier properties in the intact animal. The difficulty is that methods for obtaining pure lung lymph have developed only in a single animal model—the sheep.

Lung Gravimetry

The other classical method for transvascular flux determination involves quantifying weight changes of the isolated, perfused lung (4,23). Typically, vascular pressures are adjusted to set the isogravimetric condition in which the lung neither gains nor loses weight. A small step increase of pressure now causes a biphasic lung weight increment attributable to an increase of vascular volume in the early phase and increased filtered volume in the late phase. Kf is interpreted as the ratio of the rate of weight increase in the late phase to magnitude of the pressure step. Though widely used, this method for Kf determination requires the assumption that the surface area of filtration is constant since this variable is not quantified.

Other Whole-Lung Methods

In the indicator dilution method, bolus injections of permeant versus nonpermeant tracers give rise to concentration transients in the lung venous effluent. These transients are analyzed for calculation of the PS product based on Equation 6 (Sec. II.A) (5). Global indicators of the lung's liquid content, such as the extravascular lung water content and the uptake of macromolecular tracers such as radioactive albumin, have been widely used to obtain qualitative as well as quantitative assessments of lung liquid balance (see Chap. 4) (24,25). Recent studies have incorporated positron emission tomography (PET) that are particularly well suited for clinical studies (see Chap. 4) (26). Pilati and Maron (27) have applied Equation 5 for σ determinations in lung. In this method, a period of high-pressure filtration is used to determine M[T] and G from the increases of plasma protein concentration and hematocrit, and CP_{avg} is taken as the final plasma protein concentration.

Single-Microvessel Method

The whole-lung methods discussed above do not account for the surface area term in the transport equations (see Eq. 1). Discrimination between surface area-sensitive hemodynamic effects from direct barrier effects of an agent is therefore often difficult. To address this problem, we developed the split-drop technique for flux quantification across a defined surface area of the optically viewed single lung microvessel (14,28). A filtration segment of known dimensions is established in a lung capillary by splitting an oil drop with an injection of a test solution of known colloid osmotic pressure (πc) (Fig. 2). Capillary pressure (Pc) is held constant. Transcapillary flux per unit area (Jv/S) is determined from the changes of test solution (split-drop) volume.

Split-drop quantifications at different Pc give the linear Jv/S-Pc relation. Rewriting the Starling equation in the form of the straight line equation,

$$Jv/S = Lp\,(\Delta P - \sigma \cdot \Delta\pi) \qquad (7)$$

gives the slope as the hydraulic conductivity, Lp and the x-intercept as the zero filtration pressure, Pzf where Pzf $= \sigma\ \Delta\pi$. Pzf determinations at different πc are applied in Equation 7 to solve for σ (14). Based on direct determinations, Pi is considered equal to zero (29). The split-drop procedure takes <1.5 min, and yields consistent repeat Lp determinations in the same vessel (14).

A major advantage of the split-drop method is that flux is quantified in vessels lacking smooth muscle (30). Hence, vasoactive and hemodynamic effects do not complicate interpretation of flux data. A derivation by Glucksberg indicates that the Jv/S determination is obtained under constant transmicrovascular force conditions (28). Hence, the measurement reflects steady-state barrier con-

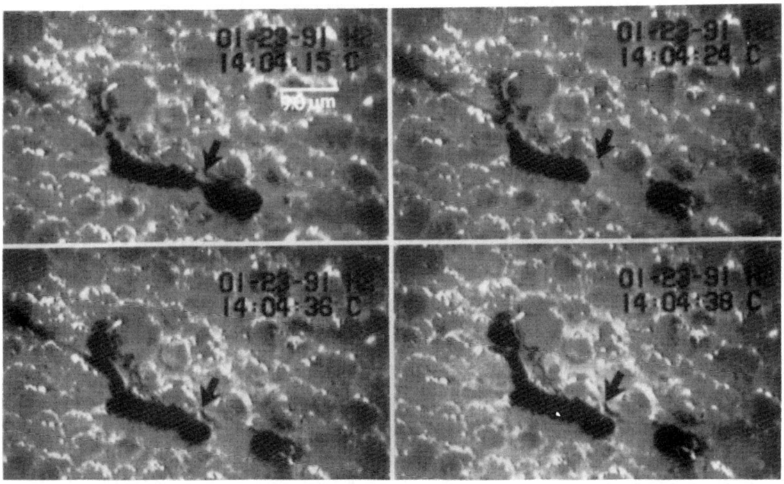

Figure 2 Steps of the split-drop technique. *Upper left.* A microvessel containing an injected oil drop is micropunctured (arrow) to inject a test solution of known πc. *Upper right.* The injection of test solution splits the oil drop. *Lower left.* To prevent leakage through puncture defects, the split-drop segment is displaced from the micropuncture site by injecting oil (arrow). *Lower right.* A positive force balance ($\Delta P > \sigma\Delta\pi$) causes flux outward from the microvessel. Outward flux is determined as progressive decrease of the test solution volume (split-drop volume). (From Ref. 14.)

ditions. The method allows quantification of time course of rapid changes in barrier properties. For example, we determined that vitronectin-induced increases in lung microvascular flux occur in 5 sec (30).

III. Properties of the Lung Microvascular Barrier

A. Barrier Structure

Membrane barrier function is determined primarily by the intercellular tight junction region (zona occludens). The width of lung endothelial tight junctions varies from 0 (completely closed) to an average of ~3 nm (31). Tight-junction ultrastructure has been determined by scanning electronmicroscopy following freeze fracture. In this approach, ultracold tissue sections fractured in the plane of the cell membrane separate into the hydrophobic outer (ectoplasmic or "E" face) and the protoplasmic inner ("P" face) faces of the membrane (32,33). Scanning electronmicroscopy of carbon-coated replicas of the fracture faces of endothelial tight junctions reveals rows of interconnected particles along grooves on the E face, together with complementary strands of particle poor ridges on the P face (Fig. 3).

Tight-junction features have been correlated with barrier function. Higher strand density and richer fiber content on the epithelial than the endothelial P face directly correlate with higher epithelial resistance to bulk transport (32,33).

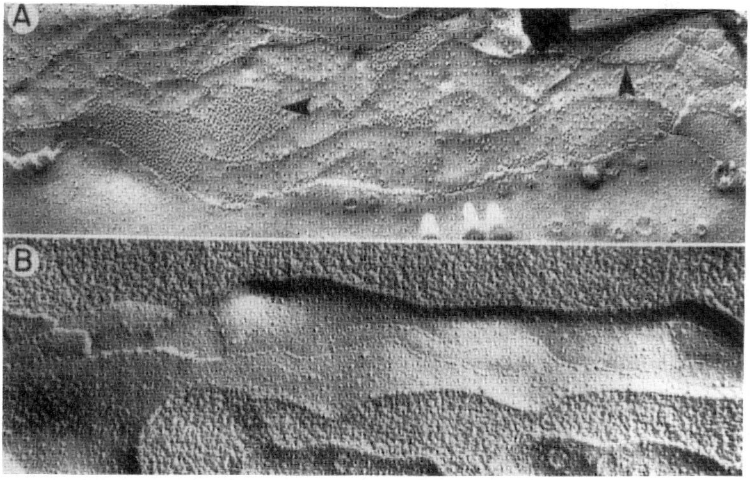

Figure 3 Freeze-fracture replicas of endothelial tight junctions from an intra-acinar pulmonary artery (A) and a pulmonary capillary (B). The capillary junction shows fewer rows of particles on the P face. (From Ref. 32.)

Walker et al. demonstrated that gaps appear in the P face ridges in association with increased lung microvascular permeability (33). Strand content is also important, as indicated in an epithelial study by Schneeberger and McCormack (34), in which tight junction permeability to colloidal lanthanum related inversely to strand density.

Based on the relative paucity of tight-junction strands and particles in pulmonary capillaries and venules versus intra-acinar arteries (Fig. 3), Schneeberger proposed that lung microvascular permeability increases at the venular end (35). This has now been confirmed by split-drop studies that indicate a 40% higher Lp and a 25% lower albumin reflection coefficient in venules than in arterioles (14). Such a gradient of lung microvascular barrier properties may result in regional unevenness of microvascular filtration, which may explain reported nonhomogeneities in the distribution of edematous regions in high-pressure edema (36,37).

B. Barrier Quantification

Using serum as the test solution in the split drop technique in rat lung, Lp is estimated as 3.4×10^{-7} mL/(scm^{2}cm H_2O)[38] and σ as 0.7. For albumin, Lp is at least 40% higher and σ 30% lower (14), indicating the higher permeability of lung microvessels to albumin than serum. As reviewed (39), similar data in previous reports indicate consensus in the σ estimate for lung.

A comparison of barrier descriptors for continuous, nonfenestrated endothelium indicates that the microvascular barrier is more permeable in lung than in systemic beds. Thus for skeletal muscle, Lp is 10 times smaller and σ is >0.9 (39,40). These differences are surprising given that the lung endothelial junctional structure shows the typical features of continuous endothelium. According to Perry (31), the higher permeability may be attributable to higher density of endothelial junctions per unit surface area in lung than in systemic beds such as skeletal muscle.

C. Barrier Regulation

Although multiple factors have been shown to increase lung microvascular permeability, the relevant cellular mechanisms are only beginning to be understood. New data point to definitive evidence for endothelial receptors in barrier regulation. Proof of receptor-mediated processes requires evidence for (1) morphological receptor identification, (2) concentration dependent effects of receptor ligation, and (3) inhibition of the receptor-mediated process by specific antireceptor antibodies. In split-drop experiments, we confirmed these conditions for the vitronectin receptor (VNR), the integrin $\alpha v\beta 3$ (30). Ligation of this receptor by multimeric vitronectin, or by the vitronectin-containing complement complex

SC5b-9, given either in purified form or as SC5b-9-enriched serum, all resulted in antibody-inhibitible increases in Lp.

The induction of endothelial signaling is indicated by the inhibition of the VNR-induced Lp effects in the presence of tyrosine kinase inhibitors. Although this result implicates protein tyrosine phosphorylation (PTP) as the critical step in VNR signaling, other receptor-mediated Lp increases involve the activation of protein kinase C (PKC). The PTP and PKC pathways may operate independently of each other in barrier regulation. This became evident in experiments in which α-thrombin-induced Lp increases were blocked by the PKC inhibitor calphostin C, but not by tyrosine kinase inhibitors (30). Conversely, the VNR-induced Lp increase was calphostin C-insensitive. New evidence from our laboratory also implicates tyrosine phosphorylation in other mechanisms of barrier deterioration—for example, in that attributable to hyperosmolarity (9). Further studies are required to determine details of proteins phosphorylated and their subsequent interactions that lead to barrier effects.

A second receptor identified in lung microvascular barrier regulation is P-selectin. Lung vascular expression of P-selectin following ischemia-reperfusion (95) and hemorrhagic shock (96) increased lung microvascular permeability as quantified, respectively, by the lung microvascular filtration coefficient, K*f*, and the extravasation of plasma protein. In each study, the evoked permeability increase was inhibited by the anti-P-selectin monoclonal antibody PB1.3. Although P-selectin is traditionally associated with the initiation of neutrophil rolling on blood vessels, these results implicate the selectin in a barrier regulatory role that may importantly contribute to the pulmonary edema of lung injury. Further studies are required to understand the detailed mechanisms of the barrier deteriorating effect of P-selectin.

D. Transport Across the Barrier

Convective Transport

As discussed above, theoretical analyses of the lung transport data indicate that transmicrovascular protein transport occurs primarily by convection (1,10,41). For albumin, convection accounts for almost all of the transport. Convective protein transport is also evident in the lymph data, in that vascular pressure elevation increases not only lymph flow but also lymph protein flux (42,43).

There are, however, puzzling aspects to the convection theory. Protein convection requires a pathway of sufficient size to accommodate plasma proteins that have an effective molecular diameter of 3 to 4 nm. Many consider the endothelial junctional route to be the favored pathway. Although the junctional width is sufficient to accommodate flow of water and small solutes of <10 kD, it approximates the protein molecular diameter. Hence, mechanisms by which proteins negotiate the pathway that is likely to be highly restrictive because of size considerations, continue to be conjectural. Moreover, although the microvascular membrane demonstrates size-dependent sieving of macromolecules (42), albumin transport exceeds the amount predicted by sieving alone.

A further confusing issue is the lack of morphological evidence for the junctional transport theory. The microvascular transport pathway of monomeric albumin, as traced with antibodies tagged with electronopaque tracers, shows no evidence of junctional albumin transport (44,45). However, the absence of morphological evidence does not preclude the possibility of junctional protein transport. Convective protein transport may occur only through preferential pathways within a given junction, or across special junctions in the endothelial membrane, such as tricellular or slit-type junctions (46,47). Such preferential pathways may be sparse and may be missed in random electronmicroscopic sections.

Caveolar Transport

The transcellular route of protein transport occurs via flask-shaped structures in the endothelial plasmalemma, the caveoli, that engulf plasma proteins and then transport them to the abluminal side of the endothelial membrane. Mechanisms of caveolar transport remain incompletely understood. Evidence for transcellular caveolar transport, which was first proposed by Palade in 1968 (48), is extensively supported by electronmicroscopic data (45), although supportive physiological data have not been reported.

Caveolar transport probably involves receptor-mediated processes. Plasma substances that lack endothelial receptors, such as immunoglobulins, are probably endocytosed and transported in the fluid phase, as shown for experimental tracers such as horseradish peroxidase. Several putative albumin-binding proteins such as gp60 (albondin), gp30, and gp18 are implicated in albumin transcytosis (49,50). Recent data from our laboratory on cultured lung endothelial cells indicate that albumin may be the critical plasma factor that initiates caveolar transport (51).

There is considerable confusion among authorities regarding the significance of the caveolar mechanism in overall liquid flux. Physiological opinion varies from the extreme view that caveolar transport is nonexistent, to one in which the mechanism is acknowledged but not considered significant for resting flux. This is because both theoretically (10,41) and according to recent data (52), the putative transcellular component of the transport is much smaller than the convective. Accordingly, the caveolar mechanism is not featured in theoretical models of lung microvascular transport.

However, a more inclusive theory may be to consider the significance of caveolar transport in the context of conditions that increase endothelial caveolar content. Caveoli capture plasma proteins in the bulk phase, so caveolar protein osmotic pressure may equal the plasma colloid osmotic pressure, πc. Therefore, enhanced interstitial release of caveolar contents may increase πi and thereby increase transmicrovascular flux. Caveolar content of alveolar capillaries increases in septal edema (53). This intriguing finding suggests that increased caveolar transport may contribute to the development of pulmonary edema.

This possibility is supported by our recent finding that active albumin transport occurs across the lung capillary. A capillary was coinfused with albumin at different concentrations together with a fluoresceinated tracer, then washed with buffer. Marked retention of pericapillary fluorescence was evident with hyperoncotic albumin (6 g/100 mL) at a concentration 50% larger than normal for rat plasma (Fig. 4), but not at normal albumin concentration (54).

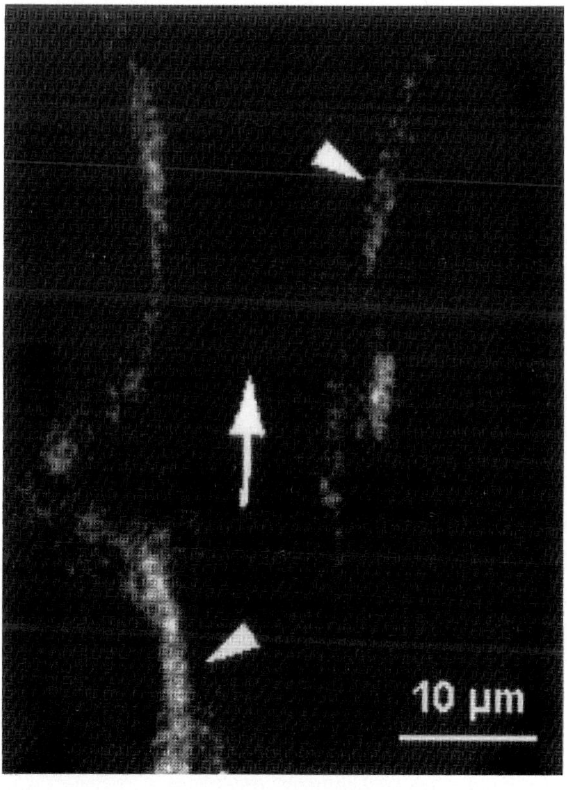

Figure 4 Active transport of fluorescent albumin in a lung venular capillary. Arrow shows direction of blood flow. Arrowheads show endothelial retention of fluorescence.

Active albumin transport into the pericapillary interstitium is implicated, because the fluorescence retention was blocked at low temperature (5 to 7°C). Evidently, high albumin concentration augmented caveolar transport of the tracer.

Also relevant is the finding that hyperoncotic albumin decreases the zero-filtration pressure, Pzf (Fig. 5) (15). By contrast, no decreases in Pzf occur with albumin at normal concentration or with hyperoncotic dextran. These findings also indicate that enhanced caveolar albumin transport at high albumin concentration increases πi and thereby decreases $\Delta\pi$; hence Pzf, which varies directly with $\Delta\pi$, decreases.

These findings indicate that active albumin transport exists across the lung capillary endothelium, and they are consistent with the transport being attributable to caveolar mechanisms. The extent to which such mechanisms promote lung liquid accumulation in lung injury requires further investigation.

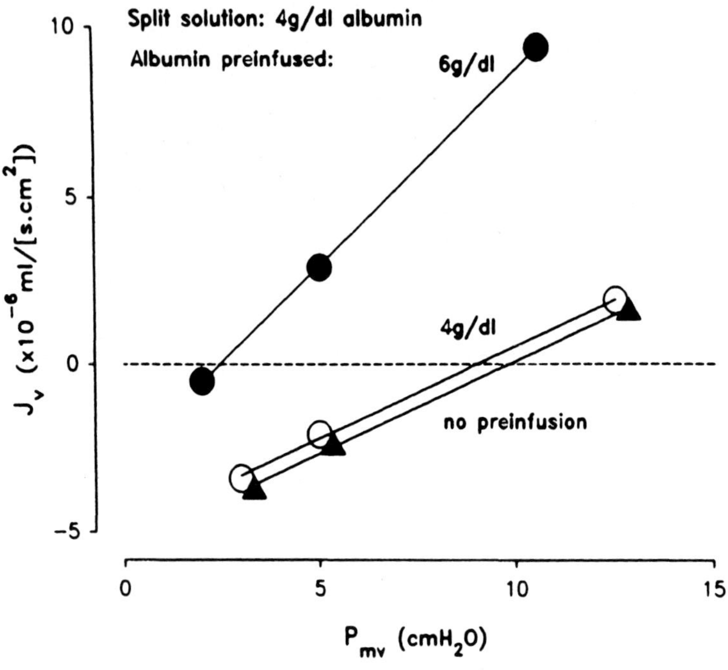

Figure 5 Split-drop data from lung venular capillaries. Jv, transvascular flux; Pmv, microvascular pressure. Hyperoncotic (6 g/dl) or normal albumin concentration (4 g/dl) was preinfused for 6 min, then split-drop determinations were made using 4 g/dl albumin as test solution. The slopes give the hydraulic conductivity. The x-intercepts give the zero-filtration pressure. (From Ref. 15.)

IV. Distribution of Filtration in the Lung Microvascular Bed

Although lung liquid formation is traditionally attributed entirely to filtration across alveolar septal capillaries, the longitudinal distribution of filtration in the septum remains unclear. Septal widening in hydrostatic edema indicates that all septal capillaries are capable of supporting filtration at high vascular pressure (36,37,55). Under conditons of stopped blood flow and high microvascular pressures, septal capillaries accounted for ~90% of total lung filtration (56,57). However, these data do not clarify the septal filtration profile that exists during normal blood flow and normal pressure distribution.

Some lung filtration coefficient (K*f*) determinations indicate that filtration may not occur across the entire lung microvascular bed. Perry calculated K*f* based on morphological determinations on endothelial junctions across the total septal capillary surface area (31). This approach, which maximizes the vascular surface area term in K*f*, overestimates lung K*f* determined by physiological methods by at least an order of magnitude, possibly to an extent that the total vascular surface area overestimates the actual surface area of filtration. A similar conclusion may be drawn from a consideration of the effective surface area of filtration, using the identity K*f*/Lp = S. Based on available data, the K*f*/Lp ratio indicates that only 16% of the lung vascular surface area supports filtration (58).

A. Lung Microvascular Pressure Profile

Micropuncture Measurements

If all other variables of the Starling equation are constant, the longitudinal fall of vascular pressure along the direction of blood flow must accompany a drop in filtration rates. To understand this filtration profile, the pressure drop across the capillary bed must be known. This critical determination is obtained by means of the micropuncture technique that alone permits direct determinations of pressure at the entry and exit portals of the septal bed, namely in the preseptal arteriole and the postseptal venule (59). Pressure measurements within the septum itself have not yet been achieved.

Most micropuncture pressure determinations indicate that a significant pressure drop exists across the alveolar septal capillary network (60–66,94). Although this pressure drop ranges between 3 and 6 cm H_2O in absolute magnitude, it accounts for 33% to 50% of the total vascular pressure drop across the lung from pulmonary artery to left atrium. In early experiments little or no pressure drop was detected in the arterial and venous segments of the isolated blood-perfused lung because vascular tone was inhibited with papaverine (60). Subsequent determinations in open-chest preparations in dog and rabbit under

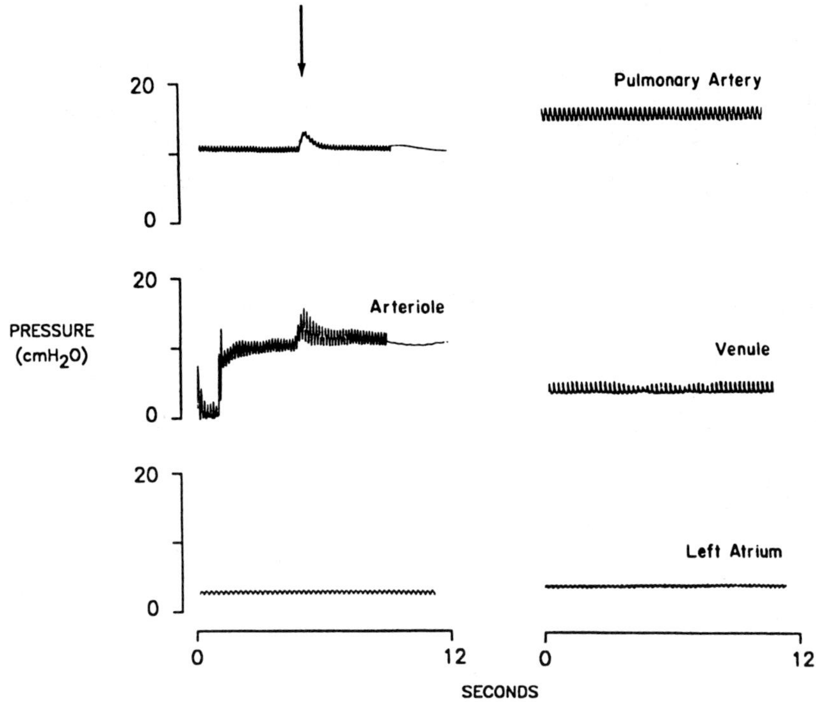

Figure 6 Lung vascular pressure measurements in the open-chested rabbit. A saline bolus was injected at the arrow. The arteriole and the venule pressures were determined by micropuncture and are, respectively, 1.5 cm H_2O below pulmonary artery, and 0.5 cm H_2O above left atrial pressures. (From Ref. 63.)

nonvasodilated conditions indicate that the pressures in the precapillary arteriole and the postcapillary venule are respectively, 2 to 3 cm H_2O below pulmonary artery pressure and 0 to 2 cm H_2O above left atrial pressure (Fig. 6) (63,66).

Since blood flow is the same in the arterial, microvascular, and venous segments, and since vascular resistance is the ratio of pressure drop to blood flow, the high microvascular pressure drop indicates that, under normal conditions, the microvascular resistance is the highest of the segmental resistances. In some species the arterial resistance is either equally high or slightly higher. The reason for the high microvascular resistance is not understood, although it may relate to pressure-induced capillary distension and the inverse relation between vascular resistance and capillary diameter. As the vascular pressure falls along the septal length, capillaries become less distended; hence, capillary diameter may progressively decrease and capillary resistance may concomitantly increase. Thus, capillary narrowing may explain the high microvascular resistance under normal conditions.

The findings of Nagasaka et al. (94) are consistent with this proposal. These authors reported that doubling of pulmonary blood flow shifts the site of maximum vascular resistance from the microvascular to the arterial and venous segments. Presumably, the high vascular pressures generated by the flow increase, distend septal capillaries, and decrease microvascular resistance (94). In the arterial and venous segments, pressure-drops increase in proportion to the increase of blood flow hence the respective segmental resistances remain unchanged. As concluded by Nagasaka et al., the net result is a decrease in overall pulmonary vascular resistance.

The relative sparsity of the septal capillary layer on the pleural face of the most superficial alveoli is of potential concern in the interpretation of lung micropressure data. However, micropunctured arterioles and venules have extensive deeper connections with capillary networks of normal vascular density (Fig. 7). Therefore despite vessel sparsity in a single superficial layer, micropressures of arterioles and venules are likely to reflect corresponding deeper pressures. Blood flow distribution determined in thinly sectioned tissue slices indicates the absence of a significant gradient of blood perfusion between superficial and deep

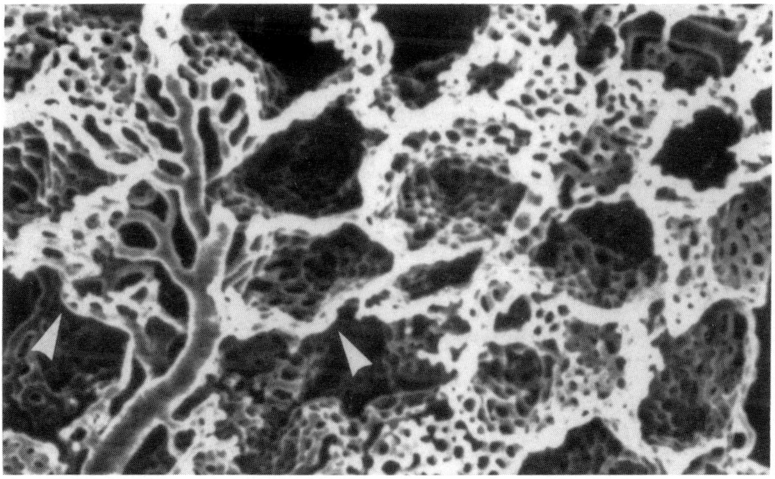

Figure 7 Elastomer cast of superficial microvascular network in rat lung seen by scanning electron microscopy. The arteriole that enters the field left below was accessible to micropuncture. Note the several deeper connections of this vessel (arrowheads).

lung layers (66), a finding that attests to the lack of significant hemodynamic differences between superficial and deep regions. Although pressure data from deep vessels are not easily accessible by micropuncture, this difficult determination has been achieved by Onizuka et al., who confirmed good agreement between superficial and deep lung microvascular pressures (67).

Occlusion Methods

Inflow and outflow occlusion methods are used for assessment of lung microvascular pressure distribution. As recently reviewed (6), the data are interpreted on an equivalent circuit model in which the lung arterial and venous segments are considered as resistive elements in series with the septal capillary bed, the region of major compliance (capacitance). In the arterial or venous segment brief flow occlusion at, respectively, the inflow or outflow end, causes instantaneous equalization of segmental pressures with the pressure at the point of highest compliance. Since the highest compliance occurs in the septal capillaries, the instantaneous equalization pressure equals septal capillary pressure. An equalization pressure transient in the venous segment is shown in the upper tracing in Figure 8 as the step pressure increase following sudden occlusion of venous outflow. The subsequent ramp increase of pressure reflects progressive increase of vascular blood volume during maintained venous occlusion.

Arterial occlusion pressure is higher than venous occlusion pressure. The difference is interpreted as the arteriole-venule pressure drop across the lung microvascular bed. This interpretation is limited by the uncertainty regarding the proximal and distal boundaries of the central compliance. As compared with the arteriole-venule pressure difference determined by micropuncture, the arterial-venous occlusion pressure difference may be similar (68) or much smaller (69).

Outflow occlusion in the presence of venular micropuncture reveals the presence of step increases in both venous and venular pressures (Fig. 8). The pressure step following outflow occlusion indicates pressure equilibration between the point of pressure measurement and the upstream region of maximal compliance. Hence, the venular transient confirms that postseptal venules are downstream of the region of maximal compliance. By a similar argument, the arteriolar pressure may lie upstream of the region. Accordingly, the arterial-venous occlusion pressure difference is likely to underestimate the septal pressure drop determined by micropuncture.

Regulation of Lung Microvascular Pressures

It has been long understood that lung microvascular pressures increase in left ventricular failure. The new understanding from the segmental studies discussed above indicates that in even in the absence of heart failure, pulmonary venular

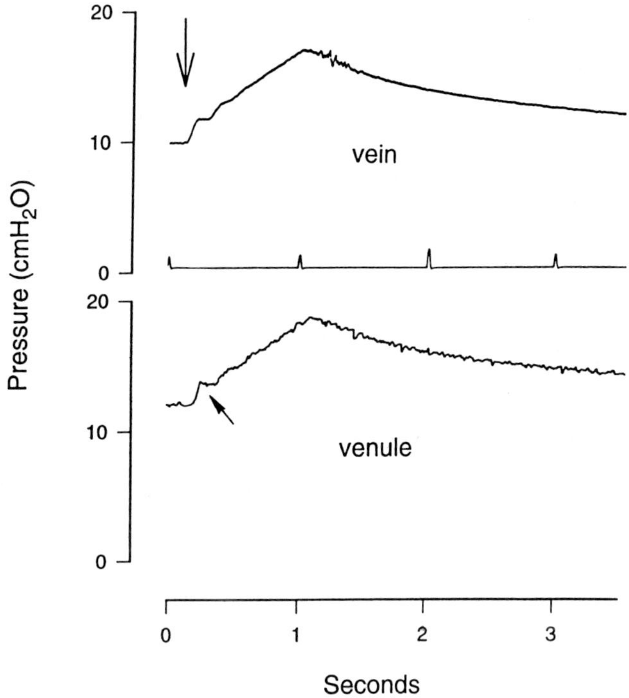

Figure 8 Lung vascular pressure transients following outflow occlusion. Large arrow indicates point of occlusion. Pressure equilibration transients seen as step pressure increases are evident both for the vein and the micropunctured venule tracings (small arrow).

constriction provides a potent mechanism for increasing lung microvascular pressures upstream of the constricting venules (97,98). Because of pressure-induced capillary distension, venular constriction also increases surface area of filtration (see Sec. II.B). This mechanism may be particularly relevant in some forms of pulmonary edema, such as neurogenic pulmonary edema (Chap. 10) and high altitude pulmonary edema (Chap. 11). However, since septal capillaries are compliant, the increase of capillary pressure may be blunted by the capillary bed and not transmitted upstream to increase the pulmonary arterial pressure. By contrast, arteriolar constriction increases all upstream pressures including the pulmonary arterial pressure, but it does not increase pressures in the microvascular bed downstream of the constriction.

By these considerations, venular constriction and increased left atrial pressure are the major predisposing factors for hydrostatic edema because they increase pressures and surface area of filtration in the lung microvascular segment. On the other hand, increase of pressures in the arterial segment alone, as in the presence of arteriolar constriction, does not predispose to pulmonary edema. Pulmonary vasoconstrictors tend to localize to either arterioles or venules as the predominant constriction site. Although a detailed discussion of these agents is outside the scope of this chapter, we may consider hypoxia to be a primary arteriolar constrictor, while major venoconstrictors include histamine and thromboxane A_2 (98–100). The content of cyclic GMP, which promotes vascular relaxation, is higher in pulmonary veins than arteries (101). This finding provides a basis for the differential vasoreactivity in lung veins versus arteries that may be significant in the regulation of venular constriction, hence lung microvascular pressures.

B. Major Filtration Site

The lung microvascular pressure profile provides a basis for interpreting the distribution of lung microvascular filtration. To identify the major filtration region, the microvascular location of the zero-filtration pressure (Pzf) must be determined, since filtration ceases beyond the point at which microvascular pressures fall below the Pzf. An estimate of this location is derived by placing the Pzf as one of the pressures in a pressure distribution diagram. Such a relation is shown in Figure 9, which plots data from rat lung for which data are available both for microvascular pressures and the Pzf (38,70). Note that of the total pulmonary artery-left atrial pressure drop, 30% occurs at the precapillary arteriole. Assuming a nearly linear pressure decrease in the capillary segment, the Pzf is achieved after a further pressure drop of 16%. This small pressure difference from the arteriole suggests that the Pzf occurs close to the septal introitus, possibly in the proximal 25% of the alveolar capillary bed. Hence according to this model, microvessels distal to the Pzf location, those comprising the bulk of the alveolar capillary bed, do not support filtration under normal conditions.

In the steady state, the lack of microvascular filtration is potentially untenable, unless specific mechanisms maintain constant perimicrovascular conditions. Prolonged absorptive flux should increase πi as interstitial proteins are concentrated by sieving. A sufficient increase of πi should inhibit absorption and establish filtration. Therefore, steady-state absorption is possible only if the πi buildup is prevented by either removal or dilution of perimicrovascular protein.

A dilutional mechanism may exist in the alveolar septal interstitium. The alveolar subfase constitutes a 0.2-μm-thick liquid layer of total volume ~5 mL, that underlies the surfactant layer (71). An active Na pump drives liquid from alveoli to the pericapillary interstitium (see Chap. 14) (72). Although the normal transalveolar flux remains unknown, alveolar instillates of Ringers-lactate generate a flux of ~10 mL/h (73). Therefore, in the normal steady state, active

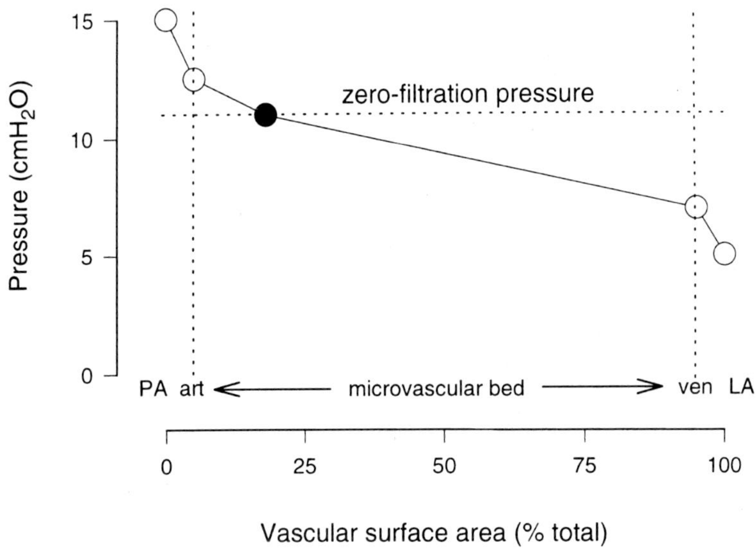

Figure 9 Vascular pressure distribution along the length of the lung microvascular bed. Pressures determined in rat lung (70) are shown for the pulmonary artery (PA), preseptal arteriole (art), postseptal venule (ven), and left atrium (LA). The zero filtration pressure (filled circle) was determined by the split-drop technique in rat lung venules (From Ref. 38).

transport may generate a transepithelial liquid flux of at least 5 mL/h from the alveolar lining phase to the pericapillary interstitium. Subsequently, the transalveolar liquid may be removed by osmotic uptake into nonfiltering alveolar capillaries. According to this theory, in the absorbing part of the alveolar septum a steady transport of transalveolar liquid dilutes perimicrovascular protein concentration and prevents increase of πi. The mechanism of replenishment of the subphase liquid remains unknown, although the source is likely to be the microvascular filtrate that is channeled partly into alveoli.

A second mechanism that sustains the absorption may be attributable to the convective removal of interstitial proteins by means of the lung interstitial pressure gradient. Such a mechanism which could abolish or minimize protein buildup, hence πi increase, is discussed below (see Sec. V.C).

V. Perimicrovascular Dynamics

A. Lung Perimicrovascular Pressures

The understanding of perimicrovascular liquid flow requires consideration of perimicrovascular pressures. Lung interstitial pressures as determined by a variety of techniques, such as the capsule, wick, and needle methods, have been reviewed and are not discussed here (4,7). The interstitial pressure relevant to lung microvascular filtration occurs in the perimicrovascular space which is uniquely accessible by micropuncture. Such determinations have been obtained in the interstitium surrounding 10- to 15-μm-diameter vessels at the alveolar septal junctions (Pjct) and in the adventitial space of 30- to 50-μm-diameter vessels (Padv) (29,74).

The main findings are:

1. At end-expiratory lung volume of 50% TLC (total lung capacity), Pjct and Padv average ~1.3 and ~0.3 cm H_2O, respectively (Fig. 10)
2. Even in severe edema the pressures increase by only 2 to 3 cm H_2O
3. Lung expansion to 80% TLC decreases both pressures (75)
4. Increase of vascular pressure by 10 cm H_2O decreases Padv (21).

These findings necessitate a reexamination of the traditional view of interstitial pressures. First, the Starling equation (see Sec. II.A) identifies the

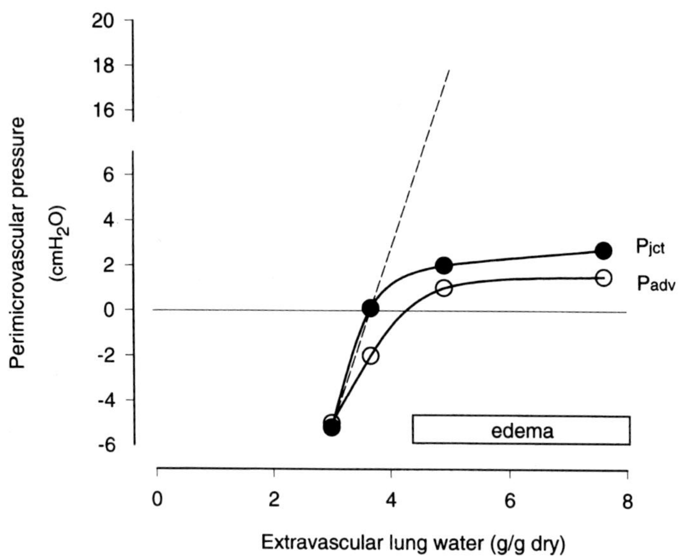

Figure 10 Lung perimicrovascular pressures. Alveolar junctional (Pjct) and microvessel adventitial (Padv) interstitial pressures were determined by micropuncture. Points at lung water ~3.9 g/g dry are baseline data. Points at lung water of 3 g/g dry obtained after lung dehydration. Dashed line shows that in the absence of increase in interstitial compliance, the rate of pressure increase in the nonedematous range predicts pressures of 18 cm H_2O at lung water of 5 g/g dry. (Adapted from Ref. 74.)

interstitial pressure as a counterfiltration force and therefore as a potential safety factor against high filtration. However, the small increases of Pjct and Padv in edema are not sufficient to provide a major counterfiltration force. Moreover, vascular pressure elevation does not increase Pjct or Padv. Therefore, the perimicrovascular interstitial pressures are not a safety factor against edema formation.

Second, lung interstitial pressures are traditonally thought to be determined directly by the alveolar pressure. However, the pressure responses to lung expansion and elevated vascular pressure, which both induce tissue distortion, attest to the dependency of Pjct and Padv on geometrical deformations of the lung matrix. Hence, we may conclude that the mechanical tension of the interstitial matrix is the principal determinant of lung interstitital pressures. The alveolar pressure is an indirect determinant of lung interstitial pressures, to the extent that it modifies matrix tension.

B. Interstitial Compliance

Although the lung matrix swells in edema, as classically seen in bronchovascular cuff formation, the swelling does not compress vessels. Accordingly, in the absence of secondary factors such as hypoxic vasoconstriction, vascular resistance does not increase in pulmonary edema (24). The swelling is explained by the water-imbibing property of interstitial matrix constituents such as hyaluronan. The lung content of hyaluronan correlates with lung water content under both normal and diseased conditions (76,77).

The lack of vascular compression in edema is attributable to the swelling-induced hyperbolic profile of the interstitial pressure-hydration curve (Fig. 10). The shape of the curve indicates that increase of lung water blunts potential increases of Pjct and Padv. This effect is attributable to the edema-induced increase of interstitial compliance which is the Δlung water/Δinterstitial pressure ratio, and is given by the inverse slope of the pressure–lung water plot. The dashed line in Figure 10 projects the protective compliance effect. If interstitial compliance were not to increase, Pjct alone could achieve levels as high as 18 cm H_2O that could clearly compress vessels. Hence, the ability of the interstitial matrix to imbibe water and increase compliance is a safety factor by which excess filtrate is retained within the matrix without compromising blood flow.

C. Interstitial Pressure Gradient

As postulated by Staub (3), the Pjct-Padv difference indicates that an interstitial pressure gradient exists in the perialveolar interstitium. The putative role of this gradient in supporting perimicrovascular liquid flow is suggested in micropuncture-imaging studies. The quantification of perimicrovascular flow was achieved by microinjection of fluorescent albumin into perimicrovascular adventia in lungs held at a normal end-expiratory volume. The albumin was convectively cleared with a half-time of ~1.2 min (Fig. 11), as consistent with a mathematical model of the perimicrovascular interstitium (78,79). Uptake of the injected interstitial liquid occurred into nonpulsatile lymphatics (Fig. 12). This is consistent with the nonpulsatility of Padv recordings and suggests that the filtrate flows passively into intial lymphatics.

We may conclude from these data that no lymphatic suction operates in the perimicrovascular interstitium and that perimicrovascular flux is driven passively by the Pjct-Padv gradient. Lung expansion to 70% total lung capacity almost totally abolishes the clearance of injected albumin from the perimicrovascular space (78). A similar lung expansion also abolishes the Pjct-Padv gradient (75,76). This association between the loss of the pressure gradient and the inhibition of perimicrovascular flow suggests that the Pjct-Padv gradient and perimicrovascular flow are causally linked.

These lung expansion data, if applicable to the breathing cycle, indicate that during inspiratory lung expansion the Pjct-Padv gradient is lost and interstitial liquid flow is impeded. The opposite may occur as lung volume decreases in expiration. Hence respiratory lung volume changes may cyclically vary the Pct-Padv gradient and thereby generate a pump-like mechanism to facilitate interstitial liquid clearance. In contrast, increase of vascular pressure by 10 cm H_2O almost doubles the pressure gradient (21). During vascular pressure increases, this effect may provide a safety mechanism for increasing liquid clearance from septal junctions into lymphatics in the microvessel adventitia.

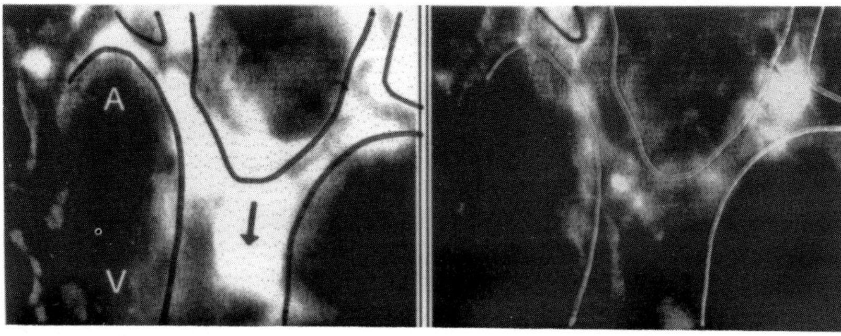

Figure 11 Images of the interstitial space adjacent to a 24-μm-diameter lung venule. Blood flow was present in the venule which is drawn in outline. *Left.* A, alveoli; V, venule. Image taken 0.5 min after 20 nl microinjection of fluorescent albumin shows fluorescence as white discoloration. *Right.* Image taken 3 min later shows removal of fluorescence. (From Ref. 78.)

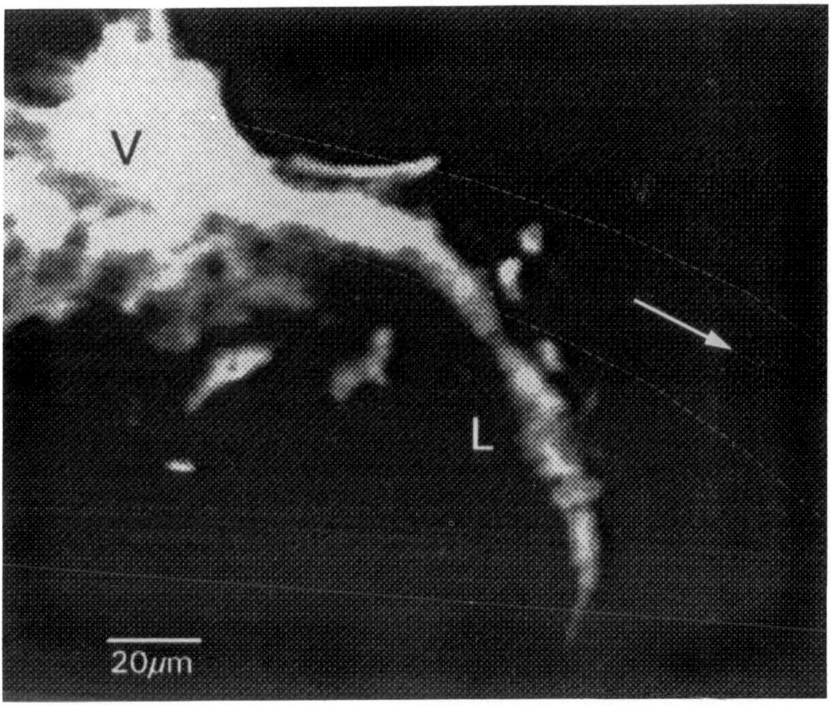

Figure 12 Lymphatic uptake of fluorescent albumin. V, venule adventia; L, lymphatic. Arrow shows direction of blood flow. Image taken ~70 μm downstream from site at which fluorescent albumin was microinjected. (From Ref. 78.)

D. Interstitial Charge

Although the lung interstitium has long been known to carry negative charge, the significance of the charge as a determinant of interstitial liquid flow is being understood only from recent experiments. Parker and colleagues determined the lung interstitial distribution volume of two positively charged tracers, LDH5 and LDH1 (80). LDH5, the more positively charged tracer, occupied a larger interstitial volume which is consistent with its expected distribution behavior in a negatively charged matrix. Lai-Fook and colleagues showed that interstitial transit of positively charged molecules across the interstitial matrix was less impeded than that of negatively charged molecules (81). Hyaluronan has been identified as the cause of the anionic impedance, because hyaluronidase treatment improves anion flow. The overall conclusion to be derived from these studies is that the lung interstitium carries a global net negative charge that excludes plasma anions from the interstitial matrix.

The ability of interstitial cations to determine the interstitial flow of charged proteins is potentially important in edema formation. In pressure- or sepsis-induced increases of filtration, loss of hyaluronan in lung lymph (82) may decrease negative charge in the lung interstitium. Conversely, upregulation of hyaluronan synthesis as part of the postinjury repair process (83) may increase interstitial negative charge. Loss of interstitial anions may reduce the interstitial anionic barrier and facilitate interstitial entry of anionic plasma proteins such as albumin that increase πi and predispose to edema.

VI. Alveolar Flooding

Clinically, the critical stage of pulmonary edema occurs when edema liquid enters the alveolar space. Traditionally, the mechanics of alveolar filling has been attributed to an "all-or-none" mechanism in which once liquid enters an alveolus, it fills either completely or not at all. This hypothesis is supported by morphological data (55) as well by a consideration of alveolar mechanics (102). Alveolar liquid pressures determined in lungs filled with different liquid volumes are also consistent with the notion that alveoli fill completely (93). However, the all-or-none hypothesis has been challenged by the proposal that alveolar filling occurs as a process of graded liquid entry into alveoli (36).

The route of alveolar liquid entry also continues to be confounding. The simplest explanation—that the liquid enters directly across epithelial junctions of the intact alveolar membrane—is unlikely because perialveolar interstitial pressures are far too low a driving force (see Sec. V.A) to overcome the high epithelial hydraulic resistance. Although the alveolar liquid is protein-rich, proteins are unlikely to be transported across epithelial junctions which are impermeable to albumin-size molecules (84). The following hypotheses are proposed.

A. Airway Entry Hypothesis

According to many investigators, edematous liquid enters airspaces across a natural "weakness" in the epithelium of the conducting airway, then flows distally into alveoli. Evidence for this mechanism is attributable to staining of airway structures by probes introduced intravascularly (85,86). In alveolar edema, protein concentrations are similar in the interstitial and alveolar liquids (87). Hence, proteins must enter the airway across a large nonrestricting pore. The precise site of liquid entry remains unknown, but proposed locations are the terminal or the respiratory bronchioles (86,87). Evidence for airway liquid entry was also recently interpreted from morphological differences of alveolar protein content (37). The airway entry hypothesis has not been tested in models of permeability edema.

B. Membrane Damage Hypothesis

According to this theory, liquid enters alveoli through breaks in the alveolar membrane. Evidence for membrane damage during pressure increases of up to 45 cm H_2O has been documented as outright breaks in alveolar membrane continuity and as formation of large epithelial blebs (36,37). Pressure increases to >52 cm H_2O induce breaks in the microvascular membrane as well (88). Walker et al. documented ultrastructural changes in tight junctions of alveolar epithelial and endothelial cells in both high-pressure and high-permeability edemas (33). These studies indicate that increases of epithelial membrane permeability may determine alveolar liquid entry.

A common feature of some of the membrane rupture studies is that edema was induced very rapidly—in 1 to 3 min (36,88). In the experiments by Bachofen et al. (36,37), not only were isolated rabbit lungs exposed to high vascular pressures but they were perfused with 6% albumin, which causes barrier deterioration in the rat lung (15). Thus their findings may be attributable to the combined effects of high pressure and increased permeability. We may conclude from these morphological data that membrane rupture provides a mechanism for alveolar flooding in forms of alveolar edema that occur very rapidly, as for example the edema caused by immune reactions (89). However, at more modest pressure elevations, to <45 cm H_2O, in which onset of alveolar edema occurs with a latency of hours, and in which alveolar membrane rupture has not been described, the membrane break hypothesis remains unsubstantiated.

VII. Conclusion

The new data lead to some new proposals concerning the physiology of lung liquid production:

1. Filtration occurs across a small fraction of the total surface area of the lung microvascular bed. The bulk of the microvascular surface area is not normally responsible for liquid production. Recruitment of this surface for filtration is likely to increase the lung's liquid burden and promote edema. This recruitment could occur through increase of barrier permeability, or through increase of the local vascular pressure to a level exceeding the zero-filtration pressure.
2. The microvascular wall's role in liquid transport is not passive. Active mechanisms are identifiable in endothelial receptor-mediated signal transduction processes that are clearly capable of modifying barrier properties.

3. Caveolar transport of plasma proteins cannot be discounted in considerations of lung liquid transport. Some new data indicate that active protein transport exists in lung capillaries and that augmentation of this transport modifies transmicrovascular flux.

4. The perimicrovascular interstitial pressure is not a safety factor against pulmonary edema. However, two new interstitial safety factors are identified. These are an interstitial pressure gradient and the interstitial compliance. The pressure gradient drives liquid flow toward lymphatics and thereby promotes liquid removal from the perimicrovascular space. The increase of interstitial compliance in edema protects against potentially deleterious increases of interstitial pressure.

5. The microphysiological approach provides a new paradigm for the cell biological investigation of the intact lung capillary. The arteriolar or venular capillary provides a platform for the study of in situ endothelial responses in lung. In a postmodern turnaround, it is becoming possible to apply methods reserved largely for cultured cells to the intact microvessel. Thus, new investigative directions include the incorporation of imaging methods to determine endothelial second messengers such as the cytosolic free Ca^{2+} concentration which is likely to affect several aspects of microvascular function (90). One of the challenges for future research is to test in intact models the hypotheses generated from current in vitro experiments in order to further the understanding of pulmonary edema.

Acknowledgments

Drs. S. Bhattacharya and H. Jerome read the manuscript. Dr. X. Ying and Ms. W. Chen helped in preparation of the manuscript. The author's cited research was supported by grants from the National Heart, Lung and Blood Institute (HL36024, HL53625), the American Heart Association, and the New York Lung Association.

References

1. Staub NC. Pathophysiology of pulmonary edema. In: Staub NC, Taylor AE, eds. Edema. New York: Raven Press, 1984:719–746.
2. Guyton AC, Lindsey AW. Effect of elevated left atrial pressure and decreased plasma protein concentration on the development of pulmonary edema. Circ Res 1959; 7:649–657.
3. Staub NC. Pulmonary edema. Physiol Rev 1974; 54:678–811.

4. Taylor AE, Parker JC. Pulmonary interstitial spaces and lymphatics. In: Geiger SR, ed. Handbook of Physiology. Bethesda, MD: Am Physiol Soc, 1984:167–230.
5. Effros RM. Pulmonary microcirculation and exchange. In: Handbook of Physiology: The Cardiovascular System IV. Bethesda, MD: Am Physiol Soc 1984. Vol. IV, Part 2 Chap. 18:865–915.
6. Dawson CA, Linehan JH, Bronikowski TA. Pressure and flow in the pulmonary vascular bed. In: Pulmonary Vascular Physiology and Pathophysiology. New York: Marcel Dekker, 1989:51–91.
7. Lai-Fook SJ. Mechanical factors in lung liquid distribution. Annu Rev Physiol 1993; 55:155–180.
8. Sadurski R, Ying X, Tsukada H, Bhattacharya S, Bhattacharya J. Diameters of juxta-capillary venules determined by an oil-drop method in rat lung. J Appl Physiol 1994; 77:718–725.
9. Ragette R, Fu CZ, Bhattacharya J. Barrier effects of hyperosmolar signalling in microvascular endothelium of rat lung. J Clin Invest 1997; 100:685–692.
10. Blake L, Staub NC. Pulmonary vascular transport in sheep a mathematical model. Microvasc Res 1976; 12:197–220.
11. Zarins CK, Rice CL, Peters RM, Virgilio RW. Lymph and pulmonary response to isobaric reduction in plasma oncotic pressure in baboons. Circ Res 1978; 43: 925–930.
12. Kramer GC, Harms BA, Bodai BI, Renkin EM, Demling RH. Effects of hypoproteinemia and increased vascular pressure on lung fluid balance in sheep. J Appl Physiol 1983; 55:1514–1522.
13. Dodek PM, Rice TW, Bonsignore MR, Yamada S, Staub NC. Effects of plasmapheresis and of hypoproteinemia on lung liquid conductance in awake sheep. Circ Res 1986; 58:269–280.
14. Qiao RL, Bhattacharya J. Segmental barrier properties of the pulmonary microvascular bed. J Appl Physiol 1991; 64:2562–2567.
15. Qiao RL, Ying X, Bhattacharya J. Hyperoncotic albumin decreases the endothelial barrier in rat lung. Am J Physiol 1993; 265:H198–H204.
16. Zadrobilek E, Schindler I, Redl G, Mauritz W, Gilly H, Sporn P, Steinbereithner K. Intravascular starling forces and extravascular lung water in advanced septic shock states. Prog Clin Biol Res 1987; 236:139–144.
17. Weaver DW, Ledserwood AM, Lucas CE, Higgins R, Bouwman DL, Johnson SD. Pulmonary effects of albumin resuscitation for severe hypovolumic shock. Arch Surg 1978; 113:387–392.
18. Rippe B, Haraldsson B. Transport of macromolecules across microvascular walls: the two-pore theory. Physiol Rev 1994; 74:163–219.
19. Patlak CS, Rapoport SI. Theoretical analysis of net tracer flux due to volume circulation in a membrane with pores of different sizes. Relation to solute drag model. J Gen Physiol 1971; 57:113–124.
20. Granger DN, Taylor AE. Permeability of intestinal capillaries to endogenous macromolecules. Am J Physiol 1980; 238:H457–H464.
21. Glucksberg MR, Bhattacharya J. Effect of vascular pressure on interstitial pressures in the isolated dog lung. J Appl Physiol 1993; 75:268–272.

22. Wolf MB, Watson PD, Scott DRC. Integral-mass balance method for determination of solvent drag reflection coefficient. Am J Physiol 1987; 253:H194–H204.
23. Gaar KA Jr, Taylor AE, Owens LJ, Guyton AC. Pulmonary capillary pressure and filtration coefficient in the isolated perfused lung. Am J Physiol 1967; 213:910–914.
24. Bhattacharya J, Nakahara K, Staub NC. The effect of edema on pulmonary blood flow in the isolated perfused dog lung lobe. J Appl Physiol 1980; 48:444–449.
25. Gorin AB, Stewart PA. Differential permeability of endothelial and epithelial barriers to albumin flux. J Appl Physiol: Respirat Environ Exercise Physiol 1979; 47:1315–1324.
26. Kaplan JD, Calandrino FS, Schuster DP. A positron emission tomographic comparison of pulmonary vascular permeability during the adult respiratory distress sydrome and pneumonia. Am Rev Respir Dis 1991; 143:150–154.
27. Pilati CF, Maron MB. A technique to measure the reflection coefficient using endogenous vascular indicators. Microvasc Res 1986; 32:255–260.
28. Bhattacharya J. Hydraulic conductivity of lung venules determined by split-drop technique. J Appl Physiol 1988; 64:2565–2567.
29. Bhattacharya J, Gropper MA, Staub NC. Interstitial fluid pressure gradient measured by micropuncture in excised dog lung. J Appl Physiol 1984; 56:271–277.
30. Tsukada H, Ying X, Fu C, et al. Ligation of the endothelial avb3 integrin increases capillary hydraulic conductivity of rat lung. Circ Res 1995; 77:651–659.
31. Perry MA. Capillary filtration and permeability coefficients calculated from measurements of interendothelial cell junctions in rabbit lung and skeletal muscle. Microvasc Res 1980; 19:142–157.
32. Schneeberger EE, Lynch RD. Structure, function, and regulation of cellular tight junctions. Am J Physiol 1992; 262:L647–L661.
33. Walker DC, MacKenzie AL, Wiggs BR, Montaner JG, Hogg JC. Assessment of tight junctions between pulmonary epithelial and endothelial cells. J Appl Physiol 1988; 64:2348–2356.
34. Schneeberger EE, McCormack JM. Intercellular junctions in upper airway submucosal glands of the rat: a tracer and freeze fracture study. Anat Rec 1984; 210: 421–433.
35. Schneeberger EE. Segmental differentiation of endothelial intercellular junctions in intra-acinar arteries and veins of the rat. Circ Res 1981; 49:1102–1111.
36. Bachofen H, Schurch S, Michel RP, Weibel ER. Experimental hydrostatic pulmonary edema in rabbit lungs. Am Rev Respir Dis 1993; 147:989–996.
37. Bachofen H, Schurch S, Weibel ER. Experimental hydrostatic pulmonary edema in rabbit lungs. Am Rev Respir Dis 1993; 147:997–1004.
38. Ishikawa S, Tsukada H, Bhattacharya J. Soluble complex of complement increases hydraulic conductivity in single microvessels of rat lung. J Clin Invest 1993; 91:103–109.
39. Parker JC, Perry MA, Taylor AE. Permeability of the microvascular barrier. In: Staub NC, Taylor AE, eds. Edema. New York: Raven Press. 1979:143–188.
40. Curry FE, Frokjaer-Jensen J. Water flow across the walls of single muscle capillaries in the frog, *Rana pipiens.* J Physiol 1984; 350:293–307.

41. Harris TR, Roselli RJ. A theoretical model of protein, fluid, and small molecule transport in the lung. J Appl Physiol 1981; 50:1–14.
42. Brigham KL. Lung lymph composition and flow in experimental pulmonary edema. In: Pulmonary Edema. Besthesda, MD: Am Physiol Soc, 1979:161–173.
43. Erdman AJ, Vaughan TR, Brigham KL, Woolverton WC, Staub NC. Effect of increased vascular pressure on lung fluid balance in unanesthetized sheep. Circ Res 1975; 37:271–284.
44. Predescu D, Horvat R, Predescu S, Palade GE. Transcytosis in the continuous endothelium of the myocardial microvasculature is inhibited by N-ethylmaleimide. Proc Natl Acad Sci USA. 1994; 91:3014–3018.
45. Ghitescu L, Bendayan M. Transendothelial transport of serum albumin: a quantitative immunocytochemical study. J Cell Biol 1992; 117:745–755.
46. Walker DC, Mackenzie A, Hosford S. The structure of the tricellular region of the endothelial tight junctions of pulmonary capillaries. Microvasc Res 1994; 48:259–281.
47. Walker DC, Mackenzie A, Hosford S. The structure of the tricellular region of the endothelial tight junctions of pulmonary capillaries. Microvasc Res 1994; 48:259–281.
48. Palade GE, Bruns RR. Structural modulations of plasmalemmal vesicles. J Cell Biol 1968; 37:633–649.
49. Schnitzer JE, Phil O. Albondin-mediated capillary permeability to albumin. J Biol Chem 1994; 269:1–11.
50. Dobrila L, Antohe F, Heltianu C, Simionescu M. Albumin binding proteins of endothelial cells identified by anti-idiotypic antibodies. Int Immunol 1992; 4: 789–796.
51. Fu CZ, Bhattacharya S, Bhattacharya J. Absence of albumin blocks fluid phase endocytosis in bovine pulmonary artery endothelial cells. Mol Biol Cell 1995; 6:297a.
52. Ying X, Qiao R, Bhattacharya J. Contribution of the intracellular pathway to microvascular albumin transport in rat lung. Microcirculation 1996; 3:110.
53. Defouw DO. Morphometric studies of endothelial vesicles of alveolar vessels in edematous lungs. Prog Appl Microcirc 1985; 9:67–79.
54. Ying X, Bhattacharya J. Counter-convective albumin transport across venular endothelium of rat lung. Faseb J 1994; A1063.
55. Staub NC, Nagano H, Pearce ML. Pulmonary edema in dogs, especially the sequence of fluid accumulation in the lungs. J Appl Physiol 1967; 22:227–240.
56. Mitzner W, Robotham JL. Distribution of interstitial compliance and filtration coefficient in canine lung. Lymphology 1979; 12:140–148.
57. Gropper MA, Bhattacharya J. Staub NC. Filtration profile in isolated zone 1 and zone 3 dog lungs at constant high alveolar pressure. J Appl Physiol 1988; 65:343–349.
58. Bhattacharya J. Sites of transendothelial liquid transport in lung microcirculation. Fed Proc 1987; 46:2502–2505.
59. Bhattacharya J, Staub NC. Direct measurement of microvascular pressure in the isolated perfused dog lung. Science 1980; 210:327–328.

60. Raj JU, Kaapa P, Hillyard R, Anderson J. Pulmonary vascular pressure profile in adult ferrets: measurements in vivo and in isolated lungs. Acta Physiol Scand 1991; 142:141–148.
61. Fike CD, Kaplowitz MR. Effect of airway and left atrial pressures on microvascular and interstitial pressures in adult lungs. J Appl Physiol 1993; 74:2112–2120.
62. Hakim TS, Kelly S. Occlusion pressures vs. micropipette pressures in the pulmonary circulation. J Appl Physiol 1989; 67:1277–1285.
63. Bhattacharya S, Glucksberg MR, Bhattacharya J. Measurement of lung microvascular pressure in the intact anesthetized rabbit by the micropuncture technique. Circ Res 1989; 64:167–172.
64. Negrini D, Gonano C, Miserocchi G. Microvascular pressure profile in intact in situ lung. J Appl Physiol 1992; 72:332–339.
65. Haworth ST, Rickaby DA, Linehan JH, Dawson CA. Subpleural pulmonary microvascular pressures in the dog lung. J Appl Physiol 1995; 79:615–622.
66. Shepard JA, Gropper MA, Nicolaysen G, Staub NC, Bhattacharya J. Microvascular pressure profile of intact dog lung measured by micropuncture. J Appl Physiol 1988; 64:874–879.
67. Onizuka M, Wagner L, Nicolaysen G, Staub NC. Micropuncture pressure in small arteries or veins of perfused rabbit lungs. J Appl Physiol 1990; 68:1838–1843.
68. Rock P, Patterson GA, Permutt S, Sylvester JT. Nature and distribution of vascular resistance in hypoxic pig lungs. J Appl Physiol 1985; 59:1891–1901.
69. Hakim TS, Dawson CA, Linehan JH. Hemodynamic responses of dog lung lobe to lobar venous occlusion. J Appl Physiol: Respirat Environ Exercise Physiol 1979; 47:145–152.
70. Bhattacharya S, Bhattacharya J. Segmental vascular responses to voltage gated calcium channel potentiation in rat lung. J Appl Physiol 1992; 73:657–663.
71. Bastacky J, Lee CYC, Goerke LJ, et al. Alveolar lining layer is thin and continuous: low-temperature scanning electron microscopy of rat lung. J Appl Physiol 1995; 79:1615–1628.
72. Matthay MA, Folkesson HG, Verkman AS. Salt and water transport across alveolar and distal airway epithelia in the adult lung. Am J Physiol (Lung Cell Mol Physiol) 1996; 270:L487–L503.
73. Matthay MA, Landolt CC, Staub NC. Differential liquid and protein clearance from the alveoli of anesthetized sheep. J Appl Physiol 1982; 53:96–104.
74. Glucksberg MR, Bhattacharya J. Effect of dehydration on interstitial pressures in the isolated dog lung. J Appl Physiol 1989; 67:839–845.
75. Bhattacharya J, Gropper MA, Shepard JM. Lung expansion and the perialveolar interstitial pressure gradient. J Appl Physiol 1989; 66:2600–2605.
76. Bhattacharya J, Cruz T, Bhattacharya S, Bray B. Hyaluronan affects extravascular water in lungs of unanesthetized rabbits. J Appl Physiol 1989; 66:2595–2599.
77. Nettelbladt O, Tengblad A, Hallgren R. Lung accumulation of hyaluronan parallels pulmonary edema in experimental alveolitis. Am J Physiol 1989; 257:L379–L384.
78. Ying X, Qiao R, Ishikawa S, Bhattacharya J. Removal of albumin microinjected in rat lung perimicrovascular space. J Appl Physiol 1994; 77:1294–1302.
79. Ford TR, Sachs JR, Grotberg JB, Glucksberg MR. Perialveolar interstitial resistance and compliance in isolated rat lung. J Appl Physiol 1991; 70:2750–2756.

80. Parker JC. Transport and distribution of charged macromolecules in lung. Adv Microcirc 1987; 13:150–159.
81. Tajaddini A, Brown LV, Lai-Fook SJ. Effect of hydration on lung interstitial permeability response to albumin and hyaluronidase. J Appl Physiol 1994; 76:578–583.
82. Lebel L, Smith L, Risberg B, Laurent TC, Gerdin B. Increased lymphatic elimination of interstitial hyaluronan during *E. coli* sepsis in sheep. Am J Physiol 1989; 256:H1524–H1531.
83. Anderson-Bray B, Sampson PM, Osman M, Giandomenico A, Turino GM. Early changes in lung tissue hyaluronan (hyaluronic acid) and hyaluronidase in bleomycin-induced alveolitis in hamsters. Am Rev Respir Dis 1991; 143: 284–288.
84. Schneeberger EE, Karnovsky MJ. The influence of entravascular fluid volume on the permeability of newborn and adult mouse lungs to ultrastructural protein tracers. J Cell Biol 1971; 49:319–334.
85. Conhaim RL. Airway level at which edema liquid enters the air space of isolated dog lungs. J Appl Physiol 1989; 67:2234–2242.
86. Zumsteg TA, Havill AM, Gee MH. Relationships among lung extravascular fluid compartments with alveolar flooding. J Appl Physiol 1982; 53:267–271.
87. Vreim CE, Staub NC. Protein composition of lung fluids in acute alloxan edema dogs. Am J Physiol 1976; 230:376–379.
88. Tsukimoto K, Matheiu-Costello O, Prediletto R, Elliott AR, West JB. Ultrastructural appearance of pulmonary capillaries at high transmural pressures. J Appl Physiol 1991; 7192:573–582.
89. Caldwell PRB, Camussi G, Brentjens JR, Andres G. Lung injury in rabbits induced by intravenous administration of heterologous polyclonal antibodies to angiotensin converting enzyme (kininase II). J Mol Cell Cardiol 1989; 21: 171–174.
90. Ying X, Minamiya Y, Fu C, Bhattacharya J. Calcium waves in lung capillary endothelium. Circ Res 1996; 79:898–908.
91. Curry FE. Mechanics and thermodynamics of transcapillary exchange. In: Renkin EM, Michel CC, eds. Handbook of Physiology: The Cardiovascular System. Microcirculation. Bethesda, MD: Am Physiol Soc. 1984: Sect 2, Vol IV, Pt 1, Chap 8:309–374.
92. Dainty J. Water relations of plant cells. Adv Bot Res 163; 1:279–326.
93. Raj JU, Conhaim RL, Bhattacharya J. Micropuncture measurement of alveolar liquid pressure in excised dog lung lobes. J Appl Physiol 1987; 62:781–784.
94. Nagasaka Y, Ishigaki M, Okazaki H, et al. Effect of pulmonary blood flow on microvascular pressure profile determined by micropuncture in perfused cat lungs. J Appl Physiol 1994; 77:1834–1839.
95. Moore TM, Khimenko P, Adkins WK, Miyasaka M, Taylor AE. Adhesion molecules contribute to ischemia and reperfusion-induced injury in the isolated rat lung. J Appl Physiol 1995; 78:2245–2252.
96. Kushimoto S, Okajima K, Uchiba M, Murakami K, Okabe H, Takatsuki K. Pulmonary vascular injury induced by hemorrhagic shock is mediated by P-selectin in rats. Thromb Res 1996; 82:97–106.

97. Bhattacharya J, Nanjo S, Staub, NC. Effect of 5-hydroxytryptamine on lung microvascular pressure: micropuncture measurements in excised dog lungs. J Appl Physiol 1982; 52:634–637.
98. Raj JU, Anderson J. Pulmonary venous responses to thromboxane A_2 analogue and atrial natriuretic peptide in lambs. Circ Res 1990; 66:496–502.
99. Nagasaka Y, Bhattacharya J, Nanjo S, Gropper M, Staub NC. Micropuncture measurement of lung microvascular pressure profile during hypoxia in cats. Circ Res 1984; 54:90–95.
100. Shirai M, Sada K, Ninomiya I. Nonuniform effects of histamine on small pulmonary vessels in cats. J Appl Physiol 1987; 62:451–458.
101. Gao Y, Zhou H, Raj JU. Endothelium-derived nitric oxide plays a larger role in pulmonarty veins than in arteries of newborn lambs. Circ Res 1995; 76:559–565.
102. Wilson TA. Effect of alveolar wall shape on alveolar water stability. J Appl Physiol 1981; 50:222–224.

2

Histopathology of Pulmonary Edema and the Acute Respiratory Distress Syndrome

KURT H. ALBERTINE

University of Utah Health Sciences Center
Salt Lake City, Utah

I. Introduction

Pulmonary edema is a common feature of acute lung injury, typified by the acute respiratory distress syndrome (ARDS). Formation of edema during the development of ARDS is the result of increased permeability of the pulmonary blood vessels. If, in the course of the injury, the alveolar epithelium is damaged, alveolar flooding can occur, resulting in abnormalities in respiratory gas exchange. The pathology of increased-permeability pulmonary edema has been appreciated for many years (1–3). Knowledge of the histopathology of pulmonary edema has proven invaluable for characterization of the process of edema liquid formation, responses of lung cells to injury, participation of inflammatory cells in the injury, and the process of edema liquid clearance.

Exciting new opportunities are available today to relate the histopathology of pulmonary edema to mediators of inflammation that may be useful predictors of either the onset of or outcome from the ARDS (4). Numerous studies have identified putative biological markers in plasma, bronchoalveolar lavage liquid collected from the distal airspaces, or pulmonary edema liquid withdrawn from the distal airspaces and airways (4,5). However, each of the compartments (vascular, distal airspace, upper airway) is composed of many cell types (an estimated 50 cell types are in the lung) (6) that may contribute to the sampled pool of biological markers. For example, the CXC chemokine epithelial cell-derived neutrophil activator 78 (ENA-78) is a biological marker of interest (7) that recently has been shown, by immunohistochemical localization in human lung tissue, to be expressed by endothelial cells and vascular smooth muscle cells, in addition to epithelial cells in the lungs of subjects who died with the ARDS or sepsis (8). The multiplicity of cell types that may express biological markers in situ provides incentive to identify how acute lung injury influences structural cells (e.g., alveolar type II epithelial cells) and mobile cells (e.g., neutrophils) in the lung.

This chapter is organized to review the structural basis of pulmonary edema in the context of the pathophysiology of pulmonary edema. First, the anatomy and physiology of solute and liquid exchange in normal lungs are compared to those of injured lungs with pulmonary edema. The histopathology of increased-permeability pulmonary edema is described for humans and experimental animals. Next, the pathogenetic mechanisms for increased-permeability pulmonary edema are described. Emphasis is given to the role played by neutrophils. Next are considered structure-function relationships for biological markers of acute lung injury that may be useful clinical predictors of injury onset or progression. Finally, the process of clearance of pulmonary edema liquid is described.

II. Solute and Liquid Movement, and Sites of Liquid Accumulation in the Lung

Filtration of solutes and liquid from pulmonary microvessels occurs in the normal lung (see Chap. 1). This has been demonstrated by collecting lymph of pulmonary origin (9,10). Based on scaled-up data derived from sheep, the flow of pulmonary lymph in the human lung has been estimated to be about 10–20 mL/hr (9).

What are the sites and pathways across which solutes and liquid move from the microvascular lumen to the interstitium of the lung? Microvascular exchange in the normal lung appears to occur predominantly from small arterioles (<100 μm in diameter), alveolar capillaries (10–12 μm in diameter), and small venules (<200 μm in diameter) (11,12). The wall of each of these vessel types consists mainly of a single layer of nonfenestrated endothelial cells, outside of which is a continuous basal lamina (Fig. 1).

Identification of the dominant pathway for solute transport (diffusion and convection) across the lung's microvasculature has been controversial (see Chap. 1). This is especially true for proteins (13), which are principally responsible for establishing the protein osmotic pressure gradient across the microvascular wall (9). The pathway for transport of small solutes, such as electrolytes, has been

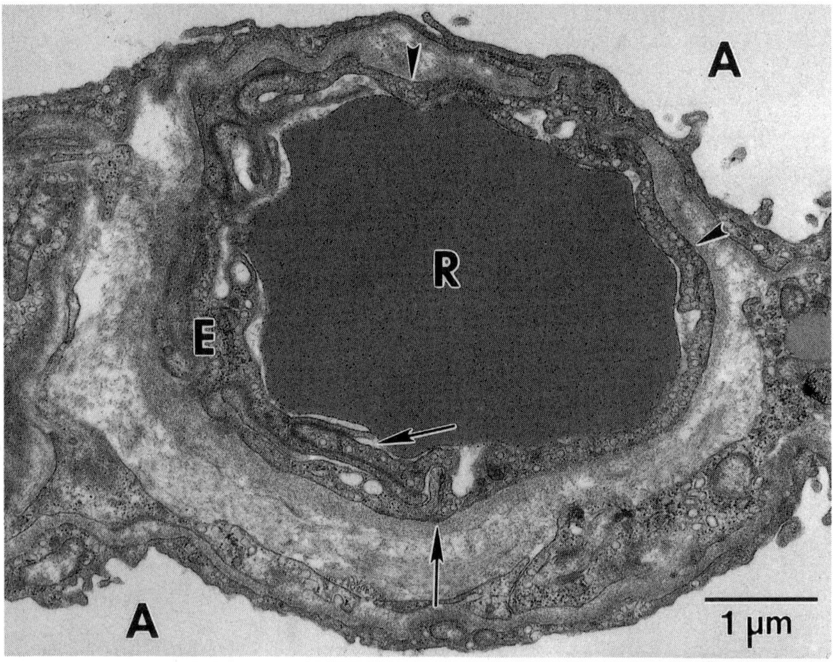

Figure 1 Transcellular transport pathways across microvascular endothelial (E) cells from a normal human lung. Intercellular channels (arrows) are visible between the capillary endothelial cells. Cytoplasmic vesicles (arrowheads) are obvious inside the endothelial cells. R, red blood cell; A, alveolus.

somewhat easier to identify. Some small solutes are transported by ion pumps (e.g., Na^+,K^+-ATPase) or ion channels (e.g., sodium or chloride channels). Other small solutes are carried along a concentration gradient (e.g., glucose) (14).

Two ultrastructural pathways for protein transport are evident in thin sections for transmission electron microscopy: intercellular channels and cytoplasmic vesicles (Fig. 1). Intercellular channels ("pores") are probably the dominant route for liquid and protein exchange in normal and edematous lungs (13,15). Schneeberger showed by the freeze-fracture technique that the arteriolar end of the pulmonary microcirculation has tighter intercellular junctions than the venular end (16,17). Her data suggest a longitudinal gradient in paracellular permeability in the lung. Curiously, Inuoe and colleagues did not find an ultrastructural gradient in intercellular junctions (18). Although there are transcellular pathways potentially available for transport, no substantive data exist to prove that cytoplasmic vesicles contribute significantly to net liquid and protein exchange across the pulmonary microvascular endothelial cells. Indeed, DeFouw and colleagues showed that endothelial cell cytoplasmic vesicles in normal and edematous lungs do not play a major role in liquid exchange (19). Alternatively, their primary role may be membrane internalization and receptor binding (20–22) (see Chap. 1 for more discussion of this issue).

The solutes and liquid that leak from the pulmonary microcirculation enter the perimicrovascular interstitial space. In the alveolar septa, this space is referred to as the alveolar wall interstitium. It is visible as the thick side of the blood-air barrier (Fig. 2), in distinction to the thin side. On the thick side of the

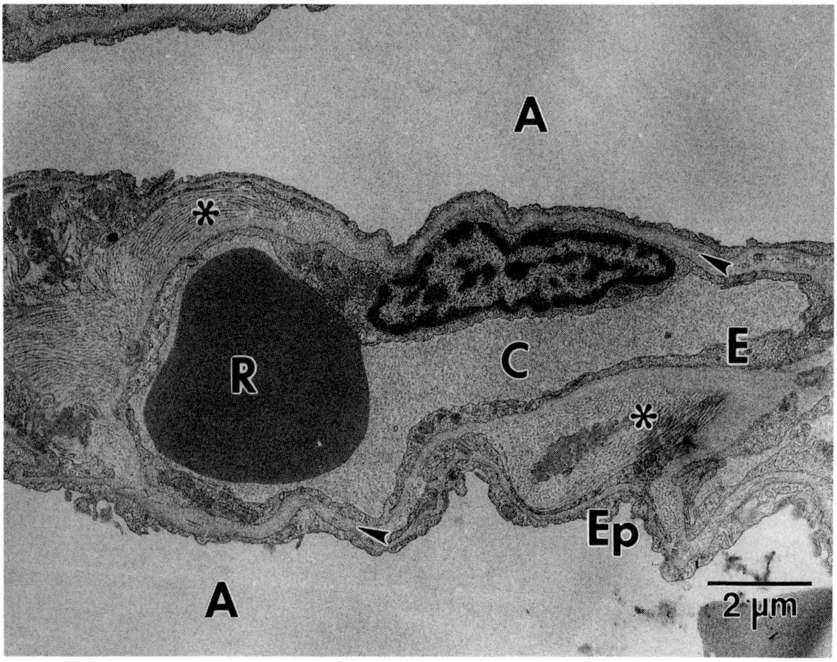

Figure 2 Ultrastructural appearance of parenchymal connective tissue from a normal human lung. The "thick" side (*) of an alveolar septum is so named because the alveolar epithelial (Ep) and capillary endothelial (E) cells, and their respective basal laminae, are separated by interstitial cells and connective tissue elements. The "thin" side (arrowheads) of an alveolar septum lacks this intervening accumulation of connective tissue elements. Therefore, the alveolar epithelial and capillary endothelial cells are separated by only their fused basal laminae. The thick and thin sides of an alveolar capillary change as the capillary (C) crosses between alveoli (A). R, red blood cell. (From Albertine KH. Structural organization and quantitative morphology of the lung. In: Cutillo AM, ed. Application of Magnetic Resonance to the Study of Lung. Armonk, NY: Futura Publishing Co, 1996; 73–114.)

blood–air barrier, the endothelial cells, epithelial cells, and their respective basal laminae are separated by connective tissue elements, such as collagen, elastin, microfibrils, interstitial cells, and proteoglycans (mainly heparan sulfate) (23–27). This intervening connective tissue space is absent along the thin side of the alveolar capillaries. Its absence reduces the width of the diffusional barrier to oxygen and carbon dioxide. The alveolar septa do not have lymphatics (28–32).

The alveolar wall interstitium is continuous with the connective tissue sheaths that surround airways and pulmonary blood vessels (and therefore are referred to as peribronchovascular connective tissue sheaths; Fig. 3), interlobular septa, and visceral pleura. We refer to all of these connective tissue spaces as "extra-alveolar" interstitium in part because the hydrostatic pressure in them is not affected by alveolar pressure. Connective tissue in the "corners" of alveolar walls is also included in the extra-alveolar interstitium because the alveolar corner interstitium is partially protected from the full effect of alveolar pressure (33–35). In this respect, the two interstitial compartments in the lung are, or are not, affected by alveolar air pressure in an analogous fashion to the alveolar and

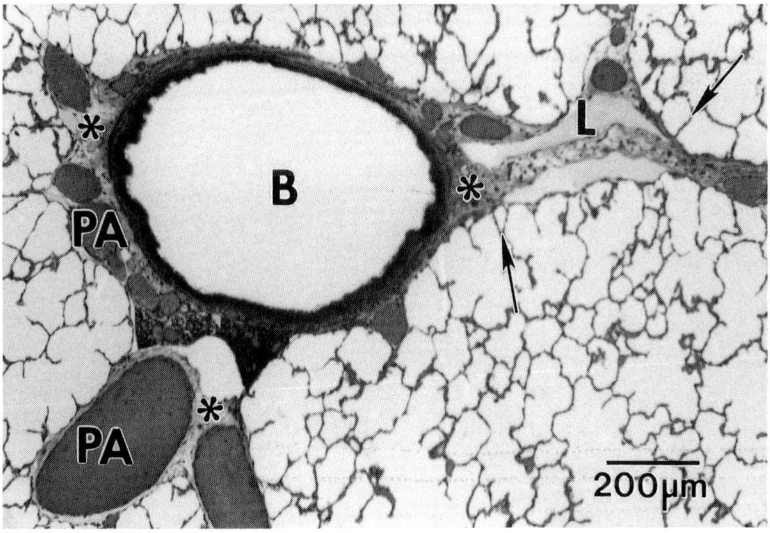

Figure 3 Histological appearance of the connective tissue spaces of a normal sheep lung. A bronchiole (B) and the surrounding pulmonary arteries (PA) are embedded in a sheath of connective tissue (*) referred to as peribronchovascular connective tissue. This connective tissue space is in series with the connective tissue in the alveolar walls (arrows). L, lymphatic.

extra-alveolar microvessels, respectively (36,37). Fibrous elements in the extra-alveolar interstitium include elastin, collagen, and reticulin. In this regard, the extra-alveolar interstitium and alveolar wall interstitium are structurally alike. However, chondroitin sulfate, rather than heparan sulfate, is the primary proteoglycan in the extra-alveolar interstitium.

Solutes and liquid that reach the peribronchovascular connective tissue sheaths may follow two pathways. One pathway is via the initial lymphatics (Fig. 4). Their wall is made solely of attenuated endothelial cells and fragmented basal lamina. The lymphatic endothelial cells have few specialized intercellular junctional complexes (31,32,38,39). These anatomical features imply that there is less resistance to solute and liquid absorption into the initial lymphatics (lymph formation) than in leakage from the pulmonary microvessels. The second pathway is a centripetal route along the peribronchovascular connective tissue sheaths themselves. That is, not all of the solutes and liquid that reach the

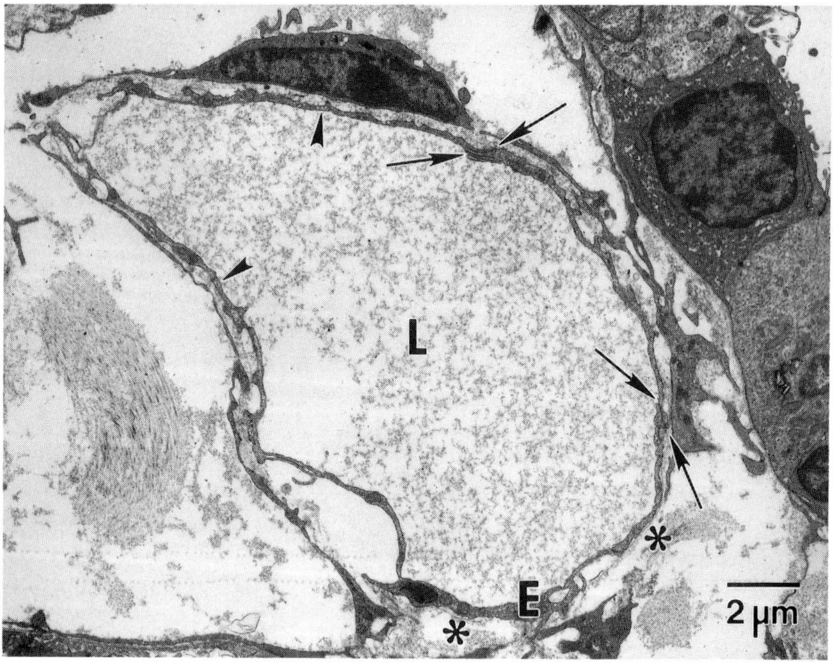

Figure 4 Initial lymphatic (L) in a peribronchovascular connective tissue sheath from a normal human lung. The lymphatic wall is composed of continuous endothelial (E) cells and fragments of basal lamina (*). Transcellular transport pathways include intercellular channels (arrows) and cytoplasmic vesicles (arrowheads).

sheaths enter the initial lymphatics. Instead, some solutes and liquid remain in the sheaths and track centrally toward the lung hilum (40,41). For example, Gee and Havill showed that the liquid in the peribronchovascular connective tissue edema cuffs represents microvascular filtrate at an earlier time than does lung lymph (42).

III. Physiology of Net Microvascular Liquid Filtration in the Lung

The factors that determine the net movement of liquid across a semipermeable barrier, such as pulmonary microvascular endothelium, are described in the Starling equation:

$$\dot{Q} = K[(P_{mv} - P_{pmv}) - \sigma(\pi_{mv} - \pi_{pmv})]$$

$\dot{Q}$ is the net filtration rate of liquid. [To completely describe net filtration for both solutes and liquid, a parallel equation for solute transport must be used (15).] K and σ refer to the liquid filtration coefficient (liquid conductance of the barrier) and protein reflection coefficient (barrier resistance to protein movement), respectively, for microvascular endothelium. P_{mv} and P_{pmv} refer to the hydrostatic pressure in microvascular (mv) and perimicrovascular (pmv) interstitial spaces, respectively. Finally, π_{mv} and π_{pmv} refer to the protein osmotic pressure (π) in the microvascular lumen and perimicrovascular interstitial space, respectively. Net liquid filtration across the pulmonary microvascular barrier is dependent on the sum of the forces in the Starling equation. As stated earlier, the sum of the forces in the lung normally exceeds zero because lung lymph flows at an estimated rate of 10–20 ml/hr from the human lung (9).

The factors in the Starling equation that contribute to liquid filtration from microvessel to interstitial space are the liquid filtration coefficient (K), the microvascular pressure (P_{mv}), and the leakiness of the microvascular barrier ($1 - \sigma$) to proteins. Countering these filtration parameters are the perimicrovascular hydrostatic pressure (P_{pmv}) and the protein osmotic pressure difference between the microvascular and perimicrovascular spaces ($\pi_{mv} - \pi_{pmv}$). Both countering parameters protect against edema formation when microvascular pressure is elevated without injury to the microvascular barrier. A more complete discussion of the physiology of liquid filtration in the lung is provided in Chapter 1.

IV. Safety Factors Against Pulmonary Edema

The large flow of filtered liquid across pulmonary microvessels would interfere with respiratory gas exchange in the lung were it not for several safety factors that maintain the respiratory gas exchange regions dry. These safety factors include a well-developed lymphatic system, a tight alveolar epithelial cell barrier, and a compliant interstitial space (Table 1) (2).

Lymphatics head the list for the microvascular and alveolar-airway barriers (Table 1) because they have loose intercellular contacts and a discontinuous basal lamina. Therefore, they provide a minimal barrier to solutes and liquid. However, the lymphatic clearance pathways in the lung are rather long and circuitous because initial lymphatics, also known as lymphatic capillaries, do not penetrate the alveolar wall interstitium (43). Instead, initial lymphatics in the lung are located in the loose connective tissue that surrounds respiratory and terminal bronchioles (42). Although it may seem surprising that initial lymphatics are not located in the alveolar wall interstitium, their absence in the pulmonary parenchyma follows the general rule in the body (43,44). Moreover, the need for peripheral distribution of lymphatic vessels to help keep the alveolar walls dry is obviated by having the alveolar wall connective tissue in series with the extra-alveolar connective tissue sheaths in which the initial lymphatic vessels are located (42).

Pulmonary blood vessels, too, act as a safety factor because their intercellular junctions are tighter than lymphatic intercellular junctions. The endothelium of blood vessels also has low conductance for liquid, small solutes, and protein. Due to the low conductance to protein in particular, protein in the vascular lumen exerts an osmotic pressure (π_{mv} in the Startling equation) that helps retain liquid in the lumen, against the driving force of microvascular hydrostatic

Table 1 Safety Factors Against Pulmonary Edema

Barrier elements	Intercellular contacts
Microvascular barrier	
Lymphatics	Loose
Blood vessels	Tight
Low liquid and small solute conductance	
Low protein conductance	
Microvascular protein osmotic pressure	
Perimicrovascular liquid pressure	
Alveolar-airway barrier	
Lymphatics	Loose
Epithelium	Extremely tight
Very low liquid and small solute conductance	
Extremely low protein conductance	
Perimicrovascular liquid and protein osmotic pressure	
Alveolar surface tension and gas pressure	
Active sodium transport	

Source: Ref. 2.

pressure (P_{mv} in the Starling equation). The latter liquid filtration force is partially counterbalanced by the perimicrovascular liquid pressure that surrounds blood vessels (P_{pmv} in the Starling equation).

The alveolar and airway epithelium is nearly impervious to all solutes, not just proteins, and it has very low liquid conductance (45–48). In fact, the alveolar epithelium is about one-tenth as permeable to solutes as the microvascular endothelium (45). Therefore, the alveolar epithelium provides a substantial barrier to the passage of interstitial liquid and protein into the alveolar airspaces. Morphologically, the restrictive behavior of the alveolar epithelial barrier is due to tight intercellular junctions (zonulae occludentes) along the intercellular contacts of the alveolar squamous (type I) and cuboidal (type II) epithelial cells, as well as among the airway cuboidal and columnar epithelial cells (49,50). Alveolar type I epithelial cells (Fig. 1), which are the predominant cell type found on the alveolar surface (51), also contain cytoplasmic vesicles, although in lesser numbers than found in microvascular endothelial cells (52).

The impervious character of the alveolar and airway epithelial cell barrier to passive liquid movement is complimented by the active ion transport capacity of the epithelium. Experiments in vitro and in vivo and clinical investigations have shown that the alveolar epithelium in adults transports excess liquid from the air spaces to the alveolar interstitium against a rising alveolar protein concentration, even when the protein concentration is greater than the protein concentration in plasma (53–59) (see Chaps. 14–17). The cell type that is primarily

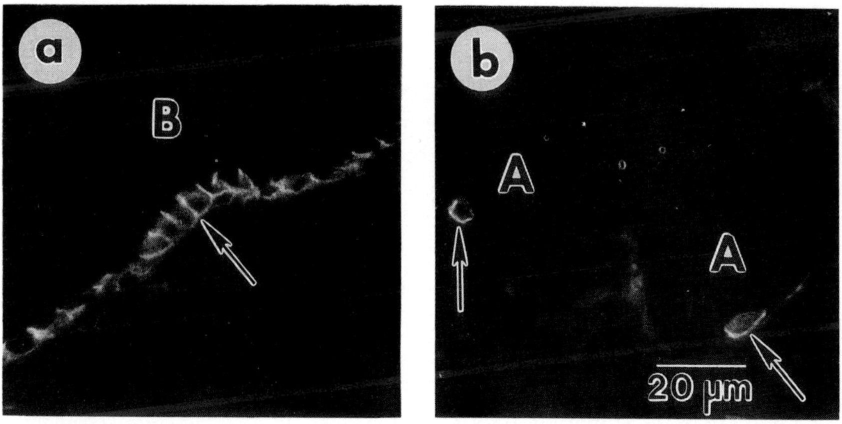

Figure 5 Localization of Na^+,K^+-ATPase protein expression in an adult sheep lung by indirect immunofluorescence microscopy. (a) Bronchiolar (B) epithelial cells are immunostained along their basolateral surface (arrow) with an anti-α_1-subunit antibody. (b) Cuboidal cells that partially line alveoli (A) have basolateral immunostaining (arrows) with an antiholoenzyme antibody (anti α_1- and β_1-subunits).

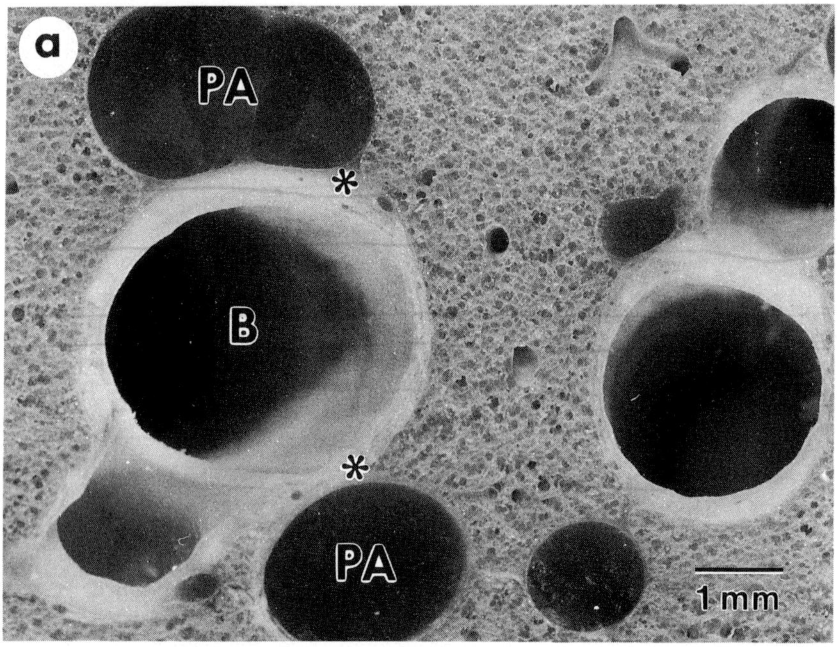

Figure 6 Appearance of the peribronchovascular (nonparenchymal) connective tissue space in frozen blocks of lung from a normal sheep (a) compared to a sheep with pulmonary edema (b). In the normal lung (a), the peribronchovascular connective tissue (*) is evident at the junction between bronchi (B) and pulmonary arteries (PA). In the edematous lung (b), on the other hand, the peribronchovascular connective tissue space is expanded enormously and is visible as peribronchovascular liquid cuffs (*). Cuff formation can occur without alveolar flooding. Froth has accumulated in an airway lumen (arrow). (From Albertine KH. Structure of the respiratory system, as related to its primary function. In: Bone R, Dantzker D, George R, Matthay R, Reynolds H, eds. Pulmonary and Critical Care Medicine. Chicago: Mosby-YearBook Publishing Co, 1993; 1–22.)

responsible for active ion transport in peripheral lung tissue is the alveolar type II epithelial cell because of its bioelectrical properties that are established by tight junctions, sodium channels on the apical surface, high concentration of Na^+,K^+-ATPase activity along the basolateral surface (Fig. 5), and numerous mitochondria in the cytoplasm (60–66) (see Chaps. 14–17). Alveolar type I epithelial cells may contribute to active ion transport as well, based on recent evidence to suggest that they may have Na^+,K^+-ATPase activity (see Chap. 16) (67).

Water transport across alveolar and airway epithelial cells may be facilitated by a molecular family of water-transporting proteins (channels). Recent studies indicate that alveolar type II epithelial cells have water channels (68).

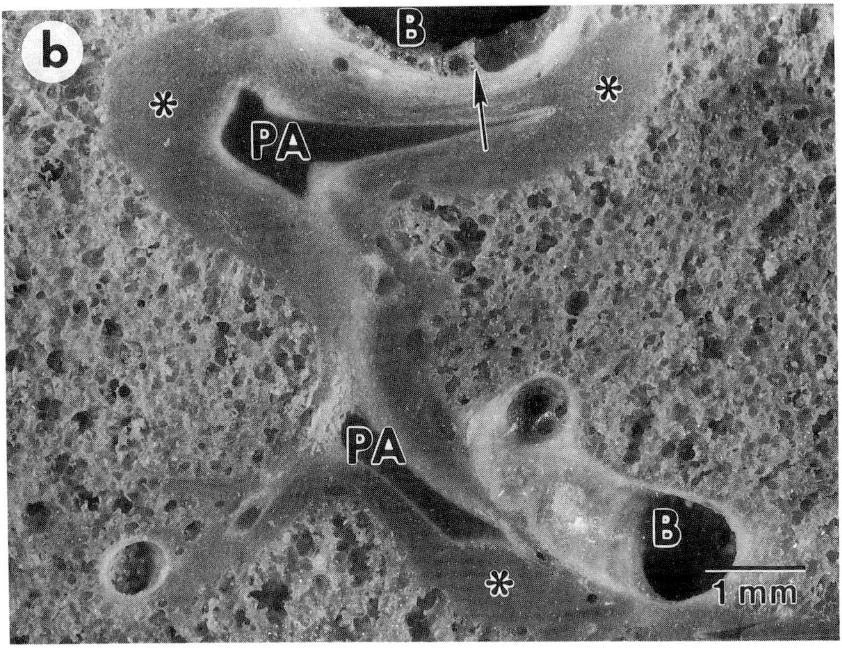

The water channels include aquaporin-1, aquaporin-4, and aquaporin-5 (68–70). These integral membrane proteins may be important in water bidirectional movement across the epithelial cells that line the lung's distal airspaces and airways (71) (see Chap. 18).

Solutes, especially ions that are actively pumped out of the airspaces by alveolar type II epithelial cells and distal airways by the lining epithelial cells, enter the alveolar wall interstitium. Liquid in the airspaces passively follows the actively pumped ions into the interstitial space. Liquid and solutes also enter the interstitium from the microvascular space. The combined interstitial liquid then flows along a hydraulic pressure gradient that exists from the alveolar wall interstitial space, through the connective tissue space at the alveolar wall junctions ("corners"), and thence to the extra-alveolar interstitial space that surrounds airways and pulmonary blood vessels. Direct micropuncture pressure measurements in the lung have shown that the hydraulic driving pressure is about 1–2 cm H_2O from the alveolar wall junctions to the extra-alveolar connective tissue sheaths that surround small airways and pulmonary blood vessels (72). Therefore, the total hydraulic driving pressure from the alveolar wall interstitial space to the peribronchovascular connective tissue sheaths where lymphatics are located may be 4–5 cm H_2O (72–74). These sheaths have a large capacity to accumulate interstitial edema liquid (Fig. 6) (75,76). The hydraulic

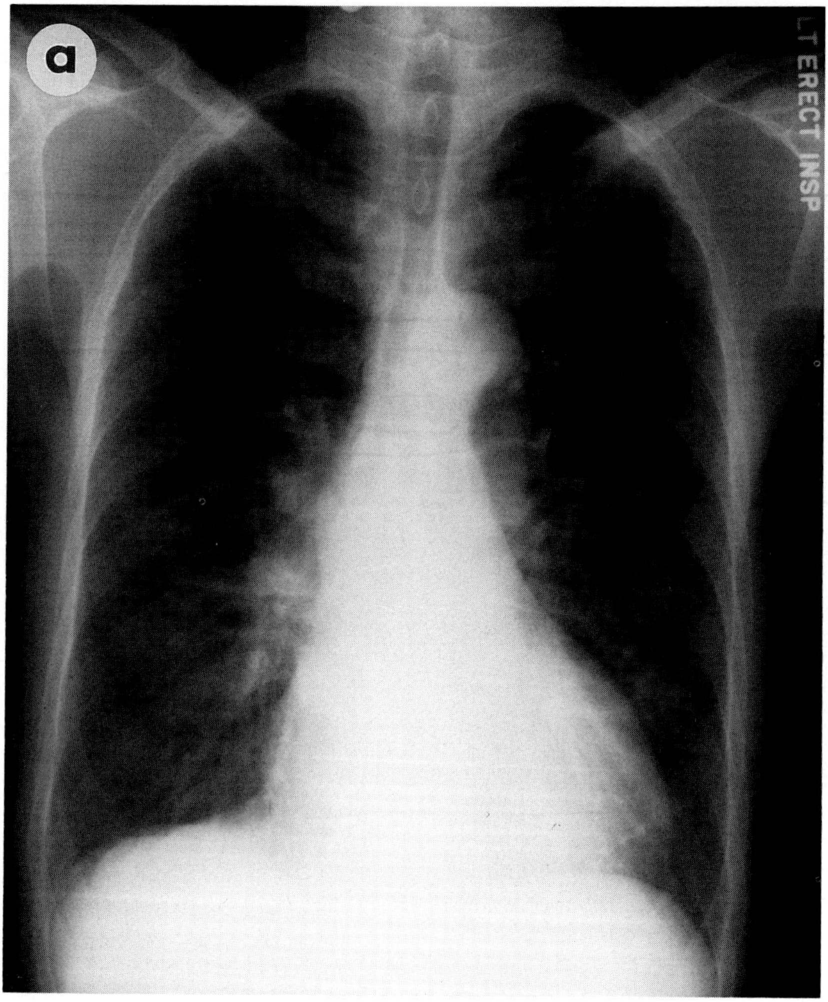

Figure 7 Plain chest roentgenograms of a patient before (a) and subsequent to developing pulmonary edema related to congestive heart failure (b). Cardiogenic pulmonary edema is characterized radiographically by opacification of the perihilar and gravity-dependent regions of the lung fields. (From Albertine KH. Structural organization and quantitative morphology of the lung. In: Cutillo AM, ed. Application of Magnetic Resonance to the Study of Lung. Armonk, NY: Futura Publishing Co, 1996; 73–114.)

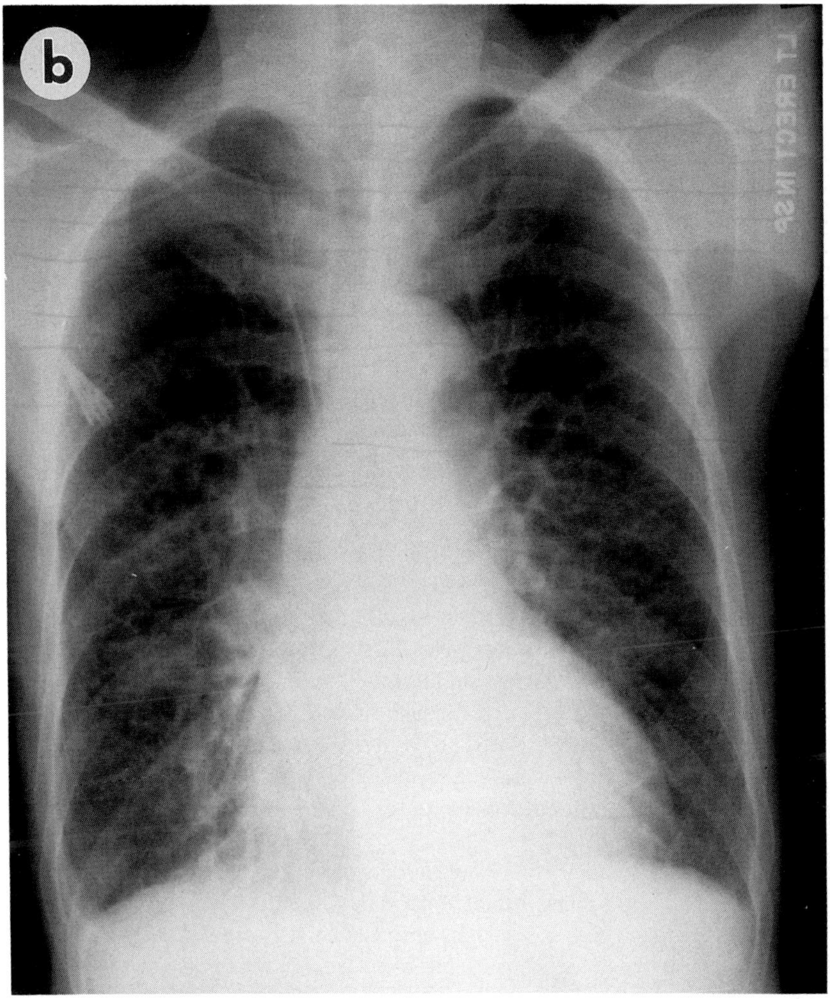

pressure gradient along the connective tissue pathways, combined with vascular pulsations, tissue movements, and pressure swings during breathing, together serve as the driving force to propel interstitial solutes and liquid away from the alveolar wall interstitium, thereby keeping it dry.

V. Pulmonary Edema

According to the Starling equation, there are two main classes of pulmonary edema: (1) increased-pressure, and (2) increased-permeability (2,9,37). In some instances, however, the two may be coincident. A third, less common form of pulmonary edema that may be considered is primary lymphatic obstruction (77).

Increased-pressure pulmonary edema is usually the result of congestive heart failure. This type of edema is primarily due to increased microvascular pressure (P_{mv} in the Starling equation) because the endothelial barrier is intact (see Chap. 5). As microvascular pressure rises, liquid filtration increases. The two safety factors against edema formation that help keep the alveoli dry are the increase in interstitial liquid volume, which raises perimicrovascular hydrostatic pressure (P_{pmv} in the Starling equation), and the increase in lung lymph flow (9). If these safety factors fail, interstitial and alveolar edema may develop. When failure occurs, the classical radiological picture is one of increased opacity in the gravity-dependent regions of the lung fields (Fig. 7).

Increased-permeability pulmonary edema, on the other hand, is a manifestation of leaky blood vessels in the lung, without evidence of congestive heart failure. Increased-permeability pulmonary edema results from decreased microvascular barrier restriction to solutes and liquid filtration (K and σ, respectively, in the Starling equation). This means that the newly formed edema liquid has a high protein concentration. Consequently, the normal gradient in protein osmotic pressure between the microvascular (π_{mv}) and perimicrovascular (π_{pmv}) compartments is lost. The loss means that another safety factor against edema formation has failed. The distribution of edema liquid is influenced by the extent of the microvascular injury. The more diffuse the permeability injury, the more uniform is the accumulation of edema liquid throughout the lung. Chest radiography usually shows bilateral and diffuse interstitial and alveolar infiltrates that progress to involve all lung zones (Fig. 8) (see Chap. 3).

The clinical hallmark of increased-permeability pulmonary edema is a high protein concentration in the alveolar edema liquid relative to plasma (78–80) (see Chap. 14). This relationship, unfortunately, is not detectable until sufficient flooding in the alveolar spaces produces edema fluid that can be collected. Therefore, alveolar flooding is a late indicator of failure of the microvascular and alveolar-airway safety factors.

In experimental animals, increased flow of protein-rich lymph from the lungs is classically interpreted to signify increased-permeability pulmonary edema (81–83). The amount of liquid filtration is excessive for the sum of pressures in the Starling equation. More specifically, the liquid filtration coefficient (K) is increased and the protein reflection coefficient (σ) is decreased, both of which indicate a loss in the integrity of the microvascular barrier (9). It is important to recall that an increase in microvascular permeability may also be accompanied by an increase in microvascular pressure.

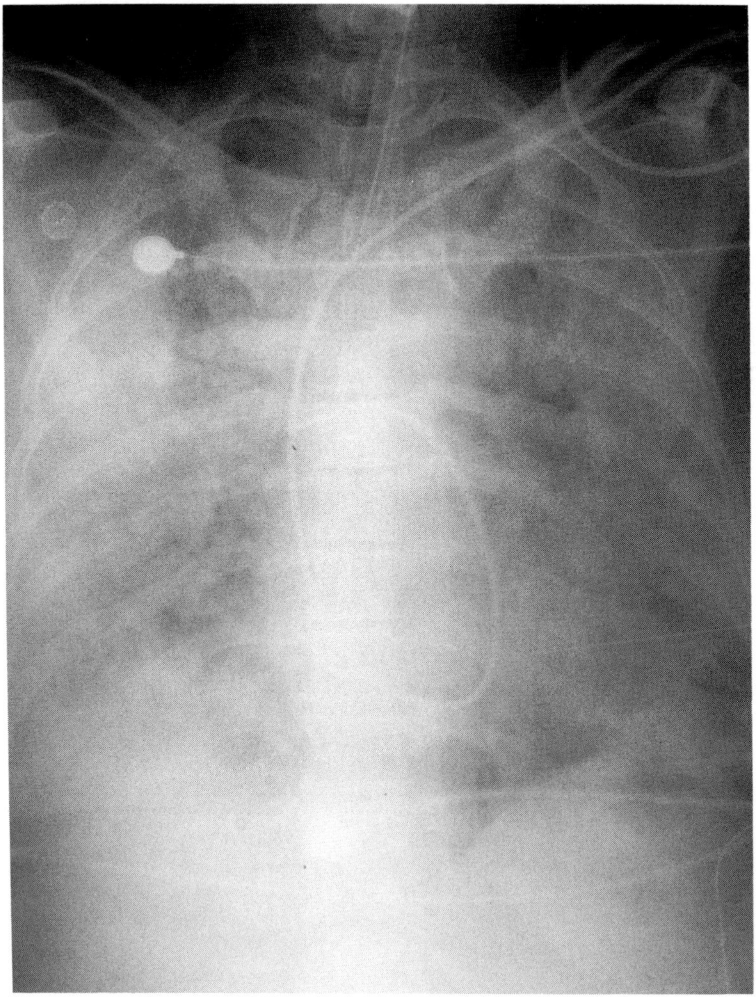

Figure 8 Plain chest roentgenogram of a patient diagnosed as having the acute respiratory distress syndrome. This syndrome is associated with fulminant pulmonary edema resulting from a generalized increase in pulmonary microvascular permeability. Therefore, most of the lung fields are opacified.

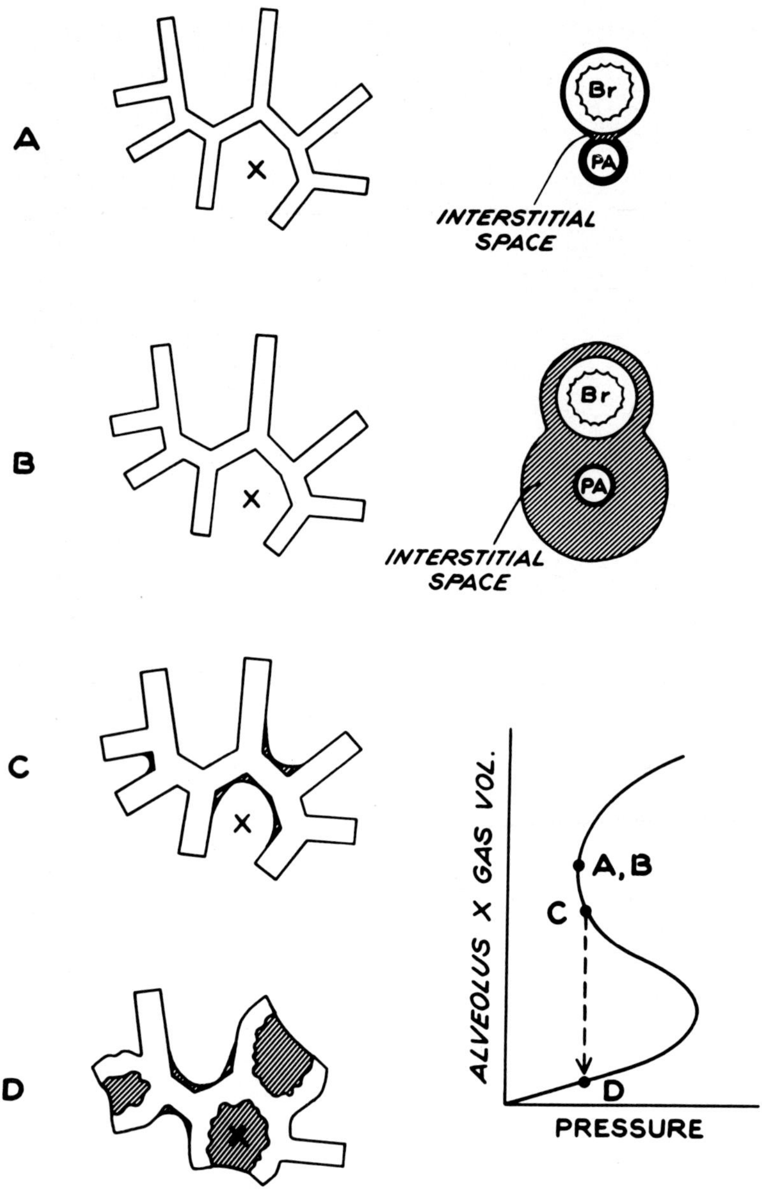

Figure 9 Schematic representation of the sequence of liquid accumulation during acute pulmonary edema. (A) Normal lung tissue in which the alveoli ("x") are empty (air-filled), alveolar walls are narrow and straight, and no excess liquid is evident in the peribronchovascular connective tissue spaces. (B) Initial liquid leak. Liquid flows to the

VI. Sequence of Edema Liquid Accumulation in the Lung

Regardless of the classification of pulmonary edema, the sequence of edema fluid accumulation in the lung, including filling of alveolar air spaces, was not fully appreciated until morphological methods were developed to follow the edema process. These methods were developed by Staub and his associates (75), who examined dog lungs that were rapidly frozen after pulmonary edema was induced by either blood and dextran transfusion (to induce increased-pressure pulmonary edema) or alloxan infusion (to cause increased-permeability pulmonary edema). Figure 9 summarizes their morphological findings.

The interstitial space in control lungs was thin where it surrounded airways and vessels, and within the alveolar walls (Fig. 9A). Alveolar wall thickness in control dogs was 4–5 μm. Connective tissue spaces in the interlobular septae and visceral pleura were also thin.

The sequence of edema liquid accumulation was (1) pulmonary edema formation in peribronchovascular connective tissue sheathes, (2) liquid accumulation in alveolar wall interstitial spaces, and (3) alveolar flooding (75,84). Mild edema was characterized by accumulation of liquid in the peribronchovascular connective tissue sheaths (Fig. 9B). Lung lymphatics located in these sheaths became distended, as they should since they represent an important safety factor against alveolar flooding. As edema became more severe, alveolar wall thickness increased to 5–7 μm, indicating early accumulation in the alveolar wall interstitium. Once edema liquid accumulation exceeded the capacity of the peribronchovascular connective tissue space and lymphatic system, further edema formation resulted in further filling of the alveolar wall interstitium (Fig. 9C). This was manifest quantitatively as increased thickness of the alveolar walls (7–9 μm). Finally, once all the safety factors against alveolar edema were overwhelmed, including the highly impermeable alveolar epithelial cell barrier,

---

peribronchovascular connective tissue spaces, forming liquid cuffs around airways and blood vessels. The alveolar walls are slightly distended but otherwise the alveoli ("x") appear normal. (C) Alveolar wall edema during more severe interstitial pulmonary edema. Leaked liquid accumulates in the alveolar wall interstitium, causing the walls to become thickened. Liquid begins to overflow into the alveoli ("x"), notably at the corners where curvature is great. (D) Alveolar flooding. Individual alveoli ("x") reach critical shape and size at which existing inflation pressure can no longer maintain alveolar stability. Alveolar gas volume rapidly passes to a lower level with much reduced curvature (see insert graph). The volume loss is associated with alveolar collapse or the volume deficit is replaced by additional alveolar edema liquid, depending on associated conditions such as alveolar surface tension and availability of edema liquid. (From Ref. 73.)

alveolar flooding ensued (Fig. 9D). Alveoli in the flooded regions were either completely liquid-filled or air-filled (Figs. 9D and 10). As Figure 10 also illustrates, large numbers of flooded alveoli can be anatomically separated from air-filled alveoli by interlobular connective tissue septae. Transition between these two states was confined to small accumulations of liquid in alveolar corners. The lack of transition stages suggested that alveolar flooding, once initiated, proceeded rapidly and completely.

Alveolar filling in severely edematous regions of the lung was associated with disappearance of air-liquid interfaces and congestion of alveolar capillaries. In the study by Staub and co-workers (75), the walls of flooded alveoli were

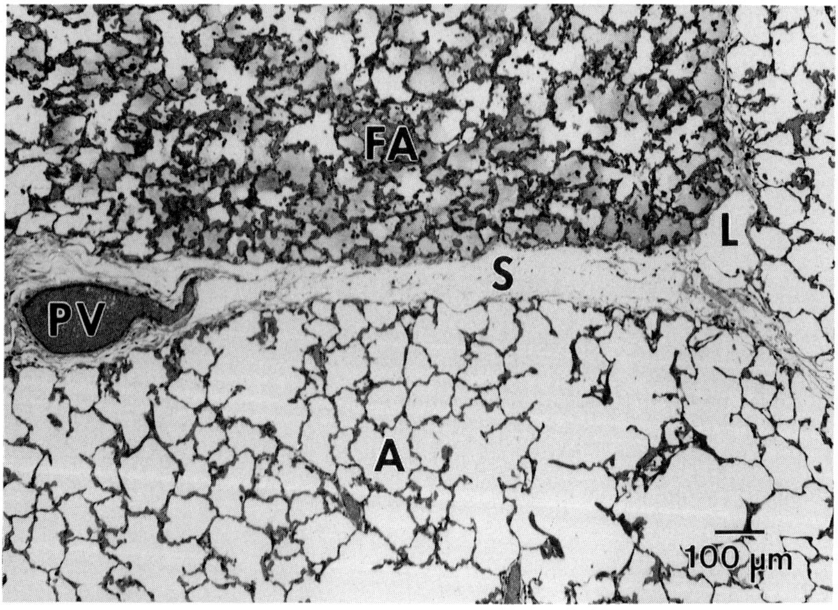

Figure 10 Histopathological appearance of inhomogeneity of alveolar size and shape in a sheep lung that developed patchy interstitial and alveolar edema during intravenous infusion of *Escherichia coli* endotoxin. Flooded alveoli (FA) are physically separated from air-filled alveoli (A) by an edematous interlobular septum (S). The flooded alveoli have protein-rich (stained) liquid in them. They are also at low volume and their walls are folded. Air-filled alveoli, by comparison, are at higher volume; consequently their walls are straighter. PV, pulmonary vein; L, lymphatic. (From Albertine KH. Structural organization and quantitative morphology of the lung. In: Cutillo AM, ed. Application of Magnetic Resonance to the Study of Lung. Armonk, NY: Futura Publishing Co, 1996; 73–114.)

slightly folded and alveolar volume appeared somewhat reduced in the rapidly frozen dog lungs. A reason for the altered shape and decreased volume of flooded alveoli was liquid filling occurred from the deepest recesses of an alveolus "up" to the opening of an alveolus into its alveolar duct or respiratory bronchiole. Therefore, the air-liquid interface was "lifted" away from the epithelium. Continued filling reduced the radius of curvature across this interface. At some point along the filling phase, a critical threshold in interfacial tension and curvature was crossed (described by the law of LaPlace) after which the existing transpulmonary pressure could not maintain stable alveolar configuration. Consequently, the alveolar walls became folded and alveolar volume decreased.

VII. Histopathology of Increased-Permeability Pulmonary Edema

A. Human Studies

Bachofen and Weibel described the structural alterations in the lungs of patients who died with complications of the ARDS (1,85). By definition, these studies were done on subjects with severe lung injury. These investigators described histopathological alterations that were classified as either acute (diffuse alveolar damage) or chronic (organizing), depending on the duration of the respiratory symptoms.

In the acute stage, corresponding to 20 hr or more of clinical symptoms, the pathological changes of diffuse alveolar damage are characterized by abundant interstitial and alveolar edema accompanied by focal damage and destruction to the microvascular and alveolar barriers. (The pathological changes in human lungs at times earlier than 20 hr are not known because of the difficulty in obtaining samples so early.) The alveolar air spaces are filled with proteinaceous liquid. Often, this liquid is hemorrhagic in appearance. By microscopic examination, the liquid in injured air spaces contains erythrocytes, leukocytes, cellular debris, fibrin strands, and globules of surfactant (Fig. 11a). Hyaline membranes, too, are seen in the alveolar spaces (Fig. 11a). These conglomerates of exudate usually blanket the alveolar surface. The current pathological term for these findings is diffuse alveolar damage.

The early structural changes in the alveolar septal interstitium, as well as cytological alterations of the epithelial and endothelial barriers, are recognizable only by transmission electron microscopy. By this method, expansion of the alveolar wall interstitium by edema liquid is detectable (Figs. 11b and 12). The edema is restricted to the thick side of the alveolar capillaries—that is, the region between the normally separated basal laminae of the endothelial and epithelial cells (refer to Fig. 1). Edema liquid does not appear to accumulate along the

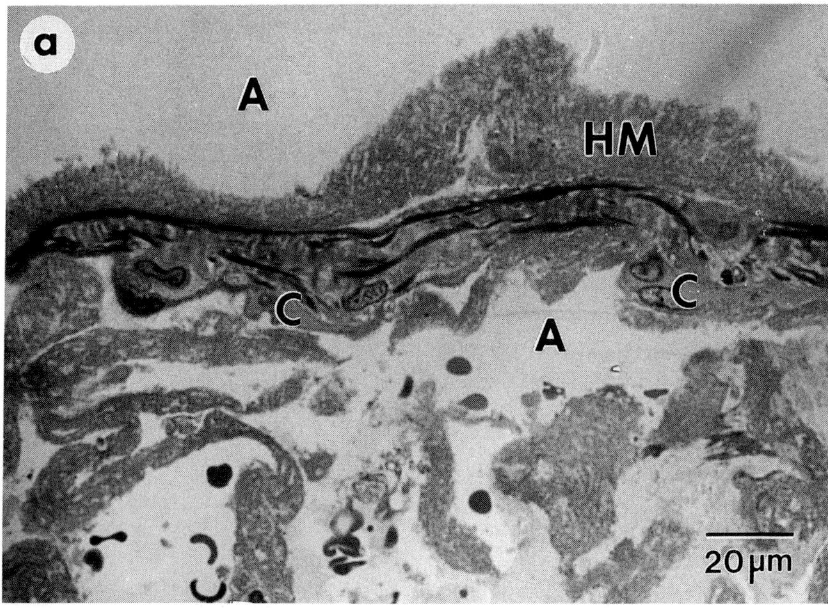

Figure 11 (a) Histological appearance of increased-permeability pulmonary edema in the lung of a 55-year-old man with acquired immune deficiency syndrome who developed the acute respiratory distress syndrome. An open lung biopsy demonstrated diffuse alveolar damage, alveolar flooding, and hyaline membrane (HM) formation in association with *Pneumocystis carinii.* The pathological findings were confirmed at autopsy. A, alveoli; C, capillary. (b) Electron micrograph of parenchyma from the same human lung. Both surfaces of the alveolar septum are lined by hyaline membranes (HM). A gap (arrow) is visible along the alveolar epithelial cell barrier. Septal width (*) is increased compared with the normal lung (see Fig. 2). A, alveoli; C, capillary. (From Ref. 2.)

thin side, thereby preserving a minimal barrier to gas exchange if the adjacent alveoli are not flooded.

Cytological changes in the alveolar epithelial and microvascular endothelial barriers are remarkably different in the human lung. Epithelial cell lesions are conspicuous. Various stages involving cytoplasmic swelling, vacuolization, bleb formation, necrosis, and/or denuding are evident. In denuded areas, the basal lamina of epithelial cells remains intact and is covered by hyaline membranes (Fig. 13a). In light of these stark changes, it should come as no surprise that the alveoli are flooded by protein-rich liquid. On the other hand, endothelial cell lesions are more subtle and appear to be inadequate structurally to explain the rapid and continuous escape of protein-rich liquid from pulmonary

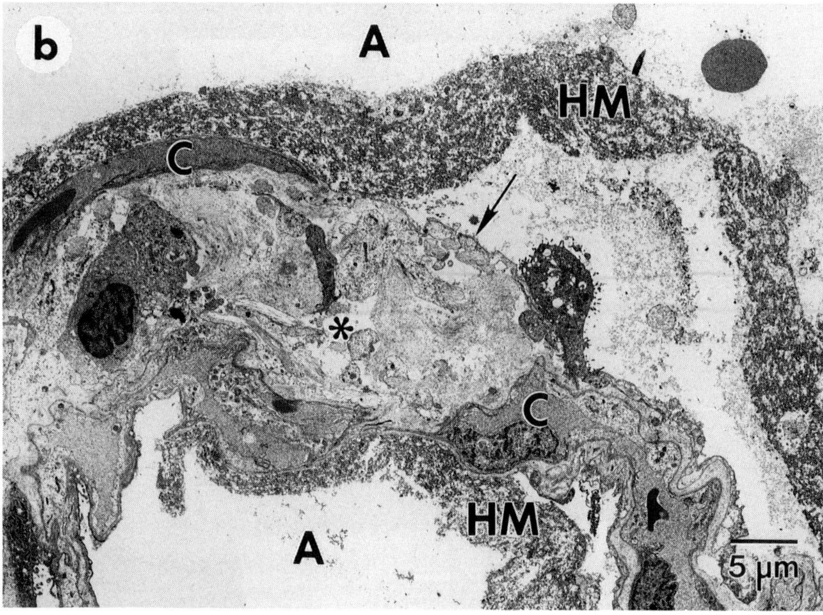

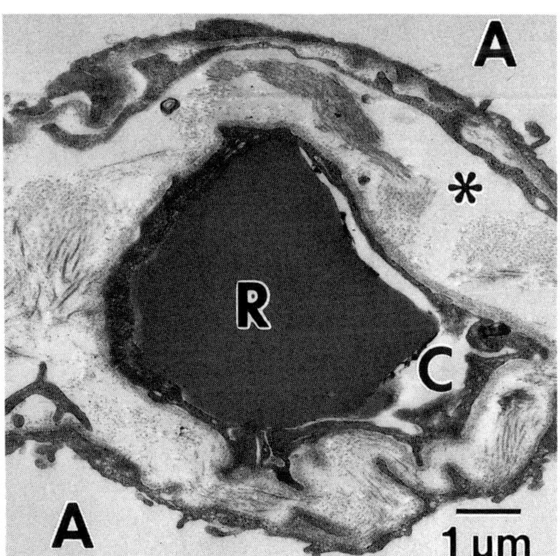

Figure 12 An alveolar septum in a human lung is expanded (*) by interstitial edema liquid. A, alveoli; C, capillary; R, red blood cell. (From Ref. 2.)

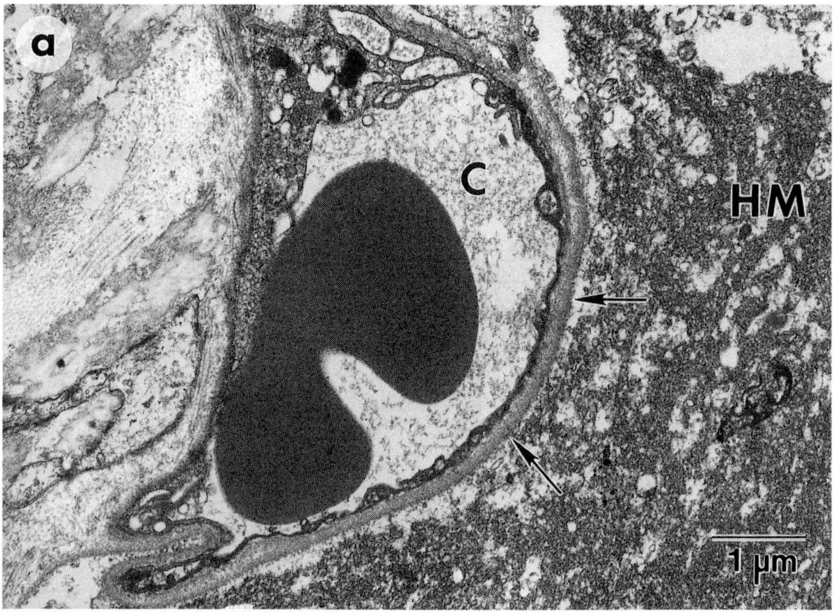

Figure 13 (a) Alveolar barrier damage during sepsis-induced increased-permeability pulmonary edema in a human lung. Epithelial cells are absent, allowing a hyaline membrane (HM) to cover the exposed basal lamina (arrows). C, capillary. (b) Microvascular barrier damage from the same human lung. Some capillary endothelial cells are severely swollen (*) while others appear normal. The alveolar barrier is devoid of epithelial cells, but its basal lamina is intact. Proteinaceous material, fibrin deposits (F), and an erythrocyte are in the alveolar space (A). (From Ref. 2.)

microvessels. Characteristic signs of endothelial cell damage are focal cytoplasmic swelling, vacuolization, and bleb formation (Fig. 13b). Occasionally, necrotic microvascular endothelial cells and denuded spaces along the microvascular lumen are seen, in which case there usually is deposition of fibrin clot.

Why the ultrastructural manifestations are so disparate between the alveolar epithelial cells and microvascular endothelial cells in severe increased-permeability pulmonary edema in humans is a mystery. It seems unlikely that a significant and sustained increase in microvascular permeability would manifest itself as decimated epithelial cells and relatively spared endothelial cells. Perhaps a better explanation is that after 20 hr or more of clinical symptoms, repair of damage to the endothelial cell barrier could already be underway.

The chronic, organizing course of increased-permeability pulmonary edema is variable. In those subjects whose lungs reabsorb the alveolar edema liquid as quickly as it forms, clinical resolution of the acute lung injury oc-

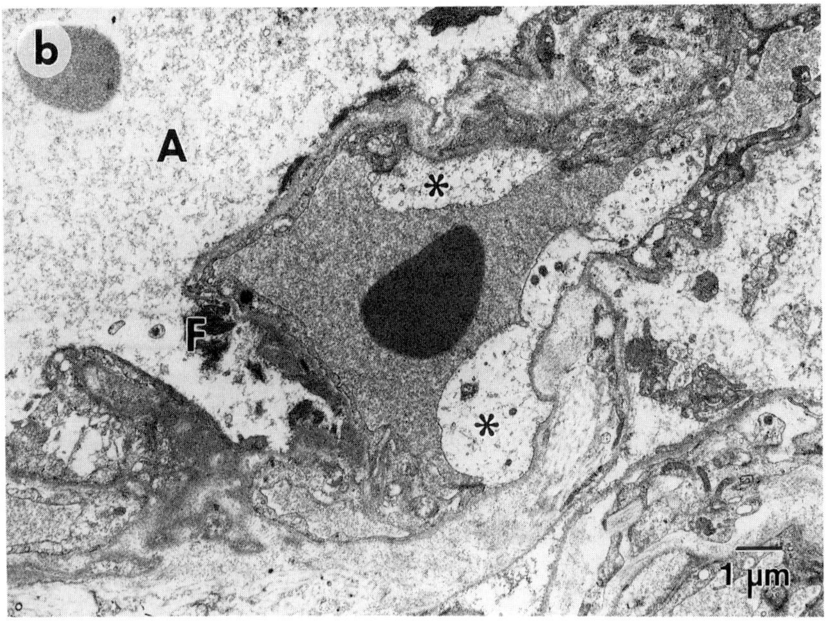

curs (58). However, many subjects who develop increased-permeability pulmonary edema are not able to clear the interstitial and alveolar edema liquid in their lungs. Among the latter subset of critically ill subjects, those who are persistently unable to clear the edema liquid and exudate develop worsening respiratory impairment and gradual fibrosing alveolitis. Bachofen and Weibel (1,85) observed that this period is characterized by proliferation of alveolar type II epithelial cells, thickening of the alveolar septa, alveolitis, and usually, progressive pulmonary fibrosis (86). A question that persists is the fate of the proliferated alveolar type II epithelial cells. Do the majority dedifferentiate into alveolar type I epithelial cells, or do many of the hyperplastic type II cells die? Recent histopathological data suggest that apoptosis may be a major pathway for removal of the excess number of alveolar type II epithelial cells during the organizing phase of diffuse alveolar damage (87,88). The fibrosis that develops can be interstitial, owing to accumulation and proliferation of cells such as lymphocytes, plasma cells, and histiocytes, or the fibrosis can be intra-alveolar. Both forms of fibrosis distort the normal alveolar architecture of the lung (89). The structural derangement of the lung parenchyma inhibits respiratory gas exchange because of loss of capillary volume (90).

Structural repair and functional resolution of the lung injury clearly do occur after increased-permeability pulmonary edema because not all affected subjects die (91). However, there still are no systematic histopathological analyses of the repair and resolution phase in humans. And there is only limited histopathological information in experimental animals. Two studies used monkeys after chronic exposure to high concentrations of inspired oxygen (92,93). The histopathological picture was one of enlarged distal airspaces, thickened alveolar walls, and interstitial fibrosis.

B. Experimental Animal Studies

Basic science investigations have provided considerable information about the ultrastructural features of increased-permeability pulmonary edema, particularly the early pathological sequelae (minutes to hours after inducing lung injury). The ultrastructural changes observed in many experimental models of acute lung injury share certain similarities, both among different models and with clinical observations. Most frequently, microvascular endothelial cell swelling, vacuolization, vesiculation, and bleb formation occur. Other microvascular changes are widened (loosened) intercellular channels, intercellular gap formation, and cellular disruption (necrosis, fragmentation, and sloughing). Similar types of epithelial cell damage are seen in some of the models, although the epithelial cells may not always show injury (94). Inflammatory cells are usually prominent.

Gap formation between contiguous endothelial cells (Fig. 14) is accepted as the ultrastructural basis for increased microvascular permeability during acute

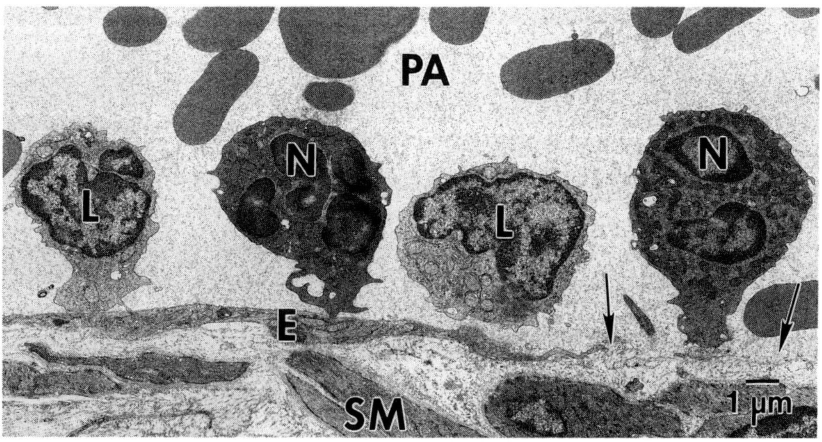

Figure 14 Effect of 1 hour of continuous venous air embolization [0.03 mL/(kg × min)] on acute lung injury in an adult sheep. A gap (arrows) is visible in the endothelial (E) barrier of a small pulmonary artery (PA). Two neutrophils (N) and two lymphocytes (L) are marginated against the endothelium. Three of the leukocytes have pseudopods extended to the endothelium. SM; smooth muscle cell. (From Ref. 2.)

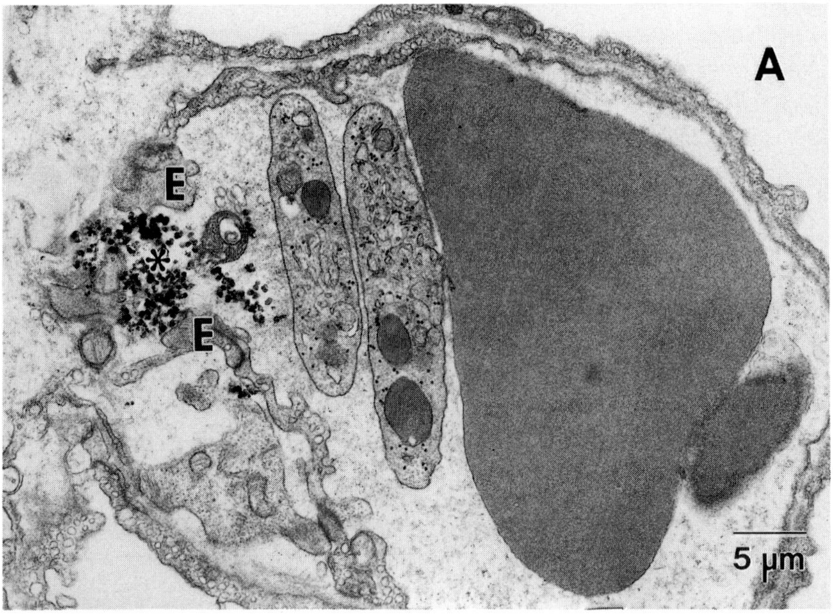

Figure 15 Alveolar capillary of a rat that was intravenously injected with colloidal carbon 3 hr after α-naphthyl thiourea (5 mg/kg body weight) was injected in the peritoneal cavity to induce acute lung injury. Carbon particles (*) lie in a gap along the "thick" side of the capillary-endothelial (E) barrier. A, alveolus. (From Ref. 2.)

inflammation, both in the lung (77,95) and in other organs and tissues (96,97). This acceptance stems from the use of vascular tracers, such as colloidal carbon (biological ink; Pelikan c11/1431a), to label the sites of increased permeability (Fig. 15). For a variety of acute inflammatory injuries to the lung, the number of intramural carbon deposits and the proportion of tracer-labeled microvessels with endothelial cell gaps are similar. Moreover, once edema is arrested, the gaps disappear. Therefore, vascular tracer studies have demonstrated the importance of endothelial cell gaps as focal and reversible lesions during increased-permeability pulmonary edema.

VIII. Pathogenesis of Increased-Permeability Pulmonary Edema

Increased-permeability pulmonary edema can be the result of either direct or indirect injury to lung tissue (77,95). Direct injury, in this context, may be the result of exposure to toxic substances. Heading the list of direct injurious agents are high concentrations of inspired oxygen (98–100), ozone (101,102), nitrogen oxides (103), ethchlorvynol (42,104), α-naphthyl thiourea (105–108), monocrotalline (109–111), alloxan (112), oleic acid (113,114), ammonium sulfate (115,116), paraquat (117–119), acid aspiration (see Chap. 8), or primary pneumonia (see Chap. 7). Indirect injury seems to require interaction between a putative inciting agent, inflammatory cells in the vascular space, and vascular endothelial cells. It is possible that indirect lung injury results from exaggeration of normal host-defense mechanisms. Among the more clinically common putative inciting agents are endotoxemia and sepsis (120–127) (see Chap. 6), microemboli of various kinds (128–132), intravascular complement activation (133–137), and hemmorrhagic shock (138–140) (see Chap. 9). Of these, the most common clinical setting is toxemia/sepsis (91).

A harbinger of acute inflammatory lung injury is accumulation of leukocytes, especially neutrophils in the lung (3,141,142). Studies in which the number of circulating neutrophils was reduced in vivo by chemical treatment or by treatment with an antineutrophil antibody have shown that neutrophils are necessary for some types of acute lung injury (125,141–146). Neutrophil depletion reduces the increase in net transvascular solute and liquid flux that is otherwise caused by different insults associated with pulmonary endothelial cell injury. However, neutrophils are not absolutely required for the development of acute lung injury because the ARDS occurs in neutropenic subjects (147,148). But we still do not know how many neutrophils are required to produce endothelial cell injury (3,143).

For neutrophil-related endothelial cell injury to be produced, secretory responses of neutrophils must be activated. Most studies have shown that reduced metabolites of oxygen released from activated neutrophils are sufficient to produce injury to endothelial cells in culture (149). Administration of free radical scavengers in prevention protocols in vivo reduces pulmonary endothelial cell injury produced by endotoxin (150), complement anaphylatoxins (151), or air emboli (152). Proteolytic enzymes from primary and secondary granules in neutrophils may also contribute to endothelial cell injury, although granule enzymes do not appear to be necessary to demonstrate injury (153).

Experiments using endothelial cell cultures have shown that a prerequisite to produce injury is contact between the activated neutrophils and endothelial cells (153). The hypothesis is that points of contact create a microenvironment between the two cell types that allows labile neutrophil activation products, such as free radicals, to act on the endothelial cell surface. As we have seen (Fig. 16a), points of contact between neutrophils and endothelial cells occur normally, particularly in alveolar capillaries, in control sheep. Neutrophils in alveolar microvessels during acute inflammatory lung injury, induced by infusion of zymosan-activated plasma, had even more cellular contact with the endothelium (Fig. 16b). Moreover, the intravascular neutrophils were vacuolated and more

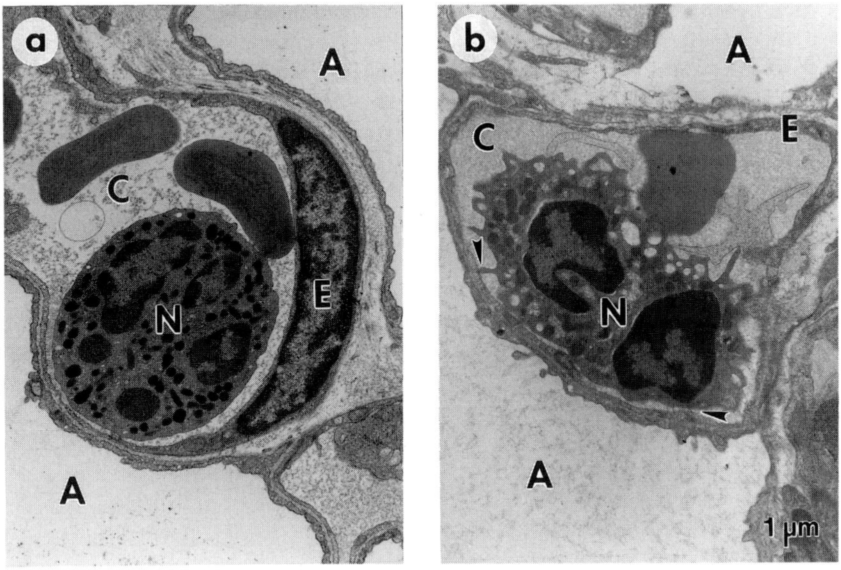

Figure 16 Effect of intravascular activation of neutrophils on their shape in situ in pulmonary microvessels. (a) Control sheep (intravenous infusion of autologous plasma). A normal neutrophil (N) in an alveolar capillary (C) is round and smooth in contour; the cytoplasm is filled with granules and nuclear lobes. E, endothelial cell; A, alveoli. (b) Thirty minutes of intravenous infusion of autologous zymosan-activated plasma. An activated neutrophil in the lumen of an alveolar capillary (C) has polarized morphology. Along the zone of neutrophil-endothelial cell (E) contact (arrowheads), the neutrophil's surface is smooth, and several points of cell-cell contact are visible. In contrast, the surface of the neutrophil that is not in contact with endothelial cells is ruffled and contains numerous clear cytoplasmic vacuoles. A, alveoli. (From Ref. 3.)

elongated than their control counterparts. Activated neutrophils in situ in the pulmonary circulation also had increased cross-sectional area (24–35% greater than control neutrophils in situ). The cross-sectional area of adherent neutrophils activated in vitro increased about 33% (154). Also evident was polarization of organelle distribution in the activated neutrophils. Cytoplasmic vacuoles congregated away from regions of neutrophil-endothelial cell contact, whereas nuclear lobes were positioned toward regions of neutrophil-endothelial cell contact. Neutrophils in control sheep lacked cytoplasmic vacuoles, and the nuclear lobes were randomly distributed in the cytoplasm. The alignment of vacuoles in the cytoplasm of activated neutrophils away from regions of neutrophil-endothelial cell contact observed in our in vivo experiments has not been described. We have reported similar polarization of vacuoles in neutrophils activated in vitro at high density where neutrophil-neutrophil interactions are prominent (155). In the latter study, the polarization of cell contents was accompanied by a general down-regulation of the biochemical changes associated with neutrophil activation. The functional significance of vacuole polarization in situ, in the context of neutrophil-related endothelial cells injury, has not been clarified.

What are the mechanisms by which neutrophils and endothelial cells interact physically in the lung? There are two schools of thought: (1) expression of adherence molecules by neutrophils and endothelial cells, and (2) changes in physical characteristics of neutrophils (3,142). Differential expression of the selectin and integrin adherence molecules by neutrophils (as well as other types of leukocytes) and endothelial cells provides a regulated process for white blood cell rolling, attachment, and directed transvascular migration (156,157). The role of adherence molecules in neutrophil-endothelial cell interaction in the lung has not been clarified because contradictory results have been obtained. Several studies have shown a role for adherence molecules in acute lung injury. Yoder and colleagues (158) showed that the transit time of complement-activated neutrophils through lung surface microvessels was increased when normal dog neutrophils were measured, but not when neutrophils from a CD11/CD18-deficient dog were measured. This result suggests that adherence proteins are necessary for retention of activated neutrophils in pulmonary capillaries in vivo. Two studies showed that acute lung injury and pulmonary edema were inhibited by treatment with an antibody to CD18, or an antibody to ICAM-1, the endothelial cell ligand for CD18 (159,160). In another study, the weight gain in isolated guinea pig lungs produced by adding neutrophils and opsonized zymosan to the perfusate was also prevented by treatment with a CD18 antibody (161). A recent study showed that inhibition of CD18 or CD11b attenuated acute lung injury after acid instillation in rabbits (162). The latter observation may be due to direct injury caused by the instilled acid. Another recent study showed that failure to express the P-selectin gene or blockade of P-selectin protected rat lungs from injury due to ischemia or transplantation (163). Other studies failed, however, to find a role played by adherence molecules or found a diminished role in the pulmonary circulation compared to the systemic circulation. Doerschuk and co-workers (164) found that anti-CD18 antibody treatment inhibited neutrophil emigration into the abdominal wall of rabbits regardless of the stimulus used (*Streptococcus,* hydrochloric acid, endotoxin, or phorbol myristate acetate). In contrast, antibody treatment had no effect on neutrophil emigration into the alveolar airspace in response to streptococcal pneumonia or hydrochloric acid, partially inhibited emigration in response to endotoxin, and abolished phorbol myristate acetate–induced emigration. Likewise, Vedder and co-workers (165) used a hemorrhage and fluid resuscitation protocol in rabbits, treating some of the rabbits with a monoclonal antibody to CD18. They found that antibody treatment improved survival and limited injury in the liver and gut. The pulmonary circulation, however, did not benefit from antibody treatment.

The aforementioned studies indicate that selectins and integrins apparently do not have the same effect on neutrophil-endothelial cell interaction in systemic and pulmonary vascular beds because the effect of antibody treatment was absolute in the abdomen whereas it was stimulus-specific in the pulmonary circulation. There is no reason to believe that the ability of neutrophils to express adherence glycoproteins depends on whether the neutrophil is located temporarily in the systemic or pulmonary circulation. An alternate explanation is that pulmonary, but not systemic, vascular endothelium is specialized to express adherence glycoproteins in a stimulus-specific manner. Although this could be the case, there are no supporting data. Recently, data have emerged to suggest that the presence of macrophages, both alveolar and intravascular, may explain what appeared to be CD18-independent neutrophil adherence and emigration in the lung (156). The hypothesis is that macrophages are the source of an as yet unidentified adherence protein. Rapidly emerging data show that different types of leukocytes utilize different adherence mechanisms to marginate and emigrate. In vitro studies have shown that monocytes, eosinophils, lymphocytes, and basophils express the very late antigen (VLA-4), whereas neutrophils lack this antigen (166–170). The ligand for VLA-4 is vascular cell adhesion molecule (VCAM-1). Another example of selective cell recruitment via specific adherence molecules is the CD11/CD18-independent emigration of lymphocytes. This selectivity appears to be related to expression of L-selectin (LECAM-1) on the surface of lymphocytes, and its ligand, E-selectin (ELAM-1), on endothelial cells. Although interactions among leukocytes with different adherence mechanisms have not been well defined, these types of interactions may provide an explanation for why neutrophil and monocyte emigration is not completely inhibited in patients whose leukocytes lack CD11/CD18 integrins.

Adherence proteins may have a different role in acute lung injury: to modulate activation and inflammatory mediator release responses of neutrophils. Specifically, neutrophil attachment via adherence proteins may augment the respiratory burst and release of other neutrophil-derived mediators of tissue injury (159,171,172). A recent study by Folkesson and Matthay (162) has provided new support of this hypothesis. They instilled acid into the airways of rabbits, some of which were treated with anti-CD18 therapy. The principal outcome of anti-CD18 therapy was reduced physiological indices of acute lung injury, without inhibition of neutrophil migration. The authors suggested that anti-CD18 therapy may be beneficial because of its ability to minimize neutrophil activation (see Chap. 8).

The inconsistency among studies of adherence molecules in the lung has prompted the search for other mechanisms to explain neutrophil-endothelial cell interaction in that organ. The low blood pressure, huge vascular surface area, long capillary segments, and different shear forces may combine to make the lung's effect on neutrophils unique. An important contribution has been made by Worthen and colleagues (173), who showed that activated neutrophils are stiffer and less deformable than quiescent neutrophils. An inference from their study is activated neutrophils become stuck in alveolar capillaries because activation changes their physical characteristics. We have shown that emigration of neutrophils in skin and into the airspace of the lung is inhibited by intravascular activation of the neutrophils (174). Decreased deformability, together with increased cross-sectional area and volume, that occur with activation may be sufficient to retard movement of activated neutrophils through alveolar capillaries and provide ample opportunity for release of toxic oxygen metabolites and proteolytic enzymes in close proximity to the endothelial cell surface.

IX. Cytokines and Chemokines Related to Pulmonary Edema

Cell-cell interactions are clearly important in the development of inflammatory lung injury. The interactions are effected, at least in part, by regulated expression of adhesion and signaling molecules (157). Signaling molecules are a diverse group of polypeptides and proteins that are linked to intracellular transduction pathways on target cells.

A number of signaling molecules for neutrophils have been implicated as mediators of inflammatory acute lung injury. Tumor necrosis factor alpha (TNF-α) and interleukin-1 beta (IL-1β) have been found in plasma and bronchoalveolar lavage samples from subjects with the ARDS (4,175). In vitro studies have shown that incubation of neutrophils with TNF-α or IL-1β stimulates neutrophil adherence to endothelium by mechanisms that depend on expression of selectins and integrins (167,176,177). Human recombinant TNF-α has been infused into awake or anesthetized sheep in several laboratories (178–181). The results show that TNF-α increased lung microvascular permeability. Immunohistochemical studies have shown that TNF-α is expressed by stimulated neutrophils in situ in the lung (182). Receptors for both cytokines are found on endothelial cells in the lung (183). Both cytokines may also amplify local inflammatory responses in the lung by inducing the expression of other signaling molecules (184), such as the neutrophil-signaling chemokines interleukin-8 (IL-8), ENA-78, neutrophil activating protein-2, granulocyte chemotactic protein-2, and the Gro homologs (α/β/γ) (185–187).

IL-8 is a prominent signaling molecule for neutrophil accumulation and activation in acute lung injury (4,185). For example, the concentration of IL-8 is elevated in bronchoalveolar lavage liquid collected from subjects with the

ARDS compared to subjects with increased-pressure pulmonary edema (188,189). A number of investigators have suggested that IL-8 concentrations in bronchoalveolar lavage liquid predict the development of the ARDS (190–193). Similar observations have been made for the related CXC chemokine, ENA-78 (7). ENA-78 was originally thought to be exclusively expressed by epithelial cells (194,195). ENA-78 activates neutrophils alone or in combination with IL-8 (8,194). A postulate is that ENA-78 is responsible for IL-8-independent chemotactic activity for neutrophils in bronchoalveolar lavage liquid from subjects with the ARDS (7).

The studies of IL-8 and ENA-78 in bronchoalveolar lavage liquid are limited by an important unknown: signaling cells that express both chemokines during the ARDS have not been identified in situ. To this end, we have used immunohistochemical methods to localize IL-8 and ENA-78 protein expression in human lung tissue (8). We compared the immunolocalization of IL-8 and ENA-78 in the lungs of subjects who met clinical criteria for the ARDS to immunolocalization in lung tissue from other subjects with nonpulmonary diseases (control, for "normal" conditions). Of 18 subjects from whom we collected lung tissue at autopsy, approximately half met clinical criteria for the ARDS/sepsis. Immunostaining with an anti-IL-8 antibody was restricted exclusively to inflammatory cells located in pulmonary blood vessels, interstitium, and air spaces of subjects (Fig. 17, Color Plate 1). Few cells were stained positively for IL-8 in "control" lungs. Whereas IL-8 immunostaining was present in one cell type in lung sections of the subjects who died with the ARDS/sepsis, immunostaining with an anti-ENA-78 antibody was prominent in endothelial cells lining the same pulmonary arteries and veins (Fig. 17, Color Plate 1). The positively stained cells were identified as endothelial cells by anti–von Willebrand staining in serial sections (Fig. 17, Color Plate 1). In many areas there were extravascular infiltrates of neutrophils around blood vessels lined by endothelial cells that reacted with the anti-ENA-78 antibody. Only rarely were endothelial cells positive for ENA-78 in lung sections from subjects who died without clinical pulmonary disease, whereas endothelial cells of arteries, veins, and microvessels in the same tissue sections were positive for von Willebrand factor. In sections of lung from patients who died with the ARDS/sepsis, hyperplastic alveolar type II epithelial cells, alveolar macrophages, neutrophils, and in some areas, vascular smooth muscle cells, were positive for ENA-78 (Fig. 17, Color Plate 1). In contrast, only occasional alveolar type II epithelial cells and alveolar macrophages were seen in lung sections from subjects who died from nonpulmonary causes.

Our findings of differential cell expression of IL-8 and ENA-78 in situ in lung tissue from subjects with the ARDS/sepsis provide an important advancement in understanding the role of these two chemokines in inflammatory lung injury. Our finding that ENA-78 is present in endothelium in situ identifies

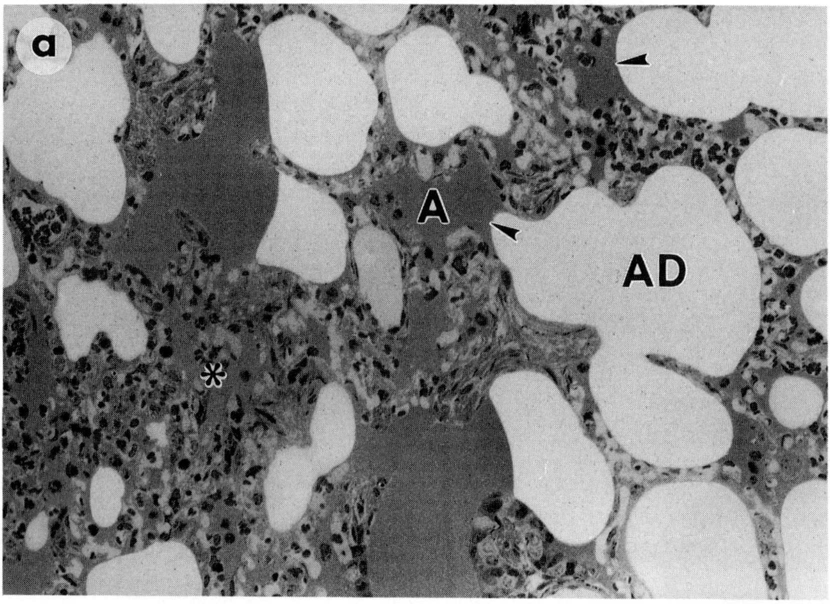

Figure 18 Histopathological features of lung tissue during resolution of alveolar "edema" liquid. Autologous serum stained with Evans blue dye was instilled bronchoscopically in adult sheep and dwelled in the lungs for 24 or 144 hr. At 24 hr (a), alveoli (A) are filled from the epithelium "up" to the opening (arrowheads) into alveolar ducts (AD). The flooded alveoli have folded walls and are at low volume (*). This configuration corresponds to Figure 9D. At 144 hr (b), the remaining liquid layer is thin and only fills the "bottom" of alveoli (arrowheads). Most of the alveoli (A) are air-inflated and at high volume. This appearance matches that depicted schematically in Figure 9C. Note that the remaining alveolar liquid is darker than that in the adjacent alveolar capillaries and in (a). This indicates that the protein concentration has increased as liquid clearance occurred. (From Albertine KH. Structural organization and quantitative morphology of the lung. In: Cutillo AM, ed. Application of Magnetic Resonance to the Study of Lung. Armonk, NY: Futura Publishing Co, 1996; 73–114.)

endothelial cells as a source of this chemokine in inflammatory lung injury. Expression of ENA-78 by endothelial cells, vascular smooth muscle cells, and epithelial cells may account for IL-8-independent mechanisms of neutrophil adhesion and accumulation in the ARDS and other conditions. Localization of the cellular distribution of signaling molecules in situ in the lung offers an important opportunity to shed new light on the role of signaling molecules in the ARDS/sepsis. So, too, will in situ localization facilitate interpretation of other biological markers in bronchoalveolar lavage liquid and plasma (4), such as

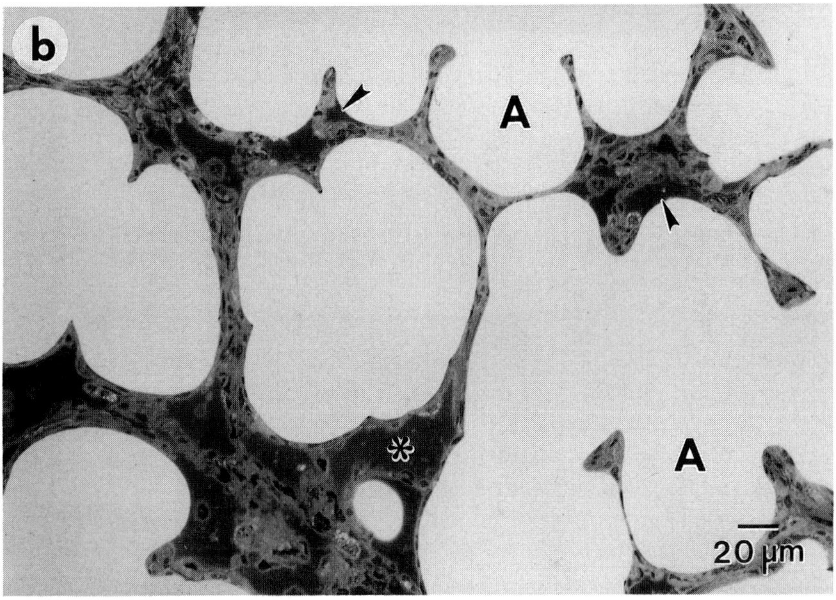

oncostatin M (196), endothelial nitric oxide synthase, inflammatory nitric oxide synthase, and endothelin-1.

X. Clearance of Lung Liquid

Resolution of alveolar edema follows the reverse course depicted in Figure 9 (57). That is, the edema liquid appears to drain "down" the alveoli. Early during the resolution phase (24 hr after filling), many of the flooded alveoli have a curved air-liquid meniscus located at the opening of alveoli into alveolar ducts. The curvature of the meniscus presumably reflects the force of airway pressure. Other flooded alveoli have a flat air-liquid meniscus, suggesting that airway pressure is too low to force air back into the flooded alveoli. The edema liquid is gradually cleared from the air spaces as ion channels and pumps located in the membranes of the airway and alveolar epithelial cells move sodium and water from the lumen to the interstitium (see Chaps. 14–18). As described earlier, the lung's epithelial cells are capable of clearing edema fluid despite a rising protein concentration in the remaining liquid (Fig. 18) (57,59). As the edema liquid recedes, its air-liquid meniscus becomes sharply curved, reflecting rising interfacial tension and transmission of airway pressure into the partially flooded alveoli. Eventually the remaining alveolar liquid fills only the corners of alveoli.

Consequently, alveolar walls become unfolded and alveolar volume returns to the normal, air-filled condition.

The clearance of edema liquid can be followed in subjects with pulmonary edema by repeatedly obtaining chest radiographs. However, chest radiography is of limited value for measuring the amount of edema liquid or its rate of resolution. It would be advantageous to follow the rate of edema liquid resolution from the clinical perspectives of patient care and management. A method that has shown promise, at least in experimental animals, is magnetic resonance imaging. Studies in rats suggest that magnetic resonance imaging measurements of changes in lung water content may be as sensitive as the gravimetric technique (197–199). Because magnetic resonance imaging is noninvasive, does not depend on ionizing radiation or radioisotopes, and can be performed on the order of seconds to minutes, fast imaging techniques could be used to repeatedly assess the spatial distribution and quantity of lung edema liquid. However, several significant problems related to peculiarities of lung anatomy limit its clinical application. The problems with imaging the lungs are the proton density (that is, the concentration of hydrogen nuclei) of inflated lung is low, air-tissue interfaces in inflated lungs perturb the magnetic fields, accumulation of water in intravascular and extravascular compartments cannot be differentiated, and causes of increased proton density, such as pulmonary edema, atelectasis, or pneumonia, cannot be differentiated thus far. Despite these current limitations, magnetic resonance imaging holds considerable promise for following and quantifying lung water (edema) distribution in disease states such as the ARDS (200) (see Chap. 4 for further discussion).

XI. Summary

Assessment of the histopathology of acute lung injury, as seen in the ARDS, has provided major insights into the processes of pulmonary edema formation and clearance. For example, it is clear that the structural design of the lung is such that the integrity of the alveolar airspaces is protected to enable adequate respiratory gas exchange even in the face of pulmonary edema. Histopathological studies also have made major contributions to our understanding of the role of inflammation in increased-permeability pulmonary edema. Today, there is a growing need and opportunity to apply immunohistochemical and in situ hybridization techniques to identify the cells in the lung that express biological markers of acute lung injury. The rationale for this growing need is twofold. First, there is promise that measurement of biological markers of acute lung injury in plasma, bronchoalveolar lavage liquid, or pulmonary edema liquid will have prognostic value for subjects who are at risk of developing the ARDS or who will die because of complications associated with the ARDS. Second, the most reliable approach to precisely determine the cell type or types that express

COLOR PLATES 2.17a–f

Figure 17 Immunohistochemical localization of inflammatory CXC chemokines in human lungs with diffuse alveolar damage at autopsy. All of the tissue sections are from subjects who died with the ARDS/sepsis.

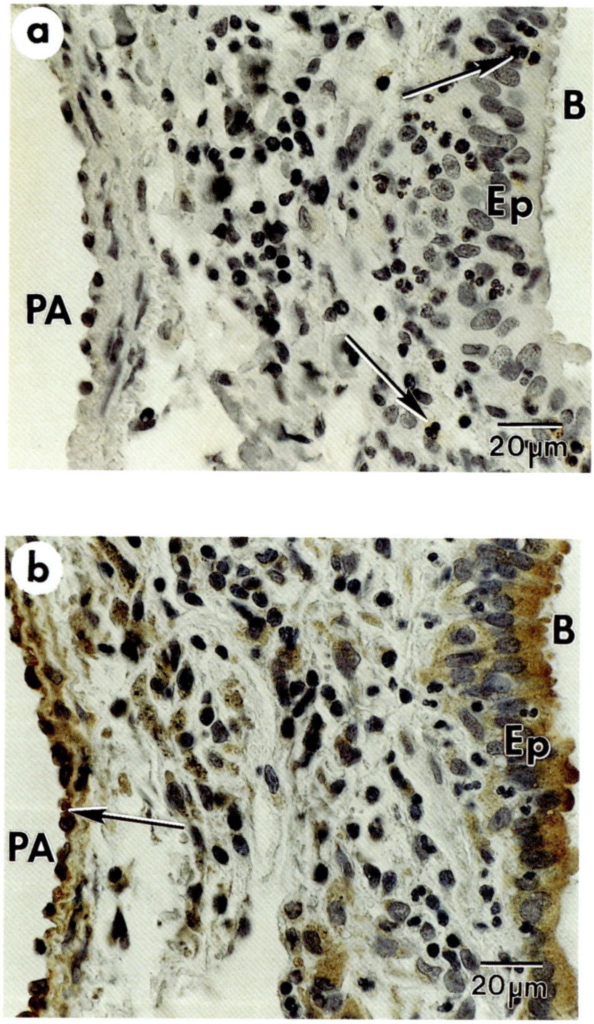

(a) An anti-IL-8 antibody immunostained some inflammatory cells (arrows) that are intercalated among the epithelial cells (Ep) of a bronchiole (B). Endothelial cells of a pulmonary artery (PA) and epithelial cells of the bronchiole are not immunostained for IL-8 protein expression. **(b)** ENA-78 immunostaining in a serial section. ENA-78 is expressed by endothelial cells (arrow) and smooth muscle cells of the pulmonary artery (PA), inflammatory cells in the perivascular interstitium, and epithelial cells (Ep) lining the bronchiole (B).

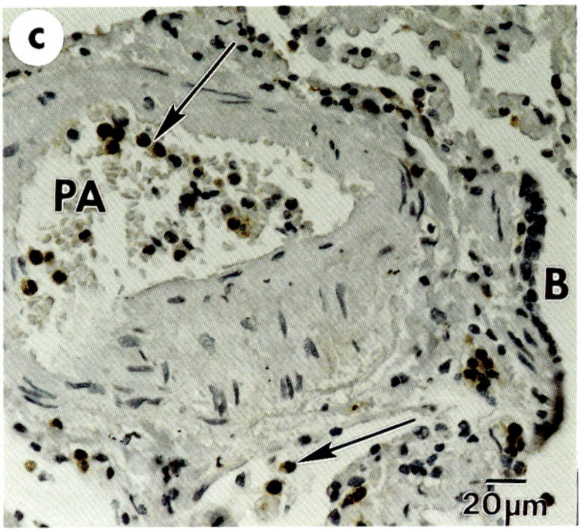

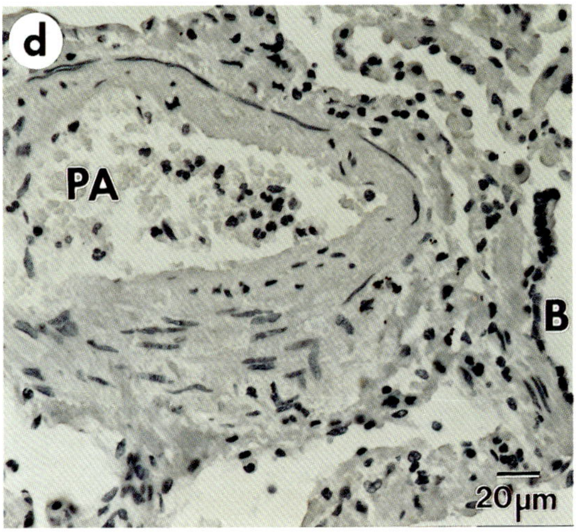

(c) IL-8 is present exclusively in inflammatory cells that are located in pulmonary blood vessels, the interstitium, and the air spaces. **(d)** Immunostaining control using an irrelevant primary antibody (insulin) that is species- and isotype-matched to the anti-IL-8 and anti-ENA-78 antibodies. There is no immunostaining with the irrelevant antibody, demonstrating specificity of the IL-8 and ENA-78 primary antibodies.

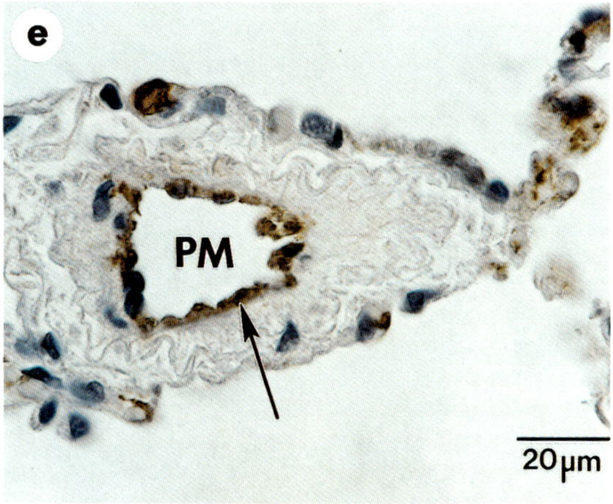

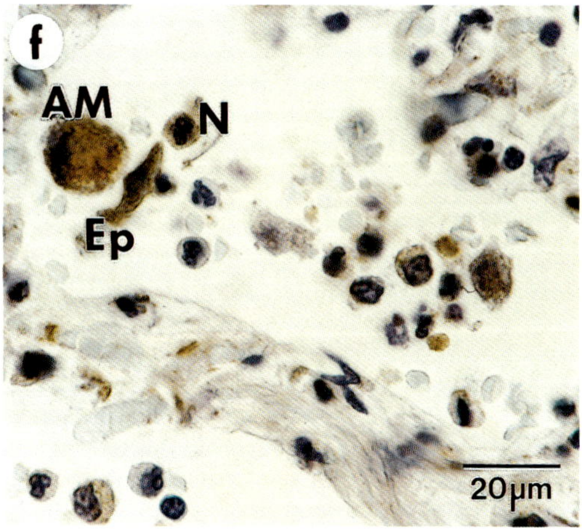

(e and f) Serial tissue sections from a patient who died with acute lobar bronchopneumonia. **(e)** ENA-78 is present in endothelial cells (arrow) of a pulmonary microvessel (PM). **(f)** ENA-78 immunostaining of inflammatory cells, notably neutrophils (N) and alveolar macrophages (AM), and desquamated airway epithelial cells (Ep) in an air space.

key biological markers in situ in the human lung are immunohistochemistry and in situ hybridization. However, for future studies to be as informative as we hope they will be, their design should include groups of subjects who are at the early phase (days) or late phase (weeks) of acute lung injury, and the major etiologies should be equally represented (sepsis, pancreatitis, aspiration, pneumonia). Careful study design and selection of analytical methods that will identify structure/function relationships may provide, for the first time, reliable means to predict the onset of the ARDS and its outcome.

Acknowledgments

I wish to thank Zhengming Wang, Nancy Chandler, and Jiancheng Sun of the Research Microscopy Facility at the University of Utah Health Sciences Center for technical assistance. Thanks are also expressed to Ms. Suzanne Irsik for secretarial assistance. Portions of this work were supported by grants from the National Institutes of Health (HL38075, S10-RR04910, S10-RR10489, HL49098, and SCOR Grant HL50153).

References

1. Bachofen M, Weibel ER. Structural alterations of lung parenchyma in the adult respiratory distress syndrome. Clin Chest Med 1982; 3:35–56.
2. Albertine KH. Ultrastructural abnormalities in increased-permeability pulmonary edema. Clin Chest Med 1985; 6:345–369.
3. Gee MH, Albertine KH. Neutrophil-endothelial cell interaction in the lung. Annu Rev Physiol 1993; 55:227–248.
4. Pittet JF, Mackersie RC, Martin TR, Matthay MA. Biological markers of acute lung injury: prognostic and pathogenetic significance. Am J Respir Crit Care Med 1997; 155:1187–1205.
5. Parsons PE, Moss M. Early detection and markers of sepsis. Clin Chest Med 1996; 17:199–212.
6. Staub NC, Albertine KH. Anatomy of the lungs. In: Murray JF, Nadel JA, eds. Textbook of Respiratory Medicine, 2nd ed. Philadelphia: WB Saunders, 1994: 3–35.
7. Goodman RB, Strieter RM, Martin DP, Steinberg KP, Milberg JA, Maunder RJ, Kunkel SL, Walz A, Hudson LD, Martin TR. Inflammatory cytokines in patients with persistence of the acute respiratory distress syndrome. Am J Respir Crit Care Med 1996; 154:602–611.
8. Imaizumi TA, Albertine KH, Jicha DL, McIntyre TM, Prescott SM, Zimmerman GA. Human endothelial cells differentially express and secrete ENA-78 and IL-8 when stimulated with inflammatory cytokines. Am J Respir Cell Mol Biol 1997; 17:181–192.

9. Staub NC. Pulmonary edema. Physiol Rev 1974; 54:678–811.
10. Albertine KH, Gee MH. Sheep lung lymph fistula preparation applied to measurements of complement-mediated pulmonary microvascular injury. In: Cantor JO, ed. Handbook of Animal Models of Pulmonary Disease. Boca Raton, FL: CRC Press, Volume II, 1989:209–229.
11. Reid L, Meyrick B. Microcirculation: definition and organization at tissue level. Ann NY Acad Sci 1982; 384:3–20.
12. Rhodin JAG. Microscopic anatomy of the pulmonary vascular bed in the cat lung. Microvasc Res 1978; 15:169–193.
13. Bundgaard M. Transport pathways in capillaries—in search of pores. Annu Rev Physiol 1980; 42:325–336.
14. Landis EM, Pappenheimer JR. Exchange of substances through the capillary walls. In: Hamilton WF, Dow P, eds. Handbook of Physiology. Section 2: Circulation. Vol. 2. Washington, DC: American Physiological Society, 1963.
15. Staub NC. The pathogenesis of pulmonary edema. Prog Cardiovasc Dis 1980; 23: 53–80.
16. Schneeberger EE, Karnovsky MJ. Substructure of intercellular junctions in freeze-fractured alveolar capillary membranes in mouse lung. Circ Res 1976; 38: 404–411.
17. Schneeberger EE. Segmental differentiation of endothelial intercellular junctions in intra-acinar arteries and veins of the rat lung. Circ Res 1981; 49:1102–1111.
18. Inuoe S, Michel RP, Hogg JC. Zonulae occludentes in alveolar epithelium and capillary endothelium of dog lungs studied with freeze-fracture technique. J Ultrastruct Res 1976; 56:215–225.
19. DeFouw DO, Cua WO, Chinard FP. Morphometric and physiological studies of alveolar microvessels in dog lungs in vivo after sustained increases in pulmonary microvascular pressures and after sustained decreases in plasma oncotic pressures. Microvasc Res 1983; 25:56–76.
20. Ryan JW, Ryan US. Pulmonary endothelial cells. Fed Proc 1977; 36:2683–2691.
21. Gillis CN, Huxtable RJ, Roth RA. Effects of monocrotaline pretreatment of rats on removal of 5-hydroxytryptamine and noradrenaline by perfused lung. Br J Pharmacol 1978; 63:435–443.
22. Johnson AR, John M, Erdos EG. Metabolism of vasoactive peptides by membrane-enriched fractions from human lung tissue, pulmonary arteries, and endothelial cells. Ann NY Acad Sci 1982; 384:72–89.
23. Yoffey JM, Courtice FC. Lymphatics, Lymph, and Lymphomyeloid Complex. London: Academic Press, 1970; 444–469.
24. Meyrick B, Reid L. Nerves in rat intra-acinar alveoli: an electron microscopic study. Respir Physiol 1971; 11:367–377.
25. Young KR Jr, Reynolds HY. Bronchoalveolar washings. Proteins and cells from normal lungs. In: Bienenstock J, ed. The Immunology of the Upper Respiratory Tract. New York: McGraw-Hill, 1984:157–173.
26. Oldmixon EH, Hoppin FG Jr. Distribution of elastin and collagen in canine lung alveolar parenchyma. J Appl Physiol 1989; 67:1941–1949.
27. Mercer RR, Crapo JD. Spatial distribution of collagen and elastin fibers in the lungs. J Appl Physiol 1990; 69:756–765.

28. Miller WS. The Lung, 2nd ed. Springfield, IL: Charles C Thomas Publishing Co, 1947.
29. von Hayek H. The Human Lung. New York: Springer-Verlag, 1960.
30. Nagaishi C. Functional Anatomy and Histology of the Lung. Baltimore, MD: University Park Press, 1972.
31. Albertine KH, Wiener-Kronish JP, Roos PJ, Staub NC. Structure, blood supply and lymphatic vessels of the sheep's visceral pleura. Am J Anat 1982; 165: 277–294.
32. Leak LV, Ferrons VJ. Lymphatics and lymphoid tissue. In: Crystal RD, West JB, Barnes PJ, Weibel ER, eds. The Lung: Scientific Foundations, 2nd ed. Philadelphia: Lippincott-Raven, 1997: Vol. 1:1129–1138.
33. Bruderman I, Somers K, Hamilton WK, Tooley WH, Butler J. Effects of surface tension on circulation in the excised lungs of dog. J Appl Physiol 1964; 19: 707–714.
34. Staub NC. Effects of alveolar surface tension on the pulmonary vascular bed. Jpn Heart J 1966; 7:386–399.
35. Nicolaysen G, Hauge A. Determinants of transvascular fluid shifts in zone I lungs. J Appl Physiol 1980; 48:256–264.
36. Howell JBL, Permutt S, Proctor DF, Riley RL. Effects of inflation of the lung on different parts of the pulmonary vascular bed. J Appl Physiol 1961; 16:71–76.
37. Staub NC. Pathophysiology of pulmonary edema. In: Staub NC, Taylor AE, eds. Edema. New York: Raven Press, 1984; 719–746.
38. Albertine KH, O'Morchoe CCC. Renal lymphatic ultrastructure and translymphatic transport. Microvasc Res 1980; 19:338–351.
39. Albertine KH, O'Morchoe CCC. An ultrastructural study of the transport pathways across arcuate, interlobar, hilar, and capsular lymphatics in the dog kidney. Microvasc Res 1981; 21:351–361.
40. Conhaim RL, Gropper MA, Staub NC. Effect of lung inflation on alveolar-airway barrier protein permeability in dog lung. J Appl Physiol 1983; 55:1249–1256.
41. Michel RP, Smith TT, Poulsen RS. Distribution of fluid in bronchovascular bundles with permeability lung edema induced by α-naphthylthiourea in dogs. A morphometric study. Lab Invest 1984; 51:97–103.
42. Gee MH, Havill AM. The relationship between pulmonary perivascular cuff fluid and lung lymph in dogs with edema. Microvasc Res 1980; 19:209–216.
43. Albertine KH, Staub NC. Lymphatic system. In: Abramson DI, Dobrin PB, eds. Blood Vessels and Lymphatics in Organ Systems. Orlando, FL: Academic Press, 1984:396–401.
44. Staub NC, Albertine KH. Biology of lung lymphatics. In: Johnston M, ed. Experimental Biology of the Lymphatic Circulation. Amsterdam: Elsevier Science Publishers, 1985:305–325.
45. Gorin AB, Stewart PA. Differential permeability of endothelial and epithelial barriers to albumin flux. J Appl Physiol 1979; 47:1315–1324.
46. Egan EA. Fluid balance in the air filled alveolar space. Am Rev Respir Dis 1983; 127:S37–S39.
47. Crandall ED. Water and nonelectrolyte transport across alveolar epithelium. Am Rev Respir Dis 1983; 127:S16–S23.

48. Crandall ED, Kim KJ. Alveolar epithelial barrier properties. In: Crystal RG, West JB, Barnes PJ, Cherniack NS, Weibel ER, eds. The Lung: Scientific Foundations. New York: Raven Press, 1991: 273–287.
49. Schneeberger EE, Karnovsky MJ. The ultrastructural basis of alveolar-capillary membrane permeability to peroxidase used as a tracer. J Cell Biol 1968; 37: 781–793.
50. Schneeberger EE, Karnovsky MJ. The influence of intravascular fluid volume on the permeability of newborn and adult mouse lungs to ultrastructural protein tracers. J Cell Biol 1971; 49:319–334.
51. Weibel ER. Design and structure of the human lung. In: Fishman AP, ed. Pulmonary Diseases and Disorders. New York: McGraw-Hill, 1980.
52. DeFouw DO, Berendsen PB. Morphologic changes in isolated perfused dog lungs after acute hydrostatic edema. Circ Res 1978; 43:72–82.
53. Goodman BE, Crandall ED. Dome formation in primary cultured monolayers of alveolar epithelial cells. Am J Physiol 1982; 243 (Cell Physiol 12):C96–C100.
54. Matthay MA, Landolt CC, Staub NC. Differential liquid and protein clearance from the alveoli of anesthetized sheep. J Appl Physiol 1982; 53:96–104.
55. Mason RJ, Williams MC, Widdicombe JH, Sanders MJ, Misfeldt DS, Berry CC. Transepithelial transport by pulmonary alveolar type II cells in primary culture. Proc Natl Acad Sci USA 1982; 79:6033–6037.
56. Matthay MA, Berthiaume Y, Staub NC. Long-term clearance of liquid and protein from the lungs of unanesthetized sheep. J Appl Physiol 1985; 59: 928–934.
57. Berthiaume Y, Albertine KH, Grady M, Fick G, Matthay MA. Protein clearance from the air spaces and lungs of unanesthetized sheep over 144 h. J Appl Physiol 1989; 67:1887–1897.
58. Matthay MA, Wiener-Kronish JP. Intact epithelial barrier function is critical for the resolution of alveolar edema in humans. Am Rev Respir Dis 1990; 142:1250–1257.
59. Sakuma T, Okaniwa G, Nakada T, Nishimura T, Fujimura S, Matthay MA. Alveolar fluid clearance in the resected human lung. Am J Respir Crit Care Med 1994; 150:305–310.
60. Schneeberger EE, McCarthy KM. Cytochemical localization of $Na^{+}K^{+}$-ATPase in rat type II pneumocytes. J Appl Physiol 1986; 60:1584–1589.
61. Walker SR, Williams MC, Benson B. Immunocytochemical localization of the major surfactant apoproteins in type II cells, Clara cells, and alveolar macrophages of rat lung. J Histochem Cytochem 1986; 34:1137–1148.
62. Basset G, Crone C, Saumon G. Significance of active ion transport in transalveolar water absorption: a study on isolated rat lung. J Physiol (Lond) 1987; 384: 311–324.
63. Cheek JM, Kim KJ, Crandall ED. Tight monolayers of rat alveolar epithelial cells: bioelectric properties and active sodium transport. Am J Physiol 1989; 256:C688–C693.
64. Crone C, Saumon G, Basset G. News from the alveoli. News in Physiol Sci (NIPS) 1990; 5:50–53.

65. Ballard ST, Schepens SM, Falcone JC, Meininger GA, Taylor AE. Regional bioelectric properties of porcine airway epithelium. J Appl Physiol 1992; 73:2021–2027.
66. Al-Bazzaz FJ. Regulation of Na and Cl transport in sheep distal airways. Am J Physiol 267 (Lung Cell Mol Physiol 11) 1994; L193–L198.
67. Ridge KM, Rutschman DH, Factor P, Katz AI, Bertorello AM, Sznajder JI. Differential expression of Na^+,K^+-ATPase isoforms in rat alveolar cells. Am J Physiol (Lung) 1997; 273:L246–L255.
68. Folkesson HG, Matthay MA, Hasegawa H, Kheradmand F, Verkman AS. Transcellular water transport in lung alveolar epithelium through mercury-sensitive water channels. Proc. Natl Acad Sci USA 1994; 91:4970–4974.
69. Hasegawa H, Ma T, Skach W, Matthay MA, Verkman AS. Molecular cloning of a mercurial-insensitive water channel expressed in selected water-transporting tissue. J Biol Chem 1994; 269:5497–5500.
70. Raina S, Preston GM, Guggino WB, Agre P. Molecular cloning and characterization of an aquaporin cDNA from salivary, lacrimal, and respiratory tissue. J Biol Chem 1995; 270:1908–1912.
71. Matthay MA, Folkesson HG, Verkman AS. Salt and water transport across alveolar and distal airway epithelia in the adult lung. Am J Physiol 270 (Lung Cell Mol Physiol 14) 1996; L487–L503.
72. Bhattacharya J, Gropper MA, Staub NC. Interstitial fluid pressure gradient measured by micropuncture in excised dog lung. J Appl Physiol 1984; 56:271–277.
73. Bhattacharya J, Staub NC. Direct measurement of microvascular pressures in the isolated perfused dog lung. Science 1980; 210:327–328.
74. Bhattacharya JH, Nanjo S, Staub NC. Micropuncture measurement of lung microvascular pressure during 5-HT infusion. J Appl Physiol 1982; 52:634–637.
75. Staub NC, Nagano H, Pearce ML. Pulmonary edema in dogs, especially the early sequence of fluid accumulation in lungs. J Appl Physiol 1967; 22:227–240.
76. Michel RP. Lung microvascular permeability to dextran in α-naphthylthiourea-induced edema. Sites of filtration, patterns of accumulation, and effects of fixation. Am J Pathol 1985; 119:474–484.
77. Hurley JV. Current views on the mechanisms of pulmonary oedema. J Pathol 1978; 125:59–79.
78. Anderson RR, Holliday RL, Driedger AA. Documentation of pulmonary capillary permeability in the adult respiratory distress syndrome accompanying human sepsis. Am Rev Respir Dis 1979; 119:869–877.
79. Fein A, Grossman RF, Jones JG. The value of edema fluid protein measurement in patients with pulmonary edema. Am J Med 1979; 67:32–38.
80. Staub NC. Pulmonary edema: physiologic approaches to management. Chest 1978; 74:559–564.
81. Brigham KL, Woolverton WC, Blake LH, Staub NC. Increased sheep lung vascular permeability caused by *Pseudomonas* bacteremia. J Clin Invest 1974; 54:792–804.
82. Ohkuda K, Nakahara K, Binder A, Staub NC. Venous air emboli in sheep: reversible increase in lung microvascular permeability. J Appl Physiol 1981; 51:887–894.

83. Johnson A, Tahamont MV, Kaplan JE, Malik AB. Lung fluid balance after pulmonary embolization: effects of thrombin vs. fibrin aggregates. J Appl Physiol 1982; 52:1565–1570.
84. Conhaim RL, Lai-Fook SJ, Eaton A. Sequence of interstitial liquid accumulation in liquid-inflated sheep lung lobes. J Appl Physiol 1989; 66:2659–2666.
85. Bachofen M, Weibel ER. Alterations of the gas exchange apparatus in adult respiratory insufficiency associated with septicemia. Am Rev Respir Dis 1977; 116:589–615.
86. Thurlbeck WM, Thurlbeck SM. Pulmonary effects of paraquot poisoning. Chest 1976; 69 (Suppl):276–280.
87. Bardales RH, Xie S-S, Schaefer RF, Hsu S-M. Apoptosis is a major pathway responsible for the resolution of type II pneumocytes in acute lung injury. Am J Pathol 1996; 149:845–852.
88. Guinee D Jr, Fleming M, Hayashi T, Woodward M, Zhang J, Walls J, Koss M, Ferrans V, Travis W. Association of p53 and WAF-1 expression with apoptosis in diffuse alveolar damage. Am J Pathol 1996; 149:531–538.
89. Pratt PC, Vollmer RT, Shelburne JD, Crapo JD. Pulmonary morphology in a multihospital collaborative extracorporeal membrane oxygenation project. I. Light microscopy. Am J Pathol 1979; 95:191–214.
90. Gehr P, Bachofen M, Weibel ER. The normal human lung: ultrastructure and morphometric estimation of diffusion capacity. Respir Physiol 1978; 32:121–140.
91. Sloane PJ, Gee MH, Gottlieb JE, Albertine KH, Peters SP, Burns JR, Machiedo G, Fish JE. A multicenter registry of patients with acute respiratory distress syndrome: physiology and outcome. Am Rev Respir Dis 1992; 146:419–426.
92. Kapanci Y, Weibel ER, Kaplan HP, Robinson FR. Pathogenesis and reversibility of the pulmonary lesions of oxygen toxicity in monkeys. 2. Ultrastructural and morphometric studies. Lab Invest 1969; 20:101–108.
93. Coalson JJ, Winter V, deLemos RA. Decreased alveolarization in baboon survivors with bronchopulmonary dysplasia. Am J Respir Crit Care Med 1995; 152: 640–646.
94. Wiener-Kronish JP, Albertine KH, Matthay MA. Differential responses of the endothelial and epithelial barriers of the lung in sheep to *E. coli* endotoxin. J Clin Invest 1991; 88:864–875.
95. Hurley JV. Types of pulmonary microvascular injury. Ann NY Acad Sci 1982; 384:269–286.
96. Cotran RS. The delayed and prolonged vascular leakage in inflammation. II. An electron microscopic study of the vascular response after thermal injury. Am J Pathol 1965; 46:589–620.
97. Cotran RS, Suter ER, Majno G. The use of colloidal carbon as a tracer in vascular injury. Vasc Dis 1967; 4:107–127.
98. Bowden DH, Adamson IYR, Wyatt JP. Reaction of lung cells to a high concentration of oxygen. Arch Pathol 1968; 86:671–675.
99. Bowden DH, Adamson IYR. Endothelial regeneration as a marker of the differential vascular responses in oxygen-induced pulmonary oedema. Lab Invest 1974; 30:350–357.

100. Kistler GS, Caldwell PRB, Weibel ER. Development of fine structural damage to alveolar and capillary lining cells in oxygen-poisoned rat lungs. J Cell Biol 1967; 32:605–628.
101. Bils RF. Ultrastructural alterations of alveolar tissue of mice. III. Ozone. Arch Environ Health 1970; 20:468–480.
102. Plopper CG, Dunworth DL, Tyler WS. Pulmonary lesions in rats exposed to ozone. Am J Pathol 1973; 71:375–386.
103. Brown RF, Clifford WE, Marrs TC, Cox RA. The histopathology of rat lung following short term exposures to mixed oxides of nitrogen (Nox). Br J Exp Pathol 1983; 64:579–593.
104. Dearden LC, Glauser FL, Smeltzer D. The effect of ethchlorvynol on pulmonary ultrastructure in dogs. Am J Pathol 1977; 87:525–536.
105. Teplitz C. The ultrastructural basis for pulmonary pathophysiology following trauma. Pathogenesis of pulmonary oedema. J Trauma 1968; 8:700–714.
106. Cunningham AL, Hurley JV. Alpha-naphthyl-thiourea-induced pulmonary oedema in the rat: a topographic and electron-microscope study. J Pathol 1972; 106: 25–35.
107. Machado DC, Bohm GM, Padovan PA. Comparative study of the ultrastructural alterations in the pulmonary vessels of rats treated with alpha naphthylthiourea (ANTU) and ammonium sulphate. J Pathol 1977; 121:205–212.
108. Havill AM, Gee MH, Washburne JD, Premkumar A, Otlaviano R, Flynn JT, Spath JA Jr. α-Naphthylthiourea produces dose-dependent lung vascular injury in sheep. Am J Physiol 1982; 243:H505–H511.
109. Hurley JV, Jago MV. Pulmonary oedema in rats given dehydromonocrotaline: a topographic and electron-microscope study. J Pathol 1975; 117:23–32.
110. Plestina R, Stoner HB. Pulmonary oedema in rats given monocrotaline pyrrole. J Pathol 1972; 106:235–250.
111. Plestina R, Stoner HB, Jones G, Butler WH, Matlocks AR. Vascular changes in the lungs of rats after the intravenous injection of pyrrole carbamates. J Pathol 1977; 121:9–18.
112. Cottrell TS, Levine OR, Senior RM, Wierar J, Spiro D, Fishman AP. Electron microscopic alterations at the alveolar level in pulmonary edema. Circ Res 1967; 21:783–798.
113. Dickey BF, Thrall RS, McCormick JR, Ward PA. Oleic-acid-induced lung injury in the rat. Failure of indomethacin treatment or complement depletion to ablate lung injury. Am J Pathol 1981; 103:376–383.
114. Spragg RG, Abraham JL, Loomis WH. Pulmonary platelet disposition accompanying acute oleic acid-induced pulmonary injury. Am Rev Respir Dis 1982; 126:553–557.
115. Hayes JA, Shiga A. Ultrastructural changes in pulmonary oedema produced experimentally with ammonium sulphate. J Pathol 1970; 100:281–286.
116. Busch RH, Buschbom RL, Cannon WC, Lauhala KE, Miller FJ, Graham JA, Smith LG. Effects of ammonium sulfate aerosol exposure on lung ultrastructure of normal and elastase-impaired rats and guinea pigs. Environ Res 1984; 33: 454–472.

117. Sykes BI, Purchase IFH, Smith LL. Pulmonary ultrastructure after oral and intravenous dosage of paraquat to rats. J Pathol 1977; 121:233–241.
118. Dearden LC, Fairshter RD, McRae DM, Smith WR, Glauser FL, Wilson AF. Pulmonary ultrastructure of the late aspects of human paraquat poisoning. Am J Pathol 1978; 93:667–680.
119. Torre C, Varetto L, Pavanelli PL, Belliardo F. Lung morphology in experimental acute paraquat poisoning. SEM observations. Am J Forens Med Pathol 1984; 5: 125–129.
120. Finegold MJ. Interstitial pulmonary edema—an electron microscopic study of the pathology of staphylococcal enterotoxaemia in rhesus monkeys. Lab Invest 1967; 16:912–924.
121. Coalson JJ, Hinshaw B, Guenter CA. The pulmonary ultrastructure in septic shock. Exp Mol Pathol 1970; 12:84–103.
122. Pietra GG, Szidon JP, Carpenter HA, Fishman AP. Bronchial venular leakage during endotoxin shock. Am J Pathol 1974; 77:387–401.
123. Pingleton WW, Coalson JJ, Guenter CA. Significance of leukocytes in endotoxin shock. Exp Mol Pathol 1975; 22:183–194.
124. Hasan FM, Teplitz C, Farrugia R, Huan E, Schwartz S. Lung function and structure after *Escherichia coli* endotoxin in rabbits: effect of dose and rate of administration. Circ Shock 1984; 13:1–19.
125. Heflin AC, Brigham KL. Prevention by granulocyte depletion of increased lung vascular permeability of sheep lung following endotoxemia. J Clin Invest 1981; 68:1253–1260.
126. Meyrick B, Brigham KL. Acute effects of *Escherichia coli* endotoxin on the pulmonary microcirculation of anesthetized sheep. Structure-function relationships. Lab Invest 1983; 48:458–470.
127. Rojas J, Larsson LE, Hellerqvist CG, Brigham KL, Gray ME, Stahlman MT. Pulmonary hemodynamic and ultrastructural changes associated with group B streptococcal toxemia in adult sheep and newborn lambs. Pediatr Res 1983; 17: 1002–1008.
128. Saldeen T. The microembolism syndrome. Microvasc Res 1976; 11:227–259.
129. Moosavi H, Utell MJ, Hyde RW, Fahey PJ, Peterson BT, Donnelly J, Jensen KD. Lung ultrastructure in noncardiogenic pulmonary edema induced by air embolization in dogs. Lab Invest 1981; 45:456–464.
130. Albertine KH, Wiener-Kronish JP, Koike D, Staub NC. Quantification of damage by air emboli to lung microvessels in anesthetized sheep. J Appl Physiol 1984; 57:1360–1368.
131. Clark MC, Flick MR. Permeability pulmonary edema caused by venous air embolism. Am Rev Respir Dis 1984; 129:633–635.
132. Niehaus GD, Saba TM, Edmonds RH, Dillon BC. Leukocyte involvement in pulmonary localization of blood-borne microparticulates: relationship to altered lung fluid balance. Circ Shock 1984; 12:95–105.
133. Craddock PR, Hammerschmidt DE, Moldow O, Yamada O, Jacob HS. Granulocyte aggregation as a manifestation of membrane interactions with complement: possible role in leukocyte margination, microvascular occlusion, and endothelial damage. Semin Hematol 1979; 16:140–147.

134. Caldwell PRB, Wigger HJ, Fernandez LT, D'Alisa RM, Tse-Eng D, Butler VP Jr. Lung injury induced by antibody fragments to angiotensin-converting enzyme. Am J Pathol 1981; 105:54–63.
135. Henson PM, Larsen GL, Webster RO, Mitchell BC, Goins AJ, Henson JE. Pulmonary microvascular alterations and injury induced by complement fragments: synergistic effect of complement activation, neutrophil sequestration, and prostaglandins. Ann NY Acad Sci 1982; 384:287–300.
136. Till GO, Johnson KJ, Kunkel R, Ward PA. Intravascular activation of complement and acute lung injury. Dependency on neutrophils and toxic oxygen metabolites. J Clin Invest 1982; 69:1126–1135.
137. Meyrick B, Brigham KL. The effect of a single infusion of zymosan-activated plasma on the pulmonary microcirculation of sheep. Structure-function relationships. Am J Pathol 1984; 114:32–45.
138. Ratliff NB, Wilson JW, Hackel DB, Martin AM Jr. The lung in hemorrhagic shock. II. Observations on alveolar and vascular ultrastructure. Am J Pathol 1970; 58: 353–373.
139. Ratliff NB, Wilson JW, Mikat E, Hackel DB, Graham TC. The lung in hemorrhagic shock. IV. The role of neutrophilic polymorphonuclear leukocytes. Am J Pathol 1971; 65:325–334.
140. Michel RP, LaForte M, Hogg JC. Physiology and morphology of pulmonary microvascular injury with shock and reinfusion. J Appl Physiol 1981; 50:1227–1235.
141. Staub NC, Schultz EL, Albertine KH. Leucocytes and pulmonary microvascular injury. Ann NY Acad Sci 1982; 384:332–342.
142. Hogg JC, Doerschuk CM. Leukocyte traffic in the lung. Annu Rev Physiol 1995; 57:97–114.
143. Albertine KH. Lung injury and neutrophil density during air embolization in sheep after leukocyte depletion with nitrogen mustard. Am Rev Respir Dis 1988; 138: 1444–1453.
144. Barie PS, Tahamont MV, Malik AB. Prevention of increased pulmonary vascular permeability after pancreatitis by granulocyte depletion in sheep. Am Rev Respir Dis 1982; 126:904–908.
145. Flick MR, Perel A, Staub NC. Leukocytes are required for increased microvascular permeability after microembolization in sheep. Circ Res 1981; 48:344–351.
146. Tahamont MV, Malik AB. Granulocytes mediate the increase in pulmonary vascular permeability after thrombin embolism. J Appl Physiol 1983; 54:1489–1495.
147. Maunder RJ, Hackman RC, Riff E, Albert RK, Springmeyer SC. Occurrence of the adult respiratory distress syndrome in neutropenic patients. Am Rev Respir Dis 1986; 133:313–316.
148. Ognibene FP, Martin SE, Parker MM, Schlesinger T, Reach P, Burch C, Shelhamer JH, Parrillo JE. Adult respiratory distress syndrome in patients with severe neutropenia. N Engl J Med 1986; 315:547–551.
149. Kaslovsky RA, Gibbs L, Malik AB. Neutrophils from chronic granulomatous disease fail to increase endothelial permeability. Am J Physiol 1991; 261: H1226–1230.

150. Bernard GR, Lucht WD, Niedermeyer ME, Snapper JR, Ogletree ML, Brigham KL. Effect of *N*-acetylcysteine on pulmonary response to endotoxin in the awake sheep and upon in vitro granulocyte function. J Clin Invest 1984; 73:1772–1784.
151. Perkowski SZ, Havill AM, Flynn JT, Gee MH. Role of intrapulmonary release of eicosanoids and superoxide anion as mediators of pulmonary dysfunction and endothelial injury in sheep with intermittent complement activation. Circ Res 1983; 53:574–583.
152. Milligan SA, Hoeffel JM, Goldstein IM, Flick MR. Effect of catalase on endotoxin induced acute lung injury in unanaesthetized sheep. Am Rev Respir Dis 1989; 137:420–428.
153. Shasby DM, Shasby SS, Peach MJ. Granulocytes and phorbol myristate acetate increase permeability to albumin of cultured endothelial monolayers and isolated perfused lungs: role of oxygen radicals and granulocyte adherence. Am Rev Respir Dis 1983; 127:72–76.
154. Albertine KH, Rosolia DL, Peters SP, Gee MH. Neutrophil activation in vivo in the lung during ZAP infusion is characterized by changes in physical and cytochemical properties of neutrophils. J Appl Physiol 1993; 74:1361–1373.
155. Peters SP, Cerasoli F Jr, Albertine KH, Gee MH, Berd D, Ishihara Y. "Autoregulation" of human neutrophil activation in vitro: regulation of phorbol myristate acetate-induced neutrophil activation by cell density. J Leukoc Biol 1990; 47: 457–474.
156. Harlan JM, Winn RK, Vedder NB, Doerschuk CM, Rice CL. In vivo models of leukocyte adherence to endothelium. In: JM Harlan, DY Liu, eds. Adhesion: Its Role in Inflammatory Disease. New York: Freeman, 1992; 6:117–150.
157. Zimmerman GA, McIntyre TM, Prescott SM. Cell-to-cell communication. In: Crystal RD, West JB, Barnes PJ, Weibel ER, eds. The Lung: Scientific Foundations, 2nd ed. Philadelphia: Lippincott-Raven, 1997: Vol 1:289–304.
158. Yoder MC, Checkley LL, Giger U, Hanson WL, Kirk KR, Capen RL, Wagner WW Jr. Pulmonary microcirculatory kinetics of neutrophils deficient in leukocyte adhesion-promoting glycoproteins. J Appl Physiol 1990; 69:207–213.
159. Horgan MJ, Wright SD, Malik AB. Antibody against leukocyte integrin (CD18) prevents reperfusion induced lung vascular injury. Am J Physiol 1990; 259:L315–L319.
160. Horgan MJ, Ge M, Go J, Rothlein R, Malik AB. Role of ICAM 1 in neutrophil-mediated lung vascular injury after occlusion and reperfusion. Am J Physiol 1991; 261:H1578–H1584.
161. Kaslovsky RA, Horgan MJ, Lure H, McCandless BK, Gilboa N, Wright SD, Malik AB. Pulmonary edema induced by phagocytosing neutrophils: protective effect of monoclonal antibody against phagocyte CD18 integrin. Circ Res 1990; 67: 795–802.
162. Folkesson HG, Matthay MA. Inhibition of CD18 or CD11b attenuates acute lung injury after acid instillation in rabbits. J Appl Physiol 1997; 82:1743–1750.
163. Naka Y, Toda K, Kayano K, Oz MC, Pinsky DJ. Failure to express the P-selectin gene or P-selectin blockade confers early pulmonary protection after lung ischemia or transplantation. Proc Natl Acad Sci USA 1997; 94:757–761.

164. Doerschuk CM, Winn RK, Coxson HO, Harlan JM. CD18-dependent and -independent mechanisms of neutrophil emigration in the pulmonary and systemic microcirculation of rabbits. J Immunol 1990; 144:2327–2333.
165. Vedder NB, Winn RK, Rice CL, Chi EY, Arfors KE, Harlan JM. A monoclonal antibody to the adherence-promoting leukocyte glycoprotein, CD18, reduces organ injury and improves survival from hemorrhagic shock and resuscitation in rabbits. J Clin Invest 1988; 81:939–944.
166. Carlos TM, Schwartz BR, Kovach NL, Yee E, Rosa M, Osborn L, Chi-Rosso G, Newman B, Lobb R, Rosa M. Vascular cell adhesion molecule-1 mediates lymphocyte adherence to cytokine-activated cultured human endothelial cells. Blood 1990; 76:965–970.
167. Bochner BS, Luscinskas FW, Gimbrone MA Jr., Newman W, Sterbinsky SA, Derse-Anthony CP, Klunk D, Schleimer RP. Adhesion of human basophils, eosinophils, and neutrophils to interleukin 1-activated human vascular endothelial cells: contributions of endothelial cell adhesion molecules. J Exp Med 1991; 173: 1553–1556.
168. Dobrina A, Menegazzi R, Carlos TM, Nardon E, Cramer R, Zacchi T, Harlan JM, Patriarca P. Mechanisms of eosinophil adherence to cultured vascular endothelial cells. J Clin Invest 1991; 88:22–26.
169. Rice GE, Munro JM, Bevilacqua MP. Inducible cell adhesion molecule 110 (INCAM-110) is an endothelial receptor for lymphocytes. A CD11/CD18-independent adhesion mechanism. J Exp Med 1990; 171:1369–1374.
170. Walsh GM, Memod JJ, Hartnell A, Kay AB, Wardlaw AJ. Human eosinophil, but not neutrophil, adherence to IL-1-stimulated human umbilical vascular endothelial cells is alpha 4 beta 1 (very late antigen-4) dependent. J Immunol 1991; 146:3419–3423.
171. Nathan CF. Neutrophil activation on biological surfaces: massive secretion of hydrogen peroxide in response to products of macrophages and lymphocytes. J Clin Invest 1987; 80:1550–1560.
172. Nathan C, Srimal S, Farber C, Sanchez E, Kabbash L, Asch A, Gailit J, Wright SD. Cytokine-induced respiratory burst of human neutrophils: dependence on extracellular matrix proteins and CD11/CD18 integrins. J Cell Biol 1989; 109:1341–1349.
173. Worthen GS, Schwab B III, Elson EL, Downey GP. Mechanics of stimulated neutrophils: cell stiffening induces retention in capillaries. Science 1989; 245: 183–186.
174. Albertine KH, Koh YY, Peters SP, Gee MH, McKenna PJ. Activated sheep neutrophils demonstrate decreased transvascular migration in response to chemoattractants in alveolar airspaces and skin. Am Rev Respir Dis 1991; 143:A542.
175. Pugin J, Ricou B, Steinberg KP, Suter PM, Martin TR. Proinflammatory activity in bronchoalveolar lavage fluids from patients with ARDS. A prominent role for interleukin-1. Am J Respir Crit Care Med 1996; 153:1850–1856.
176. Gamble JR, Skinner MP, Bemdt MC, Vadas MA. Prevention of activated neutrophil adhesion to endothelium by soluble adhesion protein GMP140. Science 1990; 249:414–417.
177. Hakkert BC, Kuijpers TW, Leeuwenberg JFM, Van Mourik JA, Roos D. Neutrophil and monocyte adherence to and migration across monolayers of cytokine-

activated endothelial cells: the contribution of CD18, ELAM 1, and VLA-4. Blood 1991; 78:2721–2726.

178. Horvath CJ, Ferro TJ, Jesmok G, Malik AB. Recombinant tumor necrosis factor increases pulmonary vascular permeability independent of neutrophils. Proc Natl Acad Sci USA 1988; 85:9219–9223.
179. Johnson J, Meyrick B, Jesmok G, Brigham KL. Human recombinant tumor necrosis factor alpha infusion mimics endotoxemia in awake sheep. J Appl Physiol 1989; 66:1448–1454.
180. Kreil EA, Greene E, Fitzgibbon C, Robinson DR, Zapol WM. Effects of recombinant human tumor necrosis factor alpha, lymphotoxin, and *Escherichia coli* lipopolysaccharide on hemodynamics, lung microvascular permeability, and eicosanoid synthesis in anesthetized sheep. Circ Res 1989; 65:502–514.
181. Redl H, Schlag G, Lamche H, Vogel C, Paul E. TNF- and LPS-induced changes of lung vascular permeability: studies in unanesthetised sheep. Circ Shock 1990; 31:183–192.
182. Cirelli RA, Carey LA, Fisher JK, Rosolia DL, Elsasser TH, Caperna TJ, Gee MH, Albertine KH. Endotoxin infusion in anesthetized sheep is associated with intrapulmonary sequestration of leukocytes that immunohistochemically express tumor necrosis factor-α. J Leukoc Biol 1995; 57:820–826.
183. Mantovani A, Bussolino F, Introna M. Cytokine regulation of endothelial cell function: from molecular level to the bedside. Immunol Today 1997; 18:231–240.
184. Ebnet K, Kaldjian EP, Anderson AO, Shaw S. Orchestrated information transfer underlying leukocyte endothelial interactions. Annu Rev Immunol 1996; 14: 155–177.
185. Murphy PM. The molecular biology of leukocyte chemoattractant receptors. Annu Rev Immunol 1994; 12:593–633.
186. Mackay CR: Chemokines: what chemokine is that? Curr Biol 1997; 7:R384–R386.
187. Rovai LE, Herschman HR, Smith JB. Cloning and characterization of the human granulocyte chemotactic protein-2 gene. J Immunol 1997; 158:5257–5266.
188. Miller EJ, Cohen AB, Nagao S, Griffith D, Maudner RJ, Martin TR, Wiener-Kronish JP, Sticherling M, Christophers E, Matthay MA. Elevated levels of NAP-1/interleukin-8 are present in the airspaces of patients with adult respiratory distress syndrome and are associated with increased mortality. Am Rev Respir Dis 1992; 146:427–432.
189. Miller EJ, Cohen AB, Matthay MA. Increased interleukin-8 concentrations in the pulmonary edema fluid of patients with acute respiratory distress syndrome from sepsis. Crit Care Med 1996; 24:1448–1454.
190. Jorens PG, Damme JV, Backer WD, Bossaert L, Jongh RFD, Herman AG, Rampart M. Interleukin-8 in the bronchoalveolar lavage fluid from patients with the adult respiratory distress syndrome and in patients at risk for ARDS. Cytokine 1992; 4:592–597.
191. Chollet-Martin S, Montravers P, Gibert C, Elbim C, Desmonts JM, Fagon J-Y, Gougerot-Pocidalo A. High levels of interleukin-8 in the blood and alveolar spaces of patients with pneumonia and adult respiratory distress syndrome. Infect Immunol 1993; 61:4553–4559.

192. Donnelly SC, Strieter RM, Kunkel SL, Walz A, Robertson CR, Carter DC, Grant IS, Pollock AJ, Hastett C. Interleukin-8 and development of adult respiratory distress syndrome in at-risk patients. Lancet 1993; 341:643–647.
193. Torre D, Zeroli C, Giola M, Fiori GP, Minoja G, Maraggia D, Chiaranda M. Levels of interleukin-8 in patients with adult respiratory distress syndrome. J Infect Dis 1993; 167:505–506.
194. Walz A, Burgener R, Car B, Baggiolini M, Kunkel SL, Strieter RM. Structure and neutrophil-activating properties of a novel inflammatory peptide (ENA-78) with homology to interleukin 8. J Exp Med 1991; 174:1355–1362.
195. Schall TJ. The chemokines. In: Thompson A, ed. The Cytokine Handbook, 2nd ed. Orlando, FL: Academic Press, 1994;419–460.
196. Modur V, Feldhaus MJ, Weyrich AS, Jicha DL, Prescott SM, Zimmerman GA, McIntyre TM. Oncostatin M is a proinflammatory mediator: in vivo effects correlate with endothelial cell expression of inflammatory cytokines and adhesion molecules. J Clin Invest 1997; 100:158–168.
197. Skalina S, Kundel HL, Wolf G, Marshall B. The effect of pulmonary edema on proton nuclear magnetic resonance relaxation times. Invest Radiol 1984; 19:7–9.
198. Cutillo AG, Morris AH, Ailion DC, Case TA, Durney CH, Ganesan K, Watanabe F, Akhtari M. Assessment of lung water distribution by nuclear magnetic resonance. A new method for quantifying and monitoring experimental lung injury. Am Rev Respir Dis 1988; 137:1371–1378.
199. Vinitski S, Steiner RM, Wexler HR, Rifkin M. Assessment of lung water by magnetic resonance in three types of pulmonary edema. Heart Vessels 1988; 4: 88–93.
200. Cutillo AM. Application of Magnetic Resonance to the Study of Lung. Armonk, NY: Futura Publishing Co, 1996.

3

Radiographic Manifestations of Pulmonary Edema

ROBERT D. SUH

Loma Linda University Medical Center
Loma Linda, California

DENISE R. ABERLE

University of California at Los Angeles
School of Medicine
Los Angeles, California

I. Introduction

The clinical assessment of critically ill patients with pulmonary edema is often challenging, despite considerable progress in our understanding of the underlying physiologic mechanisms. Pulmonary edema is defined as an abnormal increase in extravascular lung water (1,2). As inferred from the Starling equation (detailed in Chap. 1), the three principal mechanisms of edema formation are: (1) an increased hydrostatic (microvascular) pressure gradient across the semipermeable capillary membrane; (2) a decreased fluid osmotic pressure gradient across the membrane; or (3) increased permeability of the capillary endothelial-alveolar epithelial membrane. A fourth mechanism not described by the Starling equation is the lung's ability to remove extravascular lung water and protein through its lymphatic circulation, the pleura, and along the perihilar bronchovascular interstitium (3,4). Since in most patients one or more factors may be contributory, these mechanisms have been regrouped (5,6) into two major classifications: hydrostatic edema and increased permeability edema. Hydrostatic edema (as discussed in Chap. 5) is sometimes further subdivided into cardiac edema, commonly from cardiac valvular or myocardial diseases, and renal edema, which results from intravascular volume overload as in renal insufficiency or following aggressive intravenous fluid administration (3,7,8,9). Increased permeability edema results from a wide variety of insults to the alveolar-capillary membrane and pulmonary microvasculature (discussed in Chaps. 6–12) and is often associated with the adult respiratory distress syndrome (ARDS).

To appropriately manage these patients, the differentiation between hydrostatic and increased permeability edemas is important. The projectional chest radiograph remains the primary method of assessing the presence or absence of pulmonary edema (10,11) owing to its low cost, ready availability, portability, reproducibility, and high sensitivity (8,9). Upright posteroanterior (PA) projection images are desirable in order to minimize geometric magnification of the heart and the effects of gravity on the appearances of the lung and pulmonary vasculature. However, most critically ill patients are bedridden and can tolerate

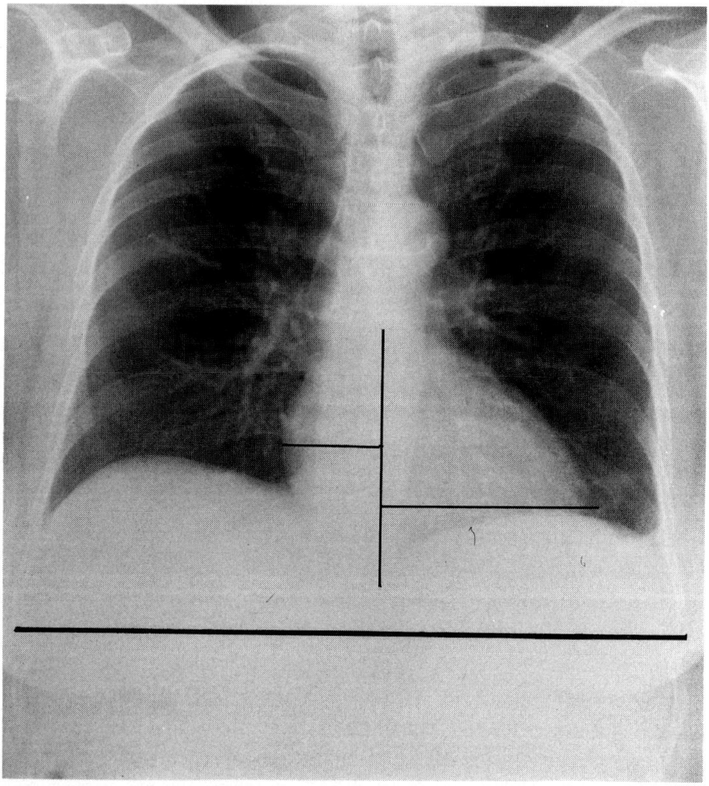

Figure 1 Normal cardiothoracic ratio: 54-year-old female. PA radiograph demonstrates normal cardiothoracic ratio, comparing the widest cardiac silhouette diameter to the widest inner thoracic diameter.

only bedside semiupright or supine radiographs in the anteroposterior (AP) projection. Because patient positioning can considerably affect radiographic findings, the use of radiopaque gravity markers is important in illustrating the position of the cassette (and patient) at the time of exposure.

Much literature has been written on the radiographic manifestations of both hydrostatic and increased permeability edemas, and the accuracy of chest radiographic differentiation (1,3,5–8). However, over the past two decades, advances in computed tomography (CT) in the form of rapid image acquisition and high-resolution techniques have made CT a potentially valuable adjunct in the evaluation and differentiation of pulmonary edema (2,6,12,13). This chapter

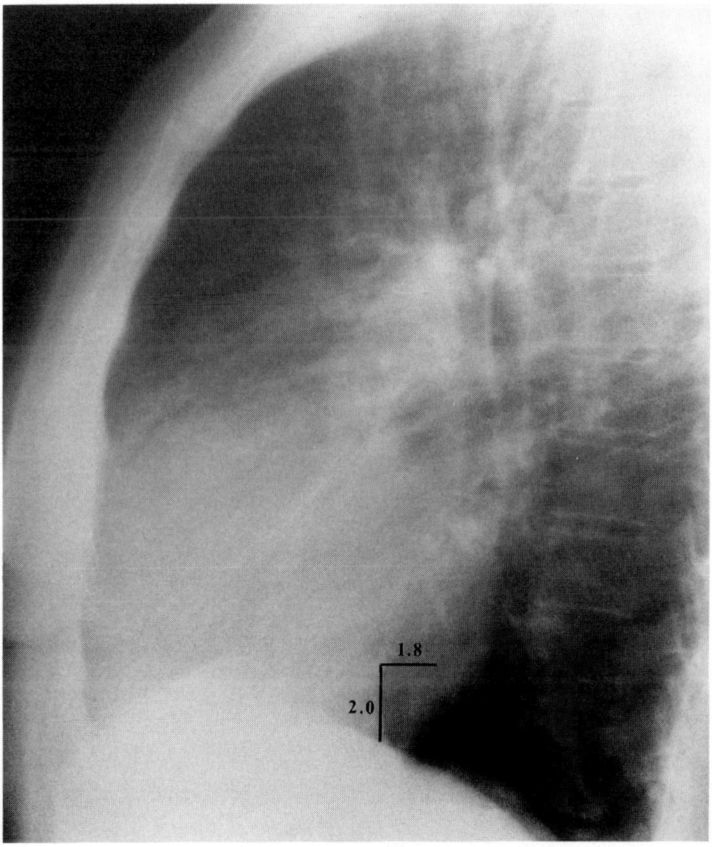

Figure 2 Hoffman-Rigler rule: 48-year-old female with congestive heart failure. Lateral radiograph shows posterior cardiac margin projecting beyond 1.8 cm posterior to the inferior vena cava shadow.

will review the chest radiographic and CT findings of hydrostatic and increased permeability pulmonary edemas, emphasizing the key points that may differentiate the two pathogenic entities. In addition, the radiographic findings in the specific conditions of high altitude, neurogenic, and postobstructive pulmonary edemas will be briefly reviewed.

II. Hydrostatic Edema: Cardiac Etiology

Hydrostatic edema of cardiac etiology is perhaps the best described pattern of edema, for which left ventricular failure is the prototype. The chest radiograph usually demonstrates some or all of the following findings: cardiac enlargement, widening of the vascular pedicle (superior mediastinum), pleural effusions, and

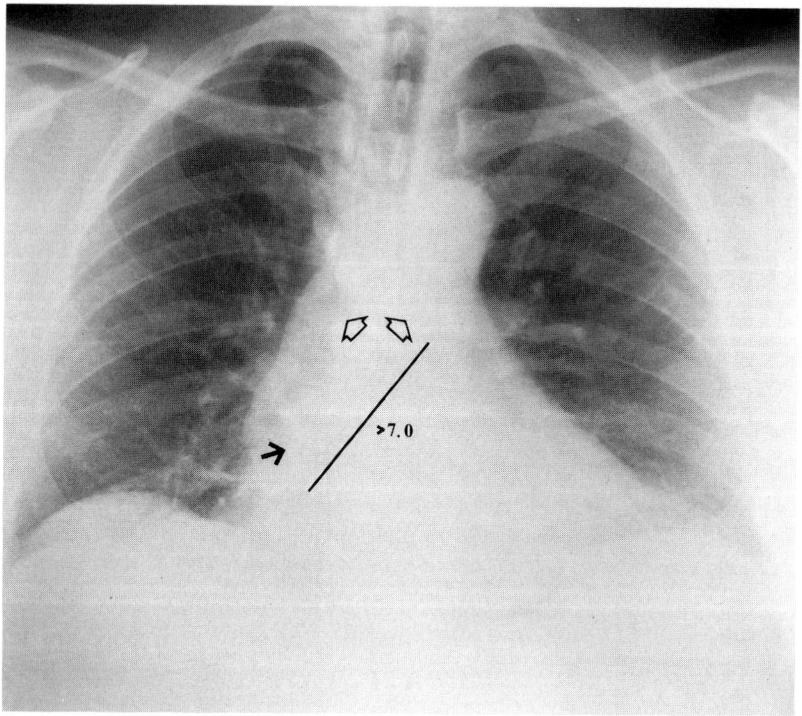

A

Figure 3 Left atrial enlargement: 64-year-old male evaluated for mediastinal mass. (A) A frontal radiograph illustrates signs of left atrial enlargement, including a right retrocardiac double density (↑), left atrial dimension > 7 cm, and carinal splaying > 75° (⇧). (B) The lateral radiograph illustrates posterior displacement of the left upper lobe bronchus (▲) due to the enlarged posterosuperior left atrial margin.

edema in the form of interstitial reticulation and, ultimately, airspace consolidation. Each of these radiographic features will be briefly reviewed.

A. Cardiac Enlargement

Cardiac enlargement is a frequent, although not invariant, finding in patients with cardiogenic edema. The normal cardiothoracic ratio, as defined on erect PA projection radiographs, has been established at < 0.55 (14). This represents the ratio of the cardiac diameter (measured as the largest sum of the most rightward and leftward margins from midline) to the inner thoracic margin at its largest diameter (Fig. 1). Depending on the etiology of the cardiac disease, there may be specific enlargement of the left ventricle or left atrium that is

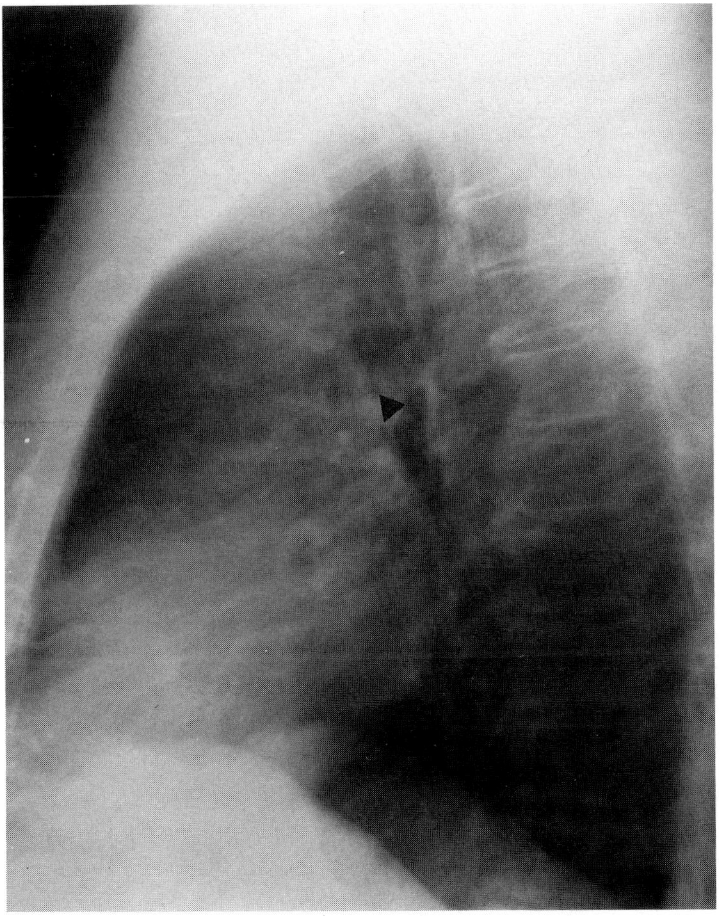

B

recognizable by alterations of the cardiac contour. Left ventricular enlargement is usually manifest as inferior, leftward displacement of the cardiac apex on frontal images. On the lateral projection, the inferoposterior margin of the cardiac silhouette is displaced posteriorly (Fig. 2). The Hoffman-Rigler rule attempts to quantify this, stating that the posterior cardiac margin should not project 1.8 cm posterior to the shadow of the inferior vena cava when measured at a point 2.0 cm above the intersection of the inferior vena cava and right

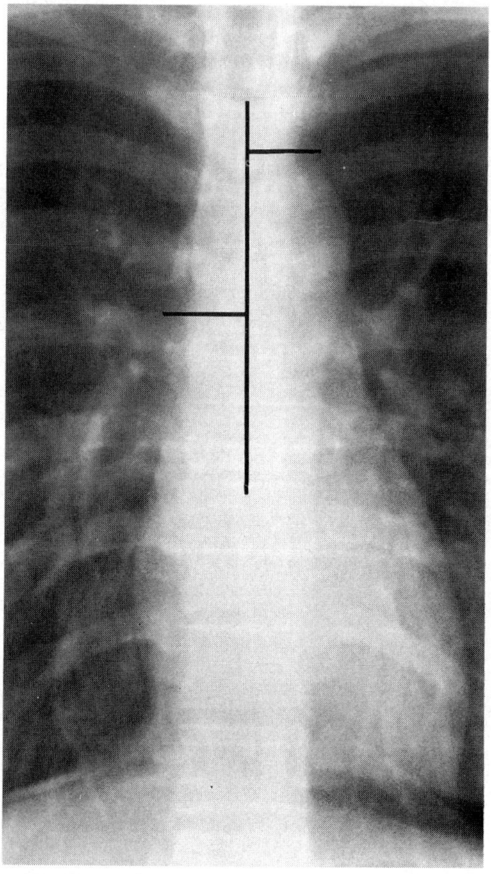

A

Figure 4 Vascular pedicle width: (A) 21-year-old female. PA radiograph shows normal vascular pedicle width. (B) 63-year-old female with renal failure. PA radiograph shows abnormally increased vascular pedicle width resulting from an increase in circulating blood volume.

hemidiaphragm (15) (Fig. 2). One exception to this rule is the presence of right ventricular enlargement, which may result in posterior displacement of the left ventricle in the absence of true left ventricular enlargement.

Left atrial enlargement is inferred from a number of radiographic signs (Fig. 3). On PA projection images the left atrial appendage may be enlarged (16), although this observation is virtually specific to rheumatic mitral valvular disease. A right retrocardiac double density has been described (14), owing to the added density of the enlarged left atrium projecting somewhat medial to the right atrial border. On frontal radiographs, left atrial size may be grossly measured as the distance from the midpoint of the left mainstem bronchus to the inferolateral margin of the left atrial shadow and is normally < 7 cm (17). In

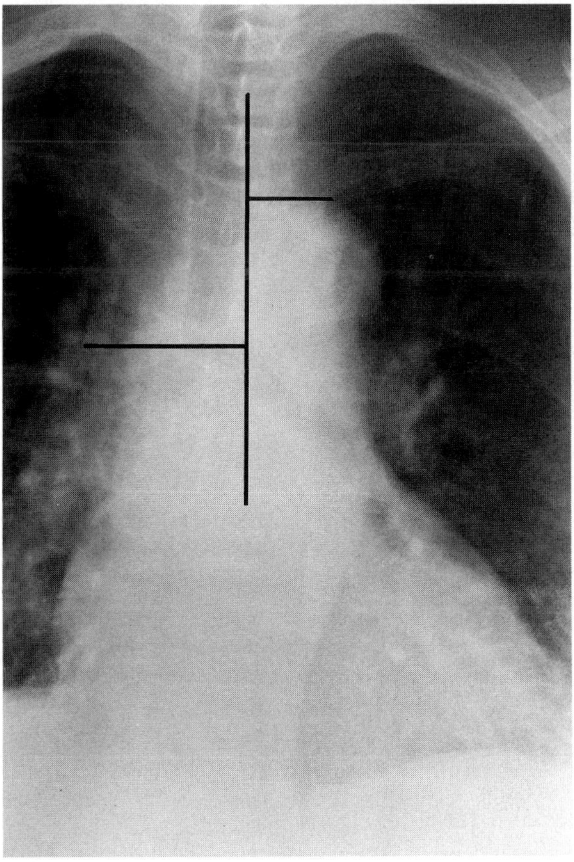

B

addition, splaying of the carina to > 75° has also been described with left atrial enlargement, although this is also seen with pericardial effusion or subcarinal masses (18). On the lateral projection, posterior displacement of the left upper lobe bronchus accompanied by convexity of the posterosuperior cardiac margin suggests left atrial enlargement (14) (Fig. 3).

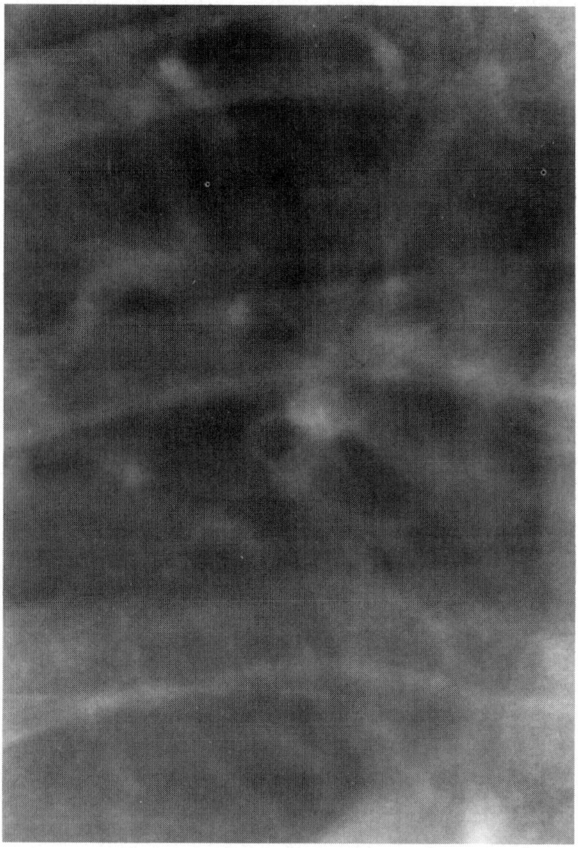

A

Figure 5 Pulmonary artery to bronchus ratios in 37-year-old female with mixed cryoglobinemia and changes in circulating blood volume. (A) Magnification view of premorbid PA radiograph illustrates the normal ABR of the anterior segmental bronchovascular bundle of the right upper lobe. (B) Subsequent frontal radiograph coincident with a pathologic increase in circulating blood volume shows an enlarging ABR with relative enlargement of the artery in the anterior segmental bronchovascular bundle.

In 1984 Milne and Pistolesi described the vascular pedicle of the superior mediastinum as the horizontal distance between the right mainstream bronchus and superior vena cava on the right margin and the left subclavian artery origin on the left mediastinal margin (19) (Fig. 4). The right margin is formed by systemic venous structures, specifically the brachiocephalic vein and superior vena cava, and is therefore distensible. In contradistinction, the left margin is defined by the much less distensible systemic arteries. In normal subjects, vascular pedicle width (VPW) averages 48 ± 5 mm on upright PA radiographs obtained at a source-to-image distance of 183 cm (72 in.). Milne et al. observed vascular pedicle enlargement greater than 53 mm in 60% of patients with cardiogenic edema and in 85% of patients with intravascular volume overload (3).

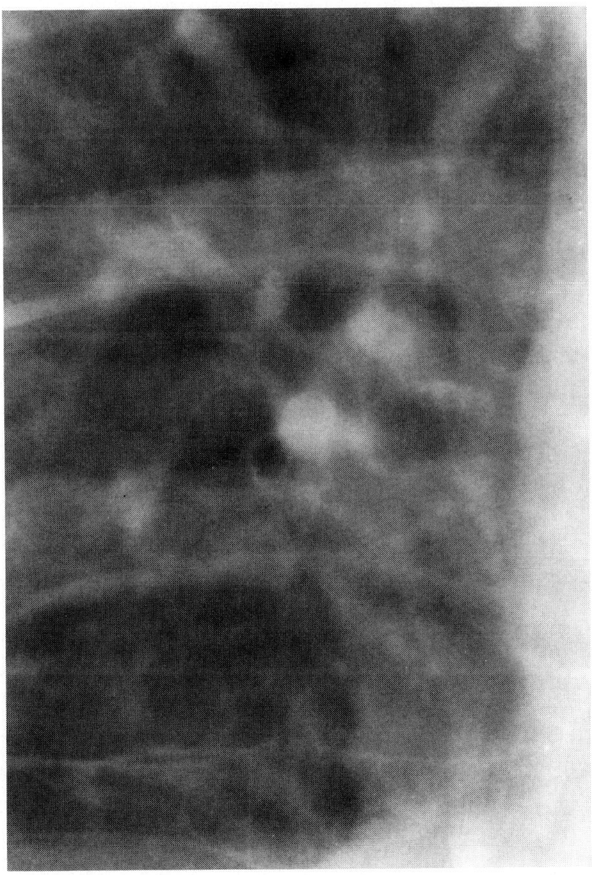

B

A number of technical factors affect the VPW, including magnification of the superior mediastinum on AP projection portable images, supine versus upright positioning, patient obliquity, and decreased lung volumes. These factors frequently compound the interpretation of portable radiographs in patients with edema and limit the utility of absolute measurements (5,7).

B. Pulmonary Circulation

Alterations of the pulmonary circulation also occur with hydrostatic edema. In the normal upright human there is an increasing gradient of lung perfusion and blood flow due to gravitational influences on the low-pressure, low-resistance pulmonary vascular bed (20,21). Reserve vessels in the upper lung zones that are normally hypoperfused can be recruited under certain physiologic conditions,

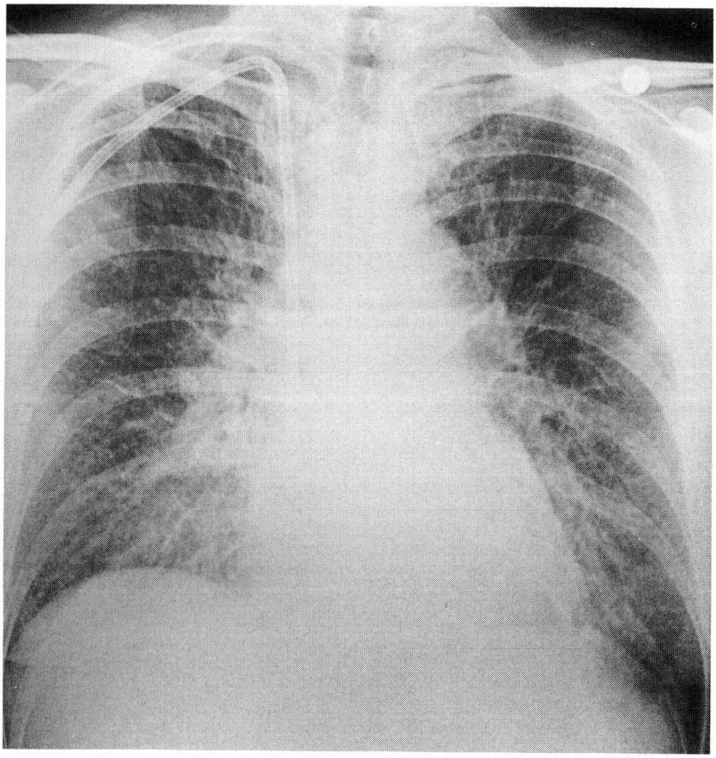

Figure 6 Interstitial edema secondary to intravascular volume overload: 54-year-old female with breast carcinoma, presenting with progressive dyspnea following aggressive fluid hydration and chemotherapy. AP radiograph shows perihilar haze, peribronchial cuffing, vascular obscuration, and interlobular septal thickening.

resulting in the phenomenon of increased flow to the upper lobes, or vascular congestion. Pulmonary vascular congestion is a spectrum ranging from equalization of flow to frank vascular redistribution, in which the size and number of upper lobes vessels exceed that of the lower lobe (22). In cardiogenic edema, vascular redistribution occurs within the context of pulmonary venous hypertension (PVH) (23). Although correlation with absolute pressure measurements is variable, PVH normally occurs when the mean pulmonary artery occlusion pressure exceeds 15 mm Hg (24–26).

Vascular redistribution is often a subjective observation based on the size differential between the apical and basal pulmonary vessels (24,27,28); however, the pulmonary artery-to-bronchus ratio (ABR) and the relationships between

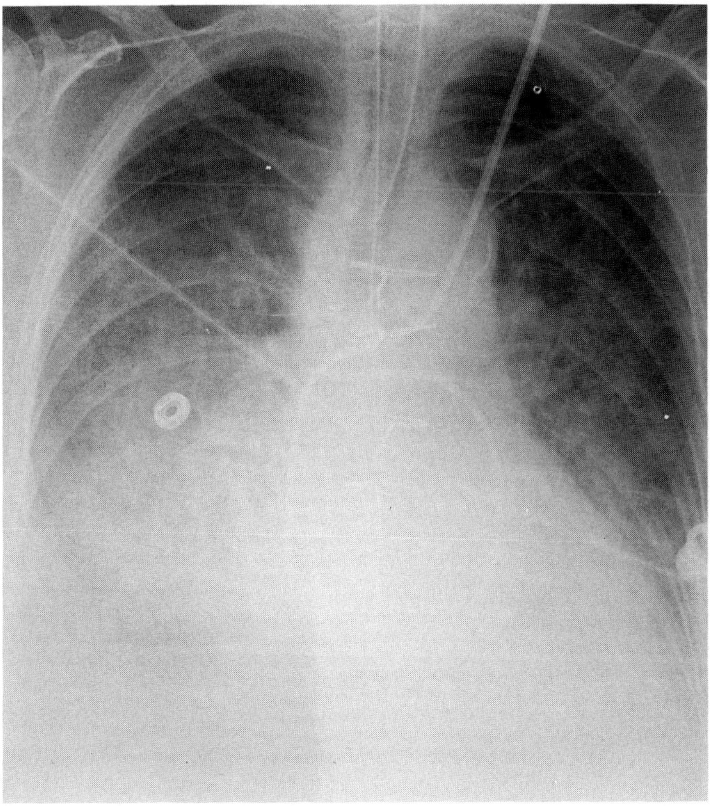

Figure 7 Cardiogenic airspace consolidation: 79-year-old female status postaortic valve replacement. A postoperative AP radiograph demonstrates pulmonary vascular congestion with interstitial and airspace edema. The airspace consolidation is greatest in the perihilar and basilar regions. Bilateral pleural effusions are also present.

upper lobe and lower lobe ratios have been used to discriminate between normal subjects, patients with cardiogenic edema, and patients with conditions of intravascular volume overload (29) (Fig. 5). In erect, normal subjects, the upper lobe ABR is smaller than the lower lobe ABR (mean values 0.85 ± 0.15 and 1.34 ± 0.25, respectively). In patients with intravascular volume overload there is balanced overcirculation of both the upper and lower lobes (ABR mean values 1.62 ± 0.31 and 1.56 ± 0.28, respectively). Finally, patients with left ventricular failure exhibit an inverted blood flow pattern with upper lobe ABRs greater than lower lobe ABRs (mean 1.50 ± 0.25 and 0.87 ± 0.20). Due to the influences of gravity on blood flow, supine radiographs are somewhat less useful in discriminating between the various types of hydrostatic edema (29).

C. Patterns of Edema

As the pulmonary intravascular capacity is exceeded, interstitial pulmonary edema results (Fig. 6). Fluid first accumulates within the peribronchovascular connective tissues, producing radiographic peribronchial cuffing and vascular obscuration (2,30,31). With further fluid accumulation, interlobular septal thick-

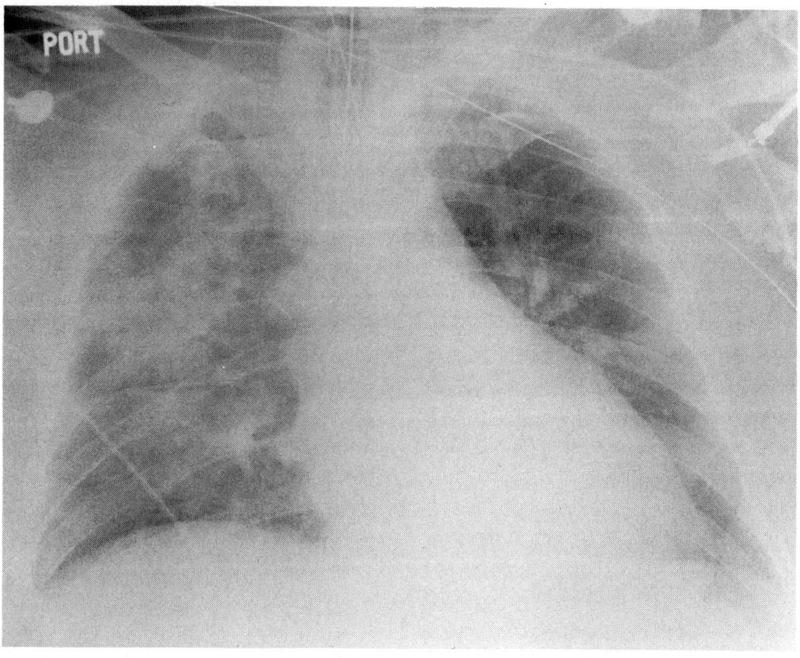

Figure 8 Asymmetric pulmonary edema: 58-year-old male with acute myocardial infarction, left ventricular failure, and mitral regurgitation. AP radiograph shows asymmetric airspace consolidation predominating in the right upper lobe.

ening becomes evident in the form of short horizontal lines in the lateral, subpleural lung bases (so-called Kerley's B-lines) (30,32). Interlobular septal thickening may also appear as 3 to 4 cm long lines radiating from the hila to the mid and upper lung zones (Kerley's A-lines). As interstitial edema progresses, the hilar vessels can be obscured by subtle increased opacification known as perihilar haze (28,32,33). Interstitial edema frequently occurs with elevated left atrial pressures between 19 and 25 mmHg (24). Interstitial fluid can accumulate within the subpleural connective tissue in communication with the interlobular septa, resulting in the appearance of fissural thickening or effusion (28,32).

Airspace consolidation will result once the interstitial compartments have been overwhelmed (Fig. 7). The distribution is most commonly bilateral within the perihilar and basilar regions, although asymmetry is not unusual due to the gravitational effects of patient positioning. Similarly, variability in the capillary bed resulting from underlying emphysema, interstitial fibrosis, or pulmonary vascular disease may give rise to markedly asymmetric patterns. A distinctive pattern of preferential right upper lobe edema has been described within the context of severe acute or chronic mitral regurgitation (34–36). In this instance, the asymmetric distribution of edema presumably relates to the more direct orientation of the right superior pulmonary veins with respect to the increased

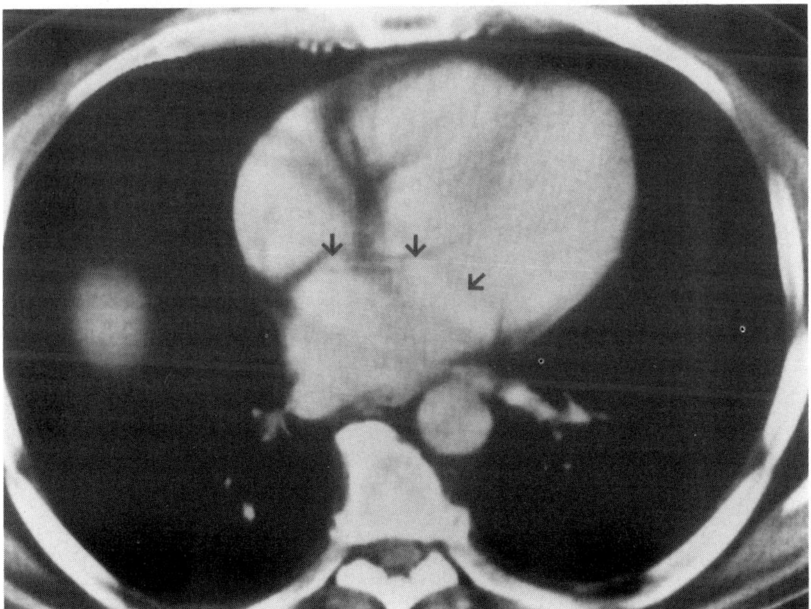

Figure 9 Left atrial enlargement: 64-year-old male evaluated for mediastinal mass. Contrast-enhanced chest CT shows left atrial enlargement (↑) in cross section.

regurgitant blood volume within the left atrium (Fig. 8). Airspace edema usually correlates roughly with left atrial pressures greater than 25 mmHg (24).

D. Associated Findings in Cardiogenic Edema

Previous studies have documented a relationship between pleural effusions and left heart failure (3,37,38). The pleura is a major route for the resolution of pulmonary edema; in experimental studies of intravascular volume overload, 40% to 50% of lung edema enters the pleural space. The presence of pleural effusion is strongly associated with elevated left atrial pressures and the degree of pulmonary edema. It has been suggested that a critical threshold of left atrial hypertension may be necessary for the formation of effusions (38).

Signs of right heart failure are also common in patients with left ventricular failure. Distension of the azygous vein beyond 1 cm is considered abnormal and has been correlated with elevated right atrial pressures, right ventricular failure, and intravascular overload (39–41). Chest wall soft tissue edema may

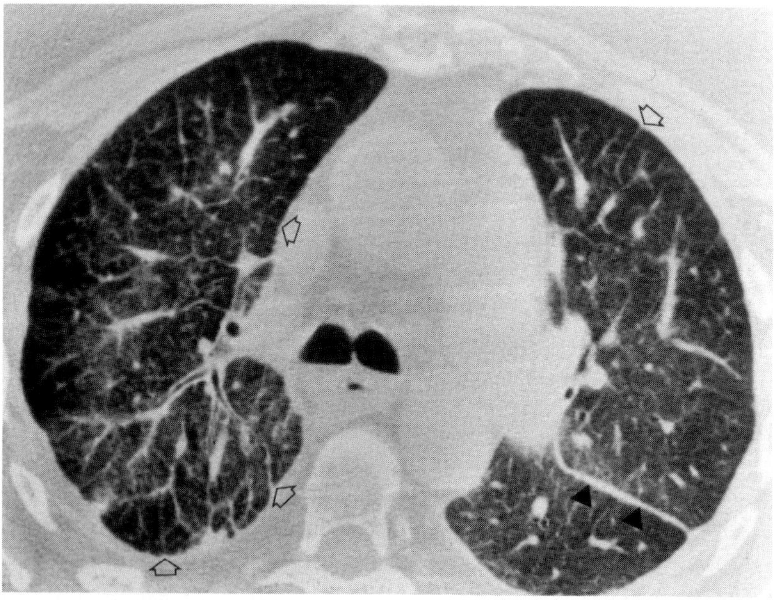

A

Figure 10 Interstitial hydrostatic edema on CT: 62-year-old female with coronary artery disease and interstitial edema. (A) HRCT demonstrates interlobular septal thickening (⇧) and fissural thickening (▲). There is increased lung attenuation (ground glass) in a predominantly centrilobular distribution. (B) On a lower cross section, peribronchial cuffing (⇧), centrilobular nodularity (▲), and reticulation are visible.

also suggest excessive extravascular third spacing of fluid from right heart disease or volume overload and is usually best appreciated by comparison of serial exams.

E. Computed Tomography in Hydrostatic Edema

Although CT imaging is not usually necessary to establish the diagnosis of cardiogenic pulmonary edema, familiarity with CT appearances is sometimes important to distinguish edema from other cardiopulmonary processes. The CT features of hydrostatic edema parallel those described on chest radiography. Overall cardiac size may be enlarged, although with CT the cross-sectional perspective facilitates the assessment of specific chamber enlargement (Fig. 9). Pulmonary vascular congestion usually effects arterial and venous enlargement in both cephalocaudal and anteroposterior directions, with enlargement of nondependent vessels analogous to cephalization on upright chest radiographs (12,13). There is also often a visible increase in the number of small centrilobular vessels, which in the lung periphery appear as centrilobular prominence (2,12).

Interstitial edema is evidenced by peribronchovascular, interlobular septal, and fissural thickening (Fig. 10) (12,42). Interstitial prominence should be

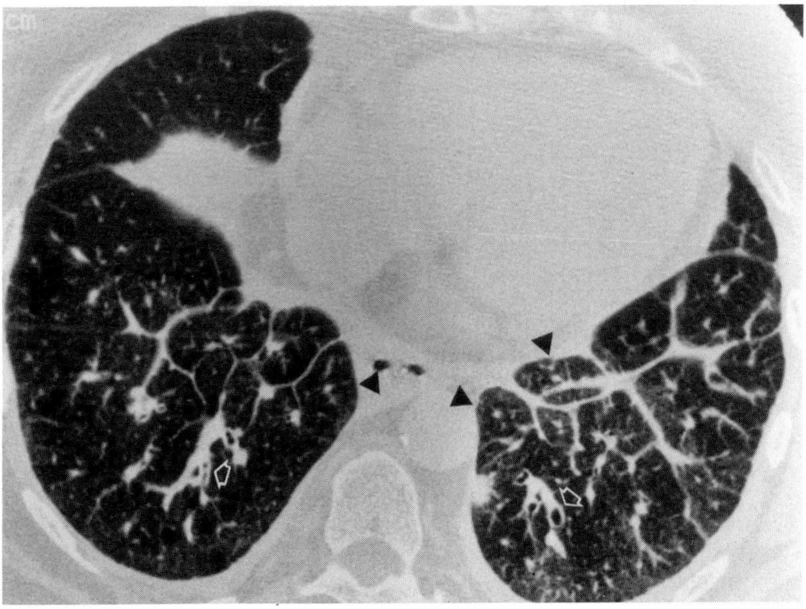

B

smooth and regular with occasional nodularity related to prominent septal veins, in contrast to lymphangitic carcinomatosis in which there is typically nodular interstitial thickening. In one study of experimental hydrostatic edema, septal thickening did not demonstrate a gravitational distribution (12). As edema progresses, patchy geographic or diffuse ground-glass opacification can appear, often showing gravitational dependence; this has been ascribed to minimal pulmonary interstitial thickening, intra-alveolar fluid layering, and increased

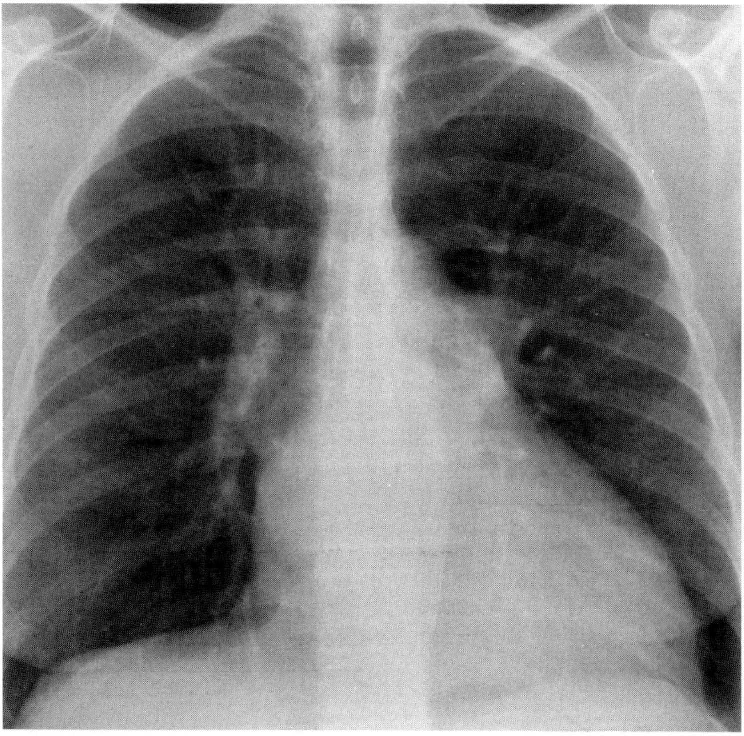

A

Figure 11 Patterns of vascular redistribution in hydrostatic edema. (A) Cephalization of pulmonary vasculature: 48-year-old female with congestive heart failure. PA radiograph shows cardiomegaly and pulmonary vascular cephalization, reflecting pulmonary venous hypertension. (B) Balanced engorgement of pulmonary vasculature: 63-year-old female with chronic renal failure. PA radiograph shows a balanced distribution of pulmonary flow with vascular engorgement of both upper and lower lobe vessels. Note the enlarged vascular pedicle width, typical of patients with an increase in circulating blood volume.

dependent perfusion (12,43). Prior CT densitometry studies have shown increased lung attenuation in hydrostatic edema, often within the central, peribronchovascular (2), and dependent portions of the lungs (44,45). Although the mechanism for the perihilar distribution is not completely understood, some investigators have postulated that this is due to mediastinal congestion and a rise in pressure, blocking liquid clearance into the mediastinum by the peribronchovascular connective tissues (4).

F. Radiographic Distinction of Hydrostatic Edemas

As stated previously, hydrostatic edema encompasses both cardiogenic and renal or intravascular volume overload states. Differences in the individual features described above may suggest one pathogenic mechanism over another, although these changes often overlap, particularly with supine portable radiography. Cardiogenic edema is classically accompanied by vascular redistribution, while in renal/overhydration edema there is balanced vascular engorgement (Fig. 11)

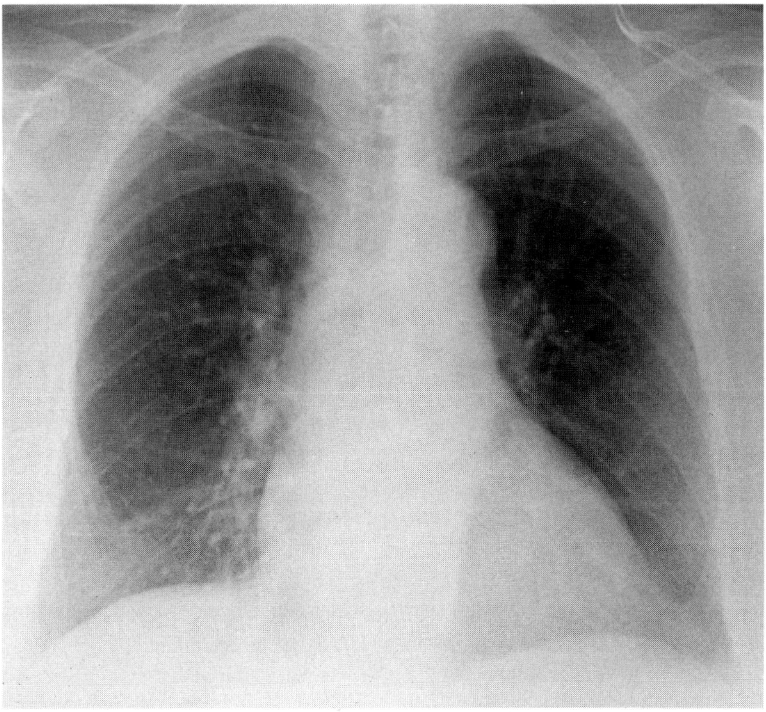

B

(3,27). Similarly, the distribution of edema in patients with cardiac edema is often basilar and roughly homogeneous along an arbitrary horizontal axis. In contrast, renal/overhydration edema has been associated with a classic "bat wing" perihilar distribution (46) (Fig. 12). Greater overlap in patterns has been described with respect to vascular pedicle width and pulmonary blood flow volume, both of which are normal or increased in cardiogenic edema (3) and typically increased in renal edema. The remaining features such as heart size, septal lines (reticulation), peribronchial cuffing, air bronchograms, and pleural effusions have not been found to distinguish the two principal types of hydrostatic edema.

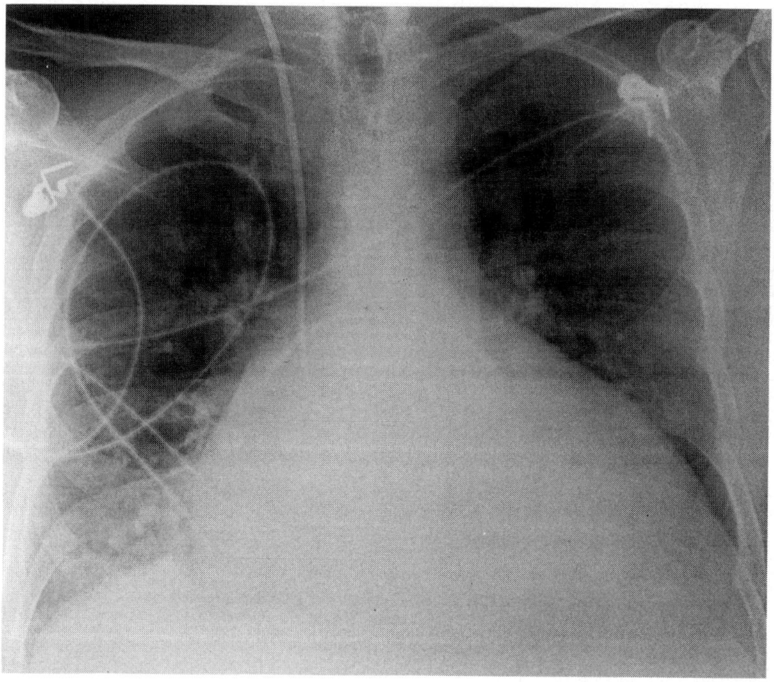

A

Figure 12 Patterns of hydrostatic pulmonary edema. (A) Airspace consolidation in severe cardiogenic edema: 65-year-old male with ischemic cardiomyopathy. AP radiograph illustrates marked cardiomegaly, pulmonary vascular redistribution, interstitial edema, and perihilar/basilar airspace edema. (B) Renal/overhydration airspace consolidation: 36-year-old male with chronic renal failure. PA radiograph shows a classic "butterfly" distribution of airspace edema.

III. Increased-Permeability Edema

Increased-permeability or lung injury edema results from numerous etiologies that share a common final pathway of pulmonary microvascular and alveolar epithelial injury. A reliable, though usually experimental, test of increased permeability edema is the finding of a high ratio of pulmonary edema to plasma protein concentration, typically exceeding 0.75, compared to a ratio of less than 0.60 for hydrostatic edema (47). The edema fluid must be sampled within the first several minutes of development because alveolar liquid clearance occurs rapidly, regardless of etiology, and results in misleading concentration of the edema fluid protein.

ARDS is a frequent clinical expression of increased capillary permeability edema and is incited by a variety of pulmonary and nonpulmonary insults. Although increased capillary permeability edema is the physiologic expression of diffuse lung injury, ARDS is operationally defined by refractory hypoxemia, decreased lung compliance resulting from diffuse microatelectasis, and the presence of diffuse parenchymal infiltrates. The pulmonary arterial occlusion

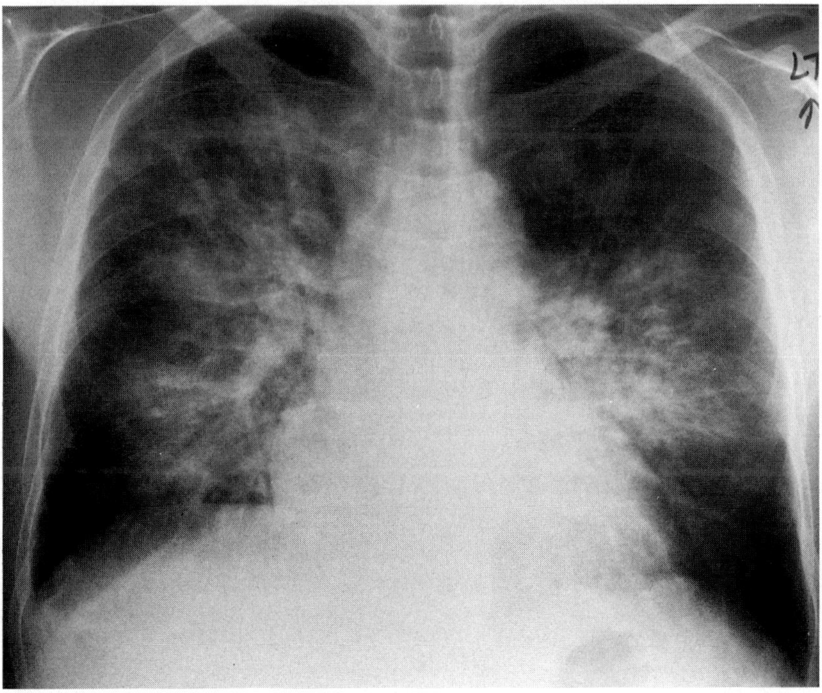

B

pressure is classically normal, although pulmonary artery pressure measurements are not a prerequisite for the diagnosis of ARDS. Some transient states of increased-permeability edema exist, and will be briefly addressed below. The chest radiographic features of increased permeability edema are best understood within the context of three stages (48,49), each of which corresponds to a distinct pathologic stage in the evolution of lung injury.

Stage I, or radiographically latent capillary leak edema, occurs during the first several hours after the inciting insult, usually before the initiation of mechanical ventilation. Although evidence of the inciting event such as aspiration may be seen, radiographs are often normal or reveal relatively subtle abnormalities (6,48). Prior to the initiation of positive pressure ventilation, lung volumes may be decreased, reflecting diffuse microatelectasis. The microatelectasis may relate to abnormalities of surfactant and the promotion of decreased lung compliance (49). Since only a small amount of extravascular lung water is present, subtle peribronchovascular obscuration or ground-glass opacification may be present (Fig. 13).

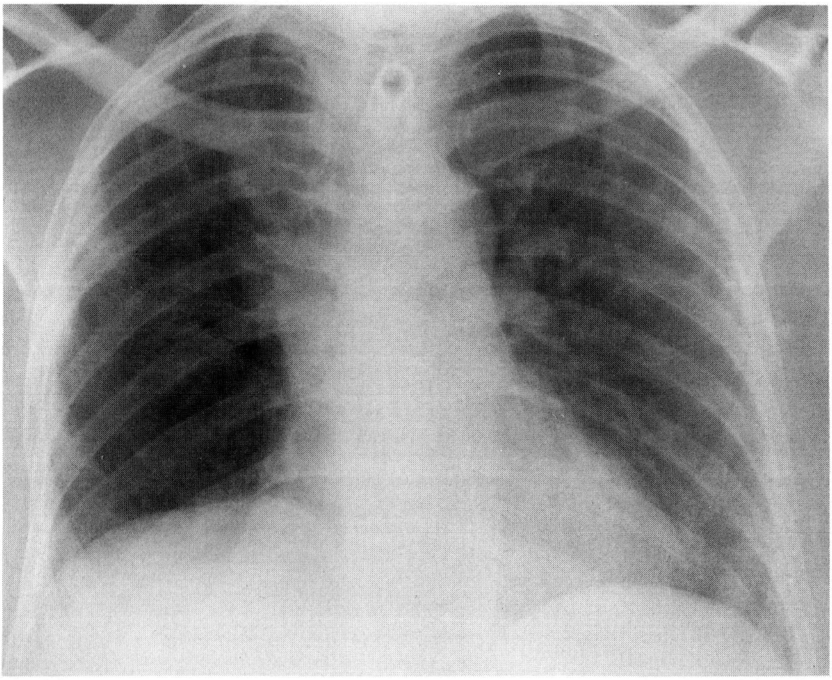

Figure 13 ARDS, Stage I: 48-year-old female with postoperative sepsis. AP radiograph shows decreased lung volumes with patchy areas of ground-glass opacification, somewhat more conspicuous in the left lung.

Within 24 hours of diffuse lung injury, stage II acute ARDS is seen (47). At this stage, the accumulation of increased extravascular water across the injured capillary endothelial-alveolar epithelial membrane culminates in the typical radiographic feature of diffuse airspace opacification. The radiographic features of this stage are probably the easiest to differentiate from those of hydrostatic edema. The airspace opacification is usually bilateral, multifocal, and peripheral (3,6,49), although marked asymmetry has been reported (Fig. 14). In patients without antecedent cardiopulmonary disease and in the absence of vigorous intravascular fluid administration, both cardiac size and vascular pedicle width should be normal (3,5). Similarly, pulmonary blood volume is normal and the distribution of pulmonary blood flow is usually normal or balanced (3). In contrast to hydrostatic edema, in which interstitial edema patterns are conspicuous, air bronchograms are very common in increased permeability edema, presumably because of diffuse microatelectasis and the direct leakage of intravascular fluid into the airspace across the injured capillary endothelial-alveolar epithelial membrane. Pleural effusions occur but are usually not a conspicuous feature of pure increased permeability edema (5,13,37). Animal studies have

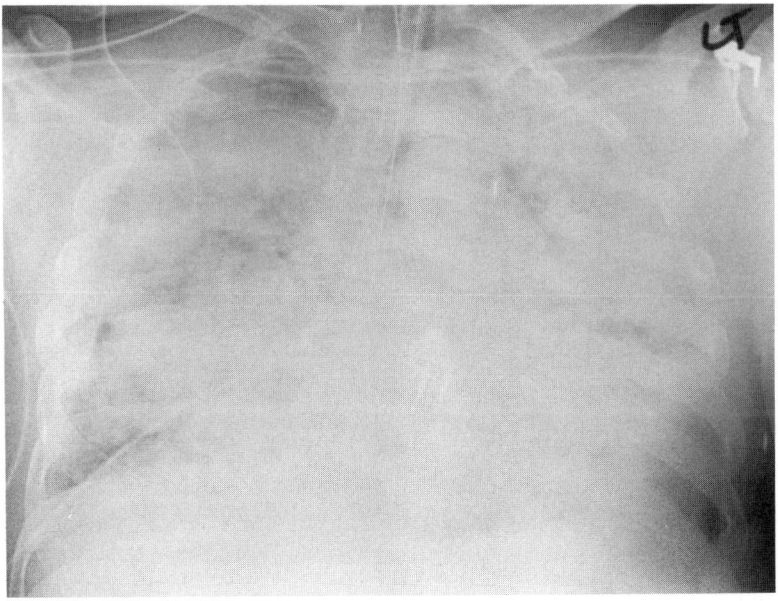

Figure 14 ARDS, Stage II: 26-year-old male with sepsis. AP radiograph shows severe diffuse, bilateral airspace consolidation with conspicuous air bronchograms. A right pleural effusion is visible along the right lateral costal margin.

shown that the effusions are exudative and form when a critical threshold of edema is reached by removal through the pleural space (37).

In situ thrombosis of the pulmonary arterial vasculature is a consistent feature in severe ARDS. Bedside balloon occlusion pulmonary angiography has confirmed the presence of intraluminal filling defects, the absence of filling of small arterial side branches, and altered microvascular background opacification (50–52). Significant vascular insult is usually expressed as elevated pulmonary arterial pressure and pulmonary vascular resistance and correlates with a high mortality rate. Experimental trials with fibrinolytic infusions have resulted in reperfusion at sites of occlusion, but fibrinolytic therapy is rarely clinically initiated because so many of these patients experience severe thrombocytopenia or have other contraindications to fibrinolytic therapy (53).

Stage III chronic ARDS usually occurs at some point during the first 3 to 7 days following injury (49). At this stage, permeability edema partially sub-

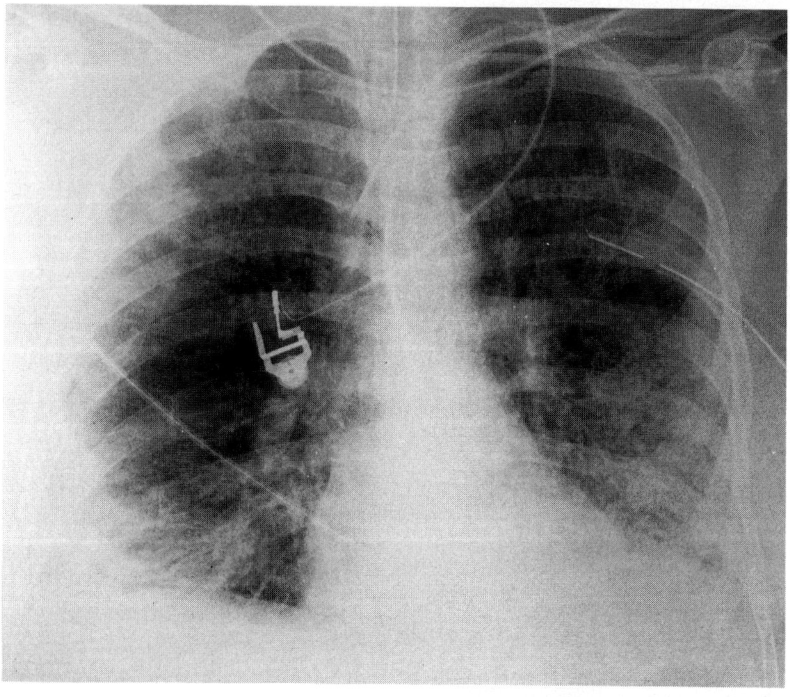

Figure 15 ARDS, Stage III: 50-year-old female with gram-negative bacterial sepsis resulting from small-bowel obstruction. AP radiograph demonstrates diffuse interstitial and ground-glass opacifications, more coalescent in the lung periphery. In chronic ARDS, parenchymal consolidation often becomes less confluent.

sides. Histologically, there is hyperplasia of type II pneumocytes, fibroblast infiltration, and the deposition of connective tissue (48). Ongoing physiologic impairment results from decreased lung compliance, diffusion impairment, destruction of the microvascular bed, and continued ventilation-perfusion imbalance. Radiographs at this stage demonstrate less confluent airspace consolidation with the development of ground-glass and interstitial opacifications (6,48,49) (Fig. 15). Moreover, areas of peripheral lucency may develop, often in those regions that were initially the most consolidated (Fig. 16). Pathologic correlations suggest that these lucent regions correspond to ischemic infarction distal to sites of pulmonary vascular occlusion. In patients maintained on high positive pressure ventilation, the ischemic zones are highly compliant and may become

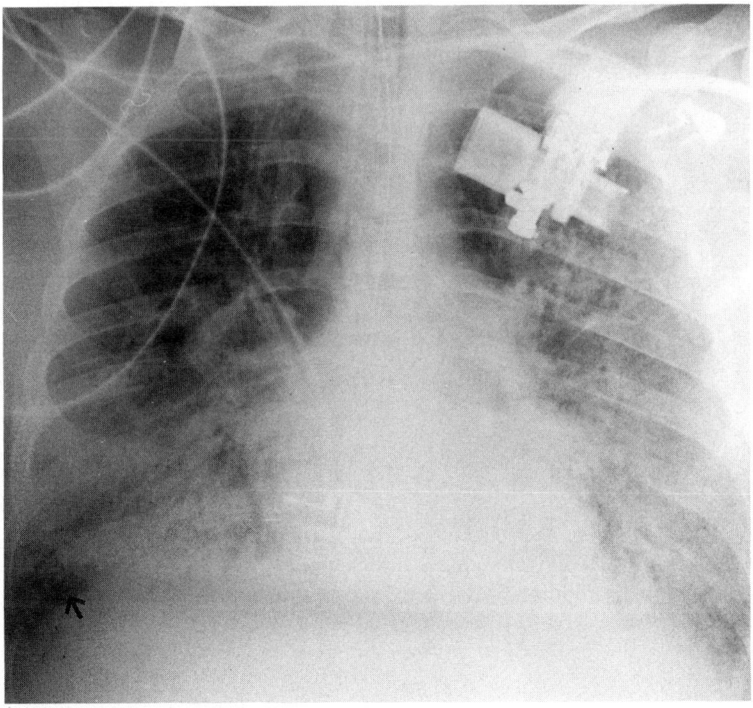

Figure 16 ARDS with air cyst formation: 27-year-old female on prolonged mechanical ventilation. AP radiograph shows patchy, asymmetric interstitial and airspace opacifications with a localized air cyst in the right costophrenic sulcus (↑). Under the influence of positive pressure ventilation, these cysts may rupture, contributing to the frequent barotraumatic complications in patients with diffuse lung injury.

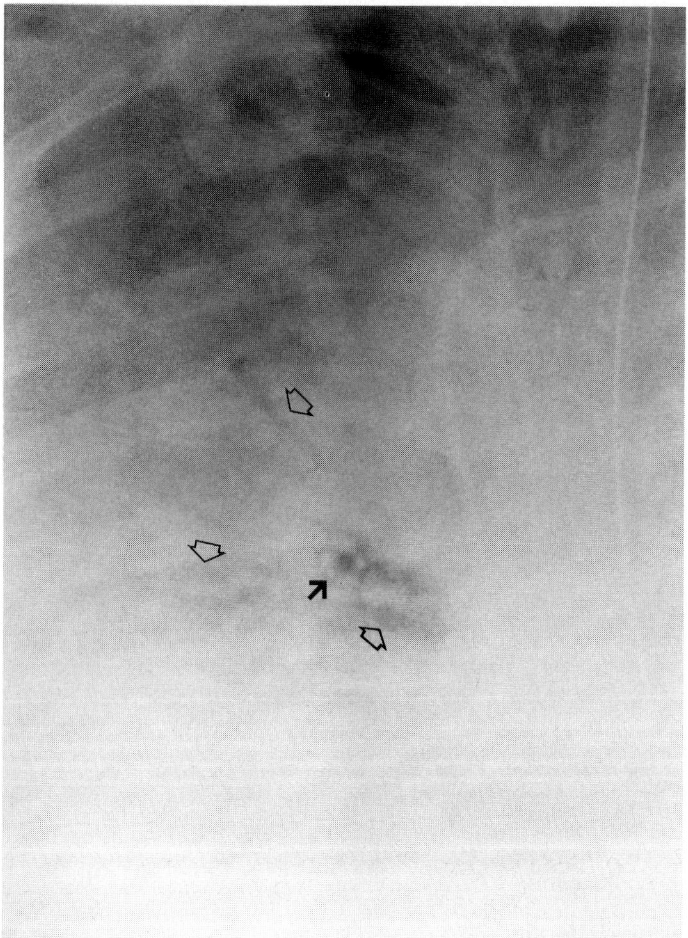

Figure 17 Pulmonary interstitial emphysema: 21-year-old female involved in a severe motor vehicle accident. Magnification view of right lung base illustrates lucent peribronchial halo (↑) with peribronchovascular extension (⇦), appearing as lucent, nontapering tram lines.

frank cysts that contribute to dead-space ventilation and barotraumatic complications.

Positive pressure ventilation and increased intra-alveolar pressure place patients with diffuse lung injury at substantial risk of barotrauma. Pulmonary interstitial emphysema is probably the initial event in most situations of extralveolar air, and occurs by rupture of alveolar walls and the dissection of air along the peribronchovascular sheaths and interlobular septa (Fig. 17) (54–56). Although often very difficult to identify, the earliest evidence of pulmonary interstitial emphysema is an increase in tissue contrast within the consolidated lung called parenchymal stippling, which renders a "salt-and-pepper" appearance to consolidations that were previously a uniform gray. The dissection of interstitial air along the more central bronchovascular bundles results in perihilar lucent streaking or, when visualized end-on, in perivascular lucent halos. Discrete air-filled cysts can occur in either intraparenchymal or subpleural locations. The size of the subpleural space enables these cysts to enlarge dramatically, leading to rupture or the development of large air collections that simulate pneumothorax (49). Pneumomediastinum, pneumothorax, and soft tissue air within the chest wall are also frequent complications of barotrauma in these patients.

A. Computed Tomography of Increased-Permeability Edema

Computed tomography (CT) has provided insights into the patterns and distribution of parenchymal consolidation in ARDS, in some instances differing from patterns suggested on projectional chest radiography. CT has helped to confirm the patchy, nonuniform patterns of consolidation in patients with diffuse lung injury. Based on observations from a number of small studies, chest radiographically latent (Stage I) ARDS may show ground-glass opacification on CT. As the disease evolves, Stage II acute ARDS demonstrates patchy, peripheral

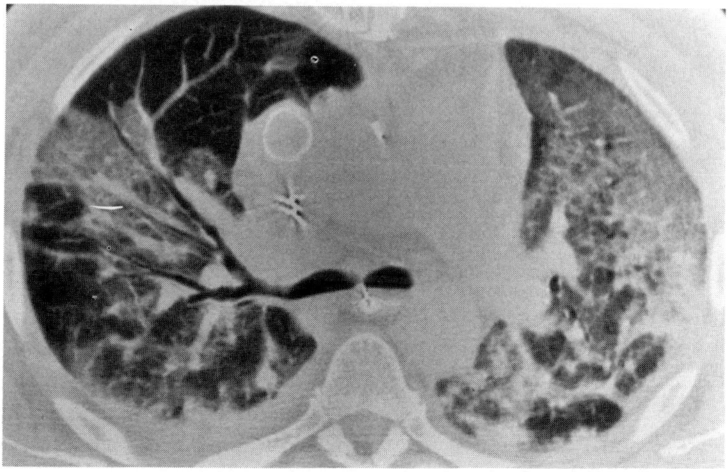

Figure 18 ARDS, Stage II: 59-year-old male with mediastinitis, status postmedian sternotomy for coronary artery bypass graft surgery and SVC graft placement. Chest CT demonstrates asymmetric ground-glass and dense airspace opacifications.

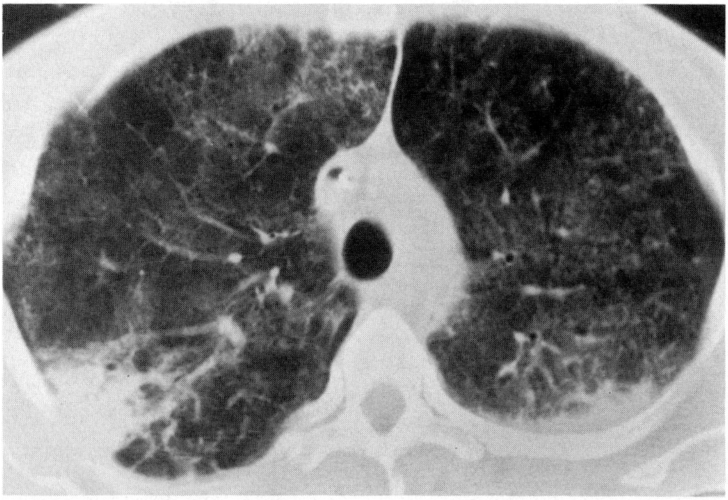

A

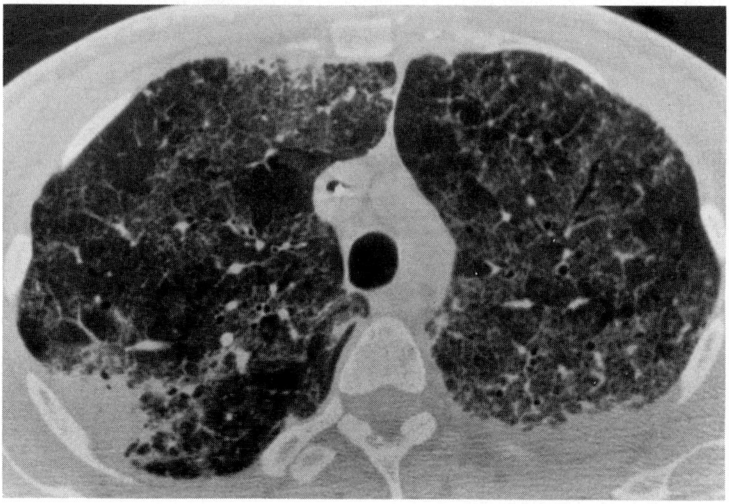

B

ground-glass or dense airspace opacification with air bronchograms (Fig. 18). The greatest consolidations tend to involve the dependent lung and have been observed to rapidly shift in distribution with patient repositioning, such that the previously less affected lung becomes densely consolidated while lung regions that were initially dependent and most consolidated become better aerated (Fig. 19) (6,57–59). Recent studies have shown that these positional shifts in consolidation occur within minutes and likely represent shifting atelectasis due to

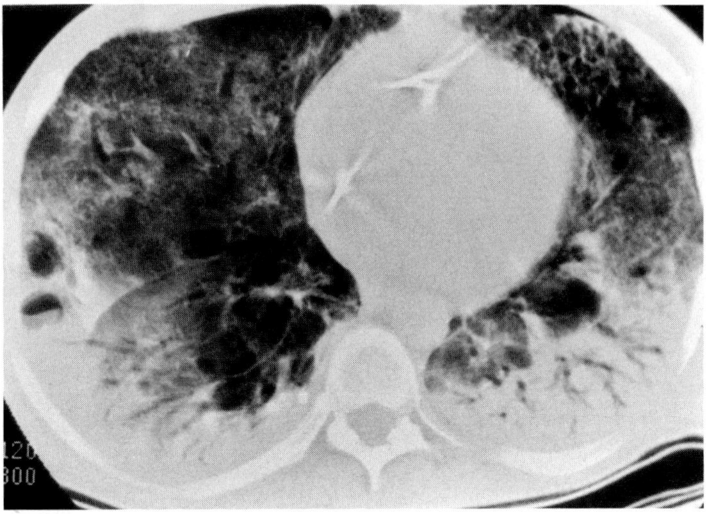

C

Figure 19 ARDS, Stage III: 50-year-old female with sepsis syndrome. (A) Conventional CT image shows asymmetric ground glass, airspace, and interstitial opacifications. (B) High-resolution CT image (1 mm thickness) at the same level better demonstrates the underlying interstitial disease as manifested by intralobular and interlobular septal thickening. Intralobular prominence appears as a fine reticular pattern, superimposed upon the larger reticular pattern of secondary lobules that results from interlobular septal prominence. (C) On lower CT images a definite, gravity-dependent distribution of dense airspace consolidation is evident, representing atelectasis of the edematous, noncompliant lung.

gravitational influences on the edematous, surfactant-deficient lung rather than the migration of pulmonary edema fluid. Pulmonary vascular dilatation and interlobular septal thickening are not prominent features of diffuse lung injury on CT.

In Stage III chronic ARDS, overall lung attenuation decreases. There is often clearance of the densest areas of opacification on CT (49). With further progression, parenchymal fibrosis results in irregular reticulation and distortion of the bronchovascular interstitial architecture. Eventual changes of prolonged ventilation and barotrauma are seen (Fig. 20). On CT, pleural effusions are much more commonly observed, and have been reported in up to 50% of patients in one series—bilateral in 28% or unilateral in 22% (13,37). Although the effusions are generally small to moderate, they are more frequent than has been appreciated on projectional radiography.

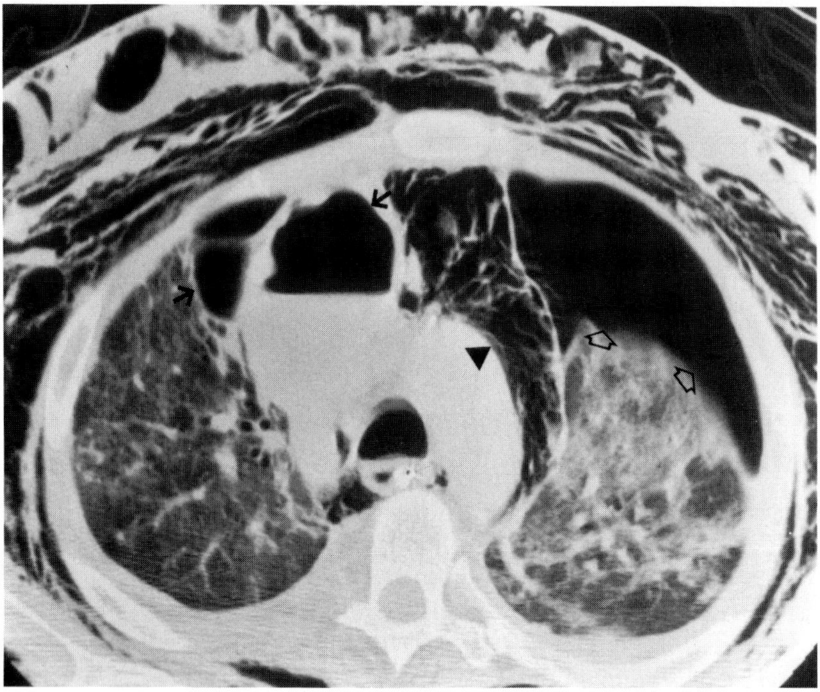

Figure 20 Barotraumatic complications of ARDS: 47-year-old male with polymicrobial sepsis. Chest CT shows multiple peripheral pneumatoceles (↑). These cysts can enlarge under the influence positive pressure ventilation, giving rise to pneumothorax (⌂), pneumomediastinum (▲), and extensive subcutaneous emphysema.

IV. Acute Postobstructive, High-Altitude, and Neurogenic Edemas

Despite recent advances and ongoing investigations, the mechanisms of postobstructive, high-altitude and neurogenic pulmonary edemas remain incompletely understood (as discussed in Chaps. 10 and 11). It is beyond the scope of this chapter to review the evidence supporting their respective pathophysiologic bases; however, their radiographic manifestations support a combination of both hydrostatic and increased permeability mechanisms. Without clinical correlation, the radiographic picture may pose confusion and difficulty in interpretation.

Acute upper airway obstruction has been associated with pulmonary edema in a variety of clinical contexts, including anesthesia, postextubation laryngospasm (60), epiglottitis (61), spasmodic croup (61), laryngotracheobronchitis (62), strangulation (28), and as part of some drownings due to laryngospasm. The radiographic appearance of acute postobstructive edema is indistinguishable from other forms of pulmonary edema, but can be suggested within the appropriate clinical context.

High-altitude pulmonary edema is a severe form of altitude sickness that generally occurs within 6 to 48 hours of ascent beyond 2500 to 4000 m. The incidence and severity of high-altitude pulmonary edema vary according to several factors, including the altitude achieved, the speed of ascent, the ambient temperature, the age of the individual, the level of physical exertion, and the individual susceptibility of the person (30). It has been described predominantly in young adults, but is known to affect sedentary, elderly individuals as well (63). Although the pathophysiology is still speculative, certain physiologic conditions are invariably present. Alveolar hypoxia is a constant finding, typically in association with relative hypoventilation, increased pulmonary vascular resistance, and pulmonary arterial hypertension (30,63,64). Alterations of the microvascular endothelium, possibly as a direct effect of hypoxia or by the release of inflammatory mediators, has also been postulated. The end result is the development of pulmonary edema having hydrostatic and increased permeability characteristics (see Chap. 11 for further discussion).

High-altitude pulmonary edema demonstrates radiographic changes similar to other forms of pulmonary edema (30), although certain observations have been described. Cardiac size remains normal, despite increasing prominence of the main pulmonary arteries (63,65) and frequent pulmonary vascular prominence (63). Pulmonary edema is manifest as multifocal, patchy parenchymal consolidations, often showing a right middle lobe predominance. The right middle lobe preference has been postulated to result from its decreased collateral ventilation, which may predispose the lobe to an accentuated pulmonary vascular response to hypoxia and higher perfusing pressures (30,64).

Neurogenic pulmonary edema occurs within the context of a variety of insults to the central nervous system (CNS) that appear to have in common a rise in intracranial pressure. Neurogenic edema can present acutely, within minutes or hours following CNS injury, or insidiously, over several days following injury (66) (see Chap. 10). Neurogenic edema demonstrates similar radiographic findings to both hydrostatic and increased permeability edemas (30,66,67) (Fig. 21). Parenchymal consolidations are often bilateral with air bronchograms; cardiac size is generally normal (30).

V. Radiographic Distinction of Pulmonary Edema

Despite best attempts to categorize radiographic findings into hydrostatic and increased permeability types, these distinctions are often subtle, if not impossible

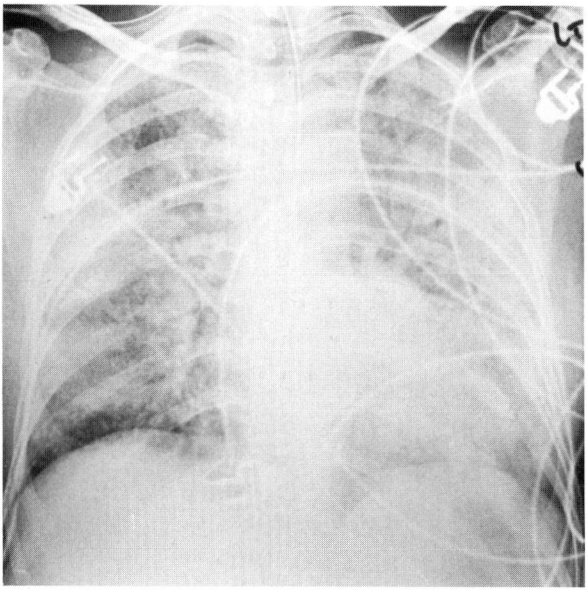

A

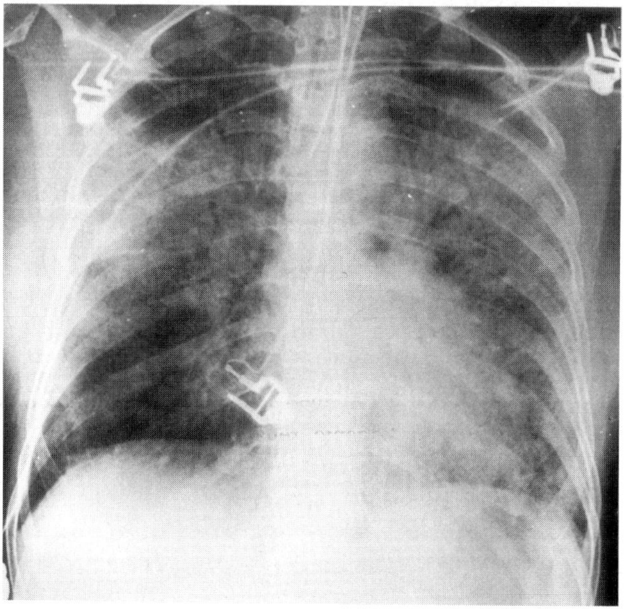

B

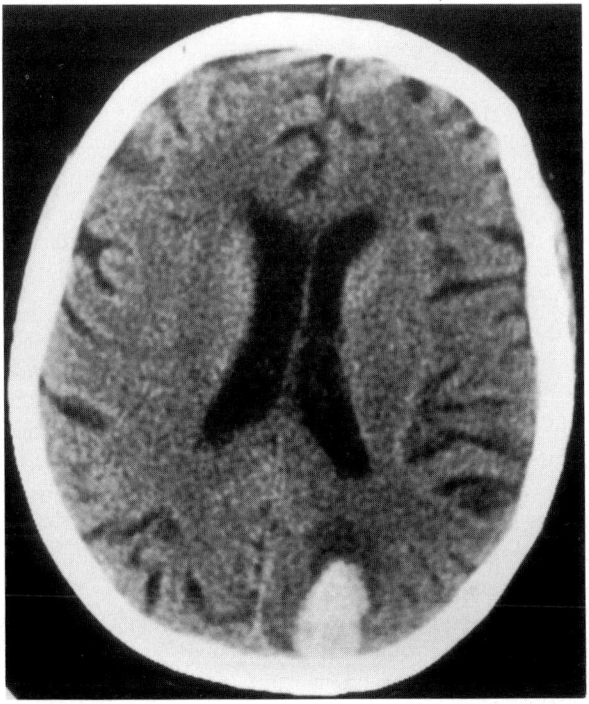

C

Figure 21 Neurogenic pulmonary edema: 45-year-old female intracranial hemorrhage. (A) Initial AP chest radiograph demonstrates diffuse asymmetric peripheral alveolar consolidation with normal cardiac size and vascular pedicle width. (B) Postintracranial hemorrhage radiograph obtained approximately 9 hours later shows marked improvement. (C) Noncontrast head CT documents focal hemorrhage within the left occipital lobe.

to make from isolated images. The accuracy of chest radiographs in distinguishing specific categories of pulmonary edema has been addressed in several studies and has been the subject of lively debates. Perhaps the best-known studies are those of Milne and colleagues (3), who classified the pattern of pulmonary edema of 119 patients into cardiogenic, renal/overhydration, and increased permeability types. An overall accuracy between 86% and 89% was reported. The authors found that the three most significant radiographic signs to distinguish edema type were the distribution of pulmonary blood flow, distribution of pulmonary edema, and vascular pedicle width. Less effective diagnostic criteria were pulmonary blood volume; the presence of septal lines, peribronchial cuffs, and air bronchograms; pleural effusions; and cardiac size. Miniati et al. (8) produced similar results using the radiographs from the same patient sample group and using each radiographic sign as input variables for computer-generated discriminate analysis.

Smith et al. (7) later studied 94 patients with pulmonary edema, but failed to reproduce the results of Milne et al. Although an overall accuracy of 83% was achieved in distinguishing hydrostatic and increased-permeability edemas on the basis of heart size and septal lines, no strategy could be formulated to differentiate cardiogenic from renal/overhydration and renal/overhydration from increased-permeability edema types. These investigators were unable to assess the distribution of pulmonary blood flow in 38% of patients and found little value in the measure of vascular pedicle width. Aberle et al. (5) achieved an overall accuracy of 70% in distinguishing hydrostatic versus increased-permeability edema types by applying previously published criteria. The distribution of edema was the single most discriminating criterion, being patchy and peripheral in 13% of patients with hydrostatic edema, but in 50% of patients with increased-permeability edema. Septal lines occurred in 67% of patients with hydrostatic edema and in 40% of patients with increased-permeability edema. As with Smith et al. (7), the distribution of pulmonary blood flow and vascular pedicle width were not useful radiographic distinctions, although enlarged cardiac size was more common in hydrostatic edema.

Although the radiographic distinctions between different edema types have been proposed, clinical information is incontrovertibly critical to diagnostic accuracy and to aid in the management of these critically ill patients. This is particularly true when findings traditionally associated with cardiogenic edema such as pleural effusions or septal lines and peribronchial cuffs reflecting interstitial edema are observed in patients with increased-permeability edema. Bedside portable radiography must often be performed with patients in supine or semi-recumbent positions, and at varying levels of inspiration, which limits the utility of many of the chest radiographic features of edemas. Furthermore, radiographic distinctions are often impossible in patients with underlying cardiopulmonary disease or when both hydrostatic and increased-permeability edema coexist.

References

1. Sibbald WJ, Cunningham DR, Chin DN. Noncardiac or cardiac pulmonary edema? a practical approach to clinical differentiation in critically ill patients. Chest 1983; 84:452–461.
2. Forster BB, Müller NL, Mayo JR, Okazawa M, Wiggs BJ, Paré PD. High-resolution computed tomography of experimental hydrostatic pulmonary edema. Chest 1992; 101:1434–1437.
3. Milne ENC, Pistolesi M, Miniati M, Giuntini C. The radiologic distinction of cardiogenic and noncardiogenic edema. AJR 1985; 144:879–894.
4. Staub NC. New concepts about the pathophysiology of pulmonary edema. J Thorac Imag 1988; 3:8–14.

5. Aberle DR, Wiener-Kronish JP, Webb WR, Matthay MA. Hydrostatic versus increased permeability pulmonary edema: diagnosis based on radiographic criteria in critically ill patients. Radiology 1988; 168:73–79.
6. Wheeler AP, Carroll FE, Bernard GR. Radiographic issues in adult respiratory distress syndrome. New Horizons 1993; 1:471–477.
7. Smith RC, Mann H, Greenspan RH, Pope CF, Sostman HD. Radiographic differentiation between different etiologies of pulmonary edema. Invest Radiol 1987; 22: 859–863.
8. Miniati M, Pistolesi M, Paoletti P, et al. Objective radiographic criteria to differentiate cardiac, renal, and injury lung edema. Invest Radiol 1988; 23: 433–440.
9. Goodman LR, Putman CE. Critical Care Imaging. 3rd ed. Philadephia: W.B. Saunders, 1992:107–127.
10. Pistolesi M, Giuntini C. Assessment of extravascular lung water. Radiol Clin North Am 1978; 16:551–574.
11. Halperin BD, Feeley TW, Mihan FG, Chiles C, Gauthaner DF, Blank NE. Evaluation of the portable chest roentgenogram for quantitating extravascular lung water in critically ill adults. Chest 1985; 88:649–652.
12. Storto ML, Kee ST, Golden JA, Webb WR. Hydrostatic pulmonary edema: high-resolution CT findings. AJR 1995; 165:817–820.
13. Goodman LR. Congestive heart failure and adult respiratory distress syndrome: new insights using computed tomography. Radiol Clin North Am 1996; 34:33–46.
14. Higgins CB. Essentials of Cardiac Radiology and Imaging. 1st ed. Philadelphia: Lippincott, 1992:1–48.
15. Hoffman RB, Rigler LG. Evaluation of left ventricular enlargement in the lateral projection of the chest. Radiology 1965; 85:93–100.
16. Green CE, Kelley MJ, Higgins CB. Etiologic significance of enlargement of the left atrial appendage in adults. Radiology 1982; 142:21–27.
17. Higgins CB, Reinke RT, Jones NE, Broderick T. Left atrial dimension on the frontal thoracic radiograph: a method for assessing left atrial enlargement. AJR 1978; 130: 251–255.
18. Chen JT. Essentials of Cardiac Roentgenology. 1st ed. Boston/Toronto: Little, Brown & Company, 1987:69–83.
19. Milne ENC, Pistolesi M, Miniati M, Giuntini C. The vascular pedicle of the heart and the vena azygos. Part I. The normal subject. Radiology 1984; 152:1–8.
20. West JB. Blood flow to the lung and gas exchange. Anesthesiology 1974; 41: 124–138.
21. West JB, Dollery CT, Naimark A. Distribution of blood flow in isolated lung: relation to vascular and alveolar pressures. J Appl Physiol 1966; 21:767–777.
22. Milne ENC. Some new concepts of pulmonary blood flow and volume. Radiol Clin North Am 1978; 16:515–536.
23. Lavender JP, Doppman J, Shawdon H, et al. Pulmonary veins in left ventricular failure and mitral stenosis. Br J Radiol 1962; 35:293–302.
24. Ravin CE. Pulmonary vascularity: radiographic considerations. J Thorac Imag 1988; 3:1–13.
25. Taveras JM, Ferrucci JT. Radiology: Diagnosis, Imaging, Intervention. Vol. 1. Philadelphia: J.B. Lippincott, 1993:(71)1–15.

26. Kostuk W, Barr JW, Simon AJ, et al. Correlations between the chest film and hemodynamics in acute myocardial infarction. Circulation 1973; 48:624–632.
27. Armstrong P, Wilson AG, Dee P, Hansell DM. Imaging of Diseases of the Chest. 2nd ed. St. Louis: Mosby, 1995:15–47.
28. Lange S, Stark P. Radiology of Chest Diseases. 1st ed. Stuttgart: Thieme, 1990: 149–163.
29. Woodring JH. Pulmonary artery-bronchus ratios in patients with normal lungs, pulmonary vascular plethora, and congestive heart failure. Radiology 1991; 179: 115–122.
30. Gropper MA, Wiener-Kronish JP, Hashimoto S. Acute cardiogenic pulmonary edema. Clin Chest Med 1994; 15:501–515.
31. Conway D, Johnson R. The nature and significance of peribronchial cuffing in pulmonary edema. Radiology 1977; 125:577–582.
32. Groskin SA. Pulmonary edema and hemorrhage. In: Groskin SA, ed. Heitzman's The Lung: Radiologic Pathologic Correlations. 3rd ed. St. Louis: Mosby, 1993: 150–172.
33. Short DS. Radiology of lung in left heart failure. Br Heart J 1956; 18:233–240.
34. Gurney JW, Goodman LR. Pulmonary edema localized in the right upper lobe accompanying mitral regurgitation. Radiology 1989; 171:397–399.
35. Grenon H, Bilodeau S. Pulmonary edema of the right upper lobe associated with acute mitral regurgitation. Can Assoc Radiol J 1994; 45:97–100.
36. Schnyder PA, Sarrag AM, Duvoisin BE, Kapenberger L, Landry MJ. Pulmonary edema associated with mitral regurgitation: prevalence of predominant involvement of the right upper lobe. AJR 1993; 161:33–36.
37. Weiner-Kronish JP, Matthay MA. Pleural effusions associated with hydrostatic and increased permeability pulmonary edema. Chest 1988; 93:852–858.
38. Weiner-Kronish JP, Matthay MA, Callen PW, Filly RA, Gamsu G, Staub NC. Relationship of pleural effusions to pulmonary hemodynamics in patients with congestive heart failure. Am Rev Respir Dis 1985; 132:1253–1256.
39. Fleischner FG, Udis SW. Dilitation of the azygos vein: a roentgen sign of venous engorgement. AJR 1952; 67:569–575.
40. Heitzman ER. Radiologic appearance of the azygos vein in cardiovascular disease. Circulation 1973; 47:628–634.
41. Pistolesi M, Milne ENC, Miniati M, Giuntini C. The vascular pedicle of the heart and the vena azygos. Part II. Acquired heart disease. Radiology 1984; 152:9–17.
42. Bessis L, Callard P, Gotheil C, Biaggi A, Grenier P. High-resolution CT of parenchymal lung disease: precise correlation with histologic findings. Radiographics 1992; 12:45–58.
43. Herold CJ, Wetzel RC, Robotham JL, et al. Measurement of pulmonary parenchymal attenuation: use of spirometric gating with quantitative CT. Radiology 1990; 175:265–274.
44. Hedlund LW, Effmann EL, Bates WM, Beck JW, Goulding PL, Putman CE. Pulmonary edema: a CT study of regional changes in lung density following oleic acid injury. J Comput Assist Tomogr 1982; 6:939–946.
45. Hedlund LW, Vock P, Effmann EL, Lischko MM, Putman CE. Hydrostatic pulmonary edema. an analysis of lung density changes by computed tomography. Invest Radiol 1984; 19:254–262.

46. Hodson CJ. Pulmonary oedema and bats-wing shadows. J Fac Radiol 1950; 1: 176–186.
47. Fein A, Grossman RF, Jones JG, et al. The value of edema fluid protein measurement in patients with pulmonary edema. Am J Med 1979; 67:32–38.
48. Greene R. Adult respiratory distress syndrome: acute alveolar damage. Radiology 1987; 163:57–66.
49. Aberle DR, Brown K. Radiologic considerations in the adult respiratory distress syndrome. Clin Chest Med 1990; 11:737–754.
50. Greene R. Pulmonary vascular obstruction in the adult respiratory distress syndrome. J Thorac Imag 1986; 1:31–38.
51. Greene R, Zapol WM, Snider MT, et al. Early bedside detection of pulmonary vascular occlusion during acute respiratory failure. Am Rev Respir Dis 1981; 124:593–601.
52. Greene R, Jantsch H, Boggis C, Strauss HW, Lowenstein E. Respiratory distress syndrome with new considerations. Radiol Clin North Am 1983; 21:699–708.
53. Greene R, Lind S, Jantsch H, et al. Pulmonary vascular obstruction in severe ARDS: angiographic alterations after IV fibrinolytic therapy. AJR 1987; 148: 501–508.
54. Unger JM, England DM, Bogust GA. Interstitial emphysema in adults: recognition and prognostic implications. J Thorac Imag 1989; 4:86–94.
55. Westcott JL, Cole SR. Interstitial pulmonary emphysema in children and adults: roentgenographic features. Radiology 1974; 111:367–378.
56. Tocina I, Westcott JL. Barotrauma. Radiol Clin North Am 1996; 34:59–81.
57. Langer M, Mascheroni D, Marcolin R, et al. The prone position in ARDS patients: a clinical study. Chest 1988; 94:103–107.
58. Maunder RJ, Shuman WP, McHugh JW, et al. Preservation of normal lung regions in the adult respiratory distress syndrome: analysis by computed tomography. JAMA 1986; 255:2463–2465.
59. Stark P, Greene R, Kott MM, et al. CT findings in ARDS. Radiologe 1987; 27: 367–369.
60. Jackson FN, Rowland V, Corssen G. Laryngoplasm-induced pulmonary edema. Chest 1980; 78:819–821.
61. Travis KW, Todres ID, Shannon DC. Pulmonary edema associated with croup and epiglottitis. Pediatrics 1977; 59:695–698.
62. DeVane GG. Acute postobstructive pulmonary edema. CRNA 1995; 6:110–113.
63. Richalet JP. High altitude pulmonary oedema: still a place for controversy? Thorax 1995; 50:923–929.
64. Schoene RB. Pulmonary edema at high altitude. Clin Chest Med 1985; 6:491–507.
65. Marticorena E, Tapia FA, Dyer J. Pulmonary edema by ascending to high altitudes. Chest 1964; 45:273–283.
66. Colice GL. Neurogenic pulmonary edema. Clin Chest Med 1985; 6:473–489.
67. Simon RP. Neurogenic pulmonary edema. Neurol Clin 1993; 11:309–323.

4

Evaluation of Pulmonary Endothelial Barrier Function

Quantifying Pulmonary Edema and Lung Injury

DANIEL P. SCHUSTER

Washington University School of Medicine
St. Louis, Missouri

I. Why Evaluate Pulmonary Barrier Function?

An important function of the pulmonary endothelium is to serve as a barrier against the abnormal extravasation of fluid and solutes from the vascular compartment into the gas-exchanging airspaces of the lungs. For over a century, Starling's "hypothesis" has served as the principal paradigm of how fluid movement is controlled across the endothelial barrier. While the original hypothesis simply suggested that the hydrostatic pressures driving fluid out of capillaries were offset by the oncotic pressures generated by proteins in blood, Starling's hypothesis has subsequently been refined, expanded, and quantified mathematically in many forms (1). When modified to account for the total surface area over which filtration might occur, as well as for "lymph flow" as a term summarizing those mechanisms responsible for returning extravasated fluid to the vascular compartment, the "Starling equation" might be written as follows:

$$EVLW = (L_p * S)[(P_c - P_i) - \sigma(\Pi_c - \Pi_c)] - \text{lymph flow} \qquad (1)$$

where $EVLW$ = extravascular lung water (mL); S = surface area (cm^2); L_p = the hydraulic conductivity for water (cm·min^{-1}mmHg^{-1}); P_c and P_i = the hydrostatic pressure within the capillary and interstitial spaces, respectively (mmHg); σ = the reflection coefficient for protein (no units); and Π_c and Π_i = the oncotic pressure within the capillary and interstitial spaces (mmHg).

According to Equation 1, *EVLW* will increase if P_c increases, *but only if changes in the other variables do not effectively compensate for the increase in* P_c. *EVLW* will also increase with lung "injury." While lung injury is often defined operationally in terms of characteristic radiographic and blood gas abnormalities (2), it can be defined more generally as any significant deterioration in lung function due to characteristic pathologic abnormalities in the lungs' normal underlying structure or architecture (2). In the case of the acute respiratory distress syndrome (ARDS), the deterioration in lung function (e.g., gas exchange, mechanics) should be linked to the characteristic pathologic changes that are referred to as "diffuse alveolar damage" (2). Thus, in ARDS, when the endothelial barrier is injured, plasma fluid and solutes "leak" into extravascular spaces. Since proteins are the principal solute responsible for the development of intravascular oncotic pressure, the flux of proteins across the endothelial barrier affects the development of *EVLW* (Eq. 1). This protein flux (or for that matter, any other solute) can be quantified with the Kedem-Katchalsky equation (3):

$$J_s = J_v(1 - \sigma)\, C_{\bar{s}} + PS(C_c - C_i) \tag{2}$$

where J_s = solute flux (mg/min); J_v is the volume flux of fluid (as described in Equation 1 after eliminating the lymph flow variable); P = permeability (cm/sec); $C_{\bar{s}}$ = the average molar concentration of solute within the membrane; and $(C_c - C_i)$ = the solute concentration gradient between the capillary and interstitium (mg/mL). $C_{\bar{s}}$ is usually assumed to simply be the average of C_c and C_i, but there is little empirical evidence to support this assumption. Note that "*S*" and "σ" are the same terms used in the Starling equation (Eq. 1). "Injury" to the endothelial barrier results in increased leakiness to both fluids (increased L_p in Eq. 1) and protein (decreased σ, and increased "*P*" from Eq. 2). Clinically, changes in these variables induced by injury always occur together. Accordingly, changes in J_s, σ, L_p $*S$, and *PS* are all taken as indicative of a change in vascular "permeability," even though, strictly speaking, "permeability" pertains only to that portion of protein flux which can be ascribed to diffusion ("*P*" in Eq. 2).

Pulmonary edema is simply an abnormal increase in *EVLW*. Generally speaking, pulmonary edema is due to either an inadequately compensated increase in P_c or "permeability," or both. An increase in P_c is usually due to heart failure, volume overload, or pulmonary venous vasoconstriction. An increase in pulmonary vascular permeability is often the result of some inflammatory process. Thus, to the extent that an increase in pulmonary vascular permeability is indicative of some form of lung injury, an evaluation of barrier function (i.e., with measurements of *EVLW*, P_c, and some index of vascular permeability) will provide useful information about the etiology of pulmonary edema (Table 1).

Table 1 Potential Reasons to Evaluate Pulmonary Endothelial Barrier Function

- As an aid to early diagnosis
- To determine natural history of injury
- To discern the etiology of pulmonary edema
- To quantify the severity of injury
- As a marker of treatment effectiveness
- To provide prognostic information about recovery

Equations 1 and 2 are most appropriate as models for the development of *interstitial* pulmonary edema. While similar equations could be written for the movement of fluid and protein from the interstitial to alveolar space, they are not very useful, since alveolar edema seems to develop by a more sudden process, termed *alveolar flooding* (4,5). However, since the development of alveolar edema is invariably associated with interstitial pulmonary edema, measuring variables in these two equations is still useful.

Since there is no reason why injury cannot be present while P_c is also elevated, *both* must be evaluated to properly define the cause of pulmonary edema. Indeed, recent experimental evidence (6–9) suggests that under some circumstances, increased P_c can not only exacerbate the development of pulmonary edema due to injury, but can actually *cause* injury as well, further obscuring the traditional simple dichotomous division of pulmonary edema into *one* of two categories: due to either increased hydrostatic pressure or increased permeability.

The normal extravascular water content of the lungs is < 500 mL (10–13). While an accumulation greater than this amount is, by definition, abnormal, symptoms and physiologic impairment do not usually develop until *EVLW* approximately doubles the normal value (14). This physiologic reserve is made possible by the interstitium, a reservoir for relatively modest amounts of excess extravascular water that can be accommodated with little derangement in gas exchange or lung mechanics (see Chap. 2). Above this amount, alveolar edema will usually develop, almost always with clinically important effects. Thus, any method that would be useful clinically must be able to detect changes in *EVLW* below the threshold of alveolar edema.

Although outcome has never been shown to be linked directly to the amount, or even continued presence, of pulmonary edema per se, the possibility that sufficiently sensitive and accurate techniques could be used to detect pulmonary edema or endothelial injury even before they became apparent clinically, or could be used to provide information about the natural history of pulmonary edema or its response to therapeutic intervention, is so inherently attractive that the effort to develop and validate such techniques still continues (Table 2). In

Table 2 Clinically Appropriate Methods to Quantify Pulmonary Edema

	Measures	Quantitation	Accuracy[a]	Reproducibility (COV)	Sensitivity[b]
CXR	LD	poor	unknown	unknown	moderate
CT	LD	excellent	unknown[c]	unknown[c]	high
NMR	TLW	fair	underestimates by 20–40%[d]	5–10%	poor[e]
PET	EVLW	excellent	underestimates by 10–15%	$<$ 5%	high
ID	EVLW	good-excellent	overestimates by 10–20%[f]	4–8%	moderate

[a]None of the methods can distinguish whether an increase in EVLW represents noncellular pulmonary edema or cellular water from an inflammatory infiltrate.
[b]Sensitivity to change.
[c]Presumably excellent, but formal studies never performed.
[d]Underestimates are primarily in normal or mildly edematous lungs.
[e]Poor sensitivity is primarily in normal or mildly edematous lungs.
[f]Overestimation is primarily in normal or mildly edematous lungs.
EVLW = extravascular lung water; TLW = total lung water (of a region on an image); LD = lung density; COV = coefficient of variation; CXR = chest x-ray; CT = computed tomography; NMR = nuclear magnetic resonance; PET = positron emission tomography; ID = indicator-dilution methods.

this chapter, the most commonly employed methods to measure *EVLW* and vascular permeability at the present time will be reviewed. The discussion will concentrate on the practical aspects of implementing clinically appropriate techniques, but will also include a brief discussion of two techniques (one for measuring lung water, the other for evaluating vascular permeability) that are often taken as the "gold standards" in their respective applications. Theoretical justifications for the models used to analyze the data generated by these methods have been published (15–17). A discussion of how to best measure P_c can be found elsewhere (18) and in Chapter 1.

II. Measurement of Lung Water

A. Gravimetrics

In experimental animals, the amount of water in the lungs can be determined quite simply (19,20) (Fig. 1). First, the lungs are excised and weighed ("gravimetrics"). This establishes the lungs' "wet" weight. The tissue is then slowly dried in an oven over a period of days and the lungs reweighed ("dry" weight). To facilitate complete drying, the lungs are often first ground up in a blender. The difference between the wet and dry weights is a direct and extremely accurate measure of lung water. To account for differences in lung size among animals or groups, the difference in wet and dry weights can be expressed as a fraction of the wet weight (i.e., wet–dry/wet) or can be normalized to the dry weight of the lung (i.e., wet–dry or W/D ratio) (21). This latter expression is particularly useful because it is quite sensitive mathematically to small changes in the fractional wet weight (e.g., a change from 80% to 90% fractional water weight is equivalent to a change in the W/D ratio from 4.0 to 9.0). Numerous studies have established that the normal lung is about 80% water, with a W/D ratio of about 4.0 (22).

The disadvantages of this approach are several (Table 3). It can only be performed in experimental animals, or in humans at autopsy or at the time of pneumonectomy—and it can only be performed once. Another disadvantage is somewhat less obvious: approximately half of the wet weight of the lung is due to blood (22). Thus, modest changes in wet weight could be due to changes in pulmonary blood volume and not to the development of pulmonary edema (by definition, defined as an increase in *extravascular* lung water). To eliminate this source of error, the blood volume of the tissue must be determined separately, usually by some labeling technique (19). The water weight of the blood is then also subtracted from the total wet weight of the lungs, producing an estimate of the *extravascular* water content of the lungs (expressed, for instance, as a "blood free" W/D ratio).

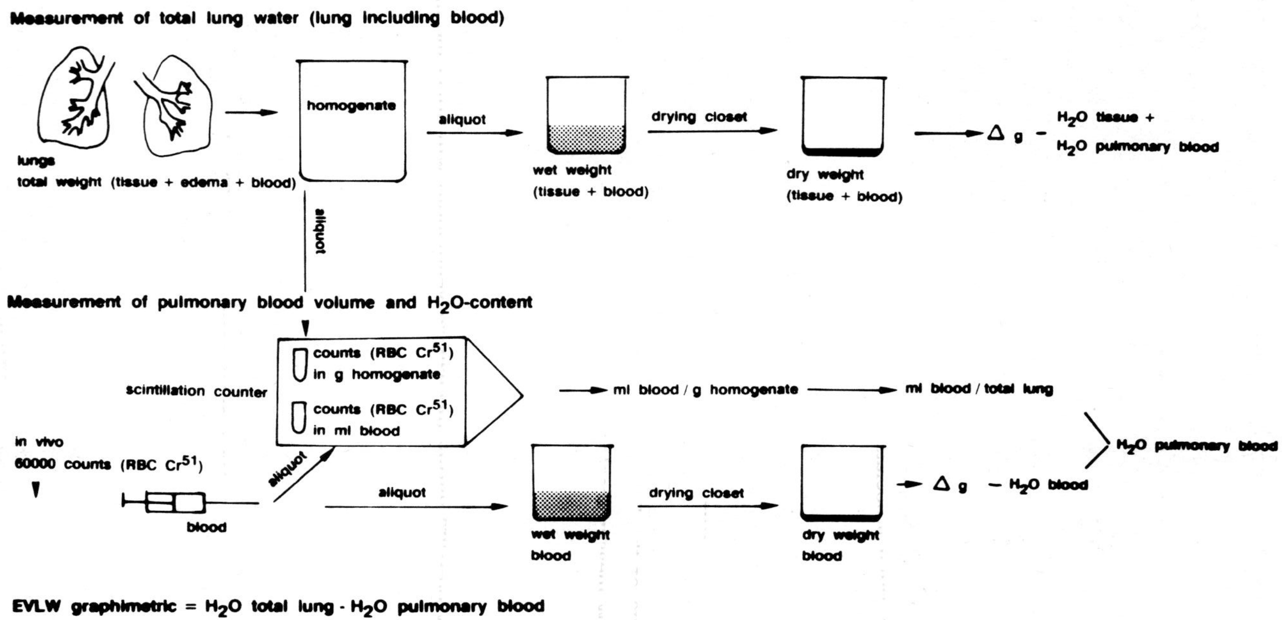

Figure 1 Schematic diagram of the gravimetric method for determining extravascular lung water in the lung. (From Ref. 19.)

Table 3 Limitations of the Gravimetric Method of Evaluating Pulmonary Edema

- Invasive and destructive
- Accuracy depends on corrections for blood content
- Increased extravascular dry weight during lung injury leads to an underestimation of EVLW
- Relationship of wet-to-dry weight ratio to EVLW is non-linear
- Cannot distinguish cellular from noncellular EVLW

With this correction, it is assumed that despite an increase in *EVLW*, the extravascular dry weight of the lung is not increased above normal. However, lung injury is often associated with both protein and red cell extravasation, leading to increased extravascular dry weight. The result is an underestimate of the change in edema accumulation (23).

B. Imaging Methods

General Comments

Each picture or volume element (i.e., pixel or voxel, respectively) in a cross-sectional image of the lungs represents a specific physical volume. Thus, the units for *EVLW* measurements within such images (or for that matter, any other variable) are those of concentration, e.g., ml *EVLW*/mL lung. Since the lung is an air-containing structure, the amount of lung *parenchyma* within each voxel can change, depending on the underlying state of lung inflation (lung volume). Therefore, anything that affects regional lung volume (e.g., atelectasis or positive end-expiratory pressure during mechanical ventilation) will affect the intensity of the measured signal in the picture element, potentially changing how one interprets the amount of *EVLW* that is present (Table 4). To quantify changes in images of *EVLW* in absolute terms, the signal over the entire organ must be integrated.

Most imaging methods for evaluating pulmonary edema (Table 2) do not estimate *EVLW* per se, but instead produce estimates of *total* water content or concentration (i.e., vascular + extravascular water). The data from such methods can be misinterpreted if the blood volume of the lungs is not constant. In

Table 4 General Limitations of Imaging Methods to Evaluate Pulmonary Edema

- Data affected by changes in regional lung inflation
- Often only evaluate lung density, not EVLW
- Cannot distinguish cellular from noncellular EVLW

contrast, when pulmonary edema is evaluated with the nuclear medicine imaging technique of positron emission tomography, it *is* possible to actually measure *EVLW,* by separately measuring the water concentration of blood and subtracting this value from the total water concentration of the lung within each image.

A problem intrinsic to all techniques used to measure *EVLW* in intact animals, including both imaging and nonimaging methods, is that the water densities of edema, blood, and inflammatory white cells are virtually identical. Thus, these components cannot be distinguished from one another strictly by how they affect *EVLW* per se. This problem becomes especially relevant as the edema of early ARDS gives way to progressive cellular infiltration, even while the alveolar edema itself begins to resolve (24).

Chest Radiography

While a roentgenographic examination of the chest is commonly used to detect whether pulmonary edema is present, to describe its overall distribution within the lung, and to evaluate associated findings to infer a probable etiology, it can also be used, at least semiquantitatively, to estimate the *amount* of pulmonary edema that is present as well. Several features of the chest radiograph make such an interpretation possible: (1) certain characteristic "signs" are associated with only modest increases in *EVLW* (perhaps as little as 30% above normal values) (25), such as pulmonary "congestion," vascular "redistribution," peribronchial cuffing, perihilar "haze," the presence of Kerley's lines, and an "interstitial" pattern to the radiographic densities); (2) as *EVLW* increases, the radiographic densities occupy a greater fraction of the total lung airspace (often, mild to moderate amounts of edema are present in gravity-dependent lung regions only, while more severe increases in *EVLW* involve both dependent and nondependent lung) (26); and (3) as edema worsens and water displaces air in any given lung region, the "density" of the "infiltrate" also worsens, becoming more and more "white."

These features are so reliable that most clinicians depend on them, virtually to the exclusion of any other approach, to determine whether the quantity of pulmonary edema in any given patient is changing or not. Even so, the overall accuracy of chest radiography is significantly limited by several technical problems, in addition to the problems common to all imaging methods discussed above (27). For one, while the accuracy of any method depends heavily on a standardized acquisition technique, clinical issues, especially those related to patient acuity, often override standardization procedures which would help ensure the accuracy and reproducibility of chest radiography as a tool for estimating *EVLW* (27,28). Thus, even though some have reported that inferences about *EVLW* accumulation by chest radiography correlate well with estimates by other techniques under very carefully controlled conditions, many others have not been able to duplicate these results, especially under conditions relevant to clinical practice (27). (See Chap. 3 for further discussion of chest radiography in patients with pulmonary edema.)

Computed Tomography

The intensity of the infiltrate on a chest radiograph, or of an image obtained by x-ray computed tomography (CT), is determined by its density. The principal advantages of using x-ray CT over conventional radiography to evaluate pulmonary edema are that the density of the infiltrates can be determined quantitatively, the spatial distribution of edema in transverse sections can be defined, and, of course, associated (but at times clinically relevant) findings can be evaluated (e.g., loculated pneumothoraces, pleural effusions, etc.). Lung density can be quantified with x-ray CT because the arbitrary Hounsfield units used for CT display can be calibrated against objects or substances of known density (e.g., air, water, bone). Experimentally, CT derived estimates of lung density increase by 69% when gravimetric measurements of lung weight increase by about 250% (29). (The differences in the percentage increase does not really indicate anything about accuracy since the units of measurement are not the same.) CT densitometry is able to detect rather modest (~50%) increases in *EVLW* in experimental animals (30).

Nuclear Magnetic Resonance (NMR) Imaging

Another approach to estimating lung water content is based on the ability to align hydrogen nuclei (protons) of water in the direction of an externally applied magnetic field (31). When a subject lays within a magnetic field and is then irradiated with electromagnetic radiation in the form of a correctly applied radio frequency pulse, "resonance" (i.e., "nuclear magnetic resonance") develops from the absorption and subsequent release of energy as the pulse is applied and discontinued. This energy can be detected with appropriately placed amplifiers, producing a signal of varying strength, depending on the strength of the magnetic field and the frequency of the radio frequency pulse. If the magnetic field is made to vary in a known fashion along the length of the subject (long axis), the strength of the magnetization will differ regionally, as will the radio frequency pulse required to detect the magnetization. For instance, if the radio frequency pulse consists of only a narrow range of frequencies and is applied 90° to the long axis, then only nuclei at a specific point along the long axis will resonate at that frequency, producing a signal corresponding to a specific transverse section through the subject. This allows the proton density to be resolved spatially, giving rise to an image in which the regional NMR signal is directly proportional to water (and therefore to lung density). With pulses at different frequencies, multiple transverse sections can be created (Fig. 2).

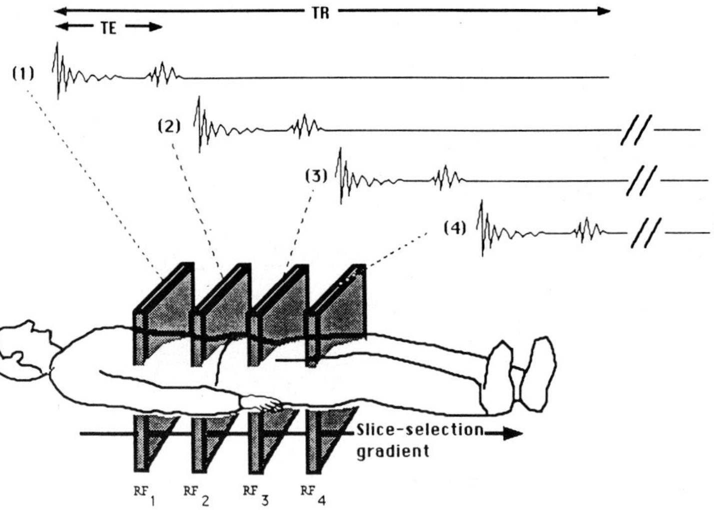

Figure 2 Production of multiple cross-sectional images slices by NMR when sequential radio-frequency pulses (RF_1, RF_2, etc), each at a different frequency, are applied in the presence of a gradient of magnetization. TR = relaxation time; TE = echo time. (From Ref. 95.)

A second radio frequency pulse, applied at 180°, will enhance the signal emanating from the resonating nuclei after the radio frequency pulse is stopped. The magnetic resonance signal therefore is often sampled some time after one or more 180° pulses. The time from the first 90° pulse to the time when the signal is sampled is called the echo delay time; accordingly, this particular NMR imaging technique employs so-called "spin-echo" pulse sequences. Although different pulse sequences are used in other NMR imaging applications, the spin-echo sequence is the only one to date that has been employed to measure lung water.

Signal intensity, detected after a spin-echo pulse sequence, varies as a function of the time it is sampled once the 90° radio frequency pulse is stopped (the "relaxation" time). The effect of the 90° pulse is to minimize the signal in the longitudinal (long-axis) direction and to maximize it in the transverse direction. As relaxation continues, the signal in the longitudinal direction increases and that in the transverse direction decreases. The rate constants describing the rate of relaxation in the longitudinal and transverse directions are referred to as T_1 and T_2, respectively. The values for these rate constants vary as a function of tissue type. Thus, by sampling the signal at different T_1 and T_2 times, visualization of different tissues in the image are emphasized ("weighted"). Generally, proton density images have been obtained with pulse sequences that minimize the effects of *both* T_1 and T_2 weighting.

An important advantage of using NMR to evaluate lung water is that the measurements can be obtained without any need for ionizing radiation; furthermore, the measurements are completely independent of any disturbance in ventilation or perfusion (unlike techniques that depend on the administration of indicators or tracers by inhalation or intravenous injection; see below).

Repeated measures of lung water by NMR vary by about 5% to 10% (32). Although there is no limit to the number of times measurements can be repeated, image acquisition times can be lengthy depending on the imaging sequence employed.

Numerous studies have reported a good correlation between NMR-determined estimates of lung water and estimates from the gold standard gravimetric method (33–37). A problem intrinsic to NMR imaging is that normal or mildly edematous lung produces relatively little signal using conventional spin-echo sequences on 1.5 Tesla imagers typically used for clinical purposes (31,37). As a result, NMR methods can underestimate true lung water in absolute terms by as much as 20% to 40% (32,38,39) (despite the good correlation with gravimetric methods). This loss of signal is due to artifacts caused by the distinct and separate magnetic susceptibilities of both air and soft tissue in the normally inflated lung. These artifacts, and therefore the loss of signal, are magnified by the strength of the external magnetic field. Recently, an imager that has only one-tenth the strength of most clinical scanners has been used along with a multiecho pulse sequence (i.e., a 90° radio frequency pulse followed by multiple 180° pulses) to minimize the effect of the air/soft tissue artifact, resulting in an excellent correlation, even in absolute terms, between NMR and gravimetrically determined lung water (40) (Fig. 3). This same NMR imaging sequence has also been successfully applied to normal volunteers (Fig. 4).

The dependency of T_1 and T_2 on tissue type also raises the theoretical possibility that NMR imaging could be used to identify differences in the *composition* of pulmonary edema generated by high intravascular pressures as opposed to increased vascular permeability (potentially allowing the edema of heart failure to be distinguished noninvasively from the edema of ARDS). Such advances have not yet materialized. However, Cutillo et al. (41) have actually reported a method of NMR image analysis that *takes advantage of* the same signal loss artifact (the one caused by the air/soft-tissue interface) that confounds the measurement of proton density in absolute terms (and therefore of lung water) in the normally inflated lung. Since the air/soft tissue interface is minimized as alveolar edema develops, the expected loss of signal is reduced. This difference in signal loss can be measured, leading to inferences about the location of the developing edema (alveolar edema causing less loss of signal than interstitial edema). To date, however, the method has only been applied to studies in rats (41).

In summary, the technique of NMR imaging continues to be developed as a quantitative tool to measure and monitor the development of pulmonary

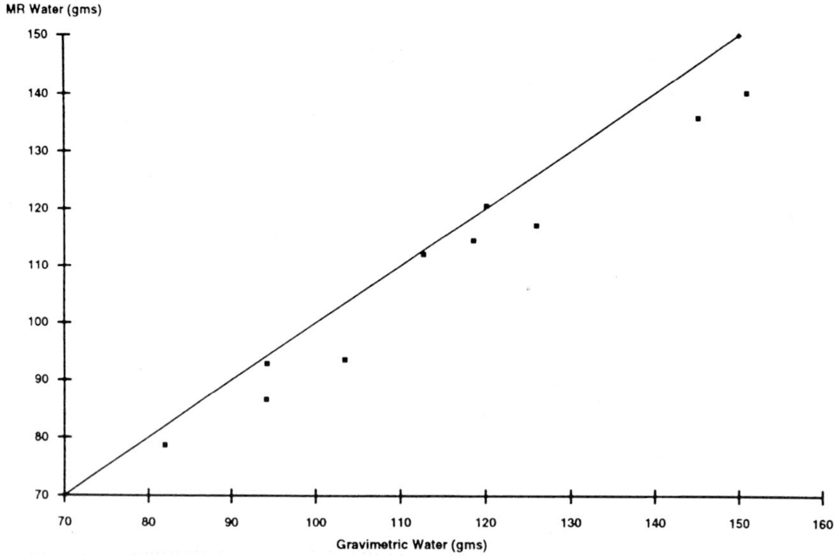

Figure 3 Correlation of lung water measurements obtained by NMR techniques with gravimetric measurements. The straight line represents the line of identity. There is an approximate 5% systematic underestimation of lung water by the NMR technique. (From Ref. 40.)

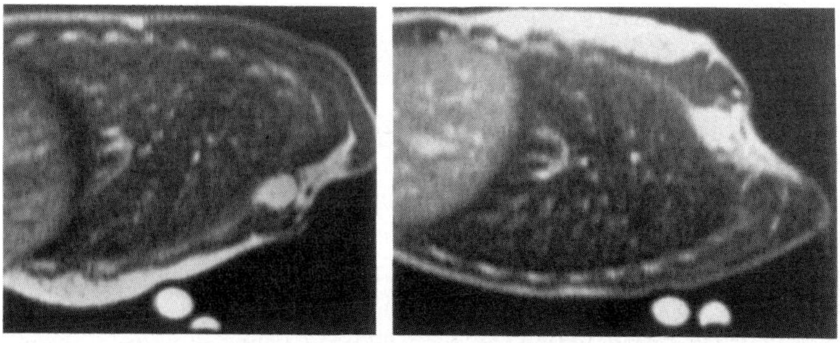

Figure 4 NMR images of a normal volunteer in the prone (left) and supine (right) positions. Higher signal (i.e., higher lung water concentration) is seen in the dependent lung in both positions. (From Ref. 40.)

Table 5 Limitations of NMR Imaging Methods to Evaluate Pulmonary Edema

- Data affected by changes in regional lung inflation
- Normal or mildly edematous lung produces little signal
- Expensive
- Complex
- Can be a lengthy procedure
- Cumbersome for ICU patients
- Cannot separate lung water into vascular and extravascular components
- Cannot distinguish cellular from noncellular EVLW

edema. Even once the technical hurdles are overcome, considerable difficulty will undoubtedly be encountered when trying to implement such methods in the critically ill patient (Table 5).

Positron Emission Tomography

EVLW can be estimated with external residue detection techniques, after separately administering radioactively labeled tracers which distribute within the total and intravascular water spaces of the lung. The radioactivity is then detected with a device like a gamma camera or a positron emission tomography (PET) scanner. Estimates of lung water can be determined by scaling the counts of activity within a lung region to activity within samples of blood (taken as the water reference).

It is difficult to obtain accurate quantitative measurements of tissue activity with most external residue detection devices for two reasons: (1) it is difficult to distinguish whether the source of activity is from lung tissue, other thoracic structures, or the chest wall; and (2) many radioactive isotopes used in nuclear medicine are of low energy. Consequently, an unknown fraction of the tissue activity is attenuated by the tissue, never arriving at the external detectors.

The first problem can be resolved with imaging devices that create transverse tomographic images (single photon emission computed tomography (SPECT or PET). The second problem can only be definitively resolved by making a measurement of the attenuation fraction in a separate scan. For all practical purposes, this can only be performed with PET imaging (42) (Fig. 5). Because PET imaging is widely held to be the "gold standard" among quantitative nuclear medicine imaging techniques, this method will be described in additional detail.

To evaluate pulmonary edema with PET, total lung water is measured first, either directly, or as estimated from tissue density measurements (42). Tissue density can also be estimated by PET imaging (42,43). When lung water is estimated from lung density measurements, a value for the water fraction of

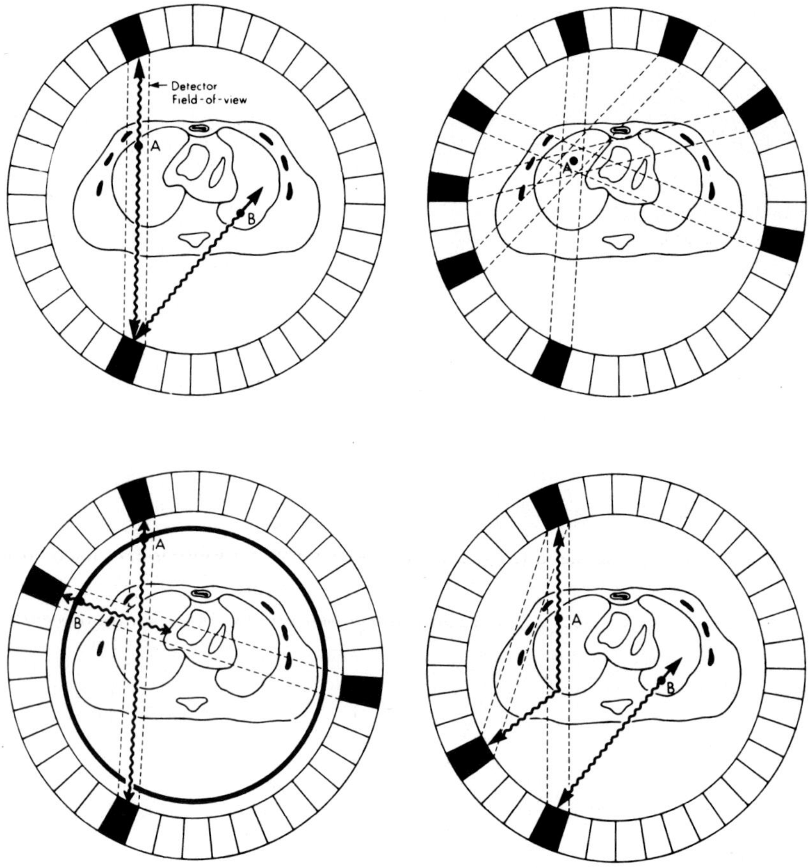

Figure 5 *Top left*: Schematic representation of a single tomographic cross section through the chest at the midventricular level, surrounded by one ring of radiation detectors. Points A and B represent sites of intrathoracic annihilation events after a positron-electron interaction; arrows represent the emitted gamma photons. Photons arriving at the darkened detectors within an allowable "coincidence window" (true coincidence) are recorded and used in later image reconstruction (e.g., event A). After event B, only one photon is detected (the other is attenuated by lung tissue). Therefore, the single annihilation photon reaching a detector is excluded from use during image reconstruction. *Top right*: Same schematic representation shown in top left. As multiple detector pairs are included, the activity emitted from the radiation source at point A is located with increasing accuracy. *Bottom left*: Same schematic representation shown in top left. However, a ring of positron-emitting activity has been added and placed between the detectors and the thorax. First, a scan is obtained without the body in the field of view. The number of coincidences registered for each detector pair is recorded. Then, the thorax is placed within the detector field and another scan obtained. The fraction of

lung tissue must be assumed (0.82 to 0.84 mL/gm). A small (~2%) correction for differences in tissue vs. blood density can also be incorporated (44).

When lung water is measured directly, a sample of sterile water is labeled with a positron-emitting isotope, such as oxygen-15 ($H_2{}^{15}O$) ($t_{1/2}$ = 2.06 min), and then administered intravenously (45). The O-15-labeled water is allowed to equilibrate with tissue water over a 3 to 4-min period. Then, the isotope's activity concentration in lung tissue is determined with a PET "scanner" or "camera," a device similar in appearance to an x-ray CT scanner. (PET scanners can detect both radiation *transmitted* through the body and radiation *emitted* from within the body. X-ray CT scanners detect only transmitted radiation.) Eventually, multiple two-dimensional images are reconstructed from the activity data using mathematical algorithms which are also similar to those used in x-ray CT. If the activity data in the PET image are scaled to simultaneously obtained activity in the blood, the image can be displayed as a quantitative regional map of lung water distribution (45).

An exactly analogous approach is used to measure the blood volume concentration in the images. In this case, O-15 (or alternatively, C-11) carbon monoxide is used instead of O-15 water. If O-15 carbon monoxide is used, trace amounts of $C^{15}O$ are inhaled as a gas, binding immediately to blood hemoglobin. After a few minutes, to allow equilibration within the body's blood volume, another PET scan is obtained. When again normalized to activity measurements in blood, the image, in this case, is a regional display of blood volume. With the assumption that 84% of blood is water (a reasonable assumption at normal hematocrits), the blood water content in a lung region can be subtracted from the total lung water concentration, yielding a derived image of *extravascular* water concentration (Fig. 6). The total time required to measure *EVLW* with

---

initial coincidences still registered by each detector pair is again recorded. For instance, a photon emitted from point A travels completely through the body, while one from point B is absorbed and attenuated by myocardium. The "attenuation fraction" is used to correct activity data from all subsequent emission scans. *Bottom right*: Same schematic representation shown in top left. In this case, however, one of the photons from event A is by chance scattered and is detected by another detector. If the two photons of event A are registered within the allowable coincidence window, a true coincidence will be recorded between those two detectors, even though event A actually occurred outside their field of view. Thus, event A will be misplaced during image reconstruction. Alternatively, if the nonattenuated single photon from event B and the nonscattered single photon from event A arrive by chance at the original detector pair within the allowable timing window, both could be used in image reconstruction even though they represent more than one event ("random coincidence"). (From Ref. 42.)

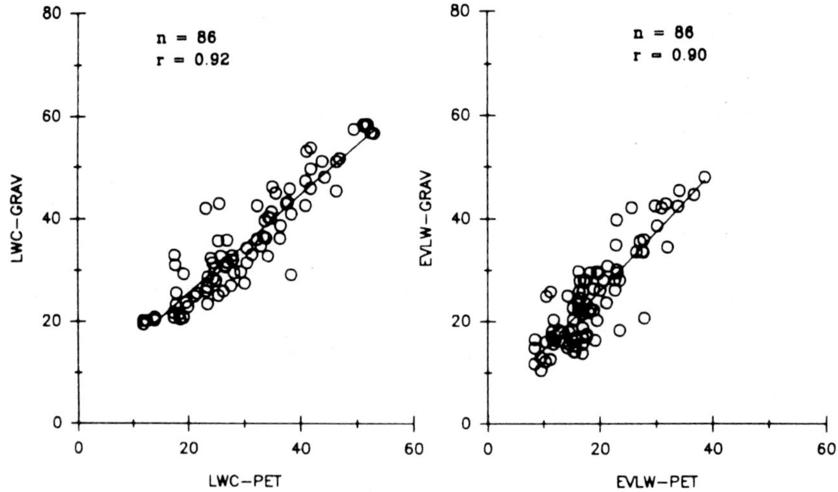

Figure 6 Correlation of total regional lung water concentration and *EVLW* measurements obtained by PET and gravimetrics. The straight line in each case represents the regression line for the multiple regional measurements obtained in 10 dogs. (From Ref. 89.)

PET is about 45 min, but repeat measurements can begin in as little as 10 to 15 min from the previous one.

To determine the blood volume concentration in lung tissue with PET, the activity within the lung regions on the images (presumably representing blood) must be normalized to activity concentration measurements from known samples of blood (42,44,45). If these samples are obtained directly via venipuncture, then a correction (~10%) can be included to account for differences in large- and small-vessel hematocrit (44). However, the actual necessity of doing so probably depends on the relative proportion of noncapillary vessels in the lung regions of interest on the PET images, since blood volume estimates using both red cell and plasma tracers are comparable, at least experimentally (implying a similar hematocrit between the blood in the images and peripheral blood samples) (45).

An alternative (to using peripheral blood samples) is to measure the activity within the blood pool of a cardiac chamber, in which case a further correction is necessary for the so-called partial volume averaging effect (~5% to 10% in humans) (44). The partial volume effect is a result of sampling structures on the PET images (e.g., the right ventricular cavity) when the dimensions are less than twice the spatial resolution of the images, as determined by the specific scanner and image reconstruction algorithms used to create the images (42).

Two previous studies showed that *EVLW* measurements by PET correlated well with *EVLW* measurements obtained by gravimetrics ($r = .86$ to .93) (Fig. 6), even though corrections for potential differences in peripheral vs. capillary hematocrit, or for differences in tissue vs. blood density were not included (46,47). Perhaps because such corrections were not incorporated, PET estimates of *EVLW* systematically underestimated the gravimetric estimates by about 10% to 15%. PET measurements, however, are highly reproducible (coefficient of variation for repeat measurements <5%) and linear ($r = .99$ for changes in lung water over a 20-fold concentration range) (47). The method also shows exquisite sensitivity: as little as 1 ml of additional extravascular water can be detected with PET (Fig. 7) (47).

Despite these impressive performance characteristics, PET imaging is expensive (like NMR) and not widely distributed among medical centers (unlike NMR) (Table 6). Positron-emitting isotopes also produce ionizing radiation (although the amounts used in any one study are quite low). As with x-ray CT or NMR imaging, the patient must be taken to the PET facility for study, an obvious problem in critically ill patients.

C. Indicator Dilution Methods

EVLW measurements can be obtained by indicator-dilution methods using either the so-called "mean transit time" or "slope-volume" approaches to analyze the temperature-time or concentration-time data (48–50). The former approach is based on a rationale similar to that used to measure cardiac output by the familiar "thermodilution" method. Two key principles underlie such techniques: (1) the mean transit time of any substance (an "indicator") through a volume of fluid depends directly on the volume itself (when the volume is small, the mean transit time is short, and vice versa); and (2) the vascular and extravascular water spaces of the lung act as two separate but contiguous volumes, separated by a semipermeable membrane. If one indicator diffuses freely between both compartments but the other does not, the two indicators will have different mean transit times through the lung (Fig. 8).

Although a variety of different indicators can be and have been used, the most clinically applicable set of indicators are administered as cold indocyanine green dye. The temperature of the green dye is the *diffusible* indicator; the green dye itself is the *nondiffusible* indicator. The dye remains within the intravascular space because it rapidly binds to serum albumin.

To implement the technique, cold green dye is injected intravenously into the right atrium. Detectors distal to the lung (e.g., within a femoral artery) then record concentration-time and temperature-time profiles (Fig. 8). The mean transit times for each indicator are computed from these data.

The volume accessible to each indicator is simply its flow through the volume (in this case, the cardiac output) multiplied by its mean transit time

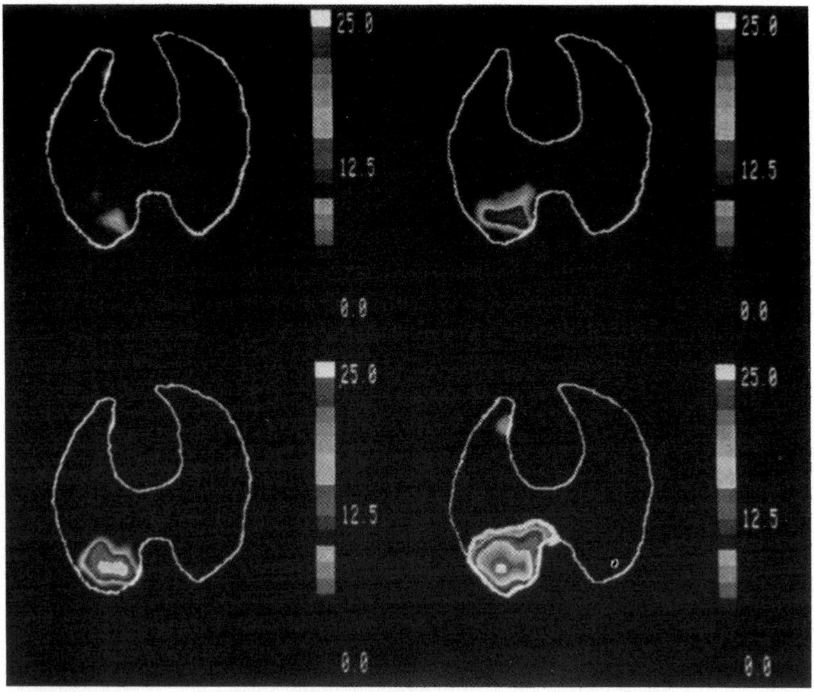

Figure 7 Subtraction PET images of change in lung water concentration from one dog. The white outline represents the chest wall and cardiac fossa borders from one tomographic image at the midventricular level. The area with the region therefore represents lung tissue. Each image represents the difference in lung water concentration before and after instillation of autologous plasma into the left caudal lobe bronchus. *Upper left*: After 1 ml plasma. *Upper right*: After an additional 4 ml plasma. *Lower left*: After an additional 5 ml plasma. *Lower right*: After an additional 10 ml plasma. Scales are in units of ml water/100 ml lung. Signal from even 1 ml of instilled plasma is seen, and a progressive increase in lung water concentration is also seen after each instillation. The region of interest used to calculate the change in lung water concentration is shown in the lower right image. (From Ref. 89.)

Table 6 Limitations of PET Imaging Methods to Evaluate Pulmonary Edema

- Data affected by changes in regional lung inflation
- Expensive
- Complex
- Relatively lengthy procedure
- Cumbersome for ICU patients
- Technology not present in most medical centers
- Cannot distinguish cellular from noncellular EVLW

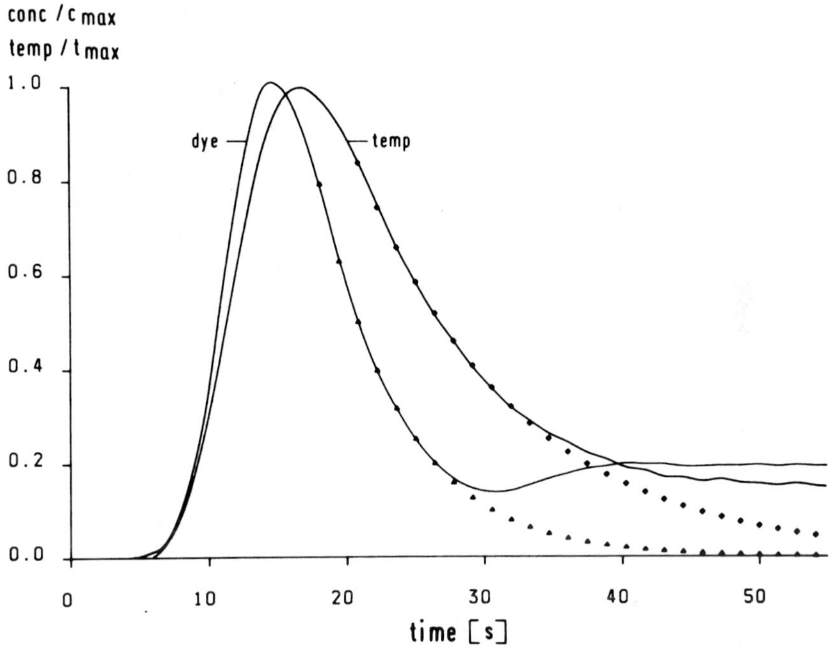

Figure 8 Thermal (temp) and indocyanine green dye indicator dilution curves. The monoexponential extrapolation is shown as dotted lines. (From Ref. 57.)

(MTT) through that volume. Since the flow for both temperature and dye is the same (cardiac output), the extravascular thermal volume (ETV) can be calculated simply as:

$$ETV = CO * (MTT_{th} - MTT_{gd}) \tag{3}$$

where MTT_{th} and MTT_{gd} are the mean transit times of the thermal and green dye indicators, respectively.

The volume of distribution for the thermal indicator is the total perfused water space between the point of injection (right atrium) and the point of detection (thermistor tip of an arterial catheter, usually placed femorally). The volume of distribution for the green dye is the blood volume between these two points. Since the extravascular water content of myocardium and nonpulmonary blood vessels is small relative to the extravascular water content of the lung, *ETV* and *EVLW* are usually considered to be equivalent variables.

While the theory underlying these measurements is well understood (48), commercially available equipment may have seriously biased the interpretation of performance in experimental and clinical settings. Since the early 1980s, most experimental and certainly virtually all studies involving thermodilution measurements of *ETV* in the United States have employed the Edwards Laboratories model 9310 Lung Water Computer. While the calculation of *ETV* from Equation 3 is superficially straightforward, accuracy depends on corrections for baseline drift, instrument response times, and recirculation artifacts (51) (see below). For instance, the usual maximum change in temperature at the femoral artery thermistor site is about 0.25°C. Obviously, small drifts in baseline could seriously interfere with the calculation of *ETV* under such circumstances if not properly detected and corrected. Thus, some early reports that cardiac output could affect estimates of *ETV* (which theoretically should *not* be true) were probably a result of the algorithms used in the Edwards Labs computer to adjust for these problems (52,53). Studies that employed alternative systems have failed to find any such cardiac output dependency (50,51,54). Likewise, it is also important to detect improper positioning of the intravascular catheters used to detect the thermal and dye signals (50,51,55).

Many studies have evaluated the accuracy of the *ETV* measurement by comparing estimates to gravimetric measurements. Effros (48) and Allison et al. (50) have both pointed out that the measurement of *ETV* is equal to *EVLW* only if one takes into account the relative transit times of the thermal indicator through red cells vs. plasma, the relative specific heats of extravascular tissue vs. plasma, the density of blood, and the fraction of extravascular mass represented by water. Without such corrections, *ETV* should consistently overestimate *EVLW* by as much as 24% in normal lungs. Interestingly, as the lungs become more edematous, a greater fraction of the extravascular mass becomes water, and the error introduced by ignoring these factors (which is the case with commercially available devices) actually goes down. To put such potential errors in perspective, however, if the normal *ETV* is about 5 mL/kg, or about 350 mL in a normal adult, a 24% error would yield an overestimate of about 72 mL. However, clinically apparent pulmonary edema usually develops with 50% to 100% increases in *EVLW,* and 5- to 10-*fold* increases in *ETV* have been reported in ARDS (56), yielding a dynamic range for *ETV* of at least 300 to 3000 mL. In this context, a 24% error at the low (normal) end is probably tolerable.

Many studies have shown that *ETV* usually (but not always) closely approximates *EVLW* (49,50). However, in general, there *has* been a tendency for *ETV* to overestimate true *EVLW* in normal lungs, and to slightly underestimate it in edematous lungs. In addition to the correction factors discussed above, the tendency for *ETV* to be greater than *EVLW* has been attributed to overestimation of the thermal mean transit time when using monoexponential extrapolation of the descending portion of the thermal curve to correct for recirculation artifacts (57) and to the inclusion of myocardial and aortic wall water content in the *ETV* calculation (57).

Overall, the correlation coefficient "*r*" for *ETV* and gravimetrically determined *EVLW* is usually at least .9, and the slope of the regression relationship usually lays between 0.9 and 1.10 (49–51). From animal data, sensitivity has been estimated to be 88% and specificity 97%, with a coefficient of variation for repeated measurements of 4% to 8% (50). However, this performance record in animals may be somewhat optimistic for the usual ICU clinical setting. Using the Edwards computer, Laggner et al. (58) reported that most consecutive measurements were within 15% of one another, although the range was +30% to −60%. Using a newer, alternative ("COLD") system, Zeravik et al. reported a coefficient of variation of only 8% (54).

The two commercially available systems (the Edwards computer and the COLD system) have also produced different results regarding the correlation of *ETV* to gravimetric measurements obtained from the lungs of organ donors. Using the Edwards computer, Mihm et al. (59) reported an excellent correlation of $r = .98$, but a systematic overestimation of true *EVLW* by almost 4 mL/kg. In contrast, using the COLD system, Sturm et al. reported an equally strong correlation coefficient with much closer absolute agreement between methods (Fig. 9) (57).

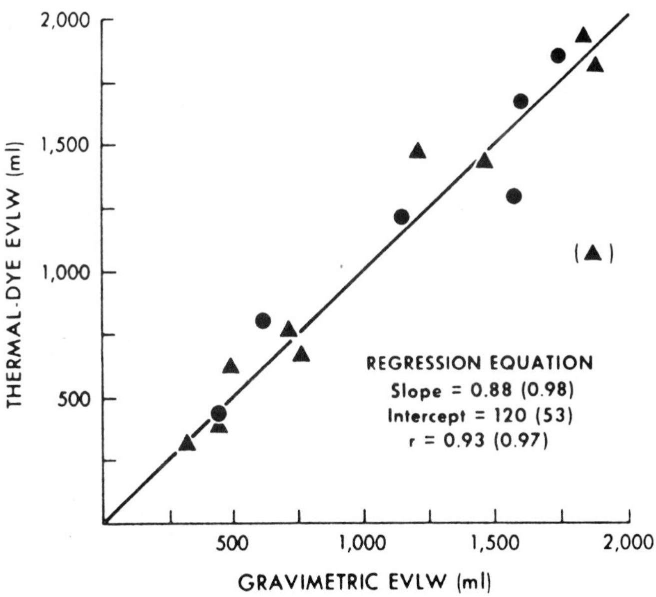

Figure 9 Comparison of the last premortem *EVLW* measurement (by double indicator "thermal-dye" technique) to the postmortem gravimetric value in 16 patients, obtained from two hospitals in California and Germany (triangles vs. circles, respectively). (From Ref. 57.)

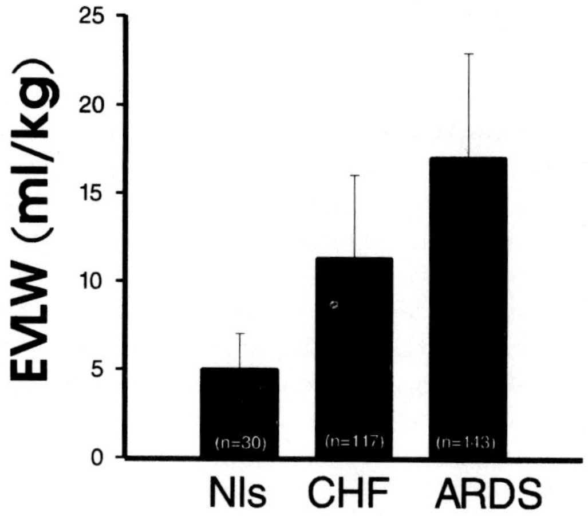

Figure 10 Average (mean ± SD) amounts of *EVLW* in patients requiring pulmonary artery catheterization without pulmonary edema (Nls), in patients with pulmonary edema and an elevated pulmonary wedge pressure (congestive heart failure, CHF), and in patients with pulmonary edema and a wedge pressure < 18 mm Hg (ARDS). Data combined from Refs. 12, 56, 60, as well as studies referred to therein.

In four studies in adults (using the Edwards system), the average value for *ETV* in normal humans has been remarkably consistent (10–13). Average values have also been reported in patients with pulmonary edema associated with both normal and elevated wedge pressures (Fig. 10) (12,56,60).

The advantages of measuring *EVLW* by the thermal-green dye double-indicator dilution method are several: the method is (superficially) simple to implement, safe, reproducible, and repeatable. On the other hand, it is somewhat invasive (it requires central venous as well as arterial catheterization) (Table 7).

Since the indicators in this technique are bloodborne, the accumulation of extravascular water in any portion of lung which is "downstream" from a large vascular obstruction cannot be detected (50). An analogous problem exists for lung regions which are poorly perfused, as a result of using positive end-

Table 7 Limitations of Indicator Dilution Methods to Evaluate Pulmonary Edema

- Results highly sensitive to instrumentation factors
- Accuracy depends on correction for indicator recirculation
- EVLW underestimated in regions with vascular obstruction or very low flow
- Commercial technology currently not available in USA
- Cannot distinguish cellular from noncellular EVLW

expiratory pressure (PEEP) (50,61), because of significant intravascular obstruction from emboli or in situ thrombosis (as has been documented to occur in ARDS), or because severe vasoconstriction from hypoxia is present. With vasoconstriction, the time required for full recovery of the thermal indicator from the lung may be so prolonged that recirculation artifacts are likely (see below) (50). (In contrast, although PET tracers are also bloodborne, measurements are made at equilibrium instead of after a single pass through the lungs. Accordingly, the PET measurements are less sensitive to hypoperfusion artifacts.)

Vascular obstruction (from PEEP or thrombosis) may cause errors because the thermal indicator cannot equilibrate within the extravascular water space if it is not delivered sufficiently close to reach that space by diffusion. The diffusion distance of water is such that this problem probably pertains only to vessels >500 μm in size (48). However, if PEEP levels are high enough to create regions of West's Zone I lung, estimates of *ETV* can actually *increase* when PEEP levels are reduced, as new lung becomes reperfused, despite no actual change in *EVLW* per se. Although this phenomenon has been documented experimentally (50), its relevance to the clinical setting is unknown.

The traditional method for determining the mean transit time of each indicator is to disregard the time-concentration curve at some point beyond which indicator recirculation begins (Fig. 8). Then, usually by a monoexponential extrapolation, further decay in the time-concentration curve is completed, and the mean transit time for the indicator is calculated from these corrected data. In regions of very low perfusion, however, the cutoff point, especially for the diffusible indicator, can occur before the curve can be correctly characterized, leading to incomplete "recovery" of the diffusible indicator and, consequently, to underestimation of the true value for *EVLW*.

With the American Edwards model 9310 lung water computer, the monoexponential decay function was determined from the downsloping portion of the thermal curve between 75% and 33% of the peak value for change in temperature from baseline (manufacturer's manual). With a newer system (COLD Z-03, Pulsion Medizintechnik, Munich, Germany), the portion of the curve used for analysis begins with the point which is 80% of the peak and continues with data until the monoexponential regression fit begins to deteriorate (representing recirculation). An alternative approach in which deconvolution algorithms are used to generate suitable transport functions for the pulmonary circulation has also been reported (62); however, this approach has not yet been incorporated into a commercially available computer.

An alternative to the "mean transit time" approach to calculating *EVLW* by the indicator-dilution technique is the so-called slope-volume method (Fig. 11). To the extent that the decay of the thermodilution curve from its peak value is indeed monoexponential, plotting it on semilogarithmic paper will yield a straight line during the decay portion of the curve, with a slope of $V/\dot{Q}$, where

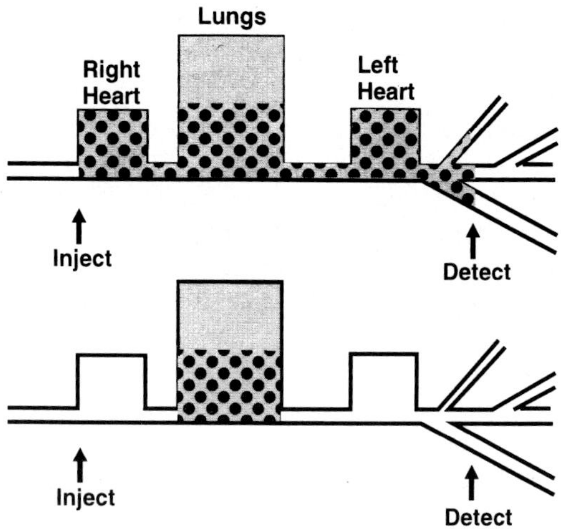

Figure 11 Schematic illustration of the theoretical difference between the mean transit and slope volume methods of determining *EVLW* by the indicator-dilution technique. *Top*: In the mean transit method, the volume of distribution for the dye indicator (circles) is less than for the thermal indicator (gray background), resulting in differences in mean transit times for the two indicators which can be used to calculate *EVLW*. *Bottom*: In the slope-volume method, the largest volume determining the slope of the linear decay portion of each dilution curve is either the blood volume of the lungs for the dye indicator (circles) or the entire lung water volume for thermal indicator (gray background). The difference is again a function of *EVLW*.

V is the volume through which the indicator is traversing and $\dot{Q}$ is the flow through that volume. Furthermore, for a set of volumes in series, the entity with the largest volume determines the slope (63,64). Thus, even though the thermal indicator traverses multiple cardiac chambers as well as the lungs, it is the lungs that determine the slope of the thermodilution curve (and, for that matter, the dye dilution curve). Therefore, *ETV* can be determined by a different mathematical approach from the same set of dilution curve data, namely as the cardiac output times the difference between slope values for the two curves (63,64). This alternative approach has been incorporated into the COLD computer system. It is used as a check on the calculation of *ETV* by the mean transit time method, since both methods are quite sensitive to a variety of artifacts related to catheter placement and positioning (50,51,55).

A variation on the slope-volume method has also been reported in which the slope of the thermodilution curve measured by the pulmonary arterial catheter is compared to that detected by the femoral arterial catheter. The former set of data allows the right heart mixing volume to be calculated, which theoretically should be closely related to the pulmonary blood mixing volume (65). As a result, it is theoretically possible to estimate *ETV* from the injection of a single indicator (thermal), as cardiac output times the difference in the slope values from the femoral arterial versus pulmonary arterial dilution curves. Such an approach is very attractive since it would not be necessary to inject a second indicator (the indocyanine green dye) nor would specialized densitometry equipment be needed to detect the dye curve. Unfortunately, the only two reports of its use in the critical care setting produced conflicting results about its accuracy when compared with double-indicator dilution calculations of *ETV* (55,66).

Although the use of indocyanine green dye and temperature change is the most common method of determining *ETV* by the double-indicator dilution technique, alternatives are still being evaluated. One promising possibility is to use hypertonic (3%) saline as the nondiffusible indicator, measuring changes in blood electrical conductivity instead of dye dilution (67,68). The obvious advantage, of course, is that one could avoid the need for using green dye.

III. Evaluation of Pulmonary Vascular Permeability

A. General Comments

The integrity of the endothelial membrane can be evaluated with measurements of several different variables: $Lp{*}S$, J_s, σ, PS or ''P'' (i.e., "true" permeability) (Eqs. 1 and 2). The techniques available to make these measurements are also rather difficult to implement, often depending on highly invasive procedures and complex mathematical models to interpret the collected data. Accordingly, these methods lack the intuitive simplicity of the gravimetric method of measuring lung water; consequently no single method has emerged as the incontrovertible "gold standard" for evaluating vascular permeability.

Most methods are based on measuring an increased concentration, accumulation, or rate of accumulation of protein in an extravascular pulmonary compartment (Table 8). These compartments may be sampled either directly (e.g., by obtaining lymph) or indirectly (e.g., by external radiation detection of labeled tracers). Usually, total protein, albumin or transferrin concentrations are measured. See Chapter 1 for a further discussion of these issues.

B. Lymph Analysis

The intravascular hydrostatic pressures that drive fluid out of pulmonary capillaries are normally slightly greater than those opposing the efflux of fluid, resulting in the formation of a small amount of lymph. From Equation 1, if vascular permeability increases (characterized by a decrease in the reflection coefficient, σ), fluid flux across the endothelial barrier will increase; this increase

Table 8 Clinically Appropriate Methods for Evaluating Pulmonary Vascular Injury

Method	Bedside?	Quantitation	Comments[a]
Edema fluid sampling	√	poor	sampling errors; potential artifacts from edema resolution
ID	√	excellent	invasive; not an assay of *protein* permeability; surface area dependent; back-diffusion artifacts
Radioaerosol	√	poor	tracer delivery artifacts; inflation artifacts; artifacts related to smoking
Radioisotopic	√[b]	good-excellent	accuracy dependent on detection system; convection vs diffusion artifacts; blood volume and surface area sensitive

[a]See text for details about each method.
[b]Range of methods includes PET which is not a bedside technique.
CXR = chest x-radiography; ID = indicator-dilution methods; PET = positron emission tomography.

in fluid flux must be balanced by an increase in lymph flow if *EVLW* is to remain constant.

Since an increase in lymph flow, along with an increase in lymph protein concentration, is an expected change when vascular permeability increases, a straightforward approach to demonstrate that vascular permeability has increased is to simply measure protein clearance (C):

$$C = \dot{Q}\left(\frac{C_L}{C_P}\right) \tag{4}$$

where $\dot{Q}$ is lymph flow, and C_L and C_P are lymph and plasma protein concentrations, respectively. To measure *C,* it is only necessary to collect lung lymph (to determine its rate of formation and protein concentration), along with simultaneous measurements of protein concentrations in plasma samples. Surgical approaches to the cannulation of lung lymphatics in experimental animals have been reported in detail (69). Chapter 6 provides examples of this experimental approach.

An alternative approach, still based on measurements in lymph, is to measure σ (Eq. 1) or ''*P*'' (Eq. 2). To do so, one set of measurements (specifically, left atrial pressure and protein concentration measurements in lymph and plasma) are made at baseline, and then repeated at a higher left atrial pressure.

These data can be used to estimate each of the variables in Equations 1 and 2 other than σ and *PS*. With more than one set of measurements, it is possible to solve the simultaneous set of equations for the two variables of interest (70).

Both approaches have important limitations (Table 9). For one, they are invasive (and accordingly, are limited to experimental animals). The surgical techniques require considerable skill; damage to the lung lymphatics will produce significant errors. Although acute surgical preparations have been used, chronic preparations are more common, allowing some "recovery" from the acute effects of invasive surgery.

A basic assumption is that lymph flow is equivalent to the filtration rate across the pulmonary endothelium, an assumption with little if any experimental support. It is also difficult to ensure that the lymph comes only from the lung, not other organs, and that it has not been altered by lymph node processing (otherwise, it would not be representative of lung interstitial fluid). Indeed, controversy over the importance of these problems has never been entirely resolved (15,17,70).

Unfortunately, conditions that alter hydrostatic pressures can potentially change vascular surface area for fluid exchange, thereby changing protein clearance in lymph (by increasing "*Q*" in Eq. 3) even without a "true" increase in vascular permeability. Likewise, "*PS*," in Equation 2, would also obviously change. Interestingly, this effect can be turned to the investigator's advantage: if hydrostatic pressures are increased to such an extent that J_v in Equation 2 is maximized (as indicated by a maximal decrease in C_L in Eq. 4), convective forces become the major determinant of protein flux. Accordingly, the "*PS*" term can be ignored and σ determined directly from Equation 2. Obviously, however, such a maneuver is likely to introduce other artifacts that will cloud data interpretation, especially during injury states.

C. Edema Fluid Sampling

The protein concentration of alveolar edema fluid can be determined from samples obtained by direct aspiration from distal airways or via bronchoalveolar lavage. In directly obtained samples, the protein concentration in the fluid should

Table 9 Limitations of Lymph Analysis Methods to Evaluate Lung Injury

- Invasive
- Assumes that lymph flow rate = filtration rate
- Accuracy assumes lymph not contaminated by non-lung sources
- Accuracy assumes lymph not processed by lymph nodes
- Results highly sensitive to changes in vascular surface area

be significantly less than that in plasma if the endothelial barrier is intact and continues to truly function as a semipermeable membrane (edema-to-plasma protein ratio <0.65). However, with injury, the concentration of protein in the edema fluid should approach that of plasma (ratio >0.75) (71–74). Patients with values between 0.65 and 0.75 are not readily classified.

The technique for obtaining alveolar edema fluid by direct aspiration is straightforward, although not always successful. A suction catheter with a 14- to 18-gauge catheter attached is blindly advanced through an endotracheal tube until it reaches a "wedged" position. Fluid is collected with gentle suction, into a standard suction trap, sometimes after several attempts, and sometimes only after patient repositioning. In some instances, all maneuvers are unsuccessful and no fluid at all is obtained.

While this method is safe, quick, noninvasive, and inexpensive, it can only be performed in intubated patients. Also, it underestimates injury at times, since proteins in the alveolar space which precipitate into hyaline membranes will not be represented in the fluid sample. Furthermore, as the edema resolves, the protein concentration in the remaining fluid will increase (72) (see Chap. 14). Since edema may begin to resolve within hours of the onset of injury, the direct sampling method should lose specificity with time. In general, the measurements of protein concentration from directly sampled alveolar fluid can be used to differentiate hydrostatic from permeability forms of pulmonary edema only when the samples are obtained within several hours of the onset of injury (Table 10).

While a threshold value of 0.75 for the edema-to-plasma protein ratio may indicate that injury is present, there is no evidence that the actual value above 0.75 will correlate with the *severity* of injury to the alveolar-capillary membrane. However, since injury interferes with the size selectivity of the endothelial barrier, an analysis of the edema fluid composition for protein size might indicate greater injury as size selectivity was lost (75,76). Once again, greatest specificity would be expected at early times after the onset of pulmonary edema, since alveolar proteins are also cleared in a size-dependent fashion (77).

A modification to direct sampling is to obtain the edema fluid via bronchoalveolar lavage. With this approach, three to five aliquots of 30 to 50 mL

Table 10 Limitations of Direct Sampling of Alveolar Edema to Evaluate Lung Injury

- Can be difficult to reliably obtain fluid
- Can only be performed in intubated patients
- Most accurate when performed within several hours of onset of injury
- Not useful as an index of severity of injury
- Results not specific for lung injury associated with ARDS

saline are instilled either via a blindly positioned catheter (72) or via a bronchoscope positioned under direct visualization (78–80). Although most studies report that the protein concentration in BAL fluid of ARDS patients is higher than that in non-ARDS patients (78–80), the sensitivity and specificity of this approach have never been determined. It might be predicted that both would suffer because it would be nearly impossible to control for the effects of dilution caused by BAL, in different studies or patients.

A problem with all these studies is that the test (i.e., protein concentration of alveolar edema fluid) has not been applied to an unselected and unbiased group of patients with pulmonary edema. Rather, patients are *first* chosen because they fit preconceived clinical criteria for heart failure, volume overload, lung injury, etc., and *then* the results of the edema fluid are analyzed in these predetermined groups. This methodologic approach obscures the true sensitivity and specificity (and thus the positive and negative predictive values) of the method. Nevertheless, a finding that the edema-to-plasma protein concentration ratio is high is strong evidence that some degree of lung injury is present.

D. Indicator-Dilution Methods

This class of techniques can be used to evaluate permeability across the endothelial barrier as well as *EVLW* (16). As with other indicator-dilution methods, a diffusible and a nondiffusible indicator are injected simultaneously into the right atrium; blood is then sampled from an arterial site after a single pass of the indicators through the lungs. The choice of diffusible indicator is the key to success when using this approach. Indicators that are freely diffusible (such as the thermal indicator used to measure extravascular lung water) are fully extracted during a single pass through the lung (defined as having the same concentration in extravascular and capillary blood). Therefore, the endothelium does not provide a barrier to the uptake of that indicator; its uptake is limited strictly by how much is delivered—i.e., its uptake is "flow-limited." In contrast, the uptake through the lungs of indicators such as albumin are so limited during a single pass, even in the presence of lung injury, that they are better used as vascular indicators.

The uptake of molecules such as urea, however, are significantly but not wholly restricted during a single pass, especially when compared to the extraction of albumin or other vascular indicators. Since the uptake of urea is limited by its permeability across the endothelium (i.e., it is "barrier-limited"), it can be used to evaluate changes in vascular permeability as a result of acute injury.

To implement methods of this type, time-activity curves are generated after simultaneously injecting radioactively labeled indicators such as albumin and urea. These data are then interpreted mathematically, using one of several appropriate models of the pulmonary microcirculation. The model developed by Crone is certainly one of the most commonly used (16). Its mathematical expression is:

$$PS = -\dot{Q}\ln\,[1 - E(t)] \tag{5}$$

where PS = the permeability-surface area product, $\dot{Q}$ is blood flow through the lung (i.e., cardiac output), and $E(t)$ is the instantaneous extraction ratio of the diffusible indicator compared to the nondiffusible indicator. In this equation, the term "*PS*" is identical to that conceptualized in Equation 2.

More complicated models are possible (16); these usually account for backdiffusion of the diffusible indicator during its passage through the lung and for nonhomogeneous pulmonary perfusion, both of which can affect the time-concentration curves used for analysis.

There are several important problems when using indicator dilution methods to evaluate vascular permeability, especially in the clinical setting (Table 11). For one, the method is inherently invasive since both the central venous and peripheral arterial circulations must be cannulated. Second, the method quantifies permeability to small molecules like urea, not plasma proteins like albumin, which, because of their effect on oncotic pressure, are more relevant to understanding how and when pulmonary edema develops. Finally, *PS* measurements by indicator dilution techniques are quite sensitive to changes in vascular surface area; unfortunately, these are quite common during lung injury. Perhaps this is why some patients with obvious acute lung injury (ARDS) do not have an elevated *PS* when measured by these methods (81). Possibly, vascular beds feeding the most injured lung regions have been derecruited, leaving relatively more normal beds to be perfused by the injected indicators. Interestingly, these same patients (clinically apparent ARDS but normal *PS*) have a better prognosis than those with a measured elevation in *PS*, suggesting that vascular derecruitment may in some way affect outcome, possibly by changing the accumulation or resolution of edema (81). In any case, given these problems, indicator-dilution methods are not commonly used, even in research settings, to detect or quantify lung injury at the present time.

Table 11 Limitations of Indicator Dilution Methods to Evaluate Lung Injury

- Requires invasive instrumentation
- Requires cumbersome off-line determinations of time-concentration profiles
- Complex modeling required to account for back-diffusion of indicator
- Highly sensitive to changes in vascular surface area
- Specificity of results uncertain

E. Radioaerosol Inhalation

While lung injury may begin with a breakdown in the barrier function of the *endothelium,* it invariably progresses to include alveolar damage by the time patients present with ARDS. Therefore, attempts have been made to specifically evaluate the integrity of the alveolar epithelium as well as the endothelium. In one sense, simply documenting that the protein concentration of alveolar edema fluid is higher than that expected with hydrostatic forms of pulmonary edema (Sec. III.B) is evidence that alveolar as well as endothelial integrity has been compromised.

Another, more quantitative approach involves first administering, by inhalation, a radioactively labeled tracer as an aerosol (17). The clearance of tracer activity from the lung is then measured, usually with some external radiation detection system such as a gamma camera. Since the alveolar epithelium is normally virtually impenetrable to macromolecules, clearance of the tracer from the alveolar space is expected to be quite slow. Any significant increase in the rate of clearance, then, would be evidence for altered epithelial integrity.

Unfortunately, many unsolved problems limit the value of this approach, including inefficient delivery of tracer, inability to ensure tracer delivery to the most injured (and thus, often, the most poorly ventilated) areas, inability to quantify the amount of tracer delivered, instability of some radioactive labels on some tracers, and uncertainty about the site of clearance (e.g., airway vs. alveolus) (17) (Table 12). Most problematic of all, changes in lung inflation alone (as with positive end-expiratory pressure), for reasons which are obscure, can increase clearance rates to levels that are indistinguishable from those observed in ARDS patients (17). Smoking in otherwise healthy individuals produces a similar result (82). As a result of these various problems, this approach to quantifying lung injury is now rarely used.

F. Radioactive Tracers in Blood

Without question, measuring the time-dependent accumulation of an intravenously administered, radioactively labeled protein tracer into lung tissue is the

Table 12 Limitations of Radioaerosol Methods to Evaluate Lung Injury

- Tracer delivery to injured lung regions difficult to quantify
- Some radioactive labels unstable
- Site of clearance uncertain
- Sensitive to changes in lung inflation
- Sensitive to effects of tobacco smoking
- Results not specific for lung injury associated with ARDS

most common clinical method of determining whether the integrity of the capillary endothelial barrier has been compromised (2,83). Both albumin and transferrin (with approximately comparable molecular weights) have been used as protein tracers; technetium-99m, gallium-68, and indium-113m have been used as the radioactive labels.

After the radioactive tracer is injected intravenously, activity within lung tissue is detected and recorded for minutes to hours with one of several kinds of external radiation detection devices: probes, gamma cameras, or PET cameras have all been used successfully. Since these devices cannot distinguish whether activity within the lung tissue originates from the blood or extravascular space, similar time-activity data must be simultaneously obtained from the blood, either by measuring activity within the cardiac blood pool of the right or left ventricle with the same external detection system, or by measuring the protein activity in separately obtained blood samples (83,84). The blood volume within the lung tissue region of interest must also be determined, either by using a single protein tracer and assuming that all the protein activity at the beginning of the data collection period is intravascular (in which case one must also assume that intravascular volume does not change during the data collection period), or by using a second tracer which can be assumed to remain intravascular (usually, radioactively labeled blood cells). The former option is the one adopted during PET imaging since only one tracer can be administered at a time with this technique (42). The latter option, used during methods that employ other detection devices, is theoretically attractive since changes in intravascular volume during the data collection period can also be monitored (usually about 1 to 2 hours) (83). However, there is little reason to believe that intravascular volume in fact changes in a unidirectional manner during this brief period of time in clinically stable subjects.

Intuitively, as the microvascular barrier becomes more "leaky" to macromolecules like albumin, the rate of labeled albumin accumulation within the lung should increase (Fig. 12). This intuitive notion can be made explicit by analyzing the time-activity data as if they represented the transfer of labeled tracer between vascular and extravascular compartments. The movement of tracer between these two compartments can be represented mathematically:

$$Q(t) = [V_b B\mathrm{l}(t)] + [K_1 B\mathrm{l}(t) * e^{-k_2 t}] \tag{6}$$

where $Q(t)$ = the time-dependent amount of activity in the lung tissue (vascular plus extravascular compartments; V_b = the blood volume in the same lung tissue region; $Bl(t)$ = the time-dependent concentration of activity in blood within the lung tissue region; K_1 is equivalent to PS; and k_2 is the rate constant for activity moving from extravascular to vascular compartments (85,86).

In this model, the term K_1 (or "PS") is again identical to the same term in Equation 2. When PS is divided by the blood volume (or plasma volume, if one knows the hematocrit) within the lung region under the radiation detector

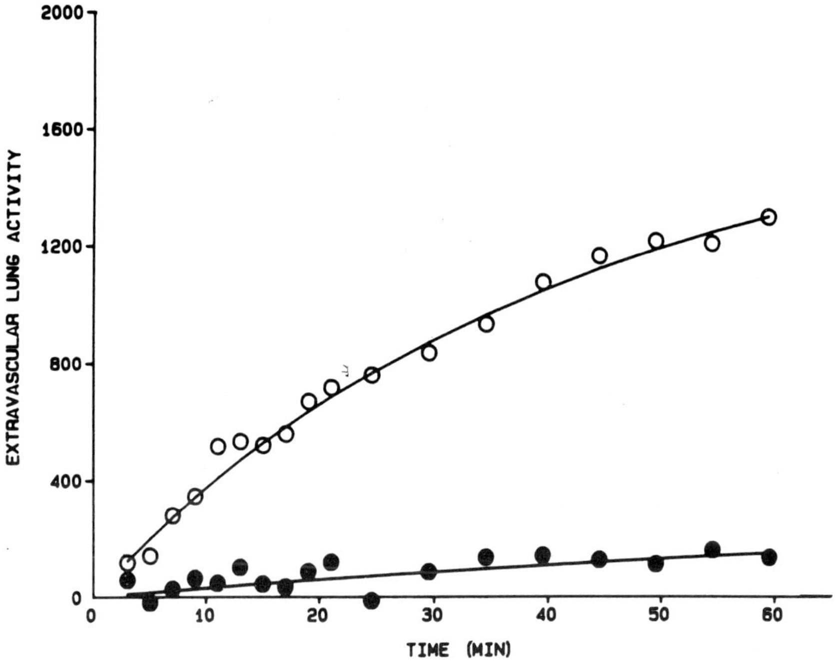

Figure 12 Illustration of the difference in the accumulation of an intravenously administered radiolabeled protein within the extravascular space of the lung under normal conditions (filled circles) and in a patient with ARDS (open circles). The greater rate of increase in the ARDS patient can be expressed mathematically as a higher value for the pulmonary transcapillary escape rate (PTCER), implying increased pulmonary vascular "permeability." (From Ref. 95.)

(83,85,86), the resulting term is referred to as the "pulmonary transcapillary escape rate" (PTCER = PS/V_b). When applied to the data in each pixel of a PET imaging study, the result is an image of pulmonary vascular "permeability." "PTCER" has the units of a rate constant (fractional time). PTCER can be derived by several different approaches mathematically by considering the mass balance of tracer between blood and lung tissue. After taking into account underlying assumptions, these various approaches are all essentially equivalent (83,85,86).

Theoretically, the measurement of *PS* should only reflect the movement of tracer by diffusion (i.e., flux due to concentration gradients, not pressure gradients, across a semipermeable membrane). However, the radioisotopic techniques used to measure PTCER (or equivalent indices) cannot in fact distinguish whether tracer movement is due to diffusion or convection ("bulk flow")

Table 13 Limitations of Using Bloodborne Radioactive Tracers to Evaluate Lung Injury

- Technology required ranges from simple to complex
- Mathematical analyses range from simple to complex
- Most methods are moderately to very expensive
- Accuracy depends on blood activity corrections
- Models usually assume passive (without convective) movement of tracer to extravascular space
- Results not specific for lung injury associated with ARDS

(Table 13). Therefore, hydrostatic pressure-driven increases in protein flux would also be detected by these techniques, and potentially misinterpreted as an increase in vascular permeability (implying, of course, that lung injury had developed). Theoretical simulation studies indicate that increased hydrostatic pressures should have little effect on indices of vascular permeability (83). However, more recent experimental evidence seems to challenge this view. Abernathy et al. (88) have shown that increased pressures *in a normal lung* will increase lymph flow more than protein flux, leading to the seemingly paradoxical result of *reduced* estimates for PTCER.

Fortunately, most (but not all) experimental studies have repeatedly shown that estimates of PTCER are *insensitive* to changes in hydrostatic pressure but are very sensitive to changes in membrane "porosity" (2,5,87). Tenfold increases in the estimate of PTCER have been measured in humans with ARDS with little or no increases detected in patients with heart failure (Fig. 13). However, whether increases in permeability and hydrostatic pressure might act synergistically to elevate PTCER has not been explored in similar detail. In addition, while increased protein flux due to increased vascular permeability may be a sine qua non of lung injury associated with ARDS, significant increases in protein flux occur in many other conditions not necessarily characterized by pulmonary edema (Fig. 13). Nevertheless, measurements of PTCER do correlate well with morphologic indices of injury (88). Thus, such measurements are a sensitive and probably accurate, even though nonspecific, marker of injury.

IV. Clinical Utility

Other than chest radiography, none of the other methods for measuring *EVLW* have been widely implemented. Even in the ICU, where necessary catheterization is often performed for clinical reasons, the indication-dilution method has not been widely incorporated into clinical practice. Undoubtedly, one reason is that no one has shown that a measurement of *EVLW* per se is needed for sound clinical decision making during the treatment of pulmonary edema; likewise, no

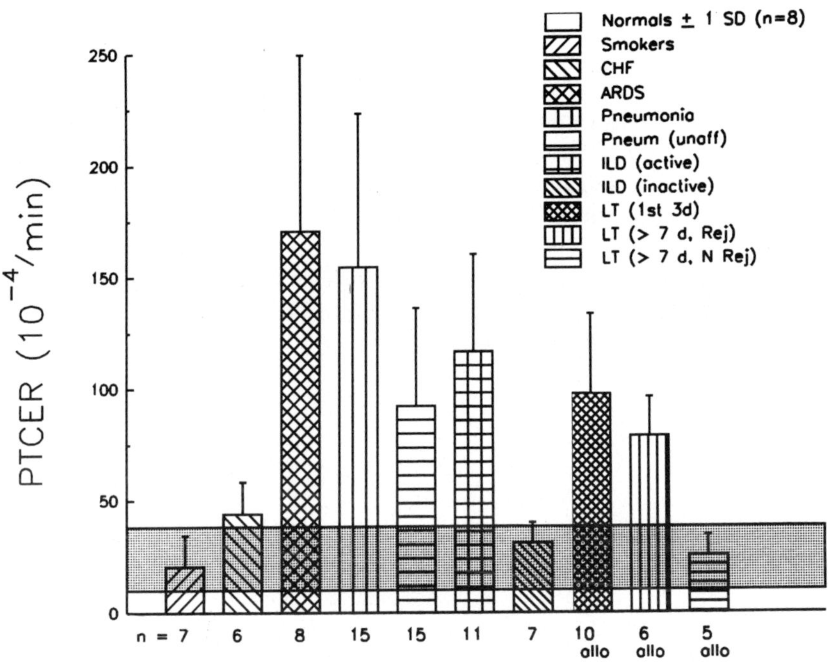

Figure 13 The pulmonary transcapillary escape rate (PTCER), an index of vascular permeability, in a variety of patient groups. Note that PTCER is in the same range of values measured in normal subjects as in the following groups of subjects: in smokers without acute illness; clinically inactive interstitial lung disease (ILD); in lung allografts (allo) in patients without clinical rejection (Rej) postlung transplantation (LT). PTCER is not significantly different from normal in patients with CHF. It is highest in patients with ARDS and in lung regions with lobar pneumonia. Other patient populations, including radiographically unaffected lung regions (unaff) in patients with pneumonia, have intermediate values. (From Ref. 2.)

one has shown that incorporating such methods into routine clinical practice will affect patient outcome. Although the *potential* value of having a quantitative measure of pulmonary edema seems obvious, and various studies have suggested how such measurements might be used in clinical decision making (57), a convincing outcome study demonstrating benefit is still needed.

Schuster and colleagues (56,89) used *EVLW* measurements in a prospective clinical trial of fluid restriction during severe pulmonary edema. They found that the fluid management protocol employed was associated with a significant decrease in *EVLW* during the time of the study compared to a control management group, and that this decrease in *EVLW* was also associated with significantly less time for mechanical ventilatory support and time in the ICU, and with favorable trends in mortality. Although this study has often been misinterpreted to mean that *EVLW* measurements should be incorporated into clinical practice, it actually shows that *EVLW* measurements might be a useful surrogate measure for mortality in clinical studies of therapy for pulmonary edema or ARDS.

At various times, some studies have found *EVLW* to correlate with prognosis (19,90), while others have not (56). Various studies have suggested that *EVLW* measurements might be useful in planning respiratory, diuretic, fluid, or other intensive care therapy (54,91,92) or in distinguishing the cause of chest x-ray infiltrates (e.g., pulmonary edema vs. atelectasis) (93). However, none of these studies have been conducted as randomized controlled trials, so the true magnitude of benefit remains in doubt.

Measurements of vascular permeability have never been incorporated into any clinical trial of therapy for pulmonary edema. It is possible that such measurements would be more useful for prognosis since they can potentially quantify severity of injury. It is possible that they might also be used as a treatment endpoint surrogate for mortality in clinical trials.

Perhaps the most immediate use of both *EVLW* and vascular permeability measurements would be to more precisely define ARDS. Based on data shown in Figures 10 and 13, it seems reasonable to suggest that ARDS could be defined as an $EVLW > 7$ mL/kg with a PTCER > four to five times the rate in normals. It would be interesting to determine whether prognosis, or outcome in clinical trials, would be more easily interpreted than data using current definitions (2).

References

1. Renkin E. Some consequences of capillary permeability to macromolecules: Starling's hypothesis reconsidered. Am J Physiol 1986; 250 (Heart Circ Physiol):H706–H710.
2. Schuster DP. What is acute lung injury? What is ARDS? Chest 1995; 107:1721–1726.
3. Kedem O, Katchalsky A. Thermodynamic analysis of the permeability of biological membranes to non-electrolytes. Biochim Biophys Acta 1958; 27:229–246.
4. Staub N. The pathogenesis of pulmonary edema. Prog Cardiovasc Dis 1980; 23: 53–80.
5. Matthay MA. Pathophysiology of pulmonary edema. Clin Chest Med 1985; 6: 301–314.
6. West JB, Mathieu-Costello O. Stress failure of pulmonary capillaries: role in lung and heart disease. Lancet 1992; 340:762–767.
7. West JB, Mathieu-Costello O. Stress failure of pulmonary capillaries in the intensive care setting. Schweizerische Medizinische Wochenschrift. J Suisse Med 1992; 122:751–757.
8. West JB, Mathieu-Costello O. Stress failure of pulmonary capillaries: role in lung and heart disease. Lancet 1992; 340:762–767.

9. West J, Mathieu-Costello O. Vulnerability of pulmonary capillaries in heart disease. Circulation 1995; 92:622–631.
10. Lewis FR, Elings VB, Sturm JA. Bedside measurement of lung water. J Surg Res 1979; 27:250–261.
11. Sivak ED, Starr NJ, Graves JW, Cosgrove DM, Borsh J, Estafanous FG. Extravascular lung water values in patients undergoing coronary artery bypass surgery. Crit Care Med 1982; 10:593–596.
12. Sibbald WJ, Warshawski FJ, Short AK, Harris J, Lefcoe MS, Holliday RL. Clinical studies of measuring extravascular lung water by the thermal dye technique in critically ill patients. Chest 1983; 83:725–731.
13. Gallagher JD, Moore RA, Kerns D, Jose AB, Botros SB, Clark DL. Effects of advanced age on extravascular lung water accumulation during coronary artery bypass surgery. Crit Care Med 1985; 13:68–71.
14. Bongard FS, Matthay M, Mackersie RC, Lewis FR. Morphologic and physiologic correlates of increased extravascular lung water. Surgery 1984; 96:395–403.
15. Taylor A, Townsley M, Korthuis R. Macromolecule transport across the pulmonary microvessel walls. Exp Lung Res 1985; 8:97–123.
16. Dawson C, Roerig D, Linehan J. Evaluation of endothelial injury in the human lung. Clin Chest Med 1989; 10:13–24.
17. Peterson BT. Permeability: theory vs. practice in lung research. Am J Physiol 1992; 262:L243–L256.
18. Cope D, Grimbert F, Downey J, Taylor A. Pulmonary capillary pressure: a review. Crit Care Med 1992; 20:1043.
19. Sturm J. Development and significance of lung water measurement in clinical and experimental practice. In: Lewis F, Pfeiffer U, eds. Practical Applications of Fiberoptics in Critical Care Monitoring. Berlin: Springer-Verlag, 1990:129–139.
20. Pearce M, Yamashita J, Beazell B. Measurement of pulmonary edema. Circ Res 1965; 16:482–488.
21. Vincent D, Lefort J, Bureau M, Dry J, Vargaftig BB. Dissociation between LPS-induced bronchial hyperreactivity and airway edema in the guinea-pig. Agents Actions 1991; 34:203–204.
22. Staub N. Pulmonary edema. Physiol Rev 1974; 54:678.
23. Julien M, Flick MR, Hoeffel JM, Murray JF. Accurate reference measurement for postmortem lung water. J Appl Physiol 1984; 56:248–253.
24. Matthay MA, Folkesson HG, Campagna A, Kheradmand F. Alveolar epithelial barrier and acute lung injury. New Horizons 1993; 1:613–622.
25. Snashall PD, Keyes SJ, Morgan BM, et al. The radiographic detection of acute pulmonary oedema. A comparison of radiographic appearances, densitometry and lung water in dogs. Br J Radiol 1981; 54:277–288.
26. Gattinoni L, Presenti A, Torresin A, et al. Adult respiratory distress syndrome profiles by computed tomography. J Thorac Imag 1986; 1:25–30.
27. Wheeler AP, Carroll FE, Bernard GR. Radiographic issues in adult respiratory distress syndrome. New Horizons 1993; 1:471–477.
28. Halperin B, Feeley T, Mihm F, Chiles C, Guthaner D, Blank N. Evaluation of the portable chest roentgenogram for quantitating extravascular lung water in critically ill adults. Chest 1985; 88:649–652.

29. Hedlund LW, Vock P, Effmann EL, Lischko MM, Putman CE. Hydrostatic pulmonary edema. An analysis of lung density changes by computed tomography. Invest Radiol 1984; 19:254–262.
30. Forster BB, Muller NL, Mayo JR, Okazawa M, Wiggs BJ, Pare PD. High-resolution computed tomography of experimental hydrostatic pulmonary edema. Chest 1992; 101:1434–1437.
31. Mayo JR. Magnetic resonance imaging of the chest. Where we stand. Radiol Clin North Am 1994; 32:795–809.
32. Cutillo AG, Morris AH, Ailion DC, et al. Assessment of lung water distribution by nuclear magnetic resonance. A new method for quantifying and monitoring experimental lung injury. Am Rev Respir Dis 1988; 137:1371–1378.
33. Morris AH, Blatter DD, Case TA, et al. A new nuclear magnetic resonance property of lung. J Appl Physiol 1985; 58:759–762.
34. Cutillo AG, Morris AH, Ailion DC, Durney CH, Case TA. Determination of lung water content and distribution by nuclear magnetic resonance imaging. J Thorac Imag 1986; 1:39–51.
35. Mayo JR, Muller NL, Forster BB, Okazawa M, Pare PD. Magnetic resonance imaging of hydrostatic pulmonary edema in isolated dog lungs: comparison with computed tomography. Can Assoc Radiol J 1990; 41:281–286.
36. Wexler HR, Nicholson RL, Prato FS, Carey LS, Vinitski S, Reese L. Quantitation of lung water by nuclear magnetic resonance imaging. A preliminary study. Invest Radiol 1985; 20:583–590.
37. Phillips DM, Allen PS, Man SF. Assessment of temporal changes in pulmonary edema with NMR imaging. J Appl Physiol 1989; 66:1197–1208.
38. Rhodes CG. Measurement of lung water using nuclear magnetic resonance imaging. Br J Radiol 1986; 59:1135–1136. Letter.
39. Cutillo A, Goodrich K, Krishnamurthy G, et al. Lung water measurement by nuclear magnetic resonance: correlation with morphometry. J Appl Physiol 1995; 79:2163–2168.
40. Mayo JR, MacKay AL, Whittall KP, Baile EM, Pare PD. Measurement of lung water content and pleural pressure gradient with magnetic resonance imaging. J Thorac Imag 1995; 10:73–81.
41. Cutillo AG, Goodrich KC, Ganesan K, et al. Alveolar air/tissue interface and nuclear magnetic resonance behavior of normal and edematous lungs. Am J Respir Crit Care Med 1995; 151:1018–1026.
42. Schuster DP. Positron emission tomography: theory and its application to the study of lung disease. Am Rev Respir Dis 1989; 139:818–840.
43. Schuster DP, Marklin GF, Mintun MA, Ter-Pogossian MM. PET measurement of regional lung density: 1. J Comput Assist Tomogr 1986; 10:723–729.
44. Rhodes C, Hughes JMB. Pulmonary studies using positron emission tomography. Eur Respir J 1995; 8:1001–1017.
45. Schuster DP, Mintun MA, Green MA, Ter-Pogossian MM. Regional lung water and hematocrit determined by positron emission tomography. J App Physiol 1985; 59:860–868.
46. Schuster DP, Marklin GF, Mintun MA. Regional changes in extravascular lung water detected by positron emission tomography. J Appl Physiol 1986; 60:1170–1178.

47. Velazquez M, Haller J, Amundsen T, Schuster DP. Regional lung water measurements with PET: accuracy, reproducibility, and linearity. J Nucl Med 1991; 32: 719–725.
48. Effros RM. Lung water measurements with the mean transit time approach. J Appl Physiol 1985; 59:673–683.
49. Sivak ED, Wiedemann HP. Clinical measurement of extravascular lung water. Crit Care Clin 1986; 2:511–526.
50. Allison RC, Carlile PV Jr, Gray BA. Thermodilution measurement of lung water. Clin Chest Med 1985; 6:439–457.
51. Pfeiffer U, Backus G, Blumel G, et al. A fiberoptics based system for integrated monitoring of cardiac output, intrathoracic blood volume, extravascular lung water, O_2 saturation, and a-v differences. In: Lewis F, Pfeiffer U, eds. Practical Applications of Fiberoptics in Critical Care Monitoring. Berlin: Springer-Verlag, 1990: 114–125.
52. Wickerts CJ, Jakobsson J, Frostell C, Hedenstierna G. Measurement of extravascular lung water by thermal-dye dilution technique: mechanisms of cardiac output dependence. Intens Care Med 1990; 16:115–120.
53. Fallon KD, Drake RE, Laine GA, Gabel JC. Effect of cardiac output on extravascular lung water estimates made with the Edwards lung water computer. Anesthesiol 1985; 62:505–508.
54. Zeravik J, Borg U, Pfeiffer UJ. Efficacy of pressure support ventilation dependent on extravascular lung water. Chest 1990; 97:1412–1419.
55. Schuster DP, Calandrino FS. Single versus double indicator dilution measurements of extravascular lung water. Crit Care Med 1991; 19:84–88.
56. Mitchell JP, Schuller D, Calandrino FS, Schuster DP. Improved outcome based on fluid management in critically ill patients requiring pulmonary artery catheterization. Am Rev Respir Dis 1992; 145:990–998.
57. Bock JC, Lewis FR. Clinical relevance of lung water measurement with the thermal-dye dilution technique. J Surg Res 1990; 48:254–265.
58. Laggner AN, Lenz K, Druml W, Kleinberger G. Reproducibility of thermal-dye lung water measurements by a lung water computer in critically ill patients. Crit Care Med 1987; 15:606–608.
59. Mihm FG, Feeley TW, Jamieson SW. Thermal dye double indicator dilution measurement of lung water in man: comparison with gravimetric measurements. Thorax 1987; 42:72–76.
60. Sibbald WJ, Short AK, Warshawski FJ, Cunningham DG, Cheung H. Thermal dye measurements of extravascular lung water in critically ill patients. Intravascular Starling forces and extravascular lung water in the adult respiratory distress syndrome. Chest 1985; 87:585–592.
61. Haider M, Schad H. Effect of positive end-expiratory airway pressure (PEEP) on extravascular thermal lung water estimation in the dog. In: Lewis F, Pfeiffer U, eds. Practical Applications of Fiberoptics in Critical Care Monitoring. Berlin: Springer-Verlag, 1990:96–104.
62. Bock J, Deuflhard P, Hoeft A, et al. Thermal recovery after passage of the pulmonary circulation assessed by deconvolution. J Appl Physiol 1988; 64:1210–1216.

63. Newman E, Merrell M, Genecin A, Monge C, Milnor W, McKeever W. The dye dilution method for describing the central circulation. An analysis of factors shaping the time-concentration curves. Circ 1951; 4:735–746.
64. Ramsey L, Puckett W, Jose A, Lacy W. Comparison of slope and mean transit time volumes by use of diffusible and non-diffusible indicators. Trans Assoc Am Phys 1961; 74:280–289.
65. Elings VB, Lewis FR. A single indicator technique to estimate extravascular lung water. J Surg Res 1982; 33:375–385.
66. Baudendistel LJ, Kaminski DL, Dahms TE. Evaluation of extravascular lung water by single thermal indicator. Crit Care Med 1986; 14:52–56.
67. Tagawa M, Okano S, Hara Y, et al. Evaluation of extravascular thermal volume in the lung in dogs with endotoxin-induced shock by double indicator dilution method using heat and sodium ions. J Vet Med Sci 1993; 55:87–91.
68. Arakawa M, Kambara K, Segawa T, Ando F, Kawada T, Ohno M. Usefulness of sodium chloride as a nondiffusible indicator in the measurement of extravascular lung thermal volume in dogs. Med Biol Eng Comput 1993; 31:S67–S72.
69. Parker R. Sheep as an Animal Model of Endotoxemia-Induced Diffuse Lung Injury. Handbook of Animal Models of Pulmonary Disease. Vol. I. Baton Rouge: CRC Press, 1989:31–46.
70. Drake RE, Laine GA. Pulmonary microvascular permeability to fluid and macromolecules. J Appl Physiol 1988; 64:487–501.
71. Matthay MA, Eschenbacher WL, Goetzl EJ. Elevated concentrations of leukotriene D4 in pulmonary edema fluid of patients with the adult respiratory distress syndrome. J Clin Immunol 1984; 4:479–483.
72. Matthay MA, Wiener-Kronish JP. Intact epithelial barrier function is critical for the resolution of alveolar edema in humans. Am Rev Respir Dis 1990; 142: 1250–1257.
73. Fein A, Grossman RF, Jones JG, et al. The value of edema fluid protein measurement in patients with pulmonary edema. Am J Med 1979; 67:32–38.
74. Sprung CL, Rackow EC, Fein IA, Jacob AI, Isikoff SK. The spectrum of pulmonary edema: differentiation of cardiogenic intermediate noncardiogenic forms of pulmonary edema. Am Rev Respir Dis 1981; 124:718–722.
75. Sprung CL, Long WM, Marcial EH, et al. Distribution of proteins in pulmonary edema. The value of fractional concentrations. Am Rev Respir Dis 1987; 136: 957–963.
76. Holter JF, Weiland JE, Pacht ER, Gadek JE, Davis WB. Protein permeability in the adult respiratory distress syndrome. Loss of size selectivity of the alveolar epithelium. J Clin Invest 1986; 78:1513–1522.
77. Hastings RH, Grady M, Sakuma T, Matthay MA. Clearance of different-sized proteins from the alveolar space in humans and rabbits. J Appl Physiol 1992; 73:1310–1316.
78. Steinberg K, Mitchell D, Maunder R, Milberg J, Whitcomb M, Hudson L. Safety of bronchoalveolar lavage in patients with the adult respiratory distress syndrome. Am Rev Respir Dis 1993; 148:556–561.
79. Steinberg K, Milberg J, Martin TRJM, Cockrill B, Hudson L. Evolution of bronchoalveolar cell populations in the adult respiratory distress syndrome. Am J Respir Crit Care Med 1994; 150:113–122.

80. Clark J, Milberg J, Steinberg K, Hudson L. Type III procollagen peptide in the adult respiratory distress syndrome: association of increased peptide levels in bronchoalveolar lavage fluid with increased risk for death. Ann Intern Med 1995; 1223: 17–23.
81. Harris T, Bernard G, Brigham K, et al. Lung microvascular transport properties measured by multiple indicator dilution methods in patients with adult respiratory distress syndrome: a comparison between patients reversing respiratory failure and those failing to reverse. Am Rev Respir Dis 1990; 141:272–280.
82. Effros RM, Mason GR, Mena I. ^{99m}Tc-DTPA aerosol deposition and clearance in COPD, interstitial disease, and smokers. J Thorac Imag 1986; 1:54–60.
83. Roselli RJ, Riddle WR. Analysis of noninvasive macromolecular transport measurements in the lung. J Appl Physiol 1989; 67:2343–2350.
84. Roselli R, Harris T. Lung fluid and macromolecular transport. In: Chang HK, Paiva M, eds. Respiratory physiology: an analytical approach. New York: Marcel Dekker, 1989:633.
85. Mintun MA, Dennis DR, Welch MJ, Mathias CJ, Schuster DP. Measurements of pulmonary vascular permeability with PET and gallium-68 transferrin. J Nucl Med 1987; 28:1704–1716.
86. Mintun MA, Warfel TE, Schuster DP. Evaluating pulmonary vascular permeability with radiolabeled proteins: an error analysis. J Appl Physiol 1990; 68:1696–1706.
87. Abernathy VJ, Pou NA, Wilson TL, Roselli RJ. Noninvasive measurements of albumin flux into lung interstitium with increased microvascular pressure. Am J Physiol 1995; 269:H288–H296.
88. Velazquez M, Weibel ER, Kuhn CD, Schuster DP. PET evaluation of pulmonary vascular permeability: a structure-function correlation. J Appl Physiol 1991; 70: 2206–2216.
89. Schuller D, Mitchell JP, Calandrino FS, Schuster DP. Fluid balance during pulmonary edema. Is fluid gain a marker or a cause of poor outcome? Chest 1991; 100:1068–1075.
90. Eisenberg PR, Hansbrough JR, Anderson D, Schuster DP. A prospective study of lung water measurements during patient management in an intensive care unit. Am Rev Respir Dis 1987; 136:662–668.
91. Laggner A, Lenz K. Lung water measurement for control of therapeutic interventions in critically ill patients. In: Lewis F, Pfeiffer U, eds. Practical Applications of Fiberoptics in Critical Care Monitoring. Berlin: Springer-Verlag, 1990:143–149.
92. Zeravik J, Eckart J, Zimmermann G, Pfeiffer U. Determination of extravascular lung water may facilitate respiratory therapy decision making. In: Lewis F, Pfeiffer U, eds. Practical Applications of Fiberoptics in Critical Care Monitoring. Berlin: Springer-Verlag, 1990:157–163.
93. Sivak E, Richmond R, O'Donoavan P, Borokowski G. Value of extravascular lung water measurements vs portable chest x-ray in the management of pulmonary edema. Crit Care Med 1983; 11:498–501.
94. Calandrino FS Jr, Anderson DJ, Mintun MA, Schuster DP. Pulmonary vascular permeability during the adult respiratory distress syndrome: a positron emission tomographic study. Am Rev Respir Dis 1988; 138:421–428.
95. Edelman RR, Hesselink JR, eds. Clinical Magnetic Resonance Imaging, Part 1—Physics and Instrumentation. Philadelphia: W.B. Saunders, 1990:20.

5

Hydrostatic Pulmonary Edema

MARY I. TOWNSLEY

University of South Alabama
Mobile, Alabama

I. Introduction

In the lung, the capillaries are arranged in an eccentric fashion along the alveolar septa, such that the alveolocapillary barrier forms both thin and thick sections, with an average thickness throughout of ~1 μm (1). Gas exchange is thought to occur primarily on the thinner side of the alveolar septum, where the endothelia and alveolar epithelial layers are separated only by their fused basement membranes. On the thicker side of the alveolocapillary barrier, the basal laminae of the endothelium and alveolar epithelium are separate, forming a finite interstitial space containing the structural elements of the septal wall (2). These features are illustrated in Figure 1. Figure 1A, a transmission electron micrograph of normal canine lung fixed by vascular perfusion, shows clearly the attenuated alveolocapillary barrier and minimal interstitial space (3). Fluid filters across the septal endothelium into the adjacent interstitium, and then percolates through the interstitium to enter initial lymphatics. Interstitial edema forms when an imbalance exists between the rate of fluid filtration (J_v) into the pulmonary interstitium and the rate of fluid exit via the lymphatic system (4–6). Figure 1B, taken from a dog after 1 month of pacing-induced heart with its associated pulmonary venous hypertension, highlights the interstitial thickening that occurs

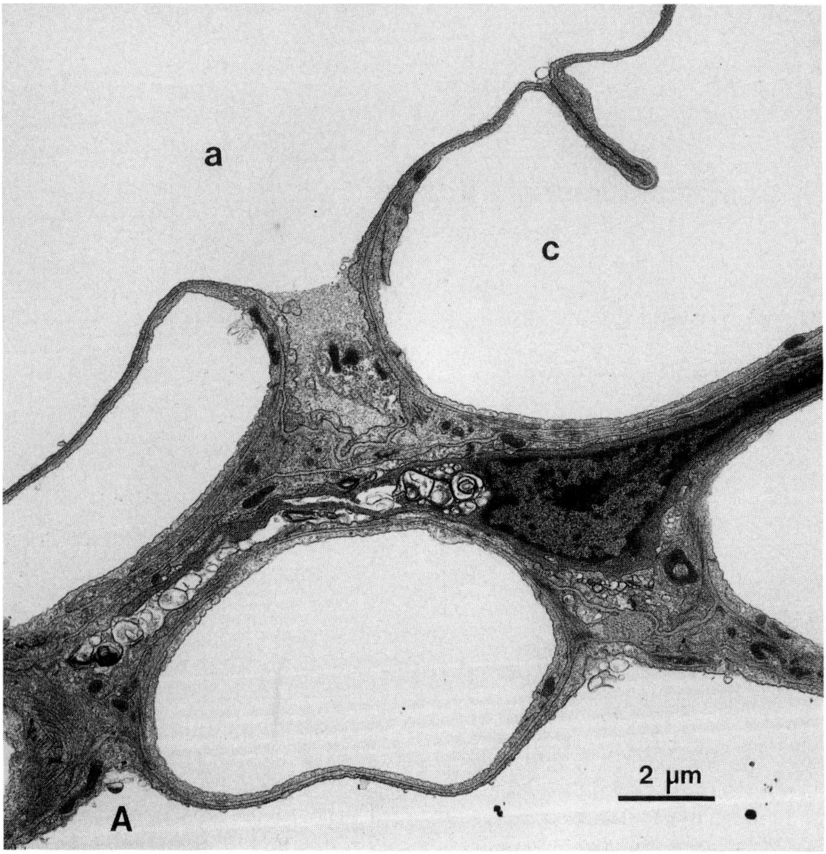

Figure 1 Electron micrographs of representative portions of the alveolar septum from control dogs (A) and those with heart failure and pulmonary venous hypertension induced by rapid ventricular pacing for 1 month (B). In each case, lung lobes were fixed by vascular perfusion at 23 cm H_2O venous pressure. After pacing, the interstitium was thickened, indicating the presence of hydrostatic edema. a, Alveolar air space; c, septal capillary lumen; i, interstitial space. (From Ref. 3.)

with hydrostatic pulmonary edema. If this scenario progresses to alveolar flooding, gas exchange is compromised.

The starting point in this chain of edemogenic events is the filtration of fluid from the intravascular to interstitial space in the lung. The magnitude of this fluid movement is dependent upon the net balance of forces across the

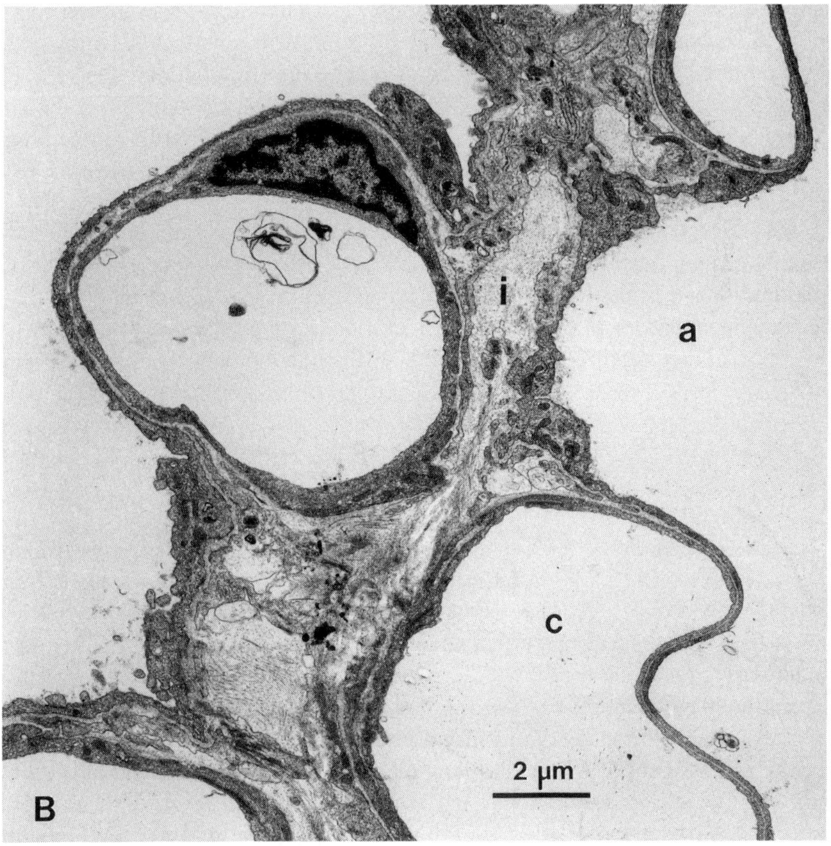

capillary barrier and capillary endothelial integrity (i.e., microvascular permeability):

$$J_v = K_{f,c}[(P_c - P_t) - \sigma_d(\pi_p - \pi_t)] \quad (1)$$

The rate of transcapillary fluid movement (J_v) is dictated by the "Starling forces": pulmonary capillary pressure (P_c), interstitial fluid pressure (P_t), and the plasma and interstitial colloid osmotic pressures (π_p and π_t, respectively). The capillary filtration coefficient ($K_{f,c}$) is the product of the endothelial hydraulic conductance (L_p) and the pulmonary capillary filtration surface area (S). Together $K_{f,c}$ and the osmotic reflection coefficient (σ_d), which describes the endothelial selectivity for total proteins, dictate the effectiveness of the transcapillary forces (4–6). From Equation 1, it is clear to see that the net Starling force balance $[(P_c - P_t) - \sigma_d (\pi_p - \pi_t)]$ represents an effective hydrostatic force promoting fluid filtration into lung interstitium. In addition, since $K_{f,c}$ is proportional to the amount of perfused exchange area in the lung (7), it should be clear that the transcapillary filtration rate can vary significantly in the lung as filtration area is recruited or derecruited. This will be true even when the net Starling force balance is constant.

Though it may not be immediately obvious, the magnitude of the transvascular protein flux (J_s) is also pertinent to this discussion of hydrostatic edema. J_s is determined in part by fluid flux which carries proteins convectively across the exchange barrier and by diffusive exchange of protein, as described in the relation first derived by Patlak et al. (8) and modified by Granger and Taylor (9):

$$J_s = \underbrace{J_v \cdot (1 - \sigma_f) \cdot C_p}_{\textit{convective flux}} + \underbrace{PS \cdot (C_p - C_t) \cdot \frac{x}{e^x - 1}}_{\textit{diffusive flux}} \tag{2}$$

σ_f is also a reflection coefficient, specifically describing the ease with which macromolecules can move in bulk flow through the membrane (a solvent drag reflection coefficient). As transcapillary fluid flow increases, σ_f approaches σ_d and at high flows the two coefficients are essentially the same (5,6,10,11). For simplicity, only a composite σ will be referred to subsequently. The permeability surface area product (PS) is the third coefficient which describes the barrier integrity, where P defines the diffusive permeability for a macromolecule. The remaining undefined variables in Equation 2 are the plasma (C_p) and interstitial fluid (C_t) protein concentrations, and the Peclet number (x), a dimensionless number describing the relative contribution of diffusive *vs* convective protein flux. The rate of protein transfer into interstitium (Eq. 2) relative to that of fluid (Eq. 1) will affect the interstitial fluid protein concentration and thus impact upon the transcapillary colloid osmotic gradient, $\sigma(\pi_p - \pi_t)$. Both the convective and diffusive components of protein flux likely contribute significantly at normal, resting pulmonary capillary pressure. However, with acute venous hypertension and the attendant increase in transvascular fluid flux, diffusive exchange dissipates and convective protein flux dominates (for a thorough review, see Reed et al. [10]). This latter effect will be particularly pertinent to the later discussion of how hydrostatic and permeability edema can be differentiated in the clinical setting.

Hydrostatic edema is specifically the result of an imbalance in the Starling forces operating across the pulmonary capillary endothelial barrier. However, many forms of lung injury are complicated by an increase in the net hydrostatic filtration force across the pulmonary exchange barrier. In this chapter an attempt will be made to dissect out these hydrostatic contributions to pulmonary edema formation. The discussion will address structures influencing fluid movement, assess the various physical factors and forces involved, contrast acute and chronic hydrostatic edema, and review the available methodologies which can be used to discriminate between hydrostatic and permeability pulmonary edema.

II. Critical Structures and Forces

A. Vascular Space—P_c and π_p

The two intravascular forces, P_c and π_p, normally oppose each other with respect to transvascular fluid filtration (see Eq. 1). P_c is dictated by the distribution of vascular resistance and compliance in the lung. A simple model of the pulmonary vasculature incorporates two resistors in series (arterial and venous resistance) and a compliance dominated by that in the capillary bed (12). Pappenheimer and Soto-Rivera (13) first showed that P_c could be calculated if the arterial (P_a) and venous (P_v) pressures, as well as the arterial (R_a) and venous (R_v) resistances of a vascular bed are known:

$$P_c = P_v + \left[\frac{R_v}{R_a + R_v} \cdot (P_a - P_v)\right] \tag{3}$$

Gaar et al. (14) first applied this relation to the isolated blood-perfused canine lung, and determined that ~40% of the total pulmonary vascular resistance was in the venous compartment. Though use of Equation 3 has been largely supplanted by direct measurement of P_c in lung (see Sec. IV), the calculation remains useful to at least estimate P_c when it cannot be directly measured or retrospectively from data in the literature. Increases in P_c induced by varied perturbations are shown in Table 1. This compilation is not meant to be exhaustive, but to highlight the fact that the intravascular filtration pressure can be increased in a number of scenarios, some long recognized and some perhaps unappreciated to date. Equation 3 predicts that if R_v increases in the lung, P_c will increase as well. Indeed this has been shown in numerous studies. Histamine, norepinephrine, and serotonin in the canine lung, for example, are effective venoconstrictor agents (15). In addition to direct vasoconstriction, one should appreciate that if blood flow through the lung (Q_b) increases, either cardiac output in vivo or perfusion flow in isolated lungs, P_c will increase even if R_v remains unchanged. This can be shown by a rearrangement of Eq. 3:

$$P_c = P_v + R_v \cdot \frac{(P_a - P_v)}{R_t} \tag{4}$$

$$P_c = P_v + R_v \cdot Q_b \tag{5}$$

The contribution of flow-induced increases in P_c is illustrated by estimates of P_c in dogs after lung resection, where flow to the remaining lung is increased

Table 1 Comparison of Changes in Pulmonary Capillary Filtration Pressure (P_c) with Active Vasoconstriction, Venous Hypertension, and Lung Injury

Model	Paradigm	Baseline	Treatment	Reference
Change in hydrostatic forces				
Dog, IL	Histamine	10.0	30.7	15
	NE	9.9	18.8	
	Serotonin	9.9	21.3	
Dog, IL	Arachidonic acid		ΔP_c15.3	185
Dog, IL	PGE_2		ΔP_c18.9	186
	$PGF_{1\alpha}$		ΔP_c12.5	
Dog, IL	NE vs. NE after propranolol			19
	—controls	ΔP_c6.2	ΔP_c8.6	
	—after heart failure	ΔP_c11.2	ΔP_c16.0	
Dog	Neurogenic pulmonary edema	10.1[a]	44.9[a]	167
Dog	Cocaine-induced edema	12.6[a]	25.0[a]	187
Rabbit	Hydrostatic edema	8.6	9.8	47
Sheep	Bicuculline seizures	15.2[a]	56.0[a]	188
Sheep	Exercise	7.3	13.9	17
	Hypoxia vs. hypoxia plus exercise	5.1	7.5	
Sheep	Overperfusion (lung resection)	12.0[a]	19.0[a]	16
	Overperfusion and hypoxia	11.9[a]	19.4[a]	
Human	Coronary artery bypass	24.9	26.1	189
	Aortic valve replacement	30.9	24.1	
	Mitral valve replacement	36.4	38.8	
Human	Renal transplant—predialysis		34.8[a]	190
	—postdialysis and diuresis		25.8[a]	

(16), or in sheep or humans with exercise (17,18) (Table 1). This physiologic response to increased flow can be complicated in some pathologic circumstances by a combination of active vasoconstriction, enhanced responses to active vasoconstriction, structural-induced increases in vascular resistance, and venous hypertension imposed by cardiac malfunction. For example, we have found that after pacing-induced heart failure in the dog, the venoconstrictor effect of norepinephrine is significantly enhanced (19). Another good example is the marked disparity between the effects of exercise-induced increase in flow on P_c in normal patients to that in patients with mitral stenosis (18) (see Table 1). One can argue successfully that the partitioning of pulmonary vascular resistance does not remain constant and thus that these estimates do not provide an *accurate* assessment of P_c in all cases. However, even if the contribution of R_v to the

Table 1 Continued

Model	Paradigm	Baseline	Treatment	Reference
Human	Rest vs. exercise—normal patients	16.5[a]	19.6[a]	18
	—patients with mitral stenosis	33.2[a]	46.2[a]	
Human	Rest vs. exercise			191
	—mild cardiomyopathy	14.1[a]	38.1[a]	
	—cardiomyopathy or IHD	34.5[a]	58.5[a]	
	—PPH	29.9[a]	34.3[a]	
Human	Veno-occlusive disease—PGI_2	54.4	64.5	26
Human	Normal controls		16.6[a]	76
	Chronic left heart failure		34.8[a]	
Human	Refractory heart failure			24
	—treatment with SNP	50.9[a]	30.6[a]	
	—nitric oxide inhalation	62.2[a]	62.6[a]	
Human	Pre-eclampsia—all patients		14.9[a]	192
	—patients with pulmonary edema		29.4[a]	
Change in permeability				
Dog, IL	Angiotensin II—controls		$\Delta P_c 1.6_c$	31
	—after heart failure		$\Delta P_c 1.9$	
Dog	Emboli	9.1	16.9	20
Dog	High-pressure ventilation	10.5[a]	23.0[a]	193
Sheep	Endotoxin	12.9[a]	27.0[a]	143
Sheep	Zymosan-activated plasma	12.5[a]	32.0[a]	23
Sheep	Thrombin	12.6[a]	28.8[a]	194
Human	HAPE—admission		20.9[a]	195
	—recovery		8.0[a]	

All pressures are in cm H_2O.
[a]P_c calculated by assuming venous resistance to be 40% of total (Eq. 3); IL isolated lung perfused at constant flow; NE, norepinephrine; SNP, sodium nitroprusside; IHD, ischemic heart disease; PPH, primary pulmonary hypertension; HAPE, high-altitude pulmonary edema.

total pulmonary vascular resistance shifts from 40% to 20%, for example, it should be clear that P_c can still be elevated compared to the baseline state if flow increases concomitantly. In support of this, Newman et al. (17) directly measured pulmonary microvascular pressure in sheep using a catheter in a fixed wedged position and found substantial increases in P_c with exercise, despite a marked fall in total pulmonary vascular resistance.

Table 1 also emphasizes the fact that there can be significant hydrostatic contributions to pulmonary edema formation in lung injury, even when that injury involves embolization of precapillary vessels. By direct measurement, we found that P_c nearly doubled after glass bead embolization in the in vivo canine lung (20). Further, the pattern of transvascular fluid versus protein transfer led us and others to suggest a hydrostatic contribution via filtration across arterial extra-alveolar vessels to the edema formation with microemboli (20,21) (see below). One would predict from the relation between hydrostatic pressure and edema formation in either normal or injured lung, that relief from active vasoconstriction would limit or reduce edema formation. Indeed, when the vasoconstrictor response to endotoxin-induced lung injury was attenuated, accumulation of edema was substantially attenuated (22). Further, with attenuation of the vasoconstrictor response to zymosan-activated plasma in sheep, the lymph flow was reduced and systemic oxygenation improved (23).

However, under some circumstances, treatment with vasodilators can actually be detrimental with respect to edema formation. In patients with refractory heart failure, though sodium nitroprusside and inhalation of nitric oxide both reduced pulmonary vascular resistance, treatment with nitric oxide did not reduce the estimated P_c (see Table 1), and pulmonary edema consequently developed as evidenced by tachypnea and rales (24). In an experimental study in lambs, PGI_2 was shown to reduce the pressor response associated with thromboxane administration, though the terminal lung water was actually increased (25). In a patient with pulmonary veno-occlusive disease, PGI_2 treatment substantially increased P_c (see Table 1), and chest radiographs subsequently showed the development of alveolar and interstitial infiltrates (26). Though PGI_2, at least, has been shown to prevent the increase in permeability associated with embolism (27), it also has been shown to oppose hypoxic pulmonary vasoconstriction (28). Thus it seems that vasodilator therapy should be approached cautiously.

The effects of active vasoconstriction and changes in flow on P_c are complicated by passive distention of the pulmonary vascular bed with acute pulmonary venous hypertension. Rippe et al. (15) evaluated these interactions in isolated, blood-perfused canine lung lobes and showed that as P_c increases with passive elevations in P_v, total pulmonary vascular resistance falls—the total pressure drop across the pulmonary circulation becomes substantially less. This response is dominated by the fall in the middle compartment resistance (encompassing the septal microvasculature), while the fall in R_v is much less dramatic. In addition, passive distension with venous pressure elevation depresses or ablates *active* vasoconstriction in the normal lung (29,30).

The benefit with respect to hydrostatic edema is that active increases in P_c during acute pulmonary venous hypertension are limited—at least P_c does not increase further. In contrast, after the development of chronic pulmonary venous hypertension in the dog, we have found passive distension to exacerbate norepinephrine-induced venoconstriction (19), but to ablate arterial vasoconstriction induced by angiotensin II (31). These disparate interactions of distension and active vasoconstriction in this chronic model imply a complex functional remodeling of pulmonary vascular smooth muscle function. The effect of venous pressure elevation on resistance in the normal lung is accompanied by a fall in total vascular compliance (15). With chronic pulmonary venous hypertension, the situation is exacerbated. We have found that after 1 month of pacing-induced heart failure in the dog, total pulmonary vascular compliance was reduced to nearly half of the normal value at comparable distending pressure and flow (19,31). These complex hemodynamic interrelationships have been reviewed in detail elsewhere (32,33).

Though P_c in the lung is generally reported as a lumped measure for the entire lobe or lung, one must keep in mind that there can be significant heterogeneity in P_c within the lung and also significant effects of vascular pressure outside of the septal exchange network. For example, due to gravitational effects on the column of blood in the lung, P_c increases by ~1 cm H_2O/cm lung distance from the apex to the base in the upright normal lung (34). This alone would tend to promote more transcapillary fluid filtration at the lung base relative to the apex. However, the gravitational effect on P_c is balanced to some extent by similar increases in P_t down the lung axis (0.6 to 0.7 cm H_2O/cm lung distance) (35). These relationships are illustrated in Figure 2. One would predict from the relation of these two hydrostatic forces alone that the net hydrostatic gradient, i.e., $(P_c - P_t)$, would be 3.5 cm H_2O greater at the lung base.

Net Starling force balance = $[(P_c\ P_t) - \sigma\ (\pi_p - \pi_t)$

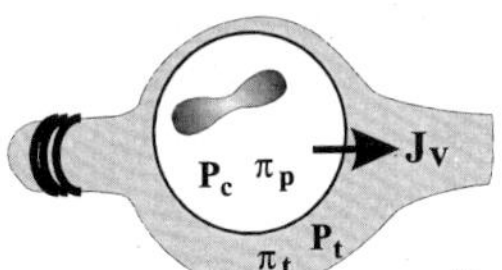

	P_c	P_t	π_t	Net
Apex:	2	-8	19	2.8
Base:	12	-1.5	15	3.1
Vertical gradient (per cm lung)	1	0.65	-0.4	

Figure 2 Schematic illustrating the Starling force balance across the pulmonary capillary exchange barrier. Absolute values (cm H_2O) for capillary pressure (P_c) interstitial fluid pressure (P_t), and interstitial fluid colloid osmotic pressure (π_t) are given as one moves from the lung apex to the base, a total distance of 10 cm in this example (data from Taylor et al. [36]). The plasma colloid osmotic pressure is assumed to be 28 cm H_2O throughout, and the reflection coefficient for total proteins is assumed to be 0.8. See text for more detail.

However, this gravitational effect is offset by changes in the remaining interstitial safety factor (π_t), as discussed below (36). An additional degree of heterogeneity is imposed by the hydrostatic gradient operating across pre- and post-capillary microvessels (extra-alveolar vessels). Iliff (37) suggested that extra-alveolar vessels up to 200 μm in diameter could contribute to fluid filtration. This is supported by the work of Bhattacharya (38), who showed that the L_p in 20- to 40-μm lung venules was similar to that in capillaries from mesentery and skeletal muscle. Filtration across extra-alveolar vessels has in fact been estimated to contribute ~25% to ~75% of the total filtrate in lung (37,39–41). Though there is marked disparity in these results, likely due to the difficulty in excluding transcapillary filtration, the notion that filtration across extra-alveolar vessels contributes to the total cannot be disputed.

Plasma protein concentration, and thus π_p, varies little under normal circumstances. However, with fluid resuscitation or volume loading via electrolyte solutions in the experimental or clinical setting, π_p will fall and transcapillary fluid filtration will increase even if P_c remains constant. Though lymph flow increases substantially with hemodilution (42–46), edema formation can still result if lymph flow does not keep pace with the filtration rate.

When edema does occur in response to an increase in the net hydrostatic force operating at the capillary exchange barrier, there can be consequences in turn for vascular and airway function. The notion that pulmonary edema impacts upon blood flow distribution in the lung has been long debated. Recently, Negrini (47) used micropuncture techniques to show that mild interstitial edema increased the pressure drop across 50 to 100 μm arterioles in rabbit lung, suggesting that vasoconstriction or compression had occurred. Interestingly, P_c actually increased slightly compared to the nonedematous state (see Table 1). Nonetheless, several lines of evidence suggest that interstitial edema at least does not alter flow distribution to any significant extent. First, we know that $K_{f,c}$ is proportional to the amount of perfused pulmonary microvascular exchange area (7). Thus, the fact that edema does not reduce $K_{f,c}$ (48) in the lung supports the lack of any edema-dependent derecruitment in the zone III lung.

Further, morphometric studies have demonstrated little if any reduction in vascular or airway diameters after edema accumulation secondary to fluid overload (49), though left atrial hypertension has been shown to result in airway edema and narrowing (50). Similarly, hydrostatic edema has been shown to result in gas trapping in the lung, presumably due to small airways closure (51), though effects on airways resistance are variable (52). Bronchial vascular engorgement, rather than edema per se, has been suggested to play a role under these circumstances. This possibility was evaluated by Wagner and Mitzner (53), who found that airway narrowing associated with left atrial pressure elevation was associated with an increase in the fraction of the airway wall occupied by vascular space. However, the airway narrowing could be abrogated with bronchodilators, despite lack of any effect on vascular engorgement, suggesting that reflex bronchoconstriction led to the narrowing. Similar engorgement of bronchial vessels, leading to airways edema and bronchoconstriction, has been observed in heart failure and pulmonary venous hypertension in humans, and has been thought to relate to the development of cardiac asthma (52). Nonetheless, alveolar edema and resultant alveolar hypoxia could potentially reduce the amount of perfused exchange area in situ. One possible mechanism is via hypoxic vasoconstriction secondary to alveolar filling. Substantial vasoconstriction per se does not derecruit exchange area in a normal lung perfused at either constant pressure or constant flow under zone III conditions (54). However, in lungs where zone II conditions dominate, derecruitment due to vasoconstriction and decreased regional blood flow could contribute to a lower $K_{f,c}$ and more importantly to a decrease in fluid filtration after lung injury (55). Several studies have shown a shift of blood flow away from dependent lung regions when alveolar edema is present (56,57).

B. Endothelial Barrier

The initial barrier to transcapillary fluid movement is the microvascular endothelial cell, with its abluminal basement membrane (Fig. 1). Net transcapillary fluid movement occurs predominantly through interendothelial junctions, or "pores." In the lung, as in many systemic vascular beds, transcapillary fluid flux is dominated by that through a numerous population of 4- to 7-nm "small" pores, which allow free passage of water and electrolytes, allow restricted movement of albumin and smaller proteins, but which prevent exchange of larger proteins. Occasional 15- to 30-nm "large" pores contribute only a small fraction to transcapillary fluid exchange, but are important with respect to the transcapillary movement of large proteins such as immunoglobulins G and M, transferrin, and α_2-macroglobulin (58). A number of comprehensive reviews have addressed at length the relation between pore size, endothelial permeability and transvascular fluid and protein fluxes, as well as detailing the range of normal values for each of these barrier coefficients (5,6,10,11). However, the relation between pore size and permeability can be generalized by saying that as the size of interendothelial pores increases, $K_{f,c}$ and PS will increase while σ will fall.

Using isolated canine lung lobes perfused under zone III conditions, we have found that $K_{f,c}$ is not altered by either hydrostatic edema (48) or acute dilution of plasma proteins to as little as 1 g/dl (59), though these perturbations will certainly increase the net Starling force balance and promote fluid filtration. Similarly, though 24 hours of hypoproteinemia in sheep increases lung lymph flow, protein permeability remains normal (43). These observations support the conclusion that edema does not alter the character of the endothelial exchange barrier, at least in the short term. With respect to effects of hydrostatic edema on the structure of the alveolocapillary barrier, Bachofen and colleagues found that though hydrostatic edema did alter the epithelial barrier (see below), endothelial perturbations and discontinuities were rare (2,60,61). Similarly, hydrostatic pulmonary edema in the canine lung did not result in any apparent change in the degree of endothelial cell vesiculation (62). Weidner et al. (63) reported that though increased intracranial hypertension in sheep resulted in hydrostatic pulmonary edema and an increase in endothelial vesicle density, no endothelial blebbing or discontinuities were observed. Overall, it seems that modest elevations in pulmonary vascular pressures and the resultant hydrostatic edema do not alter the endothelial barrier per se. Marked increases in pulmonary vascular pressure (i.e., pulmonary venous pressure >40 to 50 cm H_2O) induce both functional and structural alterations in the exchange barrier, including substantial increases in $K_{f,c}$ and, at higher pressures, frank barrier disruption (3,64–66). Since this severe hydrostatic stress actually induces a change in barrier permeability, this issue will not dealt with further here (for reviews see Townsley et al. [67]; West et al. [68,69]). Finally, whether hydrostatic edema affects *PS* per se is not clear. However, since the other barrier coefficients are not affected and since $K_{f,c}$, like *PS*, reflects the permeability of the total pulmonary exchange surface area, one could safely conclude that *PS* remains normal as well in the edematous state.

The effects of chronic pulmonary hypertension on barrier function have also been evaluated. After several days of modest left atrial pressure elevation in sheep with chronic lung lymph fistulas, the σ for endogenous total proteins was increased compared to that with acute left atrial hypertension (70,71). That is, the barrier appeared to be tighter or less permeable. While one would be tempted to conclude from this study that *chronic* venous hypertension and edema in the lung decrease microvascular permeability, more recent work by Ishibashi et al. (72) comparing σ's measured in lung using tracers and endogenous proteins strongly suggests that slow washout of endogenous interstitial proteins rather than any alteration in the exchange barrier was the cause. Moreover, we have found that after as long as 2 months of chronic heart failure and pulmonary venous hypertension induced by rapid ventricular pacing, measures of both $K_{f,c}$ and σ in the canine lung remain normal.

In parallel morphometric studies, we showed that while thickening of the endothelium and alveolar epithelium does occur in this chronic model, the basement membrane remains normal in appearance (3,19). With quite long-term venous hypertension in humans, irregular basement membrane thickening in the alveolar septum does occur (73,74), though the effects of chronic pulmonary venous hypertension on specific barrier coefficients have not been evaluated. Two studies have measured the rate of lung accumulation of radiolabeled macromolecules (also known as a protein leak index) and noted a reduction in that rate for patients with chronic venous hypertension (75,76). However, it is important to recognize that these measures of protein accumulation do not specifically allow evaluation of any barrier coefficient. The *accumulation* of protein in lung is defined by the rate of protein influx (given by J_s; Eq. 2) minus the rate at which protein leaves the lung via lymph ($C_t \cdot$ lymph flow). Given the number of unmeasured variables in this approach, these clinical data are suggestive but not definitive.

C. Interstitium—P_t and π_t

Initially, fluid that filters across the capillary endothelial barrier enters the septal interstitium, then percolates toward terminal lymphatics lying either in cuffs surrounding small airways or vessels or in the subpleural interstitium (77,78). Though resistance to fluid movement in the pulmonary interstitium is several orders of magnitude less than that across the endothelial exchange barrier (79), the interstitium nonetheless poses a barrier for fluid movement due to its biochemical composition, its three-dimensional organization, and the existence of interstitial compartments which appear to equilibrate with transcapillary filtrate at different rates (80–82). Interstitial glycosaminoglycans, including hyaluronan and the proteoglycans, impact upon fluid and protein movement (81,83). Hyaluronan, a repeating disaccharide polymer with molecular weight averaging 10^6 to 10^7 daltons, forms a large coiled, space-filling structure in the interstitium (81,84). Allen et al. (85) reported that hyaluronan is not distributed in a homogeneous fashion, but found primarily in the septal interstitium and in the peribronchial cuff area in the adult lung. The deposition of hyaluronan in the septal interstitium suggests that it could play a role in local fluid dynamics.

Bhattacharya et al. (86) reported that overall hyaluronan content in the normal rabbit lung correlated strongly with extravascular lung water (EVLW): every 100 μg/g dry weight increment in lung hyaluronan was associated with a 1 g/g dry weight increment in EVLW. Further, these investigators showed that degradation of hyaluronan via hyaluronidase reduced EVLW. There is ample evidence that the composition of the interstial matrix influences clearance of interstitial fluid into lymph. Lai-Fook et al. (87) found that hyaluronan was responsible for the majority of interstitial resistance to fluid flow. In their model of isolated pulmonary interstitium, hyaluronidase treatment increased interstitial hydraulic conductivity severalfold. In addition, local degradation and/or clearance of hyaluronan and proteoglycan aggregates in the pulmonary interstitium could play a role. Negrini et al. (88) showed that hydrostatic edema was associated with a decrease in the relative amount of high molecular weight proteoglycans in the lung, and proposed that this influenced the shift of the lung interstitium from a low compliance to a high compliance tissue. In most tissues studied, including lymph nodes, local degradation of hyaluronan occurs, a process preferentially targeted at the high-molecular-weight polymers (89–91).

However, whether similar local degradation of proteoglycans takes place in lung has not been specifically evaluated. Alternatively, new *synthesis* of proteoglycans (relative to hyaluronan) following dilution and/or washout of interstitial matrix molecules may contribute. We found that within 3 hours of saline loading and concomitant left atrial hypertension in the canine lung, uronic acid content increased by nearly 40% (46). Since uronic acid is a measure of total uronic acid containing glycosaminoglycans and proteoglycans, and further since lung hyaluronan content specifically did not change after saline loading, proteoglycan synthesis must have increased substantially. It is important to note in this regard that the molecular weight of proteoglycans is 2 or 3 orders of magnitude smaller than that of hyaluronan (81,84). Thus, saline loading and hydrostatically induced lung matrix hydration may result in a higher relative proportion of lower-molecular-weight glycosaminoglycans in the lung interstitium, thus contributing to a decrease in interstitial resistance to fluid movement. Finally, hyaluronan washout from lung interstitium into lymph with increased transcapillary fluid filtration may contribute to a fall in interstitial fluid resistance, as noted above, and facilitate ease of lymphatic filling. Basal turnover of lung hyaluronan via lymph drainage is only ~2%/day in both dogs and sheep (46,92). However, this rate increased to 15% to 18% with moderate left atrial hypertension in the canine lung (46). In the sheep lung, moderate and severe left atrial hypertension increased hyaluronan turnover to 11% and 18%/day, respectively (92).

When saline loading was coupled with increased left atrial hypertension in the canine lung, turnover increased dramatically, to 54% per day (46). In theory, filtration-induced hyaluronan washout should enhance the rate at which edema fluid can be cleared from lung. Kramer et al. (43) reported that after 24 hours of hypoproteinemia, pulmonary lymph flows remained high in sheep, despite resetting of the transcapillary hydrostatic and oncotic gradients to the basal levels, and concluded that interstitial resistance to fluid flow was decreased. This result may be due in part to filtration-induced washout of hyaluronan. Turnover of lung interstitial matrix with heart failure and chronic pulmonary venous hypertension has not been specifically evaluated. However, results of one study are suggestive: Klappacher et al. (93) reported that circulating levels of procollagen type III peptide, type I collagen telopeptide, and laminin in this patient population were significantly higher than that in patients with no evidence of heart failure.

While measures of circulating matrix components cannot be construed as a reflection of efflux from any one organ, these findings do imply that further study of lung interstitial matrix turnover in chronic hypertension may be productive. They further support the notion that there is significant turnover of interstitial collagens via lymph, in addition to that of the glycosaminoglycans.

Interstitial collagens contribute to the structural integrity of the interstitium, can limit the degree to which tissue expands, and play a role with respect to interstitial fluid pressure, P_t (81,84). In normally hydrated lung, P_t is subatmospheric by several cm H_2O. Taylor and Parker have compiled an excellent survey of studies evaluating this parameter (94). However, a great deal of heterogeneity in P_t exists within the lung. For example, there is a substantial gradient between the septal interstitium and that surrounding large pulmonary vessels (cuffs), such that fluid would preferentially flow into perivascular cuffs (94,95). In addition, due to the continuity of interstitium fluid from the lung apex to its base, there is a gravitational gradient in P_t, such that P_t increases by 0.6 to 0.7 cm H_2O/cm lung along this axis (35,36). Further, due to the interdependence of lung parenchyma, airways, and extra-alveolar vessels, P_t is responsive to changes in transpulmonary pressure—it decreases (i.e., becomes more negative) as transpulmonary pressure increases and the lung expands. This effect is most pronounced at low pulmonary venous pressure, but is partially attenuated as vascular pressure increases (96). Thus, as lung volume changes during normal rhythmic breathing, perivascular P_t will vary as well.

Initially, as fluid is filtered into the lung interstitium, P_t increases sharply, reflecting the normally low compliance of the interstitium (88,97–100). With further fluid accumulation, P_t approaches zero or becomes positive and the interstitium enters a high-compliance phase. At this point, P_t changes little despite further accumulation of fluid (88,101). Until recently, the relation between interstitial fluid volume and P_t was assumed to be a purely passive phenomenon. However, Reed and colleagues have shown that in skin and trachea, the linkage between collagens in the interstitial matrix to cells via integrins gives rise to *active* modulation of interstitial fluid pressure (102,103). As a result, during inflammation P_t decreases significantly, contributing an additional 7 to 14 cm H_2O to the total transcapillary hydrostatic pressure gradient (103,104). After burn injury in skin, the situation is much more dramatic—decreases in P_t to −200 cm H_2O have been documented (105). Based on their studies, one can hypothesize that a similar active control over P_t exists in lung interstitium, though this conclusion awaits experimental confirmation. If so, then this could provide an additional hydrostatic force promoting edema formation in the lung, particularly during lung inflammation and injury.

Accumulation of edema fluid first begins in loose perivascular and/or peribronchiolar cuffs, followed by accumulation in the septal interstitium (106,107). With moderate hydrostatic edema, septal thickening tends to accumulate preferentially on the thick side of the alveolocapillary barrier (63), though as edema progresses separation of the endo- and epithelial layers on the thin side of the septum can be observed (61). With respect to the sequence of interstitial filling, the pattern of cuff filling versus septal thickening does not appear to differ between hydrostatic and permeability edema (106). However the pattern of cuff formation per se does have species variation—filling is faster and the interstitial capacity appears to be larger in dogs than sheep (108,109). Nonetheless, there is substantial evidence that fluid cuffs in the lung equilibrate at a much slower rate with filtered fluid than does lung lymph. Using Evans' blue-labeled albumin, Gee and Havill (80) noted accumulation of the dye in lymph prior to its appearance in cuffs and, further, that cuffs surround larger pulmonary vessels filled with dye even slower than cuffs surrounding the small pulmonary vessels. This suggests that fluid can be sequestered in compartments in lung which do not equilibrate rapidly with septal or microvascular filtrate. Further, their data suggested the presence of a relatively rapid path for filtered fluid to enter lymphatics. This was indeed confirmed by the work of Ishibashi et al. (72) in the canine lung. These investigators found that radiolabeled albumin appeared in lung lymph in as little as 15 min even at low pulmonary pressures. One can envision that due to matrix organization, free fluid channels are formed which promote bulk transfer of fluid directly to initial lymphatics (81,110).

In addition to fluid movement through these pathways to lymphatics, a bulk transfer of some protein along with the fluid is promoted by charge and steric considerations which result in exclusion of proteins from a good portion of normally hydrated pulmonary interstitium. However, as pulmonary hydrostatic pressure is elevated, with the resultant hydration of the pulmonary interstitial matrix, the distribution of macromolecules in the lung interstitial matrix is altered (81,94,111). Parker et al. (42) demonstrated significant decreases in the fractional excluded volume in the lung interstitium by loading dogs with a volume of electrolyte solution equivalent to 15% of body weight. In the basal state, 38% of the pulmonary interstitial fluid volume excluded albumin. After volume expansion, interstitial fluid volume doubled while the interstitial volume, which excluded albumin, fell, such that fractional albumin exclusion decreased to 10%. Functionally, this means that as a result of hydrostatic edema the mass of interstitial protein distributes into a larger fraction of the interstitial fluid volume. This phenomenon contributes in part to the decrease in interstitial fluid protein concentration and π_t seen with hydrostatic-induced fluid filtration. Even in the normal lung, Taylor and Rippe have estimated that due to the effect of gravity on the hydrostatic forces from the apex to the base of the lung and the resultant gradient in transcapillary fluid filtration, π_t is likely to decrease by ~0.4 cm H_2O/cm lung along the same axis (95). As shown in Figure 2, the change in this interstitial safety factor subtantially blunts the gravitational effect on the hydrostatic forces (P_c and P_t), such that there is little overall change in the net Starling force balance from the apex to the base of the lung.

D. Lymphatic Drainage

Lung lymphatics are quite important for maintenance of normal interstitial fluid volume. When the volume flow of fluid filtered across the microvascular exchange network exceeds the pulmonary lymph flow, edema formation ensues. Initial lymphatics in the lung have been shown to originate around respiratory bronchioles, terminal bronchioles, and at the pleural surface, though not in the alveolar septa (77,112–114). Using light and electron microscopic techniques, these lung lymphatics have been shown to swell in edema (114). More recently, corrosion casting has been used in a series of elegant studies to demonstrate filling and possibly recruitment of *initial* lymphatics when the lung is edematous. Both the deep initial lymphatics, i.e., those originating by terminal airways and in cuffs surrounding small microvessels, as well as those on the pleural surface appeared to be more numerous after pulmonary edema was induced by hyperoxic lung injury (77,78). Since lymphatic morphology in both normal and edematous lung varies substantially, Schraufnagel (115) has suggested that lymphatic function and potential varies as well. While recruitment of initial lymphatics in hydrostatic pulmonary edema remains a plausible explanation for at least part of the resistance of the lung to hydrostatic edema, this has not been well studied to date.

As fluid is filtered into the lung interstitium, P_t increases (88,97–100). This has been thought to provide the primary driving force for filling of initial lymphatics (116). However, the forces that drive lymph flow do not appear to be entirely passive. As in other organs in the body, initial lung lymphatics drain into valved conduit lymphatics with smooth muscle, spontaneous contractile function, and autonomic innervation (94,117,118). The accessibility of mesenteric lymphatics has led to a marked expansion of our understanding of lymphatic function. Similar to ventricular contractile function, contributions of both passive filling and active contraction of collecting lymphatics to lymph flow have been recognized (117,119,120). Further, there appears to be some degree of heterogeneity in the response of collecting lymphatics to an edemogenic stress. Benoit (121) has shown that with hemodilution-induced filtration in the intestine increased flow in small collecting lymphatics dominated the overall lymph flow response. In contrast, contractile function in larger (more central) collecting lymphatics was actually depressed and limited the overall increase in lymph flow following hemodilution. In the lung, a large number of studies have clearly demonstrated an increase in lymph flow following perturbations which increase the net transcapillary Starling balance or exchange area (Eq. 1), including an increase in left atrial pressure (16,46,70–72,122–128), dilution of plasma proteins (42–46), and recruitment of filtration surface area with increased flow (16,17,126,128,129). However, it is also clear that the relative increase in lymph flow with hydrostatic edema does not always keep pace with transcapillary fluid filtration and thus edema occurs. Further, much larger increments in lung lymph flow have been observed after lung injury (130), which raises the question of whether neurogenic stimulation or release of substances from lung tissue, resident macrophages, or circulating leukocytes contribute to control of lymphatic inotropic state and thus to total lymph flow during permeability edema (118,131). Taylor has postulated that such "edema-dependent lymphatic factors" may regulate the magnitude of the lymphatic safety factor against edema formation (132). To state the problem another way, we do not fully understand the factors that limit lymph flow in hydrostatic edema. Though an answer to this problem could contribute significantly to an improvement of clinical treatment for hydrostatic edema, there has been virtually no work in this area. Admittedly, since study of contractile function in intrapulmonary lung lymphatics is difficult, perhaps application of information gleaned from study of peripheral collecting lymphatics will prove more productive.

With chronic hydrostatic pulmonary edema secondary to mitral stenosis or congestive heart failure, engorged collecting lymphatics have been observed (73,133). This has led some investigators to suggest that lymph flow is elevated under these conditions. However, there has been only one study that directly evaluated this assumption. Uhley et al. (134) created an arteriovenous fistula in dogs to produce heart failure and pulmonary venous hypertension. They found that after several weeks, lung lymph flow was well correlated with left atrial pressure, as would be expected. Yet lymph flow in a shunt dog with a left atrial pressure of 30 cm H_2O was more than 10-fold higher than that produced acutely with a left atrial pressure of 40 cm H_2O. We have found that the lung content of hyaluronan and uronic acid (per g dry tissue) does not change after 1 month of chronic pulmonary venous hypertension in the dog (135), though EVLW is significantly increased (3,19,31). If one were to assume that both matrix and water were evenly distributed in the lung interstitium, then one could postulate that a modest decrease in interstitial matrix concentration and an attendant decrease in resistance to fluid movement contribute to the ease of lymphatic filling under these conditions. This needs to be experimentally verified. Bleomycin-induced lung fibrosis appeared to produce a different result: hydrostatic edema was randomly distributed throughout the lung in contrast to the predominant sequestration in cuffs in normal lung, and there was greater degree of alveolar edema, suggesting that interstitial resistance to fluid movement was actually impaired (136). Given these diverse results, it seems fair to say that we do not yet know whether changes in interstitial fluid resistance could account for the magnitude of the lymph flow response seen with chronic hydrostatic edema. A mechanistic evaluation of how the interstitium and lymphatics adapt under these conditions is needed. Further, it is possible that any intrinsic changes in the interstitium and lymphatic function and/or recruitment could be offset by an elevation in central venous pressure, at least in heart failure (137). This is an important consideration, since an increase in lymphatic outflow pressure, i.e., the downstream pressure which lymphatic pumping must overcome, has been shown to decrease the efficacy of lung lymphatic function (138,139).

E. Overflow Compartments—Alveolar and Pleural Spaces

Alveolar flooding with acute pulmonary venous hypertension is a relatively late event, occurring only after extravascular lung water increases by more than ~35% (94). Alveolar filling with hydrostatic edema is quite heterogeneous, despite the fact that the entire exchange surface experiences hydrostatic stress (61,140). Several experimental approaches have been utilized in an effort to define the site for fluid movement from the lung interstitium into the alveoli. By infusing Evans' blue dye-labeled albumin in animals with hydrostatic pulmonary edema and comparing cuff fluid dye concentrations with that in airway fluid, Zumsteg et al. (141) concluded that perivascular and peribronchiolar cuffs formed a fluid reservoir but did not directly empty into the airspace. In a similar study, Egan et al. (142) perfused lungs with ^{131}I-albumin to study movement of fluid and macromolecules into alveoli in hemodynamic pulmonary edema. However, they also instilled ^{125}I-albumin, blue dextran, and a small molecular weight tracer (labeled cyancobalamin) into the airways. Interestingly, they showed an influx of ^{131}I-albumin into the airspace, while the ^{125}I-albumin and dextran were merely diluted by alveolar fluid accumulation and did not move into the vascular space. They concluded that discontinuities in airway epithelium led to airway filling with proteinaceous fluid, but did not define the specific site of such leakage.

Using transmission electron microscopy, Bachofen and colleagues (2,60,61) found in hydrostatic edema that epithelial blebs and frank lesions or discontinuities occurred only in lung regions with alveolar edema. The alveolar epithelium exhibited marked plasticity, in that intact blebs constraining proteinaceous fluid were quite large in some cases. Both the alveolar fluid volume fraction and that of the epithelial blebs increased from the apical to the basal portion of the lung. They concluded that the discontinuities per se were the site for leakage of interstitial fluid into the alveolar space in hydrostatic edema. (It is important to note that the frequency of epithelial breaks in hydrostatic pulmonary edema is much less than that produced by frank lung injury, even with a comparable degree of edema formation [57].)

Conhaim came to a different conclusion as to the source of the leak after tracing the path by which fluorescent albumin entered the airspace in hydrostatic edema (143). In contrast to the scenario proposed by Bachofen and colleagues, his work suggested that fluid leaked from the interstitium across the airway epithelium at the level of the alveolar ducts and respiratory bronchioles, but not via the alveolar septal epithelium. An understanding of how alveolar fluid is formed is complicated by the fact that active fluid *reabsorption* from the alveolar space occurs even in the adult lung (144–146), driven by active sodium reabsorption across type II pneumocytes (144–149). It is possible that active reabsorption of alveolar fluid is limited to lung areas with intact epithelium. This could give rise to the pattern of epithelial breaks in experimental hydrostatic edema (2,60,61), such that in areas with intact epithelium, alveolar edema would be resolved yet in areas with discontinuities alveoli would remain filled. In fact, a relatively intact alveolar epithelial barrier is known to be critical for resolution of alveolar edema in humans (150) and in sheep with experimental alveolar edema (151).

The pleural space also acts as an overflow compartment in some cases of hydrostatic pulmonary edema. Fluid filters across the visceral pleura, depending on the transpleural balance of Starling forces and the permeability of this barrier (152–155), in a manner analogous to transcapillary fluid filtration (Eq. 1). This fluid is cleared from the pleural space via lymphatics, though the arrangement is different from that in lung. A submesothelial network of lymphatic lacunae are connected to the pleural space via lymphatic stomata arrayed over the parietal pleural surface (155). Normally, this drainage is quite effective, leaving only a small steady-state volume of pleural fluid, ranging from 0.4 to 2.5 ml/kg in various species (155). Pleural effusion as an overflow pathway in edema appears to be recruited only when pulmonary lymphatic capacity is overwhelmed and alveolar flooding has already occurred, in either acute or chronic pulmonary venous hypertension. Several factors may be involved, including increases in the net Starling force balance across the visceral pleura (both acute and chronic) and increases in central venous pressure which may impair lymphatic drainage (chronic). In dogs with chronic heart failure, the incidence of pleural effusion is variable (19,134,156,157), suggesting that other mechanisms may play a role.

Thus, both the alveolar and pleural spaces represent potential overflow pathways recruited apparently when the interstitial compartment is filled to capacity during hydrostatic edema. This scenario is reminiscent of the "filtration secretion" seen in the intestine with hydrostatic edema (158), suggesting that there may be similarity with respect to mechanism as well.

III. Safety Factors Against Hydrostatic Edema

The interstitial and lymphatic safety factors form a first line of defense against edema formation. When P_c is elevated in the normal lung, the increased volume of fluid delivered across the capillary wall dilutes interstitial proteins with a resultant decrease in π_t: thus the net colloid osmotic gradient, i.e., $\sigma(\pi_p - \pi_t)$, increases. Further, the addition of fluid volume to the septal interstitium initially causes an increase in P_t, and a resultant decrease in the net transcapillary hydrostatic gradient, $(P_c - P_t)$. Finally, the increase in P_t provides a driving force for an increase in lymph flow. These traditional Starling forces each contribute significantly to the total safety factor in lung, as shown in Figure 3, and together can offset significant acute increases in pulmonary vascular pressures. Guyton

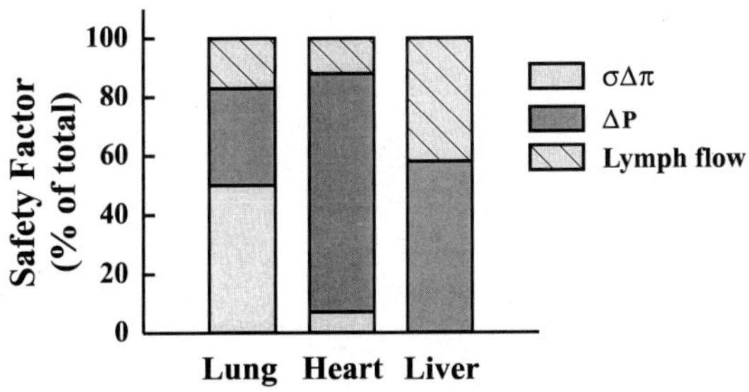

Figure 3 Contributions of the effective transcapillary colloid osmotic pressure gradient ($\sigma\Delta\pi$), the net transcapillary hydrostatic pressure gradient (ΔP), and lymph flow to the total safety factor against hydrostatic edema are compared for lung, heart, and liver. (Data from Ref. 212.)

and Lindsey (159) showed that edema was prevented in the normal canine lung in vivo at left atrial pressures (i.e., the effective pulmonary venous pressure) up to ~24 mmHg. Taylor et al. (36) have estimated the safety factor against hydrostatic edema afforded by these adjustments is equivalent to ~21 mmHg. Thus, substantial increases in left atrial pressure can be accommodated without edema formation. Nonetheless, when left atrial pressure is acutely elevated beyond this threshold, the lung does become edematous.

Figure 3 also compares the contribution from these three safety factors in lung to that in heart and liver. Laine et al. (160) have shown that P_t is quite high in the ventricular myocardium (~15 mmHg) due to transmission of ventricular pressure to the myocardial interstitium and the low compliance of that interstitial compartment. As a result, changes in P_t dominate the safety factor in this organ. Since the permeability of the exchange barrier to protein (σ) dictates the effectiveness of the transcapillary colloid osmotic pressure gradient, we can really consider barrier integrity as a safety factor as well. In the liver, where the endothelium offers little resistance to the movement of macromolecules, the product of $\sigma\Delta\pi$ is quite low. Thus changes in $\Delta\pi$ due to dilution of interstitial protein cannot be effective as a safety factor in this organ. In the lung, endothelial injury with a decrease in σ would similarly diminish the total safety factor against hydrostatic edema (36,159).

The importance of the lymphatic safety factor is highlighted by the observation that the rate of pulmonary edema formation is exacerbated if lung lymphatics are ligated (161) or if central venous pressure (CVP) is elevated (139,162). The loss of any one or more of these safety factors would shift the lung water vs pulmonary venous pressure curve to the left, as shown in Figure 4. Though not commonly treated as a safety factor, the reabsorption of alveolar fluid is an additional critical safety factor against the development of alveolar edema. If

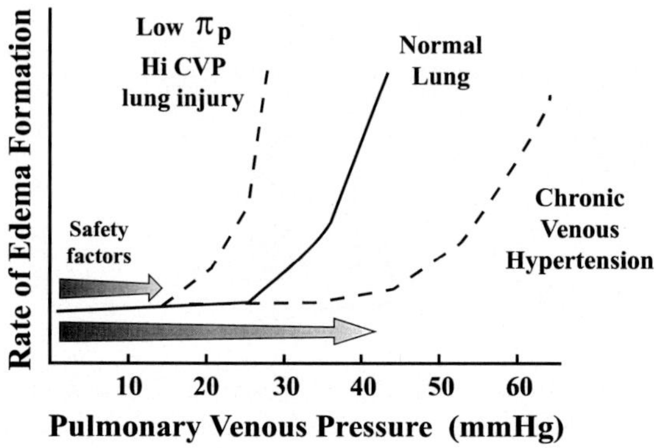

Figure 4 Rate of pulmonary edema formation is shown as a function of pulmonary venous pressure. The response in the normal lung in vivo first defined by Guyton and Lindsey (159) is compared to that after various acute or chronic perturbations. The range of venous pressure over which the safety factors are effective is highlighted in each case by the shaded arrow. See text for more detail.

this reabsorptive process were inhibited pharmacologically or if the alveolar epithelium alone were injured (150,163), the lung would have little defense against hydrostatic alveolar edema and resultant hypoxemia when the interstitial fluid capacity is filled.

With chronic pulmonary venous hypertension and chronic edema, there are adaptive changes in the lung which appear to contribute to the increased resistance to alveolar edema. We have found that the pulmonary microvascular exchange barrier becomes much more resistant to injury induced by high vascular pressure and angiotensin II (3,31). It is possible that the lung safety factor against edema is augmented by lymphatic recruitment and other interstitial adaptations in chronic venous hypertension. While this hypothesis is plausible, it remains to be confirmed experimentally. However, based on the limited experimental data available to date and given the documented resistance of this patient population to alveolar edema formation (137), the edema versus pulmonary venous pressure curve is likely shifted to the right (Fig. 4); that is, there appears to be a larger margin of safety against acute edema formation after the development of chronic pulmonary venous hypertension.

IV. Assessment of Hydrostatic Edema

In this section, various methods used to evaluate hydrostatic edema will be discussed. The methods are grouped into those used specifically to document the presence of edema (outlined in Table 2) and those used to differentiate hydrostatic from permeability edema (Table 3). Again, these compilations are not meant to be exhaustive, but to bring to the reader's attention studies in which the techniques have been applied and in which the methodology is clearly presented. With even a cursory glance at these tables, it should be evident that the investigator evaluating hydrostatic edema in the laboratory has a much wider array of experimental tools to choose from and can, in many cases, specifically dissect permeability from hydrostatic mechanisms. In contrast, the clinician or clinical investigator is limited by the paucity of specific noninvasive methods to evaluate pulmonary microvascular permeability as well as by concerns as to the risk versus benefit of measuring P_c (see below), and thus must be much more cautious in interpreting data obtained at the bedside.

The measurement or detection of edema per se is relatively straightforward. Methods available are given in Table 2. The simplest measures are gravimetric, i.e., total tissue water (TTW) or lung wet/dry weight ratio (W/D). Note that TTW is just the W/D corrected for dry weight. These measures are complicated by the inclusion of blood, both residual intravascular blood and that extravasated in the case of injury. The gravimetric measurement of extravascular lung water (EVLW) is an improvement due to correction of the lung water content for blood water (164,165). Further, one can derive the blood-free dry weight and the residual blood volume from this measure, both of which can prove useful (3,19). However, these measures cannot be taken to the bedside, since they require lung biopsy. The introduction of a double indicator dilution technique, using thermal and dye transients, allowed rapid, sequential measures of lung water in both the laboratory and at the bedside (166,167). However, this

Table 2 Evaluation of Edema Formation

Measure	Model	Method	Applied clinically?	References
W/D or TTW	EX	Gravimetric measure	No	46,163
EVLW	EX	Gravimetric measure, excludes blood	No	164,165
	IL, in vivo	Thermal-dye double indicator	Yes	166,167
Noninvasive	in vivo	Radiography	Yes	168,169,196
		Computed tomography	Yes	170,171
		Magnetic resonance imaging	Yes	173,174

W/D, ratio of wet lung weight to dry weight; TTW, total tissue water; EVLW, extravascular lung water; EX, excised lung; IL, isolated perfused lung.

Table 3 Measures Used to Differentiate Hydrostatic Versus Permeability Pulmonary Edema

Measure	Model	Method	Applied clinically?	References
Microvascular permeability				
$K_{f,c}$	IL	Zero-time extrapolation	No	197,198
	IL, in vivo	Step-increase in P_c	No	199,200
	IL	Split-drop measure of L_p	No	38
σ	IL	Filtration volumes technique	No	201,202
	IL	Osmotic transient	No	203
	in vivo	Lymphatic washdown	No	71,124,127
	IL, in vivo	Slope technique	No	10,72
PS	IL	Radiolabeled protein uptake	No	204
	in vivo	Maximal diffusion technique with endogenous or radiolabeled protein	No	10,72
Clearance[a]	in vivo	Endogenous proteins in lymph	No	72,123,129,151,205
	IL, in vivo	Radiolabeled protein uptake	No	72
	in vivo	Noninvasive clearance of labeled proteins	Yes	75,76
Starling forces				
P_c	IL, in vivo	Micropuncture	No	47,206,207
	IL	Occlusion pressure	No	12,208,209
	in vivo	Swan-Ganz pressure transients or wedge pressure	Yes	176,189
P_t	IL, in vivo	Wicks, micropuncture	No	99,210,211
π_p	IL, in vivo	Osmometer, calculate from C_p	Yes	180
π_t	IL	Micropuncture sampling of interstitial fluid	No	181
Airway fluid sampling				
C_{af}	in vivo	Ratio of proteins in airway fluid vs. plasma	Yes	150,183,184

[a]Note that measures of protein clearance or protein accumulation in lung do not specifically evaluate a barrier coefficient. See text for discussion of methodologic considerations.

C_{af}, concentration of proteins in airway fluid; IL, isolated perfused lung.

technique requires pulmonary arterial catheterization and thus is subject to the same concerns as addressed for the measure of P_c (see below).

Finally, a number of noninvasive imaging techniques are available. Chest radiographs allow assessment of the severity and distribution of edema. Milne et al. (168) devised a scoring system to aid in the differentiation of hydrostatic from permeability edema from radiographs, incorporating assessment of cardiac size, the distribution of edema, pleural effusion, interstitial changes such as septal lines and peribronchial cuffing, and distribution of pulmonary blood flow and volume. Subsequently, Aberle et al. (169) correlated the diagnosis based on an edema score from the chest radiograph with that based on evaluation of airway fluid protein concentration in patients with severe pulmonary edema. They concluded that few radiographic signs were specific for hydrostatic edema. The single most discriminating radiographic parameter was the appearance of patchy, peripheral edema, a sign that appeared relatively infrequently in patients who were diagnosed as having hydrostatic edema based on their alveolar edema fluid protein analysis (see Chap. 3 for further details).

Computed tomography (CT) has also been used as a noninvasive means of monitoring the distribution and severity of pulmonary edema, yet one providing a greater degree of resolution and sensitivity. In experimental hydrostatic pulmonary edema in isolated canine lung lobes, CT illustrated the dominant peribronchial and perihilar fluid accumulation, though with high resolution the peribronchial cuffing was seen to involve perivascular cuffs as well (170). The authors concluded that this cuffing highlighted a key interstitial clearance pathway independent of lymphatic clearance, since the lymphatics are ligated in this model. In humans with pulmonary edema secondary to established cardiac disease, interlobular septal thickening, peribronchovascular cuffing, and increased vascular diameters were seen via high-resolution CT (171). Interestingly, the distribution of hydrostatic edema was shown to be localized in one case to the right upper and middle lobes rather than the predicted central and gravitational pattern. While the resolution afforded by this technique is appealing, some have stressed that CT cannot be used as a routine approach (172). Similarly, magnetic resonance imaging has been used in the experimental setting (173,174), though the results suggest that this technique will not be able to discriminate between hydrostatic and permeability edema when only small to moderate amounts of edema fluid are formed (173) (see Chaps. 3 and 4 for further details).

It should be clear that quantitation of edema fluid will not allow discrimination between hydrostatic and permeability edema. To determine the cause of the edema requires measurement of either the hydrostatic forces involved, the permeability of the endothelial barrier, or, preferably, both. Unfortunately, specific measures of the permeability coefficients that characterize the exchange barrier—i.e., $K_{f,c}$, σ, and *PS*—can only be applied in the experimental laboratory. There are a variety of techniques, some better suited to the isolated lung lobe and other applicable to the in situ lung, as shown in Table 3. Since these have been reviewed in extensive detail elsewhere (6,11,175) as well as in Chapter 4, little will be added here. Several methodologic details should be mentioned, however. First, the investigator must keep in mind the fact that measures of $K_{f,c}$ and *PS* reflect surface area as well as permeability. As a result, area must be held constant to ensure an interpretable parameter, by keeping the lung in zone III for example. Similarly, recruitment of exchange area in vivo secondary to increased cardiac output or elevated venous pressure or derecruitment due to vasoconstriction can complicate interpretation of lymph protein flux (126). Thus, the lymphatic washdown technique (71,124,127), the slope method (10,72), and the maximal diffusion technique (10,72) to determine σ are better suited.

In contrast to these measures, the clearance of proteins in lung lymph (the product of lymph flow and C_1) or accumulation of protein in lung (evaluated using noninvasive imaging techniques) are more problematic, since they do not yield a measure of any specific barrier coefficient. In both cases, more definitive information can be gleaned if the measure is repeated at several levels of pulmonary venous pressure. Under these conditions, the slope of the clearance or accumulation relation to pressure is reflective of σ (10). This is aided by the fact that diffusive protein flux dissipates as transvascular fluid flux increases (see Reed et al. [10] for more detail). Further, the measure of protein accumulation will underestimate transvascular protein flux due to rapid efflux of protein from the lung into lymph (72). So these must be interpreted cautiously and in the light of concomitant hemodynamic measurements.

Measurement of the various Starling forces will yield definitive information regarding the net hydrostatic force balance. However, these are not without problem either. P_c can be measured directly via micropuncture, though this is relegated to the subpleural vasculature and thus may not reflect the global situation in the pulmonary vasculature under all conditions. Occlusion pressures in the isolated lung and Swan-Ganz pressure transients or wedge pressure yield comparable estimates of P_c (176,177), and can easily be applied in isolated lung lobes or in vivo, respectively. These latter techniques will yield a lumped measure of P_c based on the overall distribution of pre- and postcapillary resistance in the lung and thus should correlate with lumped measures of edema accumulation. From a basic science standpoint, a measure of P_c is critical to determination of hydrostatic edema.

However, in the clinical setting a controversy has emerged as to whether the benefit of pulmonary artery catherization and measurement of P_c is warranted given the risks involved (178,179). In the SPRINT study of patients with acute myocardial infarction, a higher mortality was associated with pulmonary artery catheterization in patients with severe heart failure, though the authors concluded that this was likely due to variation in severity of failure between the two groups. Patients with only mild cardiac dysfunction were at no greater risk when the catheterization was included as part of the treatment regimen. Subsequently, a similarly large analysis of pulmonary artery catheterization was completed in which case matching was used to minimize problems due to variation in severity of illness between groups. In this latter study, patients who had been catheterized had an increased 30-day mortality rate compared with matched patients who did not receive a pulmonary artery catheter. The resolution of this controversy is obviously important, but it could also potentially limit the number of tools the clinician or clinical investigator has available for evaluation of hydrostatic edema.

π_p is the only one of the Starling forces that can be measured directly from a blood sample. Either plasma is placed on a membrane osmometer to read π_p directly (180) or C_p is measured using a refractometer or via a colorimetric reaction and π_p is calculated (36,94). As can be seen from Equation 1, the tendency for transcapillary fluid filtration to occur is roughly proportional to $(P_c - \pi_p)$. P_t and π_p have only been evaluated in the experimental laboratory. Both require sampling of the lung interstitium. Micropuncture has been used to sample pulmonary interstitial fluid (181), and cuff fluid has been evaluated from frozen lung sections (80). More commonly, lymph protein concentration has been taken as an estimate of interstitial fluid protein concentration (94), though this is hampered to some extent by poor mixing between interstitial compartments at low and moderate pulmonary capillary pressures (80) and washout of interstitial protein (72). Methods for measurement of P_t have been reviewed extensively by Aukland and Reed (4).

As with the occlusion and micropuncture measures of P_c, the measure of P_t yields a focal value for a parameter that has great degree of spatial and temporal heterogeneity in the lung. Neither of these latter two Starling forces can be measured directly in the clinical setting. However, sampling of alveolar edema fluid and measurement of its protein concentration (C_{af}) can yield information as to the underlying mechanism for alveolar edema. Gropper et al. (182) and Matthay et al. (150) have recommended that alveolar edema fluid be sampled shortly after intubation and preferably via suctioning from distal airways. If the ratio of C_{af} to C_p is < 0.65, the edema is of hydrostatic origin (182,183). Ratios > 0.75 are associated with noncardiogenic edema or increased permeability providing some alveolar fluid reabsorption has not already occurred (150). Sprung et al. (184) have suggested that evaluating the ratio for specific protein fractions, i.e., for albumin rather than for total proteins, is more useful in terms of identifying and dissociating hydrostatic from permeability edema.

V. Summary

Through hydrostatic pulmonary edema has traditionally been appreciated as a consequence of increased P_c, it is clear that there are a number of other contributors "hiding in the woodwork," such as passive and active changes in P_t, for example. Further, in lung injury, the change in barrier integrity leads to a diminution of the product $\sigma\Delta\pi$ (Eq. 1); thus, the hydrostatic force defined by $(P_c - P_t)$ will be that much more effective in promoting edema formation. Further, with lung injury there is often substantial active vasoconstriction, leading to an increase in P_c and thus a direct hydrostatic contribution to the edema formation. In addition, the lung interstitium and lymphatics need to be recognized as dynamic structures. Changes in their function as a result of hydrostatically mediated increases in transcapillary fluid flux can variously aid or limit clearance of edema fluid. Many measures used in both the experimental laboratory and the clinical situation to evaluate hydrostatic edema treat the lung as a homogeneous compartment. However, one must keep in mind the complexity of the lung structure, the resultant heterogeneity in the hydrostatic forces promoting fluid filtration, and the potential problems associated with deducing mechanism based on such lumped measures. Further, acute and chronic venous hypertension and edema can be quite disparate. Though chronic hydrostatic edema obviously has clinical import, the mechanisms by which the lung adapts to chronic venous hypertension and chronic hydrostatic edema have yet to be fully resolved. One hope is that we will be able to address at least some of the unanswered questions posed here in the near future. A discussion of the treatment of clinical hydrostatic edema is provided in Chapter 20.

References

1. Weibel ER. Design and morphometry of the pulmonary gas exchanger. In: Crystal RG, West JB, Barnes PJ, Weibel ER, eds. The Lung: Scientific Foundations. 2nd ed. Philadelphia: Lippincott-Raven, 1997:1147–1157.
2. Bachofen H, Bachofen M, Weibel ER. Ultrastructural aspects of pulmonary edema. J Thorac Imag 1988; 3:1–7.
3. Townsley MI, Fu Z, Mathieu-Costello O, West JB. Pulmonary microvascular permeability. Responses to high vascular pressure after induction of pacing-induced heart failure in dogs. Circ Res 1995; 77:317–325.
4. Aukland K, Reed RK. Interstitial-lymphatic mechanisms in the control of extracellular fluid volume. Physiol Rev 1993; 73:1–78.
5. Parker JC, Perry MA, Taylor AE. Permeability of the microvascular barrier. In: Staub NC, Taylor AE, eds. Edema. New York: Raven Press, 1984:143–187.
6. Taylor AE, Granger DN. Exchange of macromolecules across the microcirculation. In: Renkin EM, Michel CC, eds. Handbook of Physiology. Section 2: The Cardiovascular System. Bethesda, MD: American Physiological Society, 1984: 467–520.
7. Townsley MI, Parker JC, Korthuis RJ, Taylor AE. Alterations in hemodynamics and $K_{f,c}$ during lung mass resection. J Appl Physiol 1987; 63:2460–2466.

8. Patlak CS, Goldstein DA, Hoffman JF. The flow of solute and solvent across a two-membrane system. J Theoret Biol 1963; 5:426–442.
9. Granger DN, Taylor AE. Permeability of intestinal capillaries to endogenous macromolecules. Am J Physiol 1980; 238:H457–H464.
10. Reed RK, Townsley MI, Korthuis RJ, Taylor AE. Analysis of lymphatic protein flux data. V. Unique PS products and σ_d's at low lymph flows. Am J Physiol 1991; 261:H728–H740.
11. Rippe B, Haraldsson B. Transport of macromolecules across microvascular walls: the two-pore theory. Physiol Rev 1994; 74:163–219.
12. Linehan JH, Dawson CA, Rickaby DA. Distribution of vascular resistance and compliance in a dog lung lobe. J Appl Physiol 1982; 53:158–168.
13. Pappenheimer JR, Soto-Rivera A. Effective osmotic pressure of the plasma proteins and other quantities associated with the capillary circulation in the hindlimbs of cats and dogs. Am J Physiol 1948; 152:471–491.
14. Gaar KA, Taylor AE, Owens LJ, Guyton AC. Pulmonary capillary pressure and filtration coefficient in the isolated perfused lung. Am J Physiol 1967; 213: 910–914.
15. Rippe B, Parker JC, Townsley MI, Mortillaro NA, Taylor AE. Segmental vascular resistances and compliances in dog lung. J Appl Physiol 1987; 62:1206–1215.
16. Landolt CC, Matthay MA, Albertine KH, Roos PJ, Wiener-Kronish JP, Staub NC. Overperfusion, hypoxia, and increased pressure cause only hydrostatic pulmonary edema in anesthetized sheep. Circ Res 1983; 52:335–341.
17. Newman JH, Cochran CP, Roselli RJ, Parker RE, King LS. Pressure and flow changes in the pulmonary circulation in exercising sheep: evidence for elevated pressure. Am Rev Respir Dis 1993; 147:921–926.
18. Harris P, Segel N, Bishop JM. The relation between pressure and flow in the pulmonary circulation in normal subjects and in patients with chronic bronchitis and mitral stenosis. Cardiovasc Res 1968; 2:73–83.
19. Townsley MI, Pitts VH, Ardell JL, Zhao Z, Johnson WHJ. Altered pulmonary microvascular reactivity to norepinephrine in canine pacing-induced heart failure. Circ Res 1994; 75:347–356.
20. Townsley MI, Parker JC, Longenecker GL, Perry ML, Pitt RM, Taylor AE. Pulmonary embolism: analysis of endothelial pore sizes in canine lung. Am J Physiol 1988; 255:H1075–H1083.
21. Ehrhart IC, Hall JE, Hofman WF. Vascular pressure effects on lung edema formation after glass bead embolism. J Appl Physiol 1987; 62:1989–1996.
22. Allen SJ, Drake RE, Katz J, Gabel JC, Laine GA. Lowered pulmonary arterial pressure prevents edema after endotoxin in sheep. J Appl Physiol 1987; 63: 1008–1011.
23. Gee MH, Perkowski SZ, Havill AM, Flynn JT. Role of prostaglandins and leukotrienes in complement-initiated lung vascular injury. Chest 1983; 83(suppl): 82S–85S.
24. Bocchi EA, Bacal F, Auler JR, Carmone MJC, Bellotti G, Pileggi F. Inhaled nitric oxide leading to pulmonary edema in stable severe heart failure. Am J Cardiol 1994; 74:70–72.

25. Yoshimura K, Tod ML, Pier KG, Rubin LJ. Role of venoconstriction in thromboxane-induced pulmonary hypertension and edema in lambs. J Appl Physiol 1989; 66:929–935.
26. Davis LL, DeBoisblanc BP, Glynn CE, Ramirez C, Summer WR. Effect of prostacyclin on microvascular pressures in a patient with pulmonary veno-occlusive disease. Chest 1995; 108:1754–1756.
27. Hirose T, Aoki E, Ishibashi M, Domae M, Ikeda T, Tanaka K. The effect of prostacyclin on increased hydraulic conductivity of pulmonary exchange vessels following microembolization in dogs. Microvasc Res 1983; 26:193–204.
28. Sprague RS, Stephenson AH, Lonigro AJ. Prostaglandin I_2 supports blood flow to hypoxic alveoli in anesthetized dogs. J Appl Physiol 1984; 56:1246–1251.
29. Barman SA, Taylor AE. Effect of pulmonary venous pressure elevation on vascular resistance and compliance. Am J Physiol 1990; 258:H1164–H1170.
30. Hyman AL, Lippton HL, Kadowitz PJ. Analysis of pulmonary vascular responses in cats to sympathetic nerve stimulation under elevated tone conditions. Circ Res 1990; 67:862–870.
31. Roy BJ, Pitts VH, Townsley MI. Pulmonary vascular response to angiotensin II in canine pacing-induced heart failure. Am J Physiol 1996; 271:H222–H227.
32. Dawson CA, Linehan JH, Bronikowski TA. Pressure and flow in the pulmonary vascular bed. In: Weir EK, Reeves JT, eds. Pulmonary Vascular Physiology and Pathophysiology. New York: Marcel Dekker, 1989:51–105.
33. Dawson CA, Linehan JH. Dynamics of blood flow and pressure-flow relationship. In: Crystal RG, West JB, Barnes PJ, Weibel ER, eds. The Lung: Scientific Foundations. 2nd ed. Philadelphia: Lippincott-Raven, 1997:1503–1522.
34. Parker JC, Parker RE, Granger DN, Taylor AE. Vertical gradient in regional vascular resistance and pre to post capillary resistance ratios in the dog lung. Lymphology 1979; 12:191–200.
35. Miserocchi G, Negrini D, Gonano C. Direct measurement of interstitial pulmonary pressure in in situ lung with intact pleural space. J Appl Physiol 1990; 69: 2168–2174.
36. Taylor AE, Khimenko PL, Moore TM, Adkins WK. Fluid balance. In: Crystal RG, West JB, Barnes PJ, Weibel ER, eds. The Lung: Scientific Foundations. 2nd ed. Philadelphia: Lippincott-Raven, 1997:1549–1566.
37. Iliff LD. Extra-alveolar vessels and edema development in excised dog lungs. Circ Res 1971; 28:524–532.
38. Bhattacharya J. Hydraulic conductivity of lung venules determined by split-drop technique. J Appl Physiol 1988; 64:2562–2567.
39. Albert RK, Lakshminarayan S, Huang TW, Butler J. Fluid leaks from extra-alveolar vessels in living dog lungs. J Appl Physiol 1978; 44:759–762.
40. Mitzner W, Robotham JL. Distribution of interstitial compliance and filtration coefficient in canine lung. Lymphology 1979; 12:140–148.
41. Gropper MA, Bhattacharya J, Staub NC. Filtration profile in isolated zone I and zone 3 dog lungs at constant high alveolar pressure. J Appl Physiol 1988; 65: 343–349.
42. Parker JC, Falgout HJ, Parker RE, Granger DN, Taylor AE. The effect of fluid volume loading on exclusion of interstitial albumin and lymph flow in the dog lung. Circ Res 1979; 45:440–450.

43. Kramer GC, Harms BA, Gunther RA, Renkin EM, Demling RH. The effects of hypoproteinemia on blood-to-lymph fluid transport in sheep lung. Circ Res 1981; 49:1173–1180.
44. Kramer GC, Harms BA, Bodai BI, Renkin EM, Demling RH. Effects of hypoproteinemia and increased vascular pressure on lung fluid balance in sheep. J Appl Physiol 1983; 55:1514–1522.
45. Parker RE, Wickersham NE, Roselli RJ, Harris TR, Brigham KL. Effects of hypoproteinemia on lung microvascular protein sieving and lung lymph flow. J Appl Physiol 1986; 60:1293–1299.
46. Townsley MI, Reed RK, Ishibashi M, Parker JC, Laurent TC, Taylor AE. Hyaluronan efflux from canine lung with increased hydrostatic pressure and saline loading. Am J Respir Crit Care Med 1994; 150:1605–1611.
47. Negrini D. Pulmonary microvascular pressure profile during development of hydrostatic edema. Microcirculation 1995; 2:173–180.
48. Parker JC, Townsley MI, Cartledge JT. Lung edema increases transvascular filtration rate but not filtration coefficient. J Appl Physiol 1989; 66:1553–1560.
49. Michel RP, Zocchi L, Rossi A, Cardinal GA, Ploy-Song-Sang Y, Poulsen RS, Milic-Emili J, Staub NC. Does interstitial lung edema compress airways? A morphometric study. J Appl Physiol 1987; 62:108–115.
50. Pare PD, Yager DC, Godden DJ. Airway edema. In: Crystal RG, West JB, Barnes PJ, Weibel ER, eds. The Lung: Scientific Foundations. 2nd ed. Philadelphia: Lippincott-Raven, 1997:1355–1364.
51. Harken AH, O'Connor NE. The influence of clinically undetectable pulmonary edema on small airway closure in the dog. Ann Surg 1976; 184:183–188.
52. Szidon JP. Pathophysiology of the congested lung. Cardiol Clin 1989; 7:39–48.
53. Wagner EM, Mitzner W. Effects of bronchial vascular engorgement on airway dimensions. J Appl Physiol 1996; 81:293–301.
54. Rippe B, Allison RC, Parker JC, Taylor AE. Effects of histamine, serotonin, and norepinephrine on circulation of dog lungs. J Appl Physiol 1984; 57:223–232.
55. Shibamoto T, Parker JC, Taylor AE, Townsley MI. Derecruitment of filtration surface area in paraquat-injured isolated dog lungs. J Appl Physiol 1990; 68:1581–1589.
56. Muir AL, Hall DL, Despas P, Hogg JC. Distribution of blood flow in the lungs in acute pulmonary edema in dogs. J Appl Physiol 1972; 33:763–769.
57. Montaner JSG, Tsang J, Evans KG, Mullen JBM, Burns AR, Walker DC, Wiggs B, Hogg JC. Alveolar epithelial damage: a critical difference between high pressure and oleic acid-induced low pressure pulmonary edema. J Clin Invest 1986; 77:1786–1796.
58. Rippe BNS. Pores and intercellular junctions. In: Crystal RG, West JB, Barnes PJ, Weibel ER, eds. The Lung: Scientific Foundations. 2nd ed. Philadelphia: Lippincott-Raven, 1997:663–672.
59. Rippe B, Townsley MI, Taylor AE. Effects of plasma- and cell-free perfusates on filtration coefficient of perfused canine lungs. J Appl Physiol 1985; 58:1521–1527.
60. Bachofen H, Schurch S, Weibel ER. Experimental hydrostatic pulmonary edema in rabbit lungs. Barrier lesions. Am Rev Respir Dis 1993; 147:997–1004.
61. Wu DX, Weibel ER, Bachofen H, Schurch S. Lung lesions in experimental hydrostatic pulmonary edema: an electron microscopic and morphometric study. Exp Lung Res 1995; 21:711–730.

62. Pietra GG, Szidon JP, Leventhal MM, Fishman AP. Hemoglobin as a tracer in hemodynamic pulmonary edema. Science 1969; 166:1643–1646.
63. Weidner WJ, Jones TA, Townsley MI, DeFouw DO. Ultrastructural analysis of sheep lungs after increased intracranial pressure and development of pulmonary edema. Microcirc Endothel Lymphat 1987; 3:397–410.
64. Rippe B, Townsley MI, Thigpen J, Parker JC, Korthuis RJ, Taylor AE. Effects of vascular pressure on the pulmonary microvasculature in isolated dog lungs. J Appl Physiol 1984; 57:233–239.
65. Townsley MI, Lim EH, Sahawneh TM, Song W. Interaction of chemical and high vascular pressure injury in isolated canine lung. J Appl Physiol 1990; 69:1657–1664.
66. West JB, Tsukimoto K, Mathieu-Costello O, Prediletto R. Stress failure in pulmonary capillaries. J Appl Physiol 1991; 70:1731–1742.
67. Townsley MI, Neal CR, Michel CC. High vascular pressure injury. In: Reed RK, Rubin K, eds. Connective Tissue Biology: Integration and Reductionism. London: Portland Press. In press.
68. West JB, Mathieu-Costello O. Pulmonary blood-gas barrier: a physiological dilemma. News Physiol Sci 1993; 8:249–254.
69. West JB, Mathieu-Costello O. Vulnerability of pulmonary capillaries in heart disease. Circulation 1995; 92:622–631.
70. Parker RE, Roselli RJ, Harris TR, Brigham KL. Effects of graded increases in pulmonary vascular pressures on lung fluid balance in unanesthetized sheep. Circ Res 1981; 49:1164–1172.
71. Parker RE, Roselli RJ, Brigham KL. Effects of prolonged elevated microvascular pressure on lung fluid balance in sheep. J Appl Physiol 1985; 58:869–874.
72. Ishibashi M, Reed RK, Townsley MI, Parker JC, Taylor AE. Albumin transport across pulmonary capillary-interstitial barrier in anesthetized dogs. J Appl Physiol 1991; 70:2104–2110.
73. Kay JM, Edwards FR. Ultrastructure of the alveolar-capillary wall in mitral stenosis. J Pathol 1973; 3:239–245.
74. Lee Y. Electron microscopic studies on the alveolar-capillary barrier in the patients of chronic pulmonary edema. Jpn Circ J 1979; 43:945–954.
75. Kaplan JD, Calandrino FS, Schuster DP. A positron emission tomographic comparison of pulmonary vascular permeability during the adult respiratory distress syndrome and pneumonia. Am Rev Respir Dis 1991; 143:150–154.
76. Davies SW, Bailey J, Keegan J, Balcon R, Rudd RM, Lipkin DP. Reduced pulmonary microvascular permeability in severe chronic left heart failure. Am Heart J 1992; 124:137–142.
77. Hainis KD, Sznajder JI, Schraufnagel DE. Lung lymphatics cast from the airspace. Am J Physiol 1994; 267:L199–L205.
78. Schraufnagel DE, Basterra JL, Hainis KD, Sznajder JI. Lung lymphatics increase after hyperoxic injury: an ultrastructural study of casts. Am J Pathol 1994; 144: 1393–1402.
79. Taylor AE, Rippe B, Townsley MI, Korthuis R, Parker JC. Interstitial lung tissue fluid resistance. In: Garlick DG, Korner PI, eds. Frontiers in Physiologic Research. Canberra: Australian Academy of Sciences, 1984:147–154.

80. Gee MH, Havill AM. The relationship between pulmonary perivascular cuff fluid and lung lymph in dogs with edema. Microvasc Res 1980; 19:209–216.
81. Bert JL, Pearce RH. The interstitium and microvascular exchange. In: Renkin EM, Michel CC, eds. Handbook of Physiology. Section 2. The Cardiovascular System. Bethesda: American Physiological Society, 1984:521–547.
82. Davidson JM. Biochemistry and turnover of lung interstitium. Eur Resp J 1990; 3:1048–1068.
83. Comper WD, Laurent TC. Physiological function of connective tissue polysaccharides. Physiol Rev 1978; 58:255–315.
84. Laurent TC. Structure, function and turnover of the extracellular matrix. Adv Microcirc 1987; 13:15–34.
85. Allen SJ, Sedin EG, Jonzon A, Wells AF, Laurent TC. Lung hyaluronan during development: a quantitative and morphological study. Am J Physiol 1991; 260: H1449–H1454.
86. Bhattacharya J, Cruz T, Bhattacharya S, Bray BA. Hyaluronan affects extravascular lung water in lungs of unanesthetized rabbits. J Appl Physiol 1989; 66:2595–2599.
87. Lai-Fook SJ, Rochester NL, Brown LV. Effects of albumin, dextran, and hyaluronidase on pulmonary interstitial conductivity. J Appl Physiol 1989; 67:606–613.
88. Negrini D, Passi A, De Luca G, Miserocchi G. Pulmonary interstitial pressure and proteoglycans during development of pulmonary edema. Am J Physiol 1996; 270: H2000–H2007.
89. Fraser JRE, Kimpton WG, Laurent TC, Cahill RNP, Vakakis N. Uptake and degradation of hyaluronan in lymphatic tissue. Biochem J 1988; 256:153–158.
90. Laurent TC, Fraser JRE. Catabolism of hyaluronan. In: Henriksen JH, ed. Degradation of Bioactive Substances: Physiology and Pathophysiology. Boca Raton: CRC Press, 1991:249–265.
91. Laurent UBG, Dahl LB, Reed RK. Catabolism of hyaluronan in rabbit skin take place locally, in lymph nodes and liver. Exp Physiol 1991; 76:695–703.
92. Lebel L, Smith L, Risberg B, Gerdin B, Laurent TC. Effect of increased hydrostatic pressure on lymphatic elimination of hyaluronan from sheep lung. J Appl Physiol 1988; 64:1327–1332.
93. Klappacher G, Franzen P, Haab D, Mehrabi M, Binder M, Plesch K, Pacher R, Grimm M, Pribill I, Eichler H, Glogar HD. Measuring extracellular matrix turnover in the serum of patients with idiopathic or ischemic dilated cardiomyopathy and impact on diagnosis and prognosis. Am J Cardiol 1995; 75:913–918.
94. Taylor AE, Parker JC. Pulmonary interstitial spaces and lymphatics. In: Fishman AP, Fisher AB, eds. Handbook of Physiology. Section 3. The Respiratory System. Bethesda, MD: American Physiological Society, 1985:167–230.
95. Taylor AE, Rippe B. Pulmonary edema. In: Andreoli TE, Hoffman JF, Fanestil DD, Schultz SG, eds. Physiology of Membrane Disorders. New York: Plenum, 1986:1025–1039.
96. Smith JC, Mitzner W. Analysis of pulmonary vascular interdependence in excised dog lobes. J Appl Physiol 1980; 48:450–467.
97. Parker JC, Guyton AC, Taylor AE. Pulmonary interstitial and capillary pressures estimated from intra-alveolar fluid pressure. J Appl Physiol 1978; 44:267–276.

98. Parker JC, Allison RC, Taylor AE. Edema affects intra-alveolar fluid pressures and interdependence in dog lungs. J Appl Physiol 1981; 51:911–921.
99. Lai-Fook SJ. Perivascular interstitial fluid pressure measured by micropipettes in isolated dog lung. J Appl Physiol 1982; 52:9–15.
100. Negrini D, Capelli C, Morini M, Miserocchi G. Gravity-dependent distribution of parietal subpleural interstitial pressure. J Appl Physiol 1987; 63:1912–1918.
101. Lai-Fook SJ, Toporoff B. Pressure-volume behavior of perivascular interstitium measured in isolated dog lung. J Appl Physiol 1980; 48:939–946.
102. Reed RK, Rubin K, Wiig H, Rodt SA. Blockade of β_1-integrins in skin causes edema through lowering of interstitial fluid pressure. Circ Res 1992; 71:978–983.
103. Reed RK, Woie K, Rubin K. Integrins and control of interstitial fluid pressure. News Physiol Sci 1997; 12:42–48.
104. Koller ME, Woie K, Reed RK. Increased negativity of interstitial fluid pressure in rat trachea after mast cell degranulation. J Appl Physiol 1993; 74:2135–2139.
105. Lund T, Wiig H, Reed RK. Acute postburn edema: role of strongly negative interstitial fluid pressure. Am J Physiol 1988; 255:H1069–H1074.
106. Staub NC, Nagano H, Pearce ML. Pulmonary edema in dogs, especially the sequence of fluid accumulation in lungs. J Appl Physiol 1967; 22:227–240.
107. DeFouw DO, Ritter AB, Chinard FP. Alveolar microvessels in isolated perfused dog lungs: structural and functional studies after production of moderate and severe hydrodynamic edema. Exp Lung Res 1985; 8:67–69.
108. Conhaim RL, Lai-Fook SJ, Staub NC. Sequence of perivascular liquid accumulation in liquid-filled dog lung lobes. J Appl Physiol 1986; 60:513–520.
109. Conhaim RL, Lai-Fook SJ, Eaton A. Sequence of interstitial liquid accumulation in liquid-inflated sheep lung lobes. J Appl Physiol 1989; 66:2659–2666.
110. Granger HJ. Physicochemical properties of the extracellular matrix. In: Hargens AR, ed. Tissue Fluid Pressure and Composition. Baltimore: Williams and Wilkins, 1981:43–61.
111. Wiederhielm CA, Black LL. Osmotic interaction of plasma proteins with interstitial macromolecules. Am J Physiol 1976; 231:638–641.
112. Lauweryns JM. The blood and lymphatic microcirculation of the lung. Cardiopulm Pathol Ann 1971; 6:365–415.
113. Albertine KH, Wiener-Kronish JP, Roos PJ, Staub NC. Structure, blood supply, and lymphatic vessels of the sheep's visceral pleura. Am J Anat 1982; 165: 277–294.
114. Leak LV. The interstitial-lymphatic interface in the lung. Lymphology 1987; 20: 196–204.
115. Schraufnagel DE. Forms of lung lymphatics: a scanning electron microscopic study of casts. Anat Rec 1992; 233:547–554.
116. Taylor AE, Gibson WH, Granger HJ, Guyton AC. The interaction between intracapillary and tissue forces in the overall regulation of interstitial fluid volume. Lymphology 1973; 6:192–208.
117. Benoit JN, Zawieja DC. Gastrointestinal lymphatics. In: Johnson LR, ed. Physiology of the Gastrointestinal Tract. 3rd ed. New York: Raven Press, 1994:1669–1692.

118. Ohhashi T, Yokoyama S. Nitric oxide and the lymphatic system. Jpn J Physiol 1994; 44:327–342.
119. Ohhashi T, Azuma T, Sakaguchi M. Active and passive mechanical characteristics of bovine mesenteric lymphatics. Am J Physiol 1980; 239:H88–H95.
120. Ohhashi T, Azuma T. Sympathetic effects on spontaneous activity in bovine mesenteric lymphatics. Am J Physiol 1984; 247:H610–H615.
121. Benoit JN. Relationships between lymphatic pump flow and total lymph flow in the small intestine. Am J Physiol 1991; 261:H1970–H1978.
122. Warren MF, Drinker CK. The flow of lymph from the lungs of the dog. Am J Physiol 1942; 136:207–221.
123. Erdmann III, Vaughan JR, Brigham KL, Woolverton WC, Staub NC. Effect of increased vascular pressure on lung fluid balance in unanesthetized sheep. Circ Res 1975; 37:271–284.
124. Parker JC, Parker RE, Granger DN, Taylor AE. Vascular permeability and transvascular fluid and protein transport in the dog lung. Circ Res 1981; 48:549–561.
125. Parker JC, Crain M, Grimbert F, Rutili G, Taylor AE. Total lung lymph flow and fluid compartmentation in edematous dog lungs. J Appl Physiol 1981; 51:1268–1277.
126. Jones TA, Townsley MI, Weidner WJ. Effects of intracranial and left atrial hypertension on lung fluid balance in sheep. J Appl Physiol 1982; 52:1324–1329.
127. Townsley MI, McClure DE, Weidner WJ. Assessment of pulmonary microvascular permeability in acutely prepared sheep. J Appl Physiol 1984; 56:857–861.
128. Grimbert FA, Martin D, Parker JC, Taylor AE. Lymph flow during increases in pulmonary blood flow and microvascular pressure in dogs. Am J Physiol 1988; 255:H1149–H1155.
129. Newman JH, Butka BJ, Parker RE, Roselli RJ. Effect of progressive exercise on lung fluid balance in sheep. J Appl Physiol 1988; 64:2125–2131.
130. Brigham KL, Woolverton WC, Blake LH, Staub NC. Increased sheep lung vascular permeability caused by *Pseudomonas* bacteremia. J Clin Invest 1974; 54: 792–804.
131. Benoit JN, Zawieja DC. Effects of f-Met-Leu-Phe-induced inflammation on intestinal lymph flow and lymphatic pump behavior. Am J Physiol 1992; 262:G199–G202.
132. Taylor AE. The lymphatic edema safety factor: the role of edema dependent lymphatic factors (EDLF). Lymphology 1990; 23:111–123.
133. Grossman W, Braunwald E. Pulmonary hypertension. In: Braunwald E, ed. Heart Disease. A Textbook of Cardiovascular Medicine. Philadelphia: W.B. Saunders, 1988:783–817.
134. Uhley HN, Leeds SE, Sampson JJ, Friedman M. Role of pulmonary lymphatics in chronic pulmonary edema. Circ Res 1962; 11:966–970.
135. Townsley MI, Reed RK, Ardell JL, Laurent TC. Lung, heart and skin interstitial matrix composition following development of pacing-induced heart failure. Proc XXXII Cong Int Union Physiol Sci 1993; 323.8. Abstract.
136. Zwikler MP, Iancu D, Michel RP. Effects of pulmonary fibrosis on the distribution of edema. Morphometric analysis. Am J Respir Crit Care Med 1994; 149:1276–1285.

137. Townsley MI, Lee AK, McMillon RK, Roy BJ. Pulmonary microvascular adaptations to heart failure and pulmonary venous hypertension. In: Spinale FG, ed. Pathophysiology of Tachycardia-Induced Heart Failure. Armonk, NY: Futura Publishing Co., 1996:173–192.
138. Drake RE, Adcock DK, Scott RL, Gabel JC. Effect of outflow pressure upon lymph flow from dog lungs. Circ Res 1982; 50:865–869.
139. Laine GA, Allen SJ, Katz J, Gabel JC, Drake RE. Effect of systemic venous pressure elevation on lymph flow and lung edema formation. J Appl Physiol 1986; 61:1634–1638.
140. Seibert AF, Thompson WJ, Taylor AE, Wilborn WH, Barnard JW, Haynes JJ. Reversal of increased microvascular permeability associated with ischemia-reperfusion: role of cAMP. J Appl Physiol 1992; 72:389–395.
141. Zumsteg TA, Havill AM, Gee MH. Relationships among lung extravascular fluid compartments with alveolar flooding. J Appl Physiol 1982; 53:267–271.
142. Egan EA, Nelson RM, Gessner IH. Solute permeability of the alveolar epithelium in acute hemodynamic pulmonary edema in dogs. Am J Physiol 1977; 1:H80–H86.
143. Conhaim RL. Airway level at which edema liquid enters the air space of isolated dog lungs. J Appl Physiol 1989; 67:2234–2242.
144. Basset G, Crone C, Saumon G. Significance of active ion transport in transalveolar water absorption: a study on isolated rat lung. J Physiol 1987; 384:311–324.
145. Goodman BE, Kim K-J, Crandall ED. Evidence for active sodium transport across alveolar epithelium of isolated rat lung. J Appl Physiol 1987; 62:2460–2466.
146. Berthiaume Y, Broaddus VC, Gropper MA, Tanita T, Matthay MA. Alveolar liquid and protein clearance from normal dog lungs. J Appl Physiol 1988; 65: 585–593.
147. Olver RE, Davis B, Marin MG, Nadel JA. Active transport of Na^+ and Cl^- across the canine tracheal epithelium in vitro. Am Rev Respir Dis 1975; 112:811–815.
148. Goodman BE, Fleischer RS, Crandall ED. Evidence for active Na^+ transport by cultured monolayers of pulmonary alveolar epithelial cells. Am J Physiol 1983; 245:C78–C83.
149. Mason RJ, Williams MC, Widdicombe JH. Fluid and electrolyte transport across monolayers of alveolar type II cells in vitro. Am Rev Respir Dis 1983; 127: S24–S28.
150. Matthay MA, Wiener-Kronish JP. Intact epithelial barrier function is critical for the resolution of alveolar edema in humans. Am Rev Respir Dis 1990; 142:1250–1257.
151. Sakuma T, Pittet JF, Jayr C, Matthay MA. Alveolar liquid and protein clearance in the absence of blood flow or ventilation in sheep. J Appl Physiol 1993; 74: 176–185.
152. Kinasewitz GT, Fishman AP. Influence of alterations in Starling forces on visceral pleural fluid movement. J Appl Physiol 1981; 51:671–677.
153. Miserocchi G, Negrini D, Mortola JP. Comparative features of Starling-lymphatic interaction at the pleural level in mammals. J Appl Physiol 1984; 56:1151–1156.
154. Wiener-Kronish JP, Broaddus VC. Interrelationship of pleural and pulmonary interstitial liquid. Annu Rev Physiol 1993; 55:209–226.

155. Miserocchi G, Negrini D. Pleural space: pressures and fluid dynamics. In: Crystal RG, West JB, Barnes PJ, Weibel ER, eds. The Lung: Scientific Foundations. 2nd ed. Philadelphia: Lippincott-Raven, 1997:1217–1225.
156. Armstrong PW, Stopps TP, Ford SE, DeBold AJ. Rapid ventricular pacing in the dog: pathophysiologic studies of heart failure. Circulation 1986; 74:1075–1084.
157. Howard RJ, Stopps TP, Moe GW, Gotlieb A, Armstrong PW. Recovery from heart failure: structural and functional analysis in a canine model. Can J Physiol Pharmacol 1988; 66:1505–1512.
158. Granger DN, Kvietys PR, Perry MA, Barrowman JA. The microcirculation and intestinal transport. In: Johnson LR, ed. Physiology of the Gastrointestinal Tract. New York: Raven, 1987:1671–1697.
159. Guyton AC, Lindsey AW. Effect of elevated left atrial pressure and decreased plasma protein concentration on the development of pulmonary edema. Circ Res 1959; 7:649–657.
160. Laine GA, Allen SJ. Left ventricular myocardial edema. Lymph flow, interstitial fibrosis, and cardiac function. Circ Res 1991; 68:1713–1721.
161. Magno M, Szidon JP. Hemodynamic pulmonary edema in dogs with acute and chronic lymphatic ligation. Am J Physiol 1976; 231:1777–1782.
162. Allen SJ, Drake RE, Laine GA, Gabel JC. Effect of thoracic duct drainage on hydrostatic pulmonary edema and pleural effusion in sheep. J Appl Physiol 1991; 71:314–316.
163. Khimenko PL, Barnard JW, Moore TM, Wilson PS, Ballard ST, Taylor AE. Vascular permeability and epithelial transport effects on lung edema formation in ischemia and reperfusion. J Appl Physiol 1994; 77:1116–1121.
164. Pearce ML, Yamashita J, Beazell J. Measurement of pulmonary edema. Circ Res 1965; 16:482–488.
165. Weidner WJ. Extravascular lung water content in the domestic fowl (*Gallus domesticus*). Physiol Zool 1978; 51:267–271.
166. Mihm FG, Feeley TW, Rosenthal MH, Lewis F. Measurement of extravascular lung water in dogs using thermal-green dye indicator dilution method. Anesthesiology 1982; 57:116–122.
167. Maron MB, Holcomb PH, Dawson CA, Rickaby DA, Clough AV, Linehan JH. Edema development and recovery in neurogenic pulmonary edema. J Appl Physiol 1994; 77:1155–1163.
168. Milne ENC, Pistolesi M, Miniati M, Giuntini C. The radiologic dysfunction of cardiogenic and noncardiogenic edema. Am J Radiol 1985; 144:879–894.
169. Aberle DR, Wiener-Kronish JP, Webb WR, Matthay MA. Hydrostatic versus increased permeability pulmonary edema: diagnosis based on radiographic criteria in critically ill patients. Radiology 1988; 168:73–79.
170. Forster BB, Muller NL, Mayo JR, Okazawa M, Wiggs BJ, Pare PD. High-resolution computed tomography of experimental hydrostatic pulmonary edema. Chest 1992; 101:1434–1437.
171. Storto ML, Kee ST, Golden JA, Webb WR. Hydrostatic pulmonary edema: high-resolution CT findings. Am J Roentgenol 1995; 165:817–820.
172. Bone RC. The ARDS lung: new insights from computed tomography. JAMA 1993; 269:2134–2135.

173. Schmidt HC, Tsay D-G, Higgins CB. Pulmonary edema: an MR study of permeability and hydrostatic types in animals. Radiology 1986; 158:297–302.
174. Phillips DM, Allen PS, Man SFP. Assessment of temporal changes in pulmonary edema with NMR imaging. J Appl Physiol 1989; 66:1197–1208.
175. Taylor AE, Townsley MI, Korthuis RJ. Macromolecule transport across the pulmonary microvessel walls. Exp Lung Res 1985; 8:97–123.
176. Holloway H, Perry M, Downey JM, Taylor AE. Estimation of effective pulmonary capillary pressure in intact lungs. J Appl Physiol 1983; 54:846–851.
177. Cope DK, Grimbert FA, Downey JM, Taylor AE. Pulmonary capillary pressure: a review. Crit Care Med 1992; 20:1043–1056.
178. Zion MM, Balkin J, Rosenmann D, Goldbourt U, Reicher-Reiss H, Kaplinsky E, Behar S. Use of pulmonary artery catheters in patients with acute myocardial infarction. Analysis of experience in 5,841 patients in the SPRINT registry. Chest 1990; 98:1331–1335.
179. Connors AF, Speroff T, Dawson NV, Thomas C, Harrell FE, Wagner D, Desbiens N, Goldman L, Wu AW, Califf RM, Fulkerson WJ, Vidaillet H, Broste S, Bellamy P, Lynn J, Knaus WA. The effectiveness of right heart catheterization in the initial care of critically ill patients. JAMA 1996; 276:889–897.
180. Prather JW, Gaar KA, Guyton AC. Direct continuous recording of plasma colloid osmotic pressure of whole blood. J Appl Physiol 1968; 24:602–605.
181. Raj JU, Anderson J. Regional differences in interstitial fluid albumin concentration in edematous lamb lungs. J Appl Physiol 1992; 72:699–705.
182. Gropper MA, Wiener-Kronish JP, Hashimoto S. Acute cardiogenic pulmonary edema. Clin Chest Med 1994; 15:501–515.
183. Sprung CL, Rackow EC, Fein A, Jacob AI, Isikoff SK. The spectrum of pulmonary edema: differentiation of cardiogenic, intermediate, and noncardiogenic forms of pulmonary edema. Am Rev Respir Dis 1981; 124:718–722.
184. Sprung CL, Long WM, Marcial EH, Schein RM, Parker RE, Shomer T, Brigham KL. Distribution of proteins in pulmonary edema: the value of fractional concentrations. Am Rev Respir Dis 1987; 136:957–963.
185. Townsley MI, Korthuis RJ, Taylor AE. Effects of arachidonate on permeability and resistance distribution in canine lungs. J Appl Physiol 1985; 58:206–210.
186. Townsley MI, Korthuis RJ, Taylor AE. Specific hemodynamic effects of PGE_2 and $PGF_{1\alpha}$ in the canine lung. Prost Leuk Med 1985; 20:275–282.
187. Lang SA, Maron MB. Hemodynamic basis for cocaine-induced pulmonary edema in dogs. J Appl Physiol 1991; 71:1166–1170.
188. Simon RP, Graham B, Bayne LL, Darragh TM. Effect of pulmonary vascular pressure on lung lymph flow following seizures. Chest 1988; 93:386–389.
189. Cope DK, Allison RC, Dumond ME, Taylor AE. Changes in pulmonary capillary pressure after cardiac surgery. J Cardiothorac Anesthesiol 1988; 2:182–187.
190. Boyes R, Puri VK, Toledo L, Schneider F. Pulmonary edema in renal transplant patients. Am Surg 1987; 53:647–651.
191. Janicki JS, Weber KT, Likoff MJ, Fishman AP. The pressure-flow response of the pulmonary circulation in patients with heart failure and pulmonary vascular disease. Circulation 1985; 72:1270–1278.

192. Mabie WC, Ratts TE, Sibai BM. The central hemodynamics of severe preeclampsia. Am J Obstet Gynecol 1989; 161:1443–1448.
193. Parker JC, Hernandez LA, Longenecker GL, Peevy K, Johnson W. Lung edema caused by high peak inspiratory pressures in dogs. Am Rev Respir Dis 1990; 142: 321–328.
194. Johnson A, Lo SK, Blumenstock FA, Malik AB. CVF-induced decomplementation: effect on lung transvascular protein flux after thrombin. J Appl Physiol 1987; 62:863–869.
195. Koizumi T, Kawashima A, Kubo K, Kobayashi T, Sekiguchi M. Radiographic and hemodynamic changes during recovery from high-altitude pulmonary edema. Intern Med 1994; 33:525–528.
196. Bernard GR, Pou NA, Coggeshall JW, Carroll FE, Snapper JR. Comparison of the pulmonary dysfunction caused by cardiogenic and noncardiogenic pulmonary edema. Chest 1995; 108:798–803.
197. Drake R, Gaar KA, Taylor AE. Estimation of the filtration coefficient of pulmonary exchange vessels. Am J Physiol 1978; 234:H266–H274.
198. Drake RE, Gabel JC. Comparison of techniques to measure pulmonary capillary filtration coefficients in dogs. Microvasc Res 1981; 21:133–141.
199. Morriss AW, Drake RE, Gabel JC. Comparison of microvascular filtration characteristics in isolated and intact lungs. J Appl Physiol 1980; 48:438–443.
200. Ehrhart IC, Granger WM, Hofman WF. Filtration coefficient obtained by stepwise pressure elevation in isolated dog lung. J Appl Physiol 1984; 56:862–867.
201. Pilati CF, Maron MB. A technique to measure the reflection coefficient using endogenous vascular indicators. Microvasc Res 1986; 32:255–260.
202. Wolf MB, Watson PD, Scott DRC II. Integral mass balance method for determination of solvent-drag reflection coefficient. Am J Physiol 1987; 253:H194–H204.
203. Rippe B, Townsley MI, Parker JC, Taylor AE. Osmotic reflection coefficient for total plasma protein in lung microvessels. J Appl Physiol 1985; 58:436–442.
204. Kern DF, Levitt D, Wangensteen D. Endothelial albumin permeability measured with a new technique in perfused rabbit lung. Am J Physiol 1983; 245:H229–H236.
205. Brigham KL, Woolverton WC, Staub NC. Reversible increase in pulmonary vascular permeability after *Pseudomonas aeruginosa* bacteremia in unanesthetized sheep. Chest 1974; 65:51S–54S.
206. Shepard JM, Gropper MA, Nicolaysen G, Staub NC, Bhattacharya J. Lung microvascular pressure profile measured by micropuncture in anesthetized dogs. J Appl Physiol 1988; 64:874–879.
207. Bhattacharya S, Glucksberg MR, Bhattacharya J. Measurement of lung microvascular pressure in the intact anesthetized rabbit by the micropuncture technique. Circ Res 1989; 64:167–172.
208. Hakim TS, Michel RP, Chang HK. Partitioning of pulmonary vascular resistance in dogs by arterial and venous occlusion. J Appl Physiol 1982; 52:710–715.
209. Townsley MI, Korthuis RJ, Rippe B, Parker JC, Taylor AE. Validation of double vascular occlusion method for $P_{c,i}$ in lung and skeletal muscle. J Appl Physiol 1986; 61:127–132.

210. Goshy M, Lai-Fook SJ, Hyatt RE. Perivascular pressure measurements by wick-catheter technique in isolated dog lobes. J Appl Physiol 1979; 46:950–955.
211. Bhattacharya J, Gropper MA, Staub NC. Interstitial fluid pressure gradient measured by micropuncture in excised dog lung. J Appl Physiol 1984; 56:271–277.
212. Taylor AE, Townsley MI. Evaluation of the Starling fluid flux equation. News Physiol Sci 1987; 2:48–52.

6

Increased-Permeability Pulmonary Edema from Sepsis/Endotoxemia

IVAN M. ROBBINS
KENNETH L. BRIGHAM

Vanderbilt University Medical Center
Nashville, Tennessee

JOHN H. NEWMAN

Nashville Veterans Administration Hospital and Vanderbilt University School of Medicine
Nashville, Tennessee

I. Introduction

Pulmonary edema and sepsis are frequently encountered disorders affecting a wide range of patients and resulting in varying degrees of morbidity and mortality. These illnesses can occur separately, but frequently occur in tandem. Pulmonary edema classically has been divided into two broad categories: hydrostatic or cardiogenic and increased-permeability or noncardiogenic edema. Hydrostatic edema results from left ventricular dysfunction or other disorders that impede blood flow out of the pulmonary circulation. Increased-permeability pulmonary edema is associated with numerous insults, such as aspiration of gastric contents, multiple blood transfusions, or toxic inhalations. The acute respiratory distress syndrome (ARDS) is often equated with noncardiogenic-induced increases in extravascular lung water. The most commonly cited cause of ARDS, and the one associated with the highest mortality, is sepsis (1,2,3,4). The lung's unique status as the only organ through which the entire cardiac output must pass and its function as a pool for marginated polymorphonuclear leukocytes makes it exceptionally vulnerable to mediators and inflammatory cells activated by endotoxin.

A great deal of research has been done in an effort to elucidate the mechanisms underlying the development of sepsis-induced pulmonary edema, yet our understanding of this phenomenon remains incomplete. Much has been learned about the endothelial damage that occurs in response to endotoxin release, but, until recently, there has been little characterization of the epithelial dysfunction that must take place in order for extravascular fluid to accumulate in the airways. Most of the initial findings concerning the pathogenesis of endotoxin-induced pulmonary edema came from animal models. These changes, in turn, have been inferred to take place in humans with ARDS. However, in animal models, the precise timing of endotoxin exposure can be known with certainty whereas this is difficult to determine in humans. Furthermore, only 25% to 40% of patients meeting the diagnosis of sepsis develop clinical evidence of acute lung injury, and the interval between the development of sepsis and ARDS may be only a matter of hours (5). No reliable blood marker currently exists that will prospectively identify septic patients who develop ARDS. Levels of von Willebrand factor (6), leukotrienes B_4, C_4, and D_4 (7,8), and activated complement (217) have been analyzed in this group of patients, but none of these is a reliable predictor of subsequent lung injury. Measurement of important mediators and better characterization of the sequence of changes occurring with high-

Table 1 Effects Favoring Edema Formation in Sepsis

Hydrostatic
Elevated left atrial pressure (cardiac dysfunction, fluid overload)
Pulmonary venoconstriction
Increased cardiac output (increased surface area and pressure)
Alveolar collapse (loss of surfactant and negative interstitial pressure)
Overperfusion of patent capillary bed (loss of capillary bed)
Production of arachidonic acid metabolites
Loss of hypoxic vasoconstriction
Increased permeability
Pulmonary capillary endothelium
Alveolar epithelium
Bronchial vessels
Transcellular fluid channels
Structural damage
Loss of lymphatic drainage
Disruption of alveolar wall
Inflammatory occlusion of vascular bed
Neutrophil-mediated injury (O_2 radical formation)
Cytokine production

Source: Ref. 234.

permeability pulmonary edema in humans has been achieved in recent years. It is now well known that an intricate cascade of inflammatory mediators is activated in response to endotoxin. However, the process cannot be delineated early enough to intervene effectively and improve survival.

ARDS is a condition characterized by leaky pulmonary vasculature and abnormal accumulation of alveolar fluid, yet it would be an oversimplification to ascribe all of the dysfunction to nonhydrostatic forces. It is evident that a number of other abnormalities such as altered cardiac function and pulmonary hypertension contribute to the formation of edema. Table 1 summarizes the major factors contributing to the development of pulmonary edema in sepsis. These hemodynamic and cellular changes will be explored in more detail in this chapter.

II. Sepsis: An Overview

The sepsis syndrome is characterized by significant alterations in temperature, hypotension, tachypnea, and tachycardia in association with systemic infection and evidence of end-organ damage, including ARDS, renal dysfunction, and altered mental status. Table 2 lists major clinical and laboratory findings indicative of sepsis. Gram-negative bacteria are frequently found to be the causative organism, in part reflecting our increased ability to treat and prolong the lives of severely ill and acutely decompensated patients (9), the immunosuppressed (10),

Table 2 Clinical and Laboratory Findings Supporting High-Permeability Pulmonary Edema

Clinical
Significant elevation or decrease in temperature
High flow state with warm extremities
Bounding pulses
No evidence of left heart failure (no S3, jugular venous distension)
Evidence of underlying infection (sputum production, peritonitis, endocarditis, etc.)
Laboratory
CXR, diffuse infiltrates
ECG, usually normal with normal cardiac enzymes
PCWP < 18 mm Hg
Large increase in Qs/Qt
Significant increase or decrease in WBC
Low platelets
Positive blood, urine, sputum, or other body fluid/tissue gram stain or culture
Edema fluid/serum protein > 0.7

Source: Ref. 235.

and trauma victims (11). Endotoxin, a part of the gram-negative bacterial wall, consists of a lipid region (lipid A) and a polysaccharide region, though most of the inflammatory activity resides with lipid A (12). The host response to the appearance of endotoxin in the circulation leads to release of a series of inflammatory mediators (13). This appears to be the mechanism by which gram-negative bacteria induce physiological changes and organ dysfunction (14,15). It should be noted that gram-positive bacteria, fungi, viruses, and multiple other infectious entities are capable of producing the sepsis syndrome and diffuse lung injury.

Not surprisingly, the development of shock portends a worse prognosis in septic patients (6,16,17). Accompanying respiratory failure progressing to ARDS is associated with a mortality in excess of 90% in some studies (1,3,6). Recent data suggest that survival has improved since Ashbaugh and associates first defined the syndrome of ARDS, in 1967 (18,19,20,21). This is in large part due to better supportive care rather than improved therapies. Historically, estimates of the incidence of ARDS have been as high as 150,000 cases per year (22), though more recent studies, using stricter definitions of ARDS, have reported an incidence as low as 3.5 cases per 100,000 patients, less than one-tenth the number commonly cited (23,24,25). More studies are needed to establish the true incidence of ARDS. The factors that determine who will progress from sepsis syndrome to ARDS are unknown. In patients who develop ARDS, integrity of the epithelial barrier appears to be a key of the extent of lung injury and survival (26,27).

III. Lung Fluid Balance in Sepsis

A. Starling Forces

The factors that govern transvascular fluid movement in the lung, or for that matter, any vascular space, are represented by the Starling equation: $Q_v = K_{fc}\,[(P_c - P_i) - \sigma_d\,(\pi_c - \pi_i)]$, where Q_v is the rate at which fluid traverses the pulmonary microcirculation, K_{fc} is the capillary filtration coefficient, P_c is the capillary hydrostatic pressure, P_i is the interstitial fluid pressure, σ_d is the osmotic reflection coefficient, π_c is the colloid osmotic pressure of the plasma, and π_i is the colloid osmotic pressure of the interstitial fluid. Changes in specific variables are extremely difficult to measure accurately, even in animal models, because alterations in the hydrostatic pressure gradient will affect the oncotic pressure gradient and vice versa. Direct measurement in humans of all but π_c have not been done in the pulmonary capillaries and probably are not possible (28,29,30).

Examining the hydrostatic portion of this equation, $K_{fc}\,(P_c - P_i)$, K_{fc} represents the product of hydraulic conductivity (mL H_2O/mm Hg/g of lung) and the surface area of the pulmonary capillaries. Therefore, changes in calculated

K_{fc} may not indicate a change in membrane permeability but instead may reflect alterations in surface area and/or blood flow in the pulmonary circulation (28). P_c has not been measured directly in vivo, but it has a value somewhere between that of pulmonary arterial (PA) pressure and left arterial (LA) pressure or pulmonary artery wedge pressure (PAWP) (12,31). Due to the vertical gradient of the lung, only capillaries in zone III will have continuous blood flow; therefore the P_c for an individual capillary will depend on its location, and the overall calculated value is a mean of the pressures throughout the entire lung (32). The degree of inflation of the lungs also influences P_c—the nadir of vascular resistance; hence the lowest P_c, occurs at functional residual capacity. Interstitial pressure (P_i) is difficult to approximate, though it is generally thought to be close to zero in the normal lung. With increasing interstitial fluid accumulation, P_i increases slowly until a critical volume is reached. Beyond this point, P_i can exert a significant force opposing P_c (32). In addition, positive pressure ventilation can influence P_i in a heterogeneous manner (33,34). The net hydrostatic pressure normally favors egress of fluid out of the capillaries and into the interstitial space.

The protein osmotic pressure portion of the Starling equation, σ_d (π_c − π_i), is determined by the number of particles per unit volume so that small impermeable molecules can exert substantial oncotic force. Furthermore, π_c is not linearly related to the concentration of proteins due to the Donnan equilibrium effect (32), which means that as the plasma protein concentration increases, oncotic pressure becomes disproportionately greater. π_c can be measured accurately, but π_i can only be estimated or measured fairly crudely. σ_d plays a significant role in the movement of osmotically active particles in that it reflects the porosity of the vascular membrane; the lower the value of σ_d, the more readily molecules can traverse from the vessel lumen into the interstitium and back again. Values for σ_d range from 0, a capillary membrane permeable to all proteins, to 1, a membrane impermeable to any solutes. Normal values in the lung are reported to be about 0.7 to 0.9 (35), which limits the passage of most proteins. Furthermore, there is a unique σ for each pore size and protein molecule. Summation of the forces responsible for the oncotic pressure gradient favors movement of fluid into the interstitium because of the higher percentage of small, osmotically active proteins within the interstitium.

In the normal lung, then, hydrostatic and protein osmotic forces combine to produce slow drainage of protein poor fluid from the vascular space into the interstitium. Accumulation of fluid in the interstitial space reflects both the rapidity with which it accumulates and the ability of the lymphatic drainage system to clear the excess fluid (29). In health, interstitial fluid is easily drained back into the circulation by the pulmonary lymphatics. Lymph flow from the caudal mediastinal lymphatic in normal sheep has been measured at up to 6 mL/h (36); extrapolating to a 70-kg human predicts lung lymph flow of up to 20 mL/h. After exposure to *Pseudomonas aeruginosa,* lymph flow increases 10-fold in sheep, which would correspond to a lymph flow of 200 mL/h in septic humans (37). Sepsis and acute lung injury increase the rate of extravasation of fluid from the capillaries, which may overwhelm lymphatic capacity and cause pulmonary hypertension, favoring the formation of pulmonary edema.

In addition to lymph flow, a number of other so-called safety factors exist to initially limit alveolar flooding. The interstitial space can absorb significant amounts of fluid, approximately a 35% increase above baseline, beyond which fluid begins to accumulate in the airspaces (32). As P_c increases, forcing more fluid into the interstitial space, oncotic pressure, both in the plasma and the interstitium, is changed in a way that opposes further movement of fluid: decreased vascular fluid increases π_c, while at the same time increased extravascular fluid diminishes π_i (32). Some researchers feel the P_i is increased as well, further inhibiting movement of fluid out of the blood vessels (32). With endotoxin-induced edema, these safety factors are less effective because increased permeability of the capillaries allows edema to form at a lower P_c and minimizes the changes in oncotic pressures. Brigham and associates have shown this in a chronically instrumented, awake sheep model (38). At similar hydrostatic pressure, greater increases in lymph flow occur in sheep given endotoxin compared to those developing edema as a result of elevation in left atrial pressure alone, as shown in Figure 1.

B. Evaluation of Hydrostatic and High-Permeability Edema

Several techniques have been used to measure lung fluid accumulation in animal models and in humans with cardiogenic and noncardiogenic pulmonary edema. Few of these techniques can differentiate the two processes. *Measurement of protein concentration* in lymph has been extensively studied in animal models and used to distinguish hydrostatic from high-permeability pulmonary edema. Erdmann and colleagues collected lung lymph from awake sheep and found that sequential elevations of left atrial pressure increased microvascular pressure (P_c), eventually producing a substantial increase in lymph flow (39). As lymph flow increased, lymph/plasma protein concentration ratio fell compared to baseline. Conversely, augmented lymph flow with increased protein concentration indicates increased capillary permeability, assuming that vascular surface area has not increased. Brigham et al. exposed sheep to endotoxin and observed significant increases both in lymph flow and the lymph/plasma protein ratio (40). Increases in cardiac output and elevations in left atrial pressure both can increase surface area and account for the change in protein ratio. However, because both decrease following endotoxemia in sheep, this strongly suggests that leakage of fluid into the interstitial space occurs as a result of increased permeability. It should be noted that lung lymph represents the summation of lymph draining from a variety of different areas of the lung and that lymph collection is highly

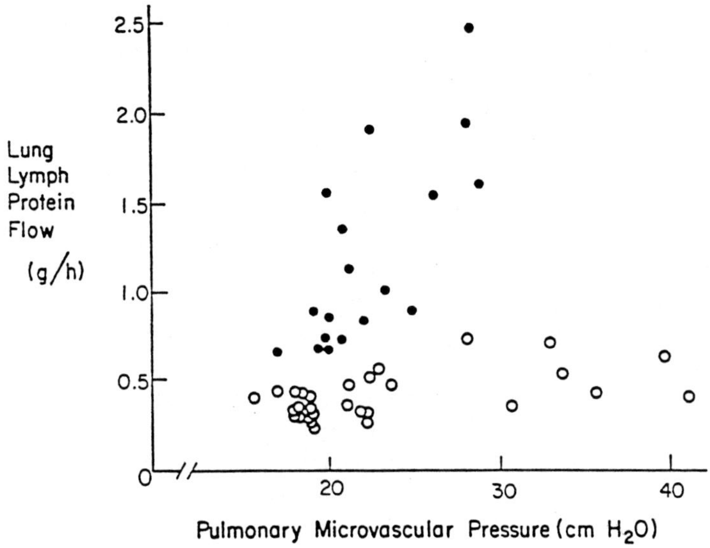

Figure 1 Steady-state lung lymph protein flow (lymph flow × lymph protein concentration) as a function of pulmonary microvascular pressure. Open circles include baseline values for each experiment and experimental observations with mechanically increased pressure. Closed circles are studies after *Pseudomonas.* Each point is averaged over at least 2 hours of steady state. Lymph protein flow after *Pseudomonas* was always higher than expected on the basis of increased pressure alone. (From Ref. 38.)

dependent on the extent of perfused vascular surface area. Furthermore, lung lymph collections in large animal models may be contaminated with lymph from extrathoracic sources (41). There is also some evidence that passage through lymph nodes may alter lymph composition (42,43).

Animal models have demonstrated that pulmonary edema accompanies this endotoxin-induced increase in lymph flow. Kuida et al. documented gross pulmonary edema in dogs given lethal doses of *E. coli* endotoxin (44). Subsequently, Snell and Ramsey showed that noncardiogenic pulmonary edema occurs in dogs given smaller doses of endotoxin (45). In a sheep model, Esbenshade et al. proved radiographically and by postmortem evaluation of lung water that pulmonary edema results from large doses of endotoxin (46). Together, these studies provide strong evidence for increased-permeability pulmonary edema in response to endotoxin in a large animal model.

Several techniques can detect alterations in permeability in humans. The easiest method to evaluate this is to compare protein concentration of alveolar edema fluid to that of plasma, the *edema fluid/plasma protein ratio.* In an intubated patient, endobronchial edema fluid is simply suctioned and protein content analyzed. Robin and colleagues showed an elevated protein concentration in edema fluid from patients with acute lung injury due to sepsis (47). Expanding upon this observation, Fein et al. calculated the ratio of edema fluid to plasma protein and used this to differentiate increased permeability from hydrostatic pulmonary edema (60). Though there is some overlap in the ratios of the two types of edema, limiting the usefulness of this analysis, one group of investigators have categorized cardiogenic edema as having an airway fluid/plasma protein ratio of < 0.5 and high-permeability pulmonary edema as having a ratio of > 0.7 (49). Others have used a cut-off of < 0.65 for hydrostatic edema (8). Employing this technique, it is assumed that edema fluid content is uniform throughout the lung and that it accurately reflects interstitial fluid content (8,48,60). Active vectorial sodium transport with water transport through transcellular water channels appears to account for the concentration of protein in edema fluid during resolution of alveolar edema (27,50,51) (see Chaps. 14–18 for further details).

Several *isotopic methods* (52,53,54,55) are available for determining transvascular movement of fluid in the lung. Various labeled tracers can be instilled directly into the airways or infused intravenously, and their rate of movement out of the airspace or the circulation, respectively, is calculated. Anderson injected ^{131}I albumin intravenously (IV) and subsequently measured levels in airway aspirates of patients with pulmonary edema (52). Greater movement of albumin from the vasculature was found in patients with ARDS compared to patients with cardiogenic pulmonary edema (Fig. 2). Scintigraphic detection of intravenous macromolecule isotopic tracers measures transvascular movement by counting external radioactivity (53,56). This technique can assess vascular permeability, is sensitive to mild increases in fluid movement across the capillary membrane, and yields information regarding both regional changes in, and severity of, vascular injury (57). In addition, alveolar epithelial permeability can be evaluated scintigraphically with aerosol administration of indicators such as Tc 99m-labeled albumin (58). Greater alveolar permeability allows for more rapid disappearance of tracer from the airway so that this may be useful in distinguishing cardiogenic from noncardiogenic edema.

Single-pass multiple indicator dilution techniques can also provide information about pulmonary microvascular permeability. Multiple tracers are given intravenously, following which, arterial blood samples are drawn to assess leakage out of the circulation during flow through the lung (54,59). Measurements of pulmonary blood flow, central volume, and lung water can be made, and by comparing the dilution curves of various tracers, a permeability-surface area product can be calculated. Shortcomings of this technique are that it is invasive, requires prolonged analysis, and is unable to fully discriminate changes in permeability from those of surface area.

The most common, least expensive method to evaluate pulmonary edema and to possibly distinguish high- from low-permeability edema, is the *chest*

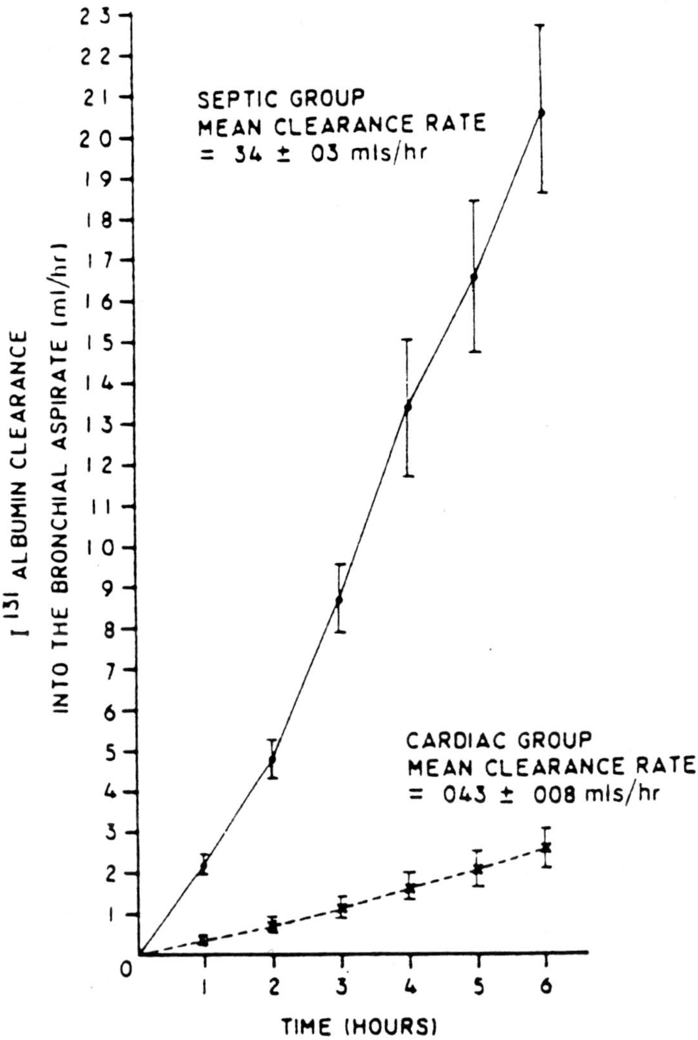

Figure 2 Comparison of the clearance of (^{131}I)albumin into bronchial secretions in patients with septic lung injury and patients with congestive heart failure. Albumin leak into the airways is increased greatly in permeability injury versus hydrostatic stress. (From Ref. 52.)

roentgenogram, which can provide information about intra- and extravascular fluid. Other major advantages of this technique include accessibility, noninvasiveness, and ability to provide information regarding distribution of edema. A number of scoring systems have been proposed to grade the degree of edema based on radiographic changes such as increase in vascular pedicle width, presence of Kerley B lines, or peribronchial cuffing (60,61,62). Fairly good correlation has been found between chest x-ray findings and other methods used to detect extravascular pulmonary water collection (60,61,63), though significant amounts of fluid (300 to 500 mL) may accumulate before changes develop on x-ray (64). In a retrospective study, a high degree of specificity in distinguishing different types of edema was obtained by Milne and associates, who evaluated chest roentgenograms in 119 patients with pulmonary edema of three etiologies—heart failure, acute lung injury, and renal failure (65). They were able to correctly differentiate the groups approximately 85% of the time. Some follow-up studies have shown a similar ability to distinguish high-permeability from cardiogenic pulmonary edema, while others have found roentgenographic studies to not be a sensitive way to differentiate the two (66,67,68) (see Chap. 3 for more details).

In patients with ARDS, attempts have been made to grade the severity of injury radiographically (69,70), but these scoring systems do not convey information about the quantity of lung fluid, which is a general limitation of x-ray evaluation of pulmonary edema. In addition, the sensitivity and specificity of the findings are low. Other important drawbacks to roentgenographic evaluation of pulmonary edema include variation in technique and quality of films, particularly in severely ill, invasively monitored, and heavily instrumented patients; changes in lung volume, which can be substantial from one film to the next in patients receiving mechanical ventilation often with the addition of positive end-expiratory pressure (PEEP) (71); and additional radiographic abnormalities due to coexisting illnesses.

New radiographic techniques for evaluating pulmonary edema include computed tomography (CT), magnetic resonance imaging (MRI) (72), and positron emission tomography (PET) (73) (see Chap. 4). However, only CT has so far demonstrated the capability to distinguish different types of pulmonary edema. Studies by Gattinoni and colleagues have shown a heterogeneous and dependent nature of infiltrates in patients with ARDS (74,75). Significant impediments to the use of these new imaging techniques are availability, expense of equipment, and need to move unstable patients; these drawbacks are not likely to be overcome in the near future.

IV. Tissue and Cellular Changes During Sepsis-Induced High-Permeability Pulmonary Edema

Lung *endothelial* damage resulting from endotoxin is well documented. Meyrick et al. studied the effect of *E. coli* endotoxin on pulmonary endothelial monolayers and on endothelial intimal explants (76,77). After 15 min of incubation with endotoxin, there was ultrastructural damage to intimal explants: dilations in intercellular junctions and ruffling of the cell membrane were noted. By 2 hours, many of the cells had lifted from the explant. Similar changes of cellular retraction and pyknosis were noted with endothelial monolayers exposed to endotoxin. The addition of serum to the culture medium leads to more severe damage, implicating a role for soluble mediators of lung injury. Furthermore, metabolic function of endothelial cells is altered by endotoxin. Increases of up to five times baseline levels of 6-keto-$PGF_{1\alpha}$, the stable plasma metabolite of the endothelial-derived eicosanoid, prostacyclin, were noted after exposure to endotoxin, indicating endothelial cell damage. Compared to control studies, there is a greater rate of equilibration of radioactive tracers across monolayers exposed to endotoxin, implying an increase in permeability. Permeability to both water, believed to traverse the endothelium through transcellular and intercellular pathways (78), and albumin, a macromolecule believed to move through the endothelium via intercellular channels only (79), was increased, providing indirect evidence for perturbation of endothelial cell membranes as well as intercellular junctions. Similar changes in endothelial structure have been noted on lung biopsy specimens taken from anesthetized, mechanically ventilated animals exposed to endotoxin (76).

Early in the course of septic lung injury, the *epithelium* appears to be more resistant than the endothelium to the insult of endotoxemia (80,81,82). Wiener-Kronish and associates evaluated the effect of *E. coli* endotoxin given to sheep both intravascularly and directly into the airways (82). They found a marked difference in the permeability of epithelial and endothelial membranes. Significant transvascular migration of proteins and accumulation of interstitial pulmonary edema was noted, but there was no increase in permeability to proteins across the epithelial barrier. In addition, alveolar liquid clearance was unaltered. Stimulation of different inflammatory responses with endotoxin given intravascularly, rather than in the airway, may account for these findings.

Other studies, however, clearly demonstrate that endotoxin injures the alveolar membrane and that this phenomenon appears to be the limiting event in the development of alveolar flooding. Pittet and associates infused live *P. aeruginosa* to 11 intact anesthetized sheep for 8 hours (81). Most of the sheep exhibited an intact, functional alveolar barrier; however, three of the sheep showed evidence of epithelial cell damage manifested by increased extravasation of protein in the airways and inability to adequately transport fluid from the alveoli. This observation has been extended to humans with ARDS (27). Patients who retained the ability to clear pulmonary edema and maintain intact epithelial function, inferred from increases in protein concentration above baseline in suctioned edema fluid, had a mortality of 22%, as opposed to 71% in patients who were not able to increase protein concentration in the edema fluid (Fig. 3).

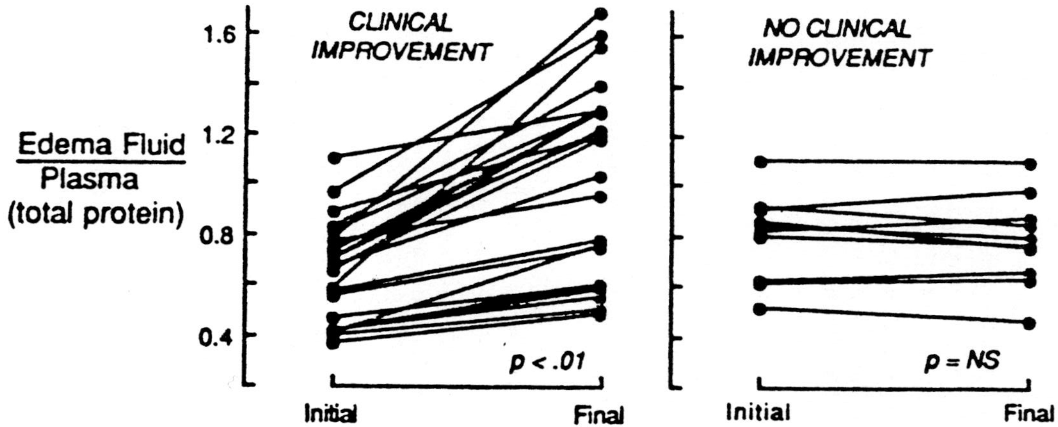

Figure 3 Individual data points are shown for the initial and final pulmonary edema fluid/plasma total protein concentration ratio in the 24 patients with clinical improvement compared to the 10 patients with no clinical improvement. The time interval between the initial and final sample was 5.3 ± 3.9 hours for the clinical-improvement group and 5.3 ± 4.7 hours for the no-clinical-improvement group. (From Ref. 27.)

Recent investigations show that a large percentage of active sodium transport, osmotically driven water movement across the alveolar epithelium occurs via *membrane water channels,* indicating a mechanism for fluid movement out of edematous alveoli and increases in edema fluid protein concentration (50,51). Endogenous release of catecholamines in response to hypotension may augment alveolar fluid removal in endotoxin-induced pulmonary edema. Pittet and colleagues have shown that, in rats with septic shock, plasma epinephrine levels increased 100-fold, accompanied by a 100% increase in liquid clearance from the airways (80). Giving propranolol, or amiloride (a sodium transport inhibitor), to the animals impeded the increase in alveolar fluid clearance. The authors concluded that large increases in endogenous catecholamines stimulate active sodium transport across the epithelial barrier, followed by passive movement of water out of the airspaces (see Chap. 14).

Morphological studies of lung specimens from patients dying of sepsis-induced ARDS reveal significant epithelial damage (26). Areas of complete epithelial destruction interspersed with areas of normal mucosa are seen on ultrastructural microscopic analysis. Interestingly, endothelial cell damage appeared less severe than that seen in the epithelium. Disruption of capillary wall integrity was rarely found. This contrasts with the findings in the above noted studies of Meyrick et al. (76,77) and may reflect species and site-specific differences in endothelial susceptibility to the effects of endotoxin (83,84). In addition, despite the unimpressive endothelial pathology, there may be significant loss of function (26,85) (see Chap. 2).

A. Neutrophils and Macrophages

Studies in both animals (76) and humans (26) reveal marked accumulation of *neutrophils* at the site of acute lung injury resulting from sepsis, which is accompanied by peripheral neutropenia (86). Macrophages, activated by endotoxin, are important in the recruitment of neutrophils to sites of injury, releasing chemoattractant mediators such as interleukin-1 (IL-1) (87). LPS injected intravenously into rats significantly increases the accumulation of neutrophils in the lung within 30 min of administration (88). Sequential lung biopsies from sheep demonstrate a threefold increase in leukocytes in the pulmonary microcirculation 15 min after injection of endotoxin (76). Evidence of neutrophil migration into the interstitium is seen as well (76). In humans with ARDS, analysis of bronchoalveolar lavage fluid demonstrates significant accumulation of neutrophils in the airways (89,90,91). How neutrophils reach the airspace has not been elucidated, but it has been shown that they can migrate across cultured pulmonary endothelial monolayers without evidence of damage to the endothelium (92,93).

Organized interaction between neutrophils and endothelial cells has been demonstrated in septic models. Endotoxin and other stimuli can induce expression of endothelial adhesion molecules such as L- and E-selectin and increase expression of intercellular adhesion molecules (ICAM-1 and ICAM-2), allowing the endothelium to bind granulocytes that have been recruited into the pulmonary microcirculation (94). Endotoxin and mediators of inflammation also activate neutrophils, thereby contributing to local injury by formation of unstable oxygen radical species and proteinases (95,96). Neutropenia in sheep, using hydroxyurea or nitrogen mustard to deplete circulating neutrophils to $< 5\%$ of baseline, markedly attenuates endotoxin induced increase in vascular permeability, reflected in decreased lung lymph protein concentration compared to normal sheep receiving endotoxin (97,98).

Some studies suggest that neutrophils may not be absolutely necessary for the development of high-permeability pulmonary edema. Winn and associates depleted leukocytes in goats using the same drugs noted above, following which high doses of *E. coli* endotoxin were infused (99). Pulmonary edema developed in animals given nitrogen mustard but was mitigated in animals given hydroxyurea. Lung injury was not directly evaluated, but was inferred from measurements of extravascular lung water. The authors concluded that neutrophils were not responsible for the development of pulmonary edema and that other effects of hydroxyurea were responsible for preventing accumulation of lung fluid. Also supporting a more limited role for direct effects of neutrophils in the generation of acute lung injury is the development of ARDS in neutropenic patients (100,101). One explanation for the discrepancy between these observations may be that neutrophils do not initiate lung injury but amplify the magnitude of injury once endothelial cells are altered by endotoxin (102). Another possibility is that there are a number of pathways through which acute lung injury can occur, involving multiple cell types and mediators. Furthermore, in septic patients, Bernard and co-workers have observed antioxidant depletion in red blood cells, normally an important scavenger of oxygen radicals, suggesting that lung injury can occur without the formation of excessive amounts of neutrophil-generated oxygen radicals (103).

B. Cytokines and Other Mediators of Lung Injury

Cytokines, a group of small signaling proteins produced by a variety of cells, are propagated in large numbers in response to infection and other disturbances in physiological homeostasis (104). An overzealous host inflammatory response appears to lead to many of the often deleterious physiological changes associated with sepsis. Tumor necrosis factor (TNF) is a cytokine secreted by macrophages and monocytes in response to LPS and other infectious and noninfectious stimuli (87,105). Over the past decade the importance of TNF in the generation of sepsis-induced acute lung injury and pulmonary edema has been extensively documented.

In 1988 Michie and associates demonstrated increased levels of TNF after intravenous administration of *E. coli* endotoxin to healthy volunteers (106). The rise in TNF levels was associated with fever, tachycardia, and other systemic responses seen with sepsis. Soon after that study, Stephens et al. injected TNF into guinea pigs and compared the physiological response to animals receiving LPS and to a control group (30). Similar degrees of increased-permeability pulmonary edema, assessed by comparing BAL fluid/plasma ratios of albumin and by direct measurement of lung water, were found in the groups that received TNF or LPS but not in the control group. Electron microscopy of lung sections from rabbits given recombinant TNF demonstrated endothelial injury and pulmonary edema similar to that seen after endotoxin infusion (107). These results suggest that TNF may play a role in acute lung injury associated with sepsis. Furthermore, Mullin and Snock have shown that leaks develop in the tight junctions between pig kidney epithelial cells exposed to TNF, leading to a breakdown of barrier function (108). These changes were inhibited by antibody to TNF, indicating that TNF is involved in the functional disruption of both the endothelium and the epithelium.

A number of studies have concluded that TNF induces neutrophil-mediated pulmonary edema and does not directly cause lung injury (30,109,110,111). Accumulation of leukocytes in the lung, as well as in other organs, occurs after administration of TNF (105). In addition, TNF is capable of activating neutrophils and promoting their adhesion to endothelial surfaces (112,113). IL-1 can act synergistically with TNF and, when given experimentally to animals and to humans, produces similar physiological changes to those seen with TNF alone (114,115). One study indicated that IL-1, not TNF, mediates neutrophil sequestration in the lung (116). Whether or not TNF acts as the primary mediator or is merely one of many players contributing to the inflammatory response responsible for endotoxin-induced pulmonary edema is not known at this time. It is evident, however, that TNF and IL-1 modulate many of the known aspects of endotoxin-induced lung injury.

Other mediators of inflammation and lung injury have been implicated in sepsis-induced ARDS. Perturbations of the coagulation system frequently occur in association with sepsis (117). Endotoxin can alter the normally antithrombotic intimal surface of the endothelium (13). Platelet-fibrin thrombi are often found in lung biopsies of patients with ARDS (118), and low platelet counts are frequently seen, which appears to correlate with mortality in sepsis (1,3). Suffredini and associates administered *E. coli* endotoxin to 19 healthy volunteers and observed an elevation in the level of tissue plasminogen activator within 1 hour of infusion. This was followed by an increase in the level of plasminogen-activator inhibitor, peaking at 5 hours and producing a pro-coagulant state (119). Increased levels of thromboxane B_2 (TxB_2), the major metabolite of thromboxane A_2 (TxA_2), a powerful vasoconstricting and platelet-aggregating cyclooxygenase product derived in large part from platelets, have been observed in animal models of endotoxemia (120,121,122). Selective inhibition of thromboxane A_2 synthesis, however, does not mitigate increases in vascular permeability (121,123,124), nor does platelet depletion alter the pulmonary vascular response to endotoxin in sheep (125).

The role of *nitric oxide* (NO) in the development of sepsis-induced lung injury is uncertain. While several studies have shown that NO is important in the development of hypotension accompanying sepsis, no direct role has been demonstrated in the lung. Nonetheless, reaction of NO with superoxide species produces peroxynitrite, a powerful oxidizing agent that can cause significant endothelial and epithelial cell injury (126). Polyclonal antibodies to nitrotyrosine, an amino acid nitrated by peroxynitrite, reveal increased staining in lung tissue specimens of patients with ARDS (127). Other studies demonstrate increased amounts of nitrotyrosine in lung sections from rats following administration of LPS (128). Together, these results indicate a possible role for endogenous NO in the generation of lung injury in ARDS.

V. Other Changes Contributing to High-Permeability Pulmonary Edema

A number of hemodynamic changes occur in septic patients and in animal models of sepsis. Following exposure to endotoxin, *pulmonary hypertension* develops in both animals and humans. Brigham and co-workers gave *E. coli* endotoxin to awake, chronically instrumented sheep and observed a two-part response consisting of an early phase of severe pulmonary hypertension followed by a more protracted phase of high vascular permeability during which PA pressure remained elevated but to a lesser degree (40) (Fig. 4). TxA_2 appears to mediate the early hypertensive response (129,130). Within 30 min following infusion of endotoxin into sheep, large increases in TxB_2 have been measured in blood and lymph samples, coinciding with substantial increases in pulmonary pressure and vascular resistance (120,121,131). Treatment with cyclo-oxygenase inhibitors reduces early hypertension but not the milder elevations of PA pressure occurring later, and, in fact, may contribute to this persistent hypertension (132). In support of this, Li et al., using a piglet model, have demonstrated a role for TxA_2, as well as TNF, in prolonged endotoxin-induced pulmonary hypertension (133).

Pulmonary hypertension is well-documented in patients with sepsis and ARDS. Independent of changes in cardiac output or PAWP, Sibbald and colleagues observed elevations of PA pressure and pulmonary vascular resistance (PVR) in 22 of 37 patients with sepsis (134). The mechanism for pulmonary hypertension in humans remains speculative. An imbalance in the release of

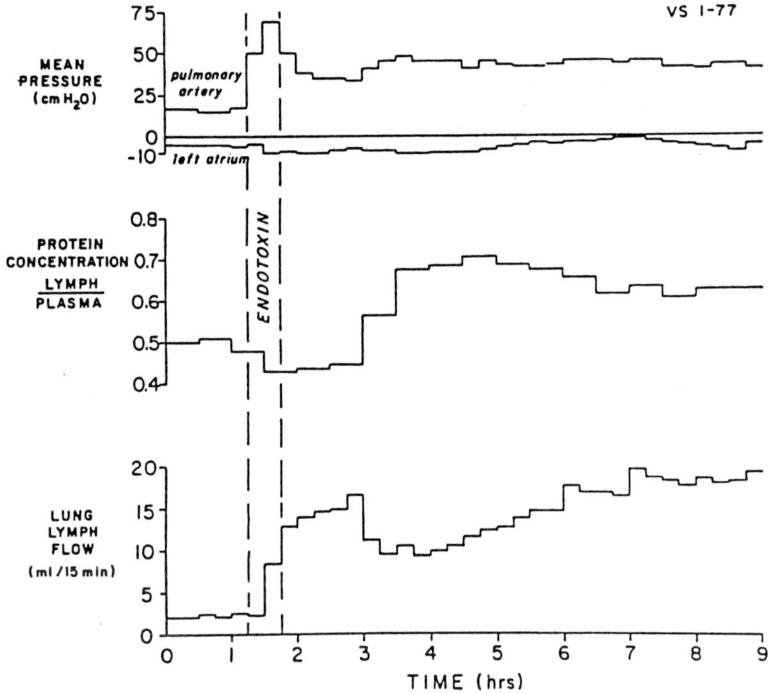

Figure 4 Effects of an intravenous infusion of *E. coli* endotoxin on pulmonary vascular pressures and lung lymph in a sheep. Late in the reaction there is high flow of protein-rich lymph at a time when pulmonary artery pressure has returned toward baseline. (From Ref. 40.)

thromboxane A_2 and PGI_2 likely plays a part, despite the fact that treatment with nonspecific cyclo-oxygenase inhibitors has not led to significant improvement in outcome in patients with ARDS. Decreases in PA pressure and improvement in oxygenation during inhalation of NO in patients with ARDS suggest that there may be a deficiency of NO in the pulmonary circulation, despite an apparent excess systemically (135). Other potential mediators of pulmonary hypertension include microthrombotic obstruction of the circulation and vasoconstriction due to autonomic nervous system activation, serotonin, or other unidentified substances (134,136,137,138).

Surfactant, synthesized by type II epithelial cells, covers the surface of the alveoli and distal airways and maintains low surface tension at the air-liquid interface, preventing collapse at low alveolar volumes. Alterations in surfactant occur in acute lung injury (18,139). Plasma proteins entering the alveolar space and polymorphonuclear leukocyte products combine to impair surfactant function (140). Abnormal surfactant with decreased amounts of phospholipid and protein has been recovered from BAL fluid in patients with ARDS (141). The inability of surfactant to function properly in this environment leads to increasing surface tension, which promotes atelectasis (142). In animal models, loss of surfactant has been shown to foster movement of fluid out of the vascular space, possibly due to the generation of very negative perimicrovascular fluid pressure in the lung as alveoli collapse (143). Though it is difficult to separate the effects of decreased surfactant in ARDS from other abnormalities, loss of vascular surface area associated with airway collapse probably contributes to pulmonary hypertension.

Importantly, *hypoxic vasoconstriction* does not seem to contribute to the pulmonary hypertension that develops with acute lung injury. In fact, there is evidence in both animals and humans that this crucial mechanism for maintaining ventilation/perfusion (V/Q) matching is lost and contributes to poor gas exchange, a defining feature of ARDS. In sheep, the PA pressure elevation associated with endotoxemia is of greater magnitude and occurs more rapidly than that which develops in response to breathing hypoxic gas mixtures (46,144). Continuous administration of 100% oxygen before and during endotoxin infusion does not prevent pulmonary hypertension from developing (144,145). Furthermore, in dogs and sheep, hypoxic vasoconstriction is inhibited for several hours following exposure to endotoxin (146,147). Even if this response were intact, hypoxic vasoconstriction becomes less effective in maintaining V/Q matching as the amount of injured lung increases (148,149). Pulmonary hypertension from any cause limits the ability of local hypoxic vasoconstriction to divert blood flow to other areas (150). In a study of 14 patients with acute, noncardiogenic respiratory failure and pulmonary edema, Brigham and associates found that survival was not associated with the amount of extravascular lung water but with the ability to maintain V/Q matching and limit perfusion to damaged or edematous areas of lung (59). Infection was the diagnosis leading to respiratory failure in eight of these patients, and reductions in lung vascular permeability-surface area, as determined by single-pass multiple tracer technique, correlated with a better outcome. These results suggest that loss of hypoxic vasoconstriction contributes to edema formation and is an important autoregulatory mechanism that is inhibited by sepsis.

Though lung lymph flow increases significantly during the early pulmonary hypertensive response to endotoxemia in sheep, lymph protein concentration decreases, suggesting capillary hypertension (40) (see Fig. 4). Parker and Brigham partitioned the pulmonary circulation of sheep into arterial and venous segments using a microwedge technique (151). They calculated vascular resistance for each segment and determined that endotoxin caused intense venoconstriction, accounting for the increased P_c and low lymph protein concentration during the early phase of sepsis. Using a two-pore mathematical model of the microvascular barrier, Bradley and co-workers measured multiple indicator dilution curves in sheep to assess permeability during the early endotoxin-induced hypertensive response (152). Their analysis showed that hemodynamic and surface changes by themselves could not explain alterations in lymph fluid protein concentration and that increases in vascular permeability did occur.

Invasive hemodynamic monitoring in septic patients reveals normal or increased cardiac output which has lead to a misconception that cardiac function is normal, or even supernormal. However, significant ventricular dysfunction has been documented in several studies. Parker et al. studied 20 patients with septic shock and found that although cardiac output was normal or elevated in all, half had an impaired left ventricular (LV) ejection fraction of $< 40\%$ assessed by radionuclide cineangiography (153). Mean end systolic and end diastolic ventricular volumes were increased in survivors, allowing stroke volume to be maintained (Fig. 5). Patients who survived, demonstrated a gradual return to normal of ejection fraction and ventricular size. The finding of reversible

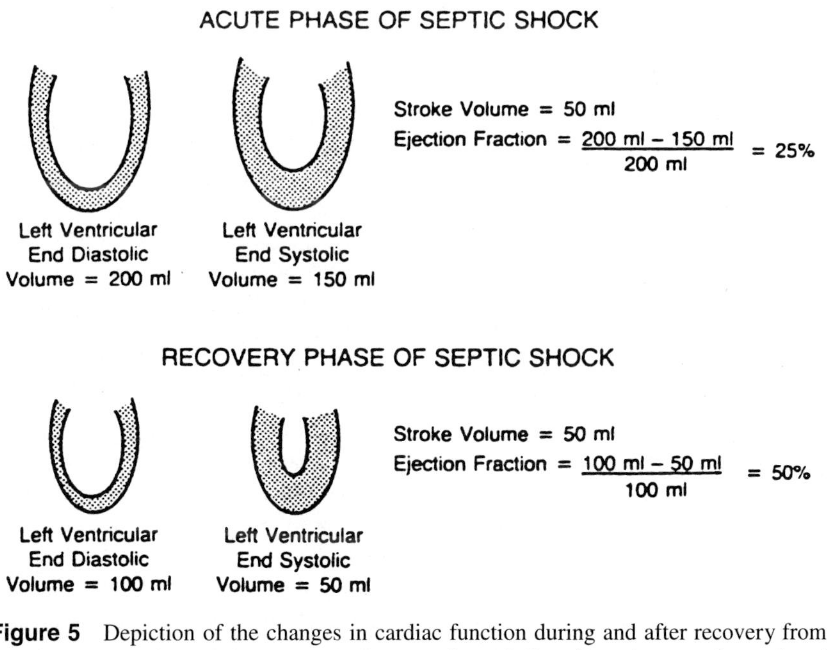

Figure 5 Depiction of the changes in cardiac function during and after recovery from septic shock. Endotoxemia causes an increase in end-diastolic volume and a reduced ejection fraction. Myocardial compliance is increased. The dysfunction occurs with both ventricles. Stroke volume is relatively unchanged. Cardiac output occurs via increased heart rate. (From Ref. 153.)

depression in cardiac function has been verified by the use of other measures of ventricular performance (154,155) and implies that greater compliance of the myocardium confers a survival advantage. The mechanism responsible for altered cardiac function in sepsis is not known. Cardiac ischemia does not occur: compared to normal subjects, angiographic evaluation of coronary arteries of patients with septic shock has demonstrated normal or increased blood flow (156). Indirect evidence points to the existence of a myocardial depressant substance (157,158), although none has been specifically identified (159).

PEEP is frequently used in mechanically ventilated patients with ARDS. It can increase PVR, and in doing so, increases right ventricular afterload. Jardin and colleagues studied the effect of PEEP on LV function and size and noted decreasing compliance as PEEP increased (160). Changes in LV compliance, in turn, alter the accuracy of PAWP readings. Other studies have confirmed that PEEP produces inaccuracies in estimating LV filling pressures (161). Although sepsis-induced pulmonary edema is classified as a high-permeability edema, it is evident that accurate calculation of hydrostatic pressures is difficult and that hydrostatic forces likely contribute to the severity of pulmonary edema in patients with ARDS.

Serum protein osmotic pressure, π_c, also affects accumulation of fluid in high-permeability edema. Nearly 40 years ago, Guyton and Lindsey examined the effect of serum protein osmotic pressure on the formation of pulmonary edema in dogs (162). In normal dogs pulmonary edema did not develop until LA pressure had been increased to more than 24 mm Hg, but when plasma protein concentration was halved, an LA pressure of only 11 mm Hg was required before extravascular fluid began to accumulate. In contrast, Rice and associates found that with PAWP held constant, infusion of *E. coli* into baboons with decreased plasma protein osmotic pressure did not result in pulmonary edema (163). Differences in techniques used to evaluate lung fluid and measure LV filling pressures and differences in the effects of endotoxin between species may account for the contradictory findings. In humans, decreases in π_c does appear to affect the accumulation of fluid in the lung (Fig. 6). Rackow et al. prospectively evaluated 76 patients with either cardiogenic or high-permeability pulmonary edema (164). They examined the plasma protein osmotic pressure-PAWP gradient and found that a decrease in the gradient identified patients who went on to develop pulmonary edema. Decreased plasma protein osmotic pressure with a normal PAWP characterized patients with high-permeability edema, and conversely, a high PAWP with normal plasma protein osmotic pressure characterized patients with cardiogenic edema. Despite the decrease in plasma protein osmotic pressure frequently seen in patients with ARDS, infusion of colloid substances does not offer advantages over volume replacement with crystalloid (165,166,167).

Whether or not sepsis-induced pulmonary edema is worsened by low protein osmotic pressure, patients with sepsis invariably have low concentrations

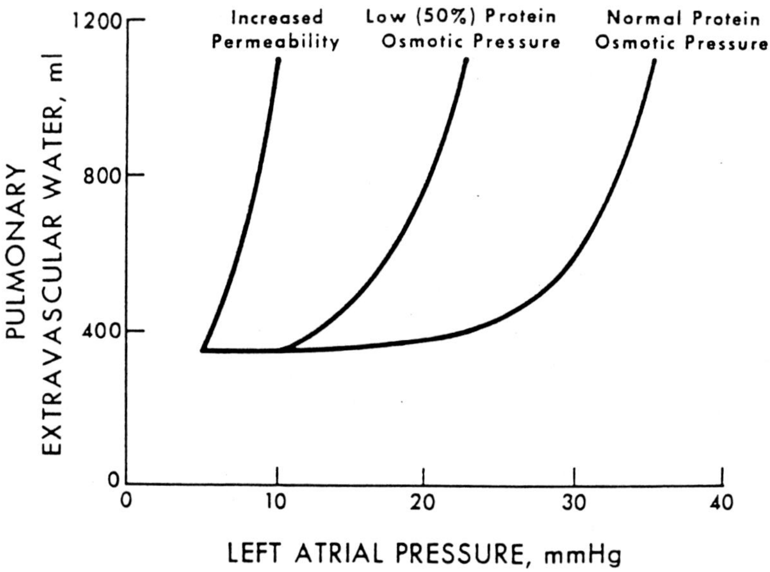

Figure 6 Pulmonary edema (extravascular lung water) as a function of left atrial pressure in the normal state and during either decreased oncotic pressure (low plasma albumin) or increased lung vascular permeability. Hypoalbuminemia and increased lung vascular permeability are features of endotoxemia that increase the likilhood of pulmonary edema. (From Ref. 233.)

of *albumin,* the major osmotic particle contributing to π_c. Moshage and coworkers have demonstrated decreases in albumin synthesis and liver albumin messenger ribonucleic acid in a rat model of turpentine-induced inflammation (168). Their findings suggest that monocyte products, especially IL-1, which may be a key mediator of the host response to endotoxemia, plays a major role in this process. In addition, increases in systemic vascular permeability may contribute to acute decreases in albumin concentration. Thrombin activation occurs during sepsis as part of the disturbances in the coagulation system, and in vitro studies demonstrated a thrombin-induced increase in permeability to albumin across monolayers of endothelial cells (169).

Patients with acute lung injury frequently require *high amounts of oxygen* to maintain an adequate oxygen saturation. High FiO_2, however, can independently produce lung injury. One hundred percent oxygen, at sea level, causes damage to the lungs of neonates, and prolonged exposure is fatal in most animal species studied (170,171). Oxygen toxicity produces interstitial swelling, influx of neutrophils, and eventually, alveolar edema (145,170,172). Mechanisms of injury include neutrophil activation and generation of oxygen radical species (173,174), increased vascular permeability, and loss of hypoxic pulmonary vasoconstriction (174). Endotoxin, administered to rats and sheep, has been demonstrated to have a protective effect against oxygen toxicity. Frank and associates exposed rats to hyperoxic gas mixtures. Increased survival and decreased lung fluid accumulation, compared to a control group, was observed in animals given a single dose of endotoxin up to 36 hours after the onset of hyperoxic exposure (174). Kobayashi et al. demonstrated a protective effect of endotoxin in sheep breathing 100% oxygen, finding that tolerance to hyperoxia was increased though ultimate progression to respiratory failure was not prevented (175). Whether septic patients with ARDS incur greater lung injury from breathing high oxygen gas mixtures or are protected from its deleterious effects is not known. However, no correlation has been shown between the amount of FiO_2 required and severity of ARDS, and patients requiring excessive amounts of oxygen for months can eventually recover near-normal lung function (170,176).

The *bronchial circulation* has not been well-studied in acute lung injury. Pietra and associates observed increased permeability in bronchial venules following endotoxin infusion in dogs (177). Colloidal carbon was injected intravenously and found on microscopy of lung sections to accumulate initially around the bronchial venules, preceding any evidence of alveolar damage by 1 hour. This study suggests that leakage of fluid across the bronchioles can contribute to extravascular fluid accumulation. The bronchial circulation is difficult to study in vivo, even in animals, but estimates of bronchial blood flow range from approximately 0.5% to 2.0% of cardiac output (178,179). This translates into an average flow of around 50 mL/min, which could significantly augment the amount of extravascular lung fluid if bronchial vessel permeability were increased. Furthermore, sepsis-associated pulmonary hypertension and loss of vascular surface area could divert additional blood flow into the bronchial circulation, increasing its importance in the development of high-permeability pulmonary edema (180).

VI. Therapies for Sepsis-Induced Pulmonary Edema

In recent years, treatment of pulmonary edema associated with sepsis has moved toward targeting specific aspects of the inflammatory response, although no clear-cut benefit from this approach has been demonstrated. This section will review some of the major features of previous and established therapies, followed by a discussion of new and experimental treatments with particular emphasis on efforts to block or modify the effects of endotoxin and the accompanying inflammatory response. A basic tenant of ARDS management is limiting pulmonary capillary pressure to avoid pulmonary edema while maintaining adequate volume for tissue perfusion. Several studies have examined fluid management, but none has documented improved survival with fluid restriction (181,182). Other studies have shown a positive correlation between increased fluid intake and weight gain and poorer outcome (183,184), though no causative effect of excessive fluid administration has been demonstrated, and, most likely, it is a marker of sicker patients (see Chap. 4).

Permissive hypercapnia, using small tidal volumes and allowing $PaCO_2$ to rise in some mechanically ventilated patients, may be prudent in order to reduce barotrauma or shear stress which may perpetuate lung injury. However, these patients often require excessive sedation and paralytics, putting them at increased risk for infection, sudden unnoticed hemodynamic decompensation, and prolonged mechanical ventilation (185). A large multicenter randomized trial to evaluate low versus high tidal volume in patients with ARDS is in progress. The treatment strategies considered above, as well as attention to comfort, prophylaxis for deep vein thrombosis, and other supportive care, are applicable not only to patients with sepsis-induced lung injury but to other critically ill patients with respiratory failure as well (see Chap. 20 for further details).

More specific to endotoxin-induced lung injury, the large influx of inflammatory mediators and cells into the lung suggested that *anti-inflammatory treatment* could prevent many of the harmful sequelae. Treatment with the nonsteroidal anti-inflammatory drug (NSAID) meclofenamate, or more selectively with thromboxane synthesis inhibitors, in sheep models of endotoxemia prevents the large increase in pulmonary artery pressure but does not prevent changes in vascular permeability, as noted earlier (120,121). Similar findings were noted in dogs treated with indomethacin prior to endotoxin infusion (186). Brigham et al. and Demling et al. both demonstrated that methylprednisolone prevented endotoxin-induced increases in vascular permeability in sheep (187,188). Subsequently, Begley and associates administered endotoxin to sheep with and without concomitant infusion of both meclofenamate and methylprednisolone (Fig. 7) and found, not surprisingly, that the combination prevented the early as well as the late-phase response to endotoxin (129).

Attempts at nonspecific anti-inflammatory therapy in humans have not met with the success found in animal models. This may in large part reflect the fact that in ARDS, unlike in animal models of sepsis-induced lung injury, patients do not receive treatment prior to the onset of endotoxemia. Once the inflammatory response is set in motion, it may not be possible to prevent lung injury. Early reports showing a benefit from treatment with steroids in septic patients (189,190) and a reduction in alveolocapillary permeability (191) were not confirmed in large, prospective, placebo-controlled trials (192,193). In another study, focusing on progression to ARDS, administration of steroids to patients with septic shock was not effective in preventing the development of

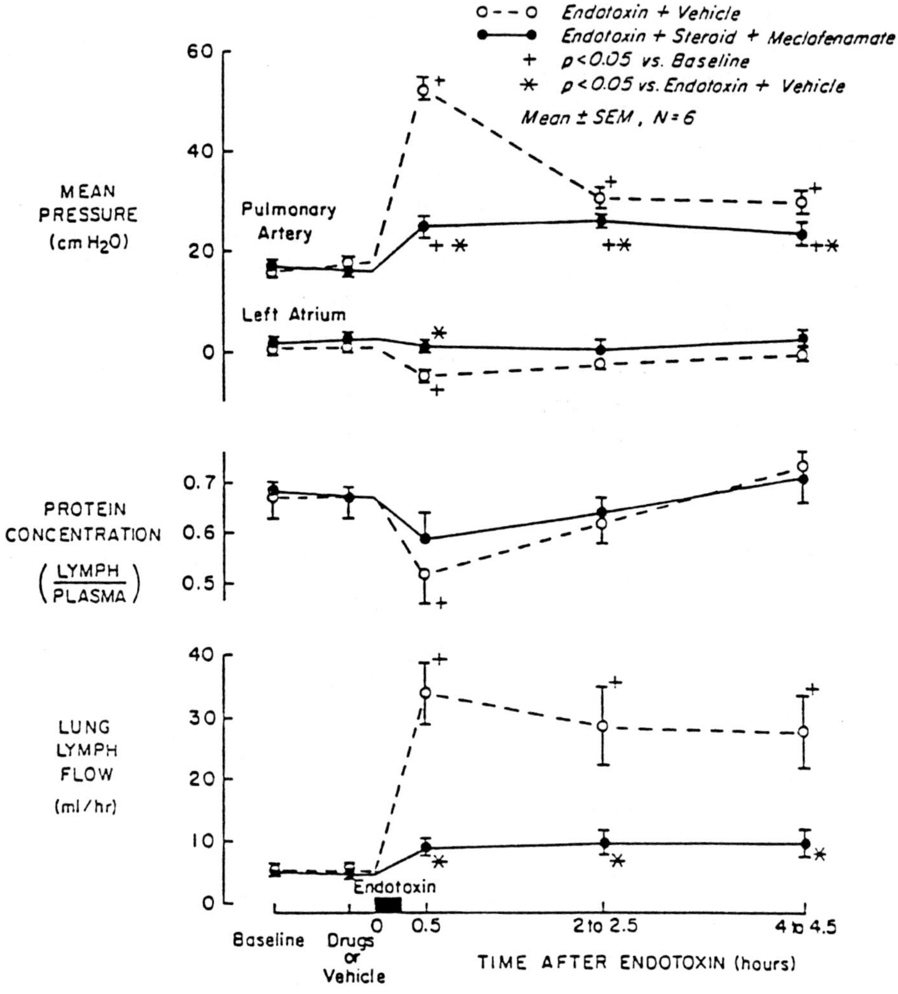

Figure 7 The effect of combined therapy with methylprednisolone and a cyclooxygenase inhibitor, meclofenamate, on the response to *E. coli* endotoxin infusion in sheep. Given separately, meclofenamate inhibits the initial response, and steroid attenuates the later response. In these experiments, combined therapy markedly diminishes the entire response. (From Ref. 129.)

ARDS (194). Evaluating the efficacy of corticosteroids in patients with established ARDS, Bernard and associates found no benefit with treatment in a randomized, double-blind, placebo-controlled study involving 99 patients (195). More recently, a large, multicenter study evaluating ibuprofen in ARDS found no improvement in survival (196).

Antioxidant therapy with N-acetyl cysteine (NAC) has been examined in patients with acute lung injury of varying degrees of severity. The one trial evaluating patients with ARDS showed no difference between the treated and placebo arms of the study either in pulmonary function during the first 7 days after enrollment or in survival at 60 days (197). *Vasodilator therapy* with PGE_1, prostacyclin, or nitroglycerin can reduce PA pressure but may worsen V/Q mismatching (198,199,200,201). The only large, randomized, placebo-controlled study of vasodilator therapy in patients with ARDS, evaluating PGE_1, did not demonstrate increased survival compared to placebo (202). As mentioned earlier, inhaled NO has been used successfully in ARDS to improve oxygenation and decrease pulmonary artery pressures (135,203,204). NO selectively dilates vasculature that is well ventilated and, in doing so, improves V/Q matching. It rapidly binds to hemoglobin and is inactivated, avoiding potentially adverse vasodilation of the systemic circulation. Studies large enough to assess impact on survival are ongoing.

Surfactant replacement therapy has been evaluated in ARDS. The success with exogenous surfactant in the treatment of newborns with respiratory distress syndrome has not been duplicated in patients with ARDS. One major difference between the two groups is that newborns have an absolute deficiency of surfactant whereas patients with ARDS have a functional abnormality (141). Additionally, a number of problems including timing of therapy, paucity of knowledge regarding optimal route of delivery or dosing interval, lack of protein in artificial surfactant, and the heterogeneous etiology of ARDS, may have contributed to the disappointing results (205). *Ventilation with perfluorocarbons,* liquids with a high affinity for oxygen and surfactant-like properties, may prove to be of benefit in the treatment of ARDS. However, limited information about efficacy in adults is available. A recent abstract evaluating liquid ventilation in nine patients with respiratory failure due to ARDS or pneumonia reported beneficial effects on gas exchange (206); more definitive information must await the results of an ongoing clinical study (see Chap. 20).

A natural target for therapy would seem to be endotoxin itself. However, a series of trials evaluating a efficacy of *monoclonal antibodies* in the treatment of sepsis have not demonstrated significant reductions in mortality (207,208, 209,210). Two studies employing a monoclonal antibody to endotoxin, E5, have been undertaken. The second of these trials showed a statistically significant decrease in the development of ARDS compared to placebo, but no survival advantage (207). Yet another trial studying septic patients with ARDS and employing the monoclonal antibody HA-1A, found no difference in resolution of respiratory failure between patients given the antibody and those given placebo (211). In light of minimal or no benefit demonstrated with these antibodies and the tremendous cost, it does not appear that therapy aimed directly at endotoxin is the panacea some envisioned. Perhaps if the development of sepsis or ARDS could be reliably predicted, and these compounds could be given as prophylaxis, efficacy would be improved.

Monoclonal antibodies directed against specific elements of the inflammatory response are being evaluated. Anticytokine therapy in the treatment of sepsis using *antibodies against TNF* and *receptor antagonists to IL-1* have been tested in clinical studies. The impetus for human trials came from animal studies demonstrating protection from septic shock with TNF antibody pretreatment (212,213). In the past 2 years, the results of three prospective, randomized, placebo-controlled multicenter trails evaluating the efficacy TNF antibodies in humans with sepsis have been published (214,215,216). None has shown a survival difference, though the most recent study did reveal more rapid improvement from shock and less multiorgan failure in survivors in the treated arm compared to placebo (215). Studies using the dimeric form of one of the two TNF receptors coupled with human IgG have been undertaken but have shown no better results. A recent Phase III multicenter trial not only failed to show a reduction in mortality, but at higher doses was associated with increased mortality (217). Methodological problems with these studies make the data difficult to interpret. For example, though reduction in TNF levels was documented after administration of antibody, inhibition of TNF was not complete.

IL-1 receptor antagonists (IL-1ra) have been evaluated in animal models. Ohlsson and colleagues showed that IL-1ra reduced endotoxin-induced neutrophil accumulation and pulmonary edema compared to rabbits given endotoxin alone (218). Mice given what normally would have been a lethal dose of endotoxin showed improved survival when administered IL-1ra (219). Results from a Phase III trial evaluating IL-1ra in humans with sepsis revealed no increase in survival (220). *Posthoc* analysis, however, did indicate a reduction in mortality in patients with evidence of end-organ failure, including patients with ARDS. Future, prospective trials will be needed to corroborate a true benefit.

A number of explanations may account for this lack of efficacy of therapy directed at specific cytokines. Difficulty in predicting the onset of ARDS continues to be a major problem, especially since anticytokine therapy is directed at early steps in the inflammatory response. Another problem is the overlapping function of cytokines so that blocking one cytokine may have little effect on the overall response. Furthermore, cytokine responses undoubtedly have beneficial functions as part of a normal response to infection, and blocking some parts of the inflammatory pathway may actually impair the host's ability to survive (104). Lastly, there are indications that cytokines function more as paracrine mediators rather than as endocrine substances and that tissue levels, rather than plasma levels, may be a more significant indicator of activity (221).

Therapeutic options that are just starting to be evaluated include *anti-cell-adhesion molecule (anti-ICAM) therapy* and *pharmacological promotion of fluid movement out of the alveoli.* As opposed to anticytokine therapy, antiadhesion therapy may allow for more selective targeting of specific organs affected by endotoxin. In rabbits given *E. coli* endotoxin, Doerschuk et al. demonstrated that administration of a monoclonal antibody to CD18, part of the endothelial leukocyte adhesion complex, effectively blocked neutrophil movement into the alveoli (222). Additional studies in pigs treated with the same antibody produced similar effects following live infusion of *P. aeruginosa* (223). This resulted in a significant decrease in lung injury compared to control animals. Monoclonal antibodies targeting ICAM-1 have also been shown to diminish acute lung injury in experimental conditions (224). Antibodies directed against selectins have been able to ameliorate sepsis-induced lung injury in pigs (225). A small Phase II trial in humans with septic shock, using antibody directed against E-selectin, indicated a beneficial effect (226). Not all of the results, however, are encouraging. Sharar and associates demonstrated that monoclonal antibody to CD18 given to rabbits injected with high doses of *Staphalococcus aureus* resulted in more subcutaneous abscess formation than in rabbits not receiving the antibody, suggesting detrimental mitigation of the host immune response (227). More preliminary data, especially concerning safety of monoclonal antibody therapy directed at specific aspects of the immune response, needs to be gathered before embarking on large-scale clinical trials (see Chap. 20 for further discussion).

The observations of Wiener-Kronish and Matthay (27) and Pittet and colleagues (80) that intact epithelial barrier function is crucial for resolution of pulmonary edema and that fluid clearance is enhanced by β-agonists, suggests some therapeutic options despite the fact that survival was not changed. Alveolar fluid absorption is increased by agents that augment cyclic adenosine monophosphate (cAMP) levels such as β-agonists or phosphodiesterase inhibitors (228). In anesthetized sheep, β-adrenergic agents increase alveolar fluid clearance when instilled into the alveoli (229). Following acid injury, aminophylline and isoproterenol moderated the degree of pulmonary edema (230). In addition, anti-inflammatory cytokines, such as IL-10, are released during sepsis. Epinephrine (231) and methylxanthines (232) potentiate IL-10 and may provide a way to augment the host's natural ability to control the extent of inflammation. Further investigations into the effects of compounds that increase cAMP seem to be warranted. Perhaps by combining therapies that prevent or limit alveolar damage with those that increase fluid removal from the alveoli, improved morbidity and mortality can be achieved in patients with sepsis-induced high-permeability pulmonary edema (see Chap. 20).

VII. Conclusion

Sepsis-induced pulmonary edema has traditionally been regarded as an increased-permeability pulmonary edema. There is no question that damage to both the endothelium and the epithelium may occur as a consequence of severe endotoxemia. Neutrophils appear to play a central role in the breakdown of the alveolar-capillary barrier through the generation of oxygen radical species. Recently, mechanisms of neutrophil recruitment and adhesion to the pulmonary vasculature and, ultimately, movement into the extravascular space, have been elucidated. Other mediators, particularly the cytokines TNF and IL-1, also have been shown to contribute to the accumulation of extravascular lung fluid characteristic of sepsis-induced pulmonary edema. It is clear, however, that many other factors are involved in the abnormal accumulation of edema fluid in sepsis. Cardiac dysfunction, pulmonary vasoconstriction, V/Q mismatching, dysfunctional surfactant, loss of microvascular surface area, and release of large numbers of vasoactive substances all promote the formation of pulmonary edema in sepsis. Thus, hydrostatic forces can augment the movement of fluid out of the lung vascular space.

Despite our improved understanding of the pathophysiological mechanisms in endotoxemia, attempts to direct therapy at specific pathways of the inflammatory response have not yet significantly affected the mortality and morbidity associated with ARDS. Inability to predict the development of clinical lung injury and provide prophylactic treatment may account for the failure to reproduce the therapeutic success seen in animal models of sepsis. Redundancy and interaction of inflammatory pathways also contributes to the limited efficacy of single therapies. It is still unknown why some patients are able to recover from the insult to the alveolar-capillary membrane while others develop fibrosis with irreversible lung damage. Perhaps with more understanding of the forces governing the movement of fluid into and out of the distal airspaces, more sophisticated therapies that attenuate but do not prevent the host response, and improved ability to predict the onset of sepsis-induced lung injury, it will be possible to apply our knowledge more effectively to clinical practice.

References

1. Fein AM, Lippmann M, Holtzman H, Eliraz A, Goldberg SK. The risk factors, incidence, and prognosis of ARDS following septicemia. Chest 1983; 83(1):40–42.
2. Fowler AA, Hamman RF, Zerbe GO, Benson KN, Hyers TM. Adult respiratory distress syndrome. Prognosis after onset. Am Rev Respir Dis 1985; 132(3): 472–478.
3. Kaplan RL, Sahn SA, Petty TL. Incidence and outcome of the respiratory distress syndrome in gram-negative sepsis. Arch Intern Med 1979; 139(8):867–869.

4. Pepe PE, Potkin RT, Reus DH, Hudson LD, Carrico CJ. Clinical predictors of the adult respiratory distress syndrome. Am J Surg 1982; 144(1):124–130.
5. Weinberg PF, Matthay MA, Webster RO, Roskos KV, Goldstein IM, Murray JF. Biologically active products of complement and acute lung injury in patients with the sepsis syndrome. Am Rev Respir Dis 1984; 130(5):791–796.
6. Rubin DB, Wiener-Kronish JP, Murray JF, Green DR, Turner J, Luce JM, Montgomery AB, Marks JD, Matthay MA. Elevated von Willebrand factor antigen is an early plasma predictor of acute lung injury in nonpulmonary sepsis syndrome. J Clin Invest 1990; 86(2):474–480.
7. Hammarstrom S. Leukotrienes. Annu Rev Biochem 1983; 52:355–377.
8. Matthay MA, Eschenbacher WL, Goetzl EJ. Elevated concentrations of leukotriene D4 in pulmonary edema fluid of patients with the adult respiratory distress syndrome. J Clin Immunol 1984; 4(6):479–483.
9. Bell RC, Coalson JJ, Smith JD, Johanson WGJ. Multiple organ system failure and infection in adult respiratory distress syndrome. Ann Intern Med 1983; 99(3): 293–298.
10. Schuster DP, Marion JM. Precedents for meaningful recovery during treatment in a medical intensive care unit. Outcome in patients with hematologic malignancy. Am J Med 1983; 75(3):402–408.
11. Fulton RL, Jones CE. The cause of post-traumatic pulmonary insufficiency in man. Surg Gynecol Obstet 1975; 140(2):179–186.
12. Bradley SG. Cellular and molecular mechanisms of action of bacterial endotoxins. Annu Rev Microbiol 1979; 33:67–94.
13. Pajkrt D, van Deventer S. The cellular response in sepsis. Current Topics in Microbiology and Immunology 1996; 216:119–132.
14. Morrison DC, Ryan JL. Bacterial endotoxins and host immune responses. Adv Immunol 1979; 28:293–450.
15. Ziegler EJ, McCutchan JA, Fierer J, Glauser MP, Sadoff JC, Douglas H, Braude AI. Treatment of gram-negative bacteremia and shock with human antiserum to a mutant *Escherichia coli.* N Engl J Med 1982; 307(20):1225–1230.
16. Rangel-Frausto MS, Pittet D, Costigan M, Hwang T, Davis CS, Wenzel RP. The natural history of the systemic inflammatory response syndrome (SIRS). A prospective study. JAMA 1995; 273(2):117–123.
17. Zimmerman GA, Morris AH, Cengiz M. Cardiovascular alterations in the adult respiratory distress syndrome. Am J Med 1982; 73(1):25–34.
18. Ashbaugh DG, Bigelow DB, Petty TL, Levine BE. Acute respiratory distress in adults. Lancet 1967; 2(7511):319–323.
19. Milberg JA, Davis DR, Steinberg KP, Hudson LD. Improved survival of patients with acute respiratory distress syndrome (ARDS): 1983–1993. JAMA 1995; 273(4):306–309.
20. Suchyta MR, Clemmer TP, Elliott CG, Orme JF Jr, Weaver LK. The adult respiratory distress syndrome. A report of survival and modifying factors. Chest 1992; 101(4):1074–1079.
21. Willms D, Nield M, Gocka I. Adult respiratory distress syndrome: outcome in a community hospital. Am J Crit Care 1994; 3(5):337–341.
22. Rinaldo JE, Rogers RM. Adult respiratory-distress syndrome: changing concepts of lung injury and repair. N Engl J Med 1982; 306(15):900–909.

23. Fowler AA, Hamman RF, Good JT, Benson KN, Baird M, Eberle DJ, Petty TL, Hyers TM. Adult respiratory distress syndrome: risk with common predispositions. Ann Intern Med 1983; 98(5:Pt 1):593–597.
24. Thomsen GE, Morris AH. Incidence of the adult respiratory distress syndrome in the state of Utah. Am J Respir Crit Care Med 1995; 152(3):965–971.
25. Villar J, Slutsky AS. The incidence of the adult respiratory distress syndrome. Am Rev Respir Dis 1989; 140(3):814–816.
26. Bachofen A, Weibel ER. Alterations of the gas exchange apparatus in adult respiratory insufficiency associated with septicemia. Am Rev Respir Dis 1977; 116(4):589–615.
27. Matthay MA, Wiener-Kronish JP. Intact epithelial barrier function is critical for the resolution of alveolar edema in humans. Am Rev Respir Dis 1990; 142(6 Pt 1):1250–1257.
28. Robin ED, Cross CE, Zelis R. Pulmonary edema. 2. N Engl J Med 1973; 288(6): 292–304.
29. Staub NC. Extravascular forces in lung affecting fluid and protein exchange. Am Rev Respir Dis 1977; 115(6 Pt 2):159–163.
30. Stephens KE, Ishizaka A, Larrick JW, Raffin TA. Tumor necrosis factor causes increased pulmonary permeability and edema. Comparison to septic acute lung injury. Am Rev Respir Dis 1988; 137(6):1364–1370.
31. Gaar KAJ, Taylor AE, Owens LJ, Guyton AC. Pulmonary capillary pressure and filtration coefficient in the isolated perfused lung. Am J Physiol 1967; 213(4): 910–914.
32. Taylor AE, Parker JC. Pulmonary interstitial spaces and lymphatics. In: Fishman A, ed. Handbook of Physiology. New York: McGraw-Hill, 1997:167–230. Pulmonary Interstitial Spaces and Lymphatics.
33. Russell JA, Hoeffel J, Murray JF. Effect of different levels of positive end-expiratory pressure on lung water content. J Appl Physiol: Respir Environ Exercise Physiol 1982; 53(1):9–15.
34. Woolverton WC, Brigham KL, Staub NC. Effect of positive pressure breathing on lung lymph flow and water content in sheep. Circ Res 1978; 42(4):550–557.
35. Parker RE, Roselli RJ, Harris TR, Brigham KL. Effects of graded increases in pulmonary vascular pressures on lung fluid balance in unanesthetized sheep. Circ Res 1981; 49(5):1164–1172.
36. Staub NC. Steady state pulmonary transvascular water filtration in unanesthetized sheep. Circ Res 1971; 28(suppl 1):135–139.
37. Staub NC. "State of the art" review. Pathogenesis of pulmonary edema. Am Rev Respir Dis 1974; 109(3):358–372.
38. Brigham KL, Woolverton WC, Blake LH, Staub NC. Increased sheep lung vascular permeability caused by pseudomonas bacteremia. J Clin Invest 1974; 54(4):792–804.
39. Erdmann AJ, Vaughan TRJ, Brigham KL, Woolverton WC, Staub NC. Effect of increased vascular pressure on lung fluid balance in unanesthetized sheep. Circ Res 1975; 37(3):271–284.
40. Brigham KL, Bowers R, Haynes J. Increased sheep lung vascular permeability caused by *Escherichia coli* endotoxin. Circ Res 1979; 45(2):292–297.

41. Drake R, Adair T, Traber D, Gabel J. Contamination of caudal mediastinal node efferent lymph in sheep. Am J Physiol 1981; 241(3):H354–H357.
42. Adair TH. Studies of lymph modification by lymph nodes. Microcirculation, Endothelium, & Lymphatics 1985; 2(3):251–269.
43. Adair TH, Moffatt DS, Paulsen AW, Guyton AC. Quantitation of changes in lymph protein concentration during lymph node transit. Am J Physiol 1982; 243(3): H351–H359.
44. Kuida H, Hinshaw LB, Gilbert RP, Visscher MB. Effect of gram-negative endotoxin on pulmonary circulation. Am J Physiol 1958; 192:335–344.
45. Snell JDJ, Ramsey LH. Pulmonary edema as a result of endotoxemia. Am J Physiol 1969; 217(1):170–175.
46. Esbenshade AM, Newman JH, Lams PM, Jolles H, Brigham KL. Respiratory failure after endotoxin infusion in sheep: lung mechanics and lung fluid balance. J Appl Physiol: Respir Environ Exercise Physiol 1982; 53(4):967–976.
47. Robin ED, Carey LC, Grenvik A, Glauser F, Gaudio R. Capillary leak syndrome with pulmonary edema. Arch Intern Med 1972; 130(1):66–71.
48. Fein A, Grossman RF, Jones JG, Overland E, Pitts L, Murray JF, Staub NC. The value of edema fluid protein measurement in patients with pulmonary edema. Am J Med 1979; 67(1):32–38.
49. Sprung CL, Rackow EC, Fein IA, Jacob AI, Isikoff SK. The spectrum of pulmonary edema: differentiation of cardiogenic, intermediate, and noncardiogenic forms of pulmonary edema. Am Rev Respir Dis 1981; 124(6):718–722.
50. Folkesson HG, Matthay MA, Frigeri A, Verkman AS. Transepithelial water permeability in microperfused distal airways. Evidence for channel-mediated water transport. J Clin Invest 1996; 97(3):664–671.
51. Folkesson HG, Matthay MA, Hasegawa H, Kheradmand F, Verkman AS. Transcellular water transport in lung alveolar epithelium through mercury-sensitive water channels. Proc Nat Acad Sci USA 1994; 91(11):4970–4974.
52. Anderson RR, Holliday RL, Driedger AA, Lefcoe M, Reid B, Sibbald WJ. Documentation of pulmonary capillary permeability in the adult respiratory distress syndrome accompanying human sepsis. Am Rev Respir Dis 1979; 119(6): 869–877.
53. Gorin AB, Kohler J, DeNardo G. Noninvasive measurement of pulmonary transvascular protein flux in normal man. J Clin Invest 1980; 66(5):869–877.
54. Harris TR, Brigham KL. The exchange of small molecules as a measure of normal and abnormal lung microvascular function. Ann NY Acad Sci 1982; 384: 417–434.
55. Tatum JL, Burke TS, Sugerman HJ, Strash AM, Hirsch JI, Fratkin MJ. Computerized scintigraphic technique for the evaluation of adult respiratory distress syndrome: initial clinical trials. Radiology 1982; 143(1):237–241.
56. Sugerman HJ, Tatum JL, Burke TS, Strash AM, Glauser FL. Gamma scintigraphic analysis of albumin flux in patients with acute respiratory distress syndrome. Surgery 1984; 95(6):674–682.
57. Dauber IM, Weil JV. Noninvasive radioisotopic assessment of pulmonary vascular protein leak. Experimental studies and potential clinical applications. Clin Chest Med 1985; 6(3):427–437.

58. Mason GR, Effros RM, Uszler JM, Mena I. Small solute clearance from the lungs of patients with cardiogenic and noncardiogenic pulmonary edema. Chest 1985; 88(3):327–334.
59. Brigham KL, Kariman K, Harris TR, Snapper JR, Bernard GR, Young SL. Correlation of oxygenation with vascular permeability-surface area but not with lung water in humans with acute respiratory failure and pulmonary edema. J Clin Invest 1983; 72(1):339–349.
60. Baudendistel L, Shields JB, Kaminski DL. Comparison of double indicator thermodilution measurements of extravascular lung water (EVLW) with radiographic estimation of lung water in trauma patients. J Trauma 1982; 22(12):983–988.
61. Laggner A, Kleinberger G, Haller J, Lenz K, Sommer G, Druml W. Bedside estimation of extravascular lung water in critically ill patients: comparison of the chest radiograph and the thermal dye technique. Intens Care Med 1984; 10(6): 309–313.
62. Sivak ED, Richmond BJ, O'Donavan PB, Borkowski GP. Value of extravascular lung water measurement vs portable chest x-ray in the management of pulmonary edema. Crit Care Med 1983; 11(7):498–501.
63. Pistolesi M, Miniati M, Milne EN, Giuntini C. The chest roentgenogram in pulmonary edema. Clin Chest Med 1985; 6(3):315–344.
64. Loyd JE, Newman JH, Brigham KL. Permeability pulmonary edema. Diagnosis and management. Arch Intern Med 1984; 144(1):143–147.
65. Milne EN, Pistolesi M, Miniati M, Giuntini C. The radiologic distinction of cardiogenic and noncardiogenic edema. AJR 1985; 144(5):879–894.
66. Aberle DR, Wiener-Kronish JP, Webb WR, Matthay MA. Hydrostatic versus increased permeability pulmonary edema: diagnosis based on radiographic criteria in critically ill patients. Radiology 1988; 168(1):73–79.
67. Rocker GM, Rose DH, Manhire AR, Pearson D, Shale DJ. The radiographic differentiation of pulmonary oedema. Br J Radiol 1989; 62(739):582–586.
68. Smith RC, Mann H, Greenspan RH, Pope CF, Sostman HD. Radiographic differentiation between different etiologies of pulmonary edema. Invest Radiol 1987; 22(11):859–863.
69. Bernard GR, Artigas A, Brigham KL, Carlet J, Falke K, Hudson L, Lamy M, Legall JR, Morris A, Spragg R. The American-European Consensus Conference on ARDS. Definitions, mechanisms, relevant outcomes, and clinical trial coordination. Am J Respir Crit Care Med 1994; 149(3 Pt 1):818–824.
70. Murray JF, Matthay MA, Luce JM, Flick MR. An expanded definition of the adult respiratory distress syndrome. (Published erratum appears in Am Rev Respir Dis 1989; 139(4):1065.) Am Rev Respir Dis 1988; 138(3):720–723.
71. Zimmerman JE, Goodman LR, Shahvari MB. Effect of mechanical ventilation and positive end-expiratory pressure (PEEP) on chest radiograph. AJR 1979; 133(5): 811–815.
72. Cutillo AG, Morris AH, Ailion DC, Durney CH, Case TA. Determination of lung water content and distribution by nuclear magnetic resonance imaging. J Thorac Imag 1986; 1(3):39–51.
73. Schuster DP, Marklin GF, Mintun MA. Regional changes in extravascular lung water detected by positron emission tomography. J Appl Physiol 1986; 60(4): 1170–1178.

74. Gattinoni L, Pelosi P, Pesenti A, Brazzi L, Vitale G, Moretto A, Crespi A, Tagliabue M. CT scan in ARDS: clinical and physiopathological insights. Acta Anaesthesiol Scand Suppl 1991; 95:87–96.
75. Gattinoni L, Pelosi P, Vitale G, Pesenti A, D'Andrea L, Mascheroni D. Body position changes redistribute lung computed-tomographic density in patients with acute respiratory failure. Anesthesiology 1991; 74(1):15–23.
76. Meyrick B, Brigham KL. Acute effects of *Escherichia coli* endotoxin on the pulmonary microcirculation of anesthetized sheep structure:function relationships. Lab Invest 1983; 48(4):458–470.
77. Meyrick BO, Ryan US, Brigham KL. Direct effects of *E. coli* endotoxin on structure and permeability of pulmonary endothelial monolayers and the endothelial layer of intimal explants. Am J Pathol 1986; 122(1):140–151.
78. Renkin EM. Multiple pathways of capillary permeability. Circ Res 1977; 41(6): 735–743.
79. Harris TR, Roselli RJ. A theoretical model of protein, fluid, and small molecule transport in the lung. J Appl Physiol: Respir Environ Exercise Physiol 1981; 50(1):1–14.
80. Pittet JF, Wiener-Kronish JP, McElroy MC, Folkesson HG, Matthay MA. Stimulation of lung epithelial liquid clearance by endogenous release of catecholamines in septic shock in anesthetized rats. J Clin Invest 1994; 94(2): 663–671.
81. Pittet JF, Wiener-Kronish JP, Serikov V, Matthay MA. Resistance of the alveolar epithelium to injury from septic shock in sheep. Am J Respir Crit Care Med 1995; 151(4):1093–1100.
82. Wiener-Kronish JP, Albertine KH, Matthay MA. Differential responses of the endothelial and epithelial barriers of the lung in sheep to *Escherichia coli* endotoxin. J Clin Invest 1991; 88(3):864–875.
83. Harlan JM, Harker LA, Reidy MA, Gajdusek CM, Schwartz SM, Striker GE. Lipopolysaccharide-mediated bovine endothelial cell injury in vitro. Lab Invest 1983; 48(3):269–274.
84. Harlan JM, Harker LA, Striker GE, Weaver LJ. Effects of lipopolysaccharide on human endothelial cells in culture. Thromb Res 1983; 29(1):15–26.
85. Albertine KH. Ultrastructural abnormalities in increased-permeability pulmonary edema. Clin Chest Med 1985; 6(3):345–369.
86. Snapper JR, Bernard GR, Hinson JMJ, Hutchison AA, Loyd JE, Ogletree ML, Brigham KL. Endotoxemia-induced leukopenia in sheep. Correlation with lung vascular permeability and hypoxemia but not with pulmonary hypertension. Am Rev Respir Dis 1983; 127(3):306–309.
87. Nathan CF. Secretory products of macrophages. J Clin Invest 1987; 79(2): 319–326.
88. Uchiba M, Okajima K, Murakami K, Okabe H, Takatsuki K. Endotoxin-induced pulmonary vascular injury is mainly mediated by activated neutrophils in rats. Thromb Res 1995; 78(2):117–125.
89. Fowler AA, Hyers TM, Fisher BJ, Bechard DE, Centor RM, Webster RO. The adult respiratory distress syndrome. Cell populations and soluble mediators in the air spaces of patients at high risk. Am Rev Respir Dis 1987; 136(5): 1225–1231.

90. Lee CT, Fein AM, Lippmann M, Holtzman H, Kimbel P, Weinbaum G. Elastolytic activity in pulmonary lavage fluid from patients with adult respiratory-distress syndrome. N Engl J Med 1981; 304(4):192–196.
91. Weiland JE, Davis WB, Holter JF, Mohammed JR, Dorinsky PM, Gadek JE. Lung neutrophils in the adult respiratory distress syndrome. Clinical and pathophysiologic significance. Am Rev Respir Dis 1986; 133(2):218–225.
92. Meyrick B, Hoffman LH, Brigham KL. Chemotaxis of granulocytes across bovine pulmonary artery intimal explants without endothelial cell injury. Tissue Cell 1984; 16(1):1–16.
93. Niedermeyer ME, Meyrick B, Parl FF, Brigham KL. Facilitation of granulocyte migration into bovine pulmonary artery intimal explants by intact viable endothelium. Am J Pathol 1984; 117(2):252–261.
94. Engelberts I, Samyo SK, Leeuwenberg JF, Van DLJ, Buurman WA. A role for ELAM-1 in the pathogenesis of MOF during septic shock. J Surg Res 1992; 53(2): 136–144.
95. Grisham MB, Everse J, Janssen HF. Endotoxemia and neutrophil activation in vivo. Am J Physiol 1988; 254(5 Pt 2):H1017–H1022.
96. Weiss SJ. Tissue destruction by neutrophils. N Engl J Med 1989; 320(6):365–376.
97. Heflin ACJ, Brigham KL. Prevention by granulocyte depletion of increased vascular permeability of sheep lung following endotoxemia. J Clin Invest 1981; 68(5): 1253–1260.
98. Hinson JMJ, Hutchison AA, Ogletree ML, Brigham KL, Snapper JR. Effect of granulocyte depletion on altered lung mechanics after endotoxemia in sheep. J Appl Physiol: Respir Environ Exercise Physiol 1983; 55(1 Pt 1):92–99.
99. Winn R, Maunder R, Chi E, Harlan J. Neutrophil depletion does not prevent lung edema after endotoxin infusion in goats. J Appl Physiol 1987; 62(1):116–121.
100. Braude S, Apperley J, Krausz T, Goldman JM, Royston D. Adult respiratory distress syndrome after allogeneic bone-marrow transplantation: evidence for a neutrophil-independent mechanism. Lancet 1985; 1(8440):1239–1242.
101. Laufe MD, Simon RH, Flint A, Keller JB. Adult respiratory distress syndrome in neutropenic patients. Am J Med 1986; 80(6):1022–1026.
102. Brigham KL, Meyrick B. Granulocyte-dependent injury of pulmonary endothelium: a case of miscommunication? Tissue Cell 1984; 16(2):137–155.
103. Bernard, GR, Swindell BB, Meredith MJ, Carroll FE, Higgins SB. Glutathione (GSH) repletion by n-acetylcysteine (NAC) in patients with the adult respiratory distress syndrome (ARDS). Am Rev Respir Dis 1989; 139(4):A221.
104. Blackwell TS, Christman JW. Sepsis and cytokines: current status. Br J Anaesthesia 1996; 77(1):110–117.
105. Beutler B, Cerami A. Cachectin: more than a tumor necrosis factor. N Engl J Med 1987; 316(7):379–385.
106. Michie HR, Manogue KR, Spriggs DR, Revhaug A, O'Dwyer S, Dinarello CA, Cerami A, Wolff SM, Wilmore DW. Detection of circulating tumor necrosis factor after endotoxin administration. N Engl J Med 1988; 318(23):1481–1486.
107. Goldblum SE, Hennig B, Jay M, Yoneda K, McClain CJ. Tumor necrosis factor alpha-induced pulmonary vascular endothelial injury. Infect Immun 1989; 57(4): 1218–1226.

108. Mullin JM, Snock KV. Effect of tumor necrosis factor on epithelial tight junctions and transepithelial permeability. Cancer Res 1990; 50(7):2172–2176.
109. Bonsignore MR, Valenti A, Spatafora M. Tumor necrosis factor-alpha does not cause lung edema in rabbits. J Appl Physiol 1992; 73(1):173–178.
110. Hocking DC, Phillips PG, Ferro TJ, Johnson A. Mechanisms of pulmonary edema induced by tumor necrosis factor-alpha. Circ Res 1990; 67(1):68–77.
111. Horgan MJ, Palace GP, Everitt JE, Malik AB. TNF-alpha release in endotoxemia contributes to neutrophil-dependent pulmonary edema. Am J Physiol 1993; 264(4 Pt 2):H1161–H1165.
112. Gamble JR, Harlan JM, Klebanoff SJ, Vadas MA. Stimulation of the adherence of neutrophils to umbilical vein endothelium by human recombinant tumor necrosis factor. Proc Natl Acad Sci USA 1985; 82(24):8667–8671.
113. Shalaby MR, Aggarwal BB, Rinderknecht E, Svedersky LP, Finkle BS, Palladino MAJ. Activation of human polymorphonuclear neutrophil functions by interferon-gamma and tumor necrosis factors. J Immunol 1985; 135(3):2069–2073.
114. Okusawa S, Gelfand JA, Ikejima T, Connolly RJ, Dinarello CA. Interleukin 1 induces a shock-like state in rabbits. Synergism with tumor necrosis factor and the effect of cyclooxygenase inhibition. J Clin Invest 1988; 81(4):1162–1172.
115. Smith JW, Urba WJ, Curti BD, Elwood LJ, Steis RG, Janik JE, Sharfman WH, Miller LL, Fenton RG, Conlon KC. The toxic and hematologic effects of interleukin-1 alpha administered in a phase I trial to patients with advanced malignancies. J Clin Oncol 1992; 10(7):1141–1152.
116. Cybulsky MI, McComb DJ, Movat HZ. Neutrophil leukocyte emigration induced by endotoxin. Mediator roles of interleukin 1 and tumor necrosis factor alpha 1. J Immunol 1988; 140(9):3144–3149.
117. Carlson RW, Schaeffer RCJ, Carpio M, Weil MH. Edema fluid and coagulation changes during fulminant pulmonary edema. Chest 1981; 79(1):43–49.
118. Saldeen T. Trends in microvascular research. The microembolism syndrome. Microvasc Res 1976; 11(2):227–259.
119. Suffredini AF, Harpel PC, Parrillo JE. Promotion and subsequent inhibition of plasminogen activation after administration of intravenous endotoxin to normal subjects. N Engl J Med 1989; 320(18):1165–1172.
120. Brigham KL, Newman, JH, Snapper, JR, Ogletree ML. Metabolites of arachidonic acid in the pathophysiology of the pulmonary circulation. In: Oates JA, ed. The Prostaglandins and the Cardiovascular System. New York: Raven Press, 1982: 357–366.
121. Brigham KL, Ogletree ML. Effects of prostaglandins and related compounds on lung vascular permeability. Bull Eur Physiopathol Respir 1981; 17(4):703–722.
122. Hales CA, Sonne L, Peterson M, Kong D, Miller M, Watkins WD. Role of thromboxane and prostacyclin in pulmonary vasomotor changes after endotoxin in dogs. J Clin Investi 1981; 68(2):497–505.
123. Hirose T, Aoki E, Domae M, Ishibashi M, Ikeda T, Tanaka K. Protective effect of a thromboxane synthetase inhibitor, OKY-1581, on increased lung vascular permeability in pulmonary microembolization in dogs. Prostaglandins Leukotrienes & Medicine 1983; 10(2):187–196.

124. Ogletree ML, Brigham KL. Arachidonate raises vascular resistance but not permeability in lungs of awake sheep. J Appl Physiol: Respir Environ Exercise Physiol 1980; 48(4):581–586.
125. Snapper JR, Hinson JM Jr, Hutchison AA, Lefferts PL, Ogletree ML, Brigham KL. Effects of platelet depletion on the unanesthesized sheep's pulmonary response to endotoxemia. J Clin Invest 1984; 74:1782–1791.
126. Beckman JS, Beckman TW, Chen J, Marshall PA, Freeman BA. Apparent hydroxyl radical production by peroxynitrite: implications for endothelial injury from nitric oxide and superoxide. Proc Natl Acad Sci USA 1990; 87(4):1620–1624.
127. Haddad IY, Pataki G, Hu P, Galliani C, Beckman JS, Matalon S. Quantitation of nitrotyrosine levels in lung sections of patients and animals with acute lung injury. J Clin Invest 1994; 94(6):2407–2413.
128. Wizemann TM, Gardner CR, Laskin JD, Quinones S, Durham SK, Goller NL, Ohnishi ST, Laskin DL. Production of nitric oxide and peroxynitrite in the lung during acute endotoxemia. J Leuk Biol 1994; 56(6):759–768.
129. Begley CJ, Ogletree ML, Meyrick BO, Brigham KL. Modification of pulmonary responses to endotoxemia in awake sheep by steroidal and nonsteroidal antiinflammatory agents. Am Rev Respir Dis 1984; 130(6):1140–1146.
130. Bowers RE, Ellis EF, Brigham KL, Oates JA. Effects of prostaglandin cyclic endoperoxides on the lung circulation of unanesthetized sheep. J Clin Invest 1979; 63(1):131–137.
131. Henry CL Jr, Ogeltree ML, Brigham KL, Hammon JW Jr. Thromboxane A_2 mediates the pulmonary vascular response to endotoxin. Surgical Forum 1984; 35: 134–136.
132. Brigham KL. Mechanisms of lung injury. Clin Chest Med 1982; 3(1):9–24.
133. Li JX, Oliver JR, Lu CY, Philips JB 3rd. Delayed thromboxane or tumor necrosis factor-alpha, but not leukotriene inhibition, attenuates prolonged pulmonary hypertension in endotoxemia. Am J Med Sci 1995; 310(3):103–110.
134. Sibbald WJ, Paterson NA, Holliday RL, Anderson RA, Lobb TR, Duff JH. Pulmonary hypertension in sepsis: measurement by the pulmonary arterial diastolic-pulmonary wedge pressure gradient and the influence of passive and active factors. Chest 1978; 73(5):583–591.
135. Rossaint R, Falke KJ, Lopez F, Slama K, Pison U, Zapol WM. Inhaled nitric oxide for the adult respiratory distress syndrome. N Engl J Med 1993; 328(6): 399–405.
136. McIntyre RC Jr, Banerjee A, Agrafojo J, Fullerton DA. Pulmonary hypertension in acute lung injury is due to impaired vasodilation with intact vascular contractility. J Surg Res 1995; 58(6):765–770.
137. Romand JA, Donald FA, Suter PM. Cardiopulmonary interactions in acute lung injury: clinical and prognostic importance of pulmonary hypertension. New Horizons 1994; 2(4):457–462.
138. Spapen H, Vincken W. Pulmonary arterial hypertension in sepsis and the adult respiratory distress syndrome. Acta Clin Belg 1992; 47(1):30–41.
139. Petty TL, Silvers GW, Paul GW, Stanford RE. Abnormalities in lung elastic properties and surfactant function in adult respiratory distress syndrome. Chest 1979; 75(5):571–574.

140. Spragg RG. Surfactant replacement for ARDS: current status. Pulmon Perspect 1996; 13(4):4–6.
141. Gregory TJ, Longmore WJ, Moxley MA, Whitsett JA, Reed CR, Fowler AA, 3d, Hudson LD, Maunder RJ, Crim C, Hyers TM. Surfactant chemical composition and biophysical activity in acute respiratory distress syndrome. J Clin Invest 1991; 88(6):1976–1981.
142. Morgan TE. Pulmonary surfactant. N Engl J Med 1971; 284(21):1185–1193.
143. Albert RK, Lakshminarayan S, Hildebrandt J, Kirk W, Butler J. Increased surface tension favors pulmonary edema formation in anesthetized dogs' lungs. J Clin Invest 1979; 63(5):1015–1018.
144. Ahmed T, Oliver WJ, Wanner A. Variability of hypoxic pulmonary vasoconstriction in sheep. Role of prostaglandins. Am Rev Respir Dis 1983; 127(1):59–62.
145. Newman JH, Loyd JE, English DK, Ogletree ML, Fulkerson WJ, Brigham KL. Effects of 100% oxygen on lung vascular function in awake sheep. J Appl Physiol: Respir Environ Exercise Physiol 1983; 54(5):1379–1386.
146. Reeves JT, Grover RF. Blockade of acute hypoxic pulmonary hypertension by endotoxin. J Appl Physiol 1974; 36(3):328–332.
147. Weir EK, Mlczoch J, Reeves JT, Grover RF. Endotoxin and prevention of hypoxic pulmonary vasoconstriction. J Lab Clin Med 1976; 88(6):975–983.
148. Thomas HM, Garrett RC. Strength of hypoxic vasoconstriction determines shunt fraction in dogs with atelectasis. J Appl Physiol: Respir Environ Exercise Physiol 1982; 53(1):44–51.
149. Zasslow MA, Benumof JL, Trousdale FR. Hypoxic pulmonary vasoconstriction and the size of hypoxic compartment. J Appl Physiol: Respir Environ Exercise Physiol 1982; 53(3):626–630.
150. Marshall BE, Marshall C, Benumof J, Saidman LJ. Hypoxic pulmonary vasoconstriction in dogs: effects of lung segment size and oxygen tension. J Appl Physiol: Respir Environ Exercise Physiol 1981; 51(6):1543–1551.
151. Parker RE, Brigham KL. Effects of endotoxemia on pulmonary vascular resistances in unanesthetized sheep. J Appl Physiol 1987; 63(3):1058–1062.
152. Bradley JD, Roselli RJ, Parker RE, Harris TR. Effects of endotoxemia on the sheep lung microvascular membrane: a two-pore theory. J Appl Physiol 1988; 64(6):2675–2683.
153. Parker MM, Shelhamer JH, Bacharach SL, Green MV, Natanson C, Frederick TM, Damske BA, Parrillo JE. Profound but reversible myocardial depression in patients with septic shock. Ann Intern Med 1984; 100(4):483–490.
154. Ognibene FP, Parker MM, Natanson C, Shelhamer JH, Parrillo JE. Depressed left ventricular performance. Response to volume infusion in patients with sepsis and septic shock. Chest 1988; 93(5):903–910.
155. Parker MM, Ognibene FP, Parrillo JE. Reversible depression of myocardial function in septic shock (SS) confirmed by a load-independent measure of ventricular performance. Clin Res 1990; 38:340A. Abstract.
156. Cunnion RE, Schaer GL, Parker MM, Natanson C, Parrillo JE. The coronary circulation in human septic shock. Circulation 1986; 73(4):637–644.
157. Parrillo JE, Burch C, Shelhamer JH, Parker MM, Natanson C, Schuette W. A circulating myocardial depressant substance in humans with septic shock. Septic

shock patients with a reduced ejection fraction have a circulating factor that depresses in vitro myocardial cell performance. J Clin Invest 1985; 76(4):1539–1553.
158. Reilly JM, Cunnion RE, Burch-Whitman C, Parker MM, Shelhamer JH, Parrillo JE. A circulating myocardial depressant substance is associated with cardiac dysfunction and peripheral hypoperfusion (lactic acidemia) in patients with septic shock. Chest 1989; 95(5):1072–1080.
159. Parrillo JE. Pathogenetic mechanisms of septic shock. N Engl J Med 1993; 328(20):1471–1477.
160. Jardin F, Farcot JC, Boisante L, Curien N, Margairaz A, Bourdarias JP. Influence of positive end-expiratory pressure on left ventricular performance. N Engl J Med 1981; 304(7):387–392.
161. Calvin JE, Driedger AA, Sibbald WJ. Does the pulmonary capillary wedge pressure predict left ventricular preload in critically ill patients? Crit Care Med 1981; 9(6):437–443.
162. Guyton AC, Lindsey AW. Effect of elevated left atrial pressure and decreased plasma protein concentration on the development of pulmonary edema. Circ Res 1959; VII:649–657.
163. Rice CL, Doroghazi PM, Kohler JP, Zarins CK, Moss GS. The effect of sepsis and reduced colloid osmotic pressure on pulmonary edema. J Surg Res 1979; 27(5):347–351.
164. Rackow EC, Fein IA, Siegel J. The relationship of the colloid osmotic-pulmonary artery wedge pressure gradient to pulmonary edema and mortality in critically ill patients. Chest 1982; 82(4):433–437.
165. Demling RH, Niehaus G, Will JA. Pulmonary microvascular response to hemorrhagic shock, resuscitation, and recovery. J Appl Physiol: Respir Environ Exercise Physiol 1979; 46(3):498–503.
166. Lowe RJ, Moss GS, Jilek J, Levine HD. Crystalloid versus colloid in the etiology of pulmonary failure after trauma—a randomized trial in man. Crit Care Med 1979; 7(3):107–112.
167. Nylander WA Jr, Hammon JW Jr, Roselli RJ, Tribble JB, Brigham KL, Bender HW Jr. Comparison of the effects of saline and homologous plasma infusion on lung fluid balance during endotoxemia in the unanesthetized sheep. Surgery 1981; 90(2):221–228.
168. Moshage HJ, Janssen JA, Franssen JH, Hafkenscheid JC, Yap SH. Study of the molecular mechanism of decreased liver synthesis of albumin in inflammation. J Clin Invest 1987; 79(6):1635–1641.
169. Garcia JG, Siflinger-Birnboim A, Bizios R, Del Vecchio PJ, Fenton JW 2d, Malik AB. Thrombin-induced increase in albumin permeability across the endothelium. J Cell Physiol 1986; 128(1):96–104.
170. Lambert I, Matthews TG, Clarke TA. Bronchopulmonary dysplasia: a longitudinal study of 23 cases. Ir J Med Sci 1991; 160(10):315–316.
171. Winter PM, Smith G. The toxicity of oxygen. Anesthesiology 1972; 37(2): 210–241.
172. Crapo JD, Freeman BA, Barry BE, Turrens JF, Young SL. Mechanisms of hyperoxic injury to the pulmonary microcirculation. Physiologist 1983; 26(3):170–176.

173. Deneke SM, Fanburg BL. Normobaric oxygen toxicity of the lung. N Engl J Med 1980; 303(2):76–86.
174. Frank L, Massaro D. Oxygen toxicity. Am J Med 1980; 69(1):117–126.
175. Kobayashi T, Shiki Y, Meyrick B, Burr IM, Newman JH. Simultaneous exposure of sheep to endotoxin and 100% oxygen. Am Rev Respir Dis 1991; 144(3): 600–605.
176. Effmann EL, Merten DF, Kirks DR, Pratt PC, Spock A. Adult respiratory distress syndrome in children. Radiology 1985; 157(1):69–74.
177. Pietra GG, Szidon JP, Carpenter HA, Fishman AP. Bronchial venular leakage during endotoxin shock. Am J Pathol 1974; 77(3):387–406.
178. Baile EM, Nelems JM, Schulzer M, Pare PD. Measurement of regional bronchial arterial blood flow and bronchovascular resistance in dogs. J Appl Physiol: Respiratory, Environmental & Exercise Physiology 1982; 53(4):1044–1049.
179. Magno MG, Fishman AP. Origin, distribution, and blood flow of bronchial circulation in anesthetized sheep. J Appl Physiol: Respir Environ Exercise Physiol 1982; 53(1):272–279.
180. Malik A, Tracy S. Bronchovascular adjustments after pulmonary embolism. J Appl Physiol 1980; 49:476.
181. Mitchell JP, Schuller D, Calandrino FS, Schuster DP. Improved outcome based on fluid management in critically ill patients requiring pulmonary artery catheterization. Am Rev Respir Dis 1992; 145(5):990–998.
182. Schuller D, Mitchell JP, Calandrino FS, Schuster DP. Fluid balance during pulmonary edema. Is fluid gain a marker or a cause of poor outcome? Chest 1991; 100(4):1068–1075.
183. Simmons RS, Berdine GG, Seidenfeld JJ, Prihoda TJ, Harris GD, Smith JD, Gilbert TJ, Mota E, Johanson WG, Jr. Fluid balance and the adult respiratory distress syndrome. Am Rev Respir Dis 1987; 135(4):924–929.
184. Sloane PJ, Gee MH, Gottlieb JE, Albertine KH, Peters SP, Burns JR, Machiedo G, Fish JE. A multicenter registry of patients with acute respiratory distress syndrome. Physiology and outcome. Am Rev Respir Dis 1992; 146(2):419–426.
185. Gentilello LM, Anardi D, Mock C, Arreola-Risa C, Maier RV. Permissive hypercapnia in trauma patients. J Trauma 1995; 39(5):846–852.
186. Fletcher JR, Ramwell PW. Modification, by aspirin and indomethacin, of the haemodynamic and prostaglandin releasing effects of *E. coli* endotoxin in the dog. Br J Pharmacol 1977; 61(2):175–181.
187. Brigham KL, Bowers RE, McKeen CR. Methylprednisolone prevention of increased lung vascular permeability following endotoxemia in sheep. J Clin Invest 1981; 67(4):1103–1110.
188. Demling RH, Smith M, Gunther R, Wandzilak T. Endotoxin-induced lung injury in unanesthetized sheep: effect of methylprednisolone. Circ Shock 1981; 8(3): 351–360.
189. Schumer W. Steroids in the treatment of clinical septic shock. Ann Surg 1976; 184(3):333–341.
190. Sprung CL, Caralis PV, Marcial EH, Pierce M, Gelbard MA, Long WM, Duncan RC, Tendler MD, Karpf M. The effects of high-dose corticosteroids in patients

with septic shock. A prospective, controlled study. N Engl J Med 1984; 311(18):1137–1143.

191. Sibbald WJ, Anderson RR, Reid B, Holliday RL, Driedger AA. Alveolo-capillary permeability in human septic ARDS. Effect of high-dose corticosteroid therapy. Chest 1981; 79(2):133–142.
192. Anonymous. Effect of high-dose glucocorticoid therapy on mortality in patients with clinical signs of systemic sepsis. The Veterans Administration Systemic Sepsis Cooperative Study Group. N Engl J Med 1987; 317(11):659–665.
193. Bone RC, Fisher CJ Jr, Clemmer TP, Slotman GJ, Metz CA, Balk RA. A controlled clinical trial of high-dose methylprednisolone in the treatment of severe sepsis and septic shock. N Engl J Med 1987; 317(11):653–658.
194. Luce JM, Montgomery AB, Marks JD, Turner J, Metz CA, Murray JF. Ineffectiveness of high-dose methylprednisolone in preventing parenchymal lung injury and improving mortality in patients with septic shock. Am Rev Respir Dis 1988; 138(1):62–68.
195. Bernard GR, Luce JM, Sprung CL, Rinaldo JE, Tate RM, Sibbald WJ, Kariman K, Higgins S, Bradley R, Metz CA, Harris TR, Brigham KL. High-dose corticosteroids in patients with the adult respiratory distress syndrome. N Engl J Med 1987; 317:1565–1570.
196. Bernard GR, Wheeler AP, Russell JA, Schein, R, Summer W, Hudson L, Steinberg KP, Fulkerson WJ, Wright PE, Carroll FE, Christman BW, DuPont WD, Higgins SB, Jiang K, Plummer WD Jr, Swindell BB. Effects of ibuprofen on the physiology, lactic acidosis and survival of sepsis syndrome. N Engl J Med 1997; 336(13):912–918.
197. Jepsen S, Herlevsen P, Knudsen P, Bud MI, Klausen NO. Antioxidant treatment with N-acetylcysteine during adult respiratory distress syndrome: a prospective, randomized, placebo-controlled study. Crit Care Med 1992; 20(7):918–923.
198. Bone RC, Balk R, Slotman G, Maunder R, Silverman H, Hyers TM, Kerstein MD. Adult respiratory distress syndrome. Sequence and importance of development of multiple organ failure. Prostaglandin E1 Study Group. Chest 1992; 101(2): 320–326.
199. Radermacher P, Santak B, Becker H, Falke KJ. Prostaglandin E1 and nitroglycerin reduce pulmonary capillary pressure but worsen ventilation-perfusion distributions in patients with adult respiratory distress syndrome. Anesthesiology 1989; 70(4): 601–606.
200. Radermacher P, Santak B, Falke KJ. Comparison of prostaglandin E1 and nitroglycerin in patients with ARDS. Prog Clin Biolog Res 1989; 301: 267–270.
201. Radermacher P, Santak B, Wust HJ, Tarnow J, Falke KJ. Prostacyclin for the treatment of pulmonary hypertension in the adult respiratory distress syndrome: effects on pulmonary capillary pressure and ventilation-perfusion distributions. Anesthesiology 1990; 72(2):238–244.
202. Holcroft JW, Vassar MJ, Weber CJ. Prostaglandin E1 and survival in patients with the adult respiratory distress syndrome. A prospective trial. Ann Surg 1986; 203(4):371–378.

203. Bigatello LM, Hurford WE, Kacmarek RM, Roberts JD Jr, Zapol WM. Prolonged inhalation of low concentrations of nitric oxide in patients with severe adult respiratory distress syndrome. Effects on pulmonary hemodynamics and oxygenation. Anesthesiology 1994; 80(4):761–770.
204. Rossaint R, Gerlach H, Schmidt-Ruhnke H, Pappert D, Lewandowski K, Steudel W, Falke K. Efficacy of inhaled nitric oxide in patients with severe ARDS. Chest 1995; 107(4):1107–1115.
205. Fulkerson WJ, MacIntyre N, Stamler J, Crapo JD. Pathogenesis and treatment of the adult respiratory distress syndrome. Arch Intern Med 1996; 156(1):29–38.
206. Hirschl RB, Pranikoff T, Wise C. Initial experience with partial liquid ventilation (PLV) in nine adult patients with severe respiratory failure. Am J Respir Cri Care 1995; 151:A427. Abstract.
207. Bone RC, Balk RA, Fein AM, Perl TM, Wenzel RP, Reines HD, Quenzer RW, Iberti TJ, MacIntyre N, Schein RM. A second large controlled clinical study of E5, a monoclonal antibody to endotoxin: results of a prospective, multicenter, randomized, controlled trial. The E5 Sepsis Study Group. (Published erratum appears in Crit Care Med 1995; 23(9):1616.) Crit Care Med 1995; 23(6): 994–1006.
208. Greenman RL, Schein RM, Martin MA, Wenzel RP, MacIntyre NR, Emmanuel G, Chmel H, Kohler RB, McCarthy M, Plouffe J. A controlled clinical trial of E5 murine monoclonal IgM antibody to endotoxin in the treatment of gram-negative sepsis. The XOMA Sepsis Study Group. JAMA 1991; 266(8):1097–1102.
209. McCloskey RV, Straube RC, Sanders C, Smith SM, Smith CR. Treatment of septic shock with human monoclonal antibody HA-1A. A randomized, double-blind, placebo-controlled trial. CHESS Trial Study Group. Ann Intern Med 1994; 121(1):1–5.
210. Ziegler EJ, Fisher CJ Jr, Sprung CL, et al. Treatment of gram-negative bacteremia and septic shock with HA-1A human monoclonal antibody against endotoxin. A randomized, double-blind, placebo-controlled trial. The HA-1A Sepsis Study Group. N Engl J Med 1991; 324(7):429–436.
211. Bigatello LM, Greene RE, Sprung CL, Panacek EA, Straube RC, Zimmerman JL, Maunder RJ, Lanken PN, Pile-Spellmann E, Stanek KS. HA-1A in septic patients with ARDS: results from the pivotal trial. Intens Care Med 1994; 20(5): 328–334.
212. Jesmok G, Lindsey C, Duerr M, Fournel M, Emerson T Jr. Efficacy of monoclonal antibody against human recombinant tumor necrosis factor in *E. coli*-challenged swine. Am J Pathol 1992; 141(5):1197–1207.
213. Tracey KJ, Fong Y, Hesse DG, Manogue KR, Lee AT, Kuo GC, Lowry SF, Cerami A. Anti-cachectin/TNF monoclonal antibodies prevent septic shock during lethal bacteraemia. Nature 1987; 330(6149):662–664.
214. Abraham E, Wunderink R, Silverman H, Perl TM, Nasraway S, Levy H, Bone R, Wenzel RP, Balk R, Allred R, Efficacy and safety of monoclonal antibody to human tumor necrosis factor alpha in patients with sepsis syndrome. A randomized, controlled, double-blind, multicenter clinical trial. TNF-alpha MAb Sepsis Study Group. JAMA 1995; 273(12):934–941.

215. Cohen J, Carlet J. INTERSEPT: an international, multicenter, placebo-controlled trial of monoclonal antibody to human tumor necrosis factor-alpha in patients with sepsis. International Sepsis Trial Study Group. Crit Care Med 1996; 24(9):1431–1440.
216. Reinhart K, Wiegand-Lohnert C, Grimminger F, Kaul M, Withington S, Treacher D, Eckart J, Willatts S, Bouza C, Krausch D, Stockenhuber F, Eiselstein J, Daum L, Kempeni J. Assessment of the safety and efficacy of the monoclonal anti-tumor necrosis factor antibody-fragment, MAK 195F, in patients with sepsis and septic shock: a multicenter, randomized, placebo-controlled, dose-ranging study. Crit Care Med 1996; 24(5):733–742.
217. Fisher CJ Jr, Agosti JM, Opal SM, Lowry SF, Balk RA, Sadoff JC, Abraham E, Schein RM, Benjamin E. Treatment of septic shock with the tumor necrosis factor receptor:Fc fusion protein. The Soluble TNF Receptor Sepsis Study Group. N Engl J Med 1996; 334(26):1697–1702.
218. Ohlsson K, Bjork P, Bergenfeldt M, Hageman R, Thompson RC. Interleukin-1 receptor antagonist reduces mortality from endotoxin shock. Nature 1990; 348(6301):550–552.
219. Alexander HR, Doherty GM, Buresh CM, Venzon DJ, Norton JA. A recombinant human receptor antagonist to interleukin 1 improves survival after lethal endotoxemia in mice. J Exp Med 1991; 173(4):1029–1032.
220. Fisher CJ Jr, Dhainaut JF, Opal SM, Pribble JP, Balk RA, Slotman GJ, Iberti TJ, Rackow EC, Shapiro MJ, Greenman RL. Recombinant human interleukin 1 receptor antagonist in the treatment of patients with sepsis syndrome. Results from a randomized, double-blind, placebo-controlled trial. Phase III rhIL-1ra Sepsis Syndrome Study Group. JAMA 1994; 271(23):1836–1843.
221. Andrejko, KM, Deutschman CS. Acute-phase gene expression correlates with intrahepatic tumor necrosis factor-α abundance but not with plasma tumor necrosis factor concentrations during sepsis/systemic inflammatory response syndrome in the rat. Crit Care Med 1996; 24(12):1947–1952.
222. Doerschuk CM, Winn RK, Coxson HO, Harlan JM. CD18-dependent and -independent mechanisms of neutrophil emigration in the pulmonary and systemic microcirculation of rabbits. J Immunol 1990; 144(6):2327–3233.
223. Walsh CJ, Carey PD, Cook DJ, Bechard DE, Fowler AA, Sugerman HJ. Anti-CD18 antibody attenuates neutropenia and alveolar capillary-membrane injury during gram-negative sepsis. Surgery 1991; 110(2):205–211.
224. Mulligan MS, Wilson GP, Todd RF, Smith CW, Anderson DC, Varani J, Issekutz TB, Miyasaka M, Tamatani T, Miyasaka M. Role of beta 1, beta 2 integrins and ICAM-1 in lung injury after deposition of IgG and IgA immune complexes. J Immunol 1993; 150(6):2407–2417.
225. Ridings PC, Windsor AC, Jutila MA, Blocher CR, Fisher BJ, Sholley MM, Sugerman HJ, Fowler AA, 3rd. A dual-binding antibody to E- and L-selectin attenuates sepsis-induced lung injury. Am J Respir Crit Care Med 1995; 152(1):247–253.
226. Friedman G, Jankowski S, Shahla M, Goldman M, Rose RM, Kahn RJ, Vincent JL. Administration of an antibody to E-selectin in patients with septic shock. Crit Care Med 1996; 24(2):229–233.

227. Sharar SR, Winn RK, Murry CE, Harlan JM, Rice CL. A CD18 monoclonal antibody increases the incidence and severity of subcutaneous abscess formation after high-dose *Staphylococcus aureus* injection in rabbits. Surgery 1991; 110(2):213–219.
228. Saumon G, Basset G. Electrolyte and fluid transport across the mature alveolar epithelium. J Appl Physiol 1993; 74(1):1–15.
229. Berthiaume Y, Staub NC, Matthay MA. Beta-adrenergic agonists increase lung liquid clearance in anesthetized sheep. J Clin Invest 1987; 79(2):335–343.
230. Mizus I, Summer W, Farrukh I, Michael JR, Gurtner GH. Isoproterenol or aminophylline attenuate pulmonary edema after acid lung injury. Am Rev Respir Dis 1985; 131(2):256–259.
231. van der Poll T, Coyle SM, Barbosa K, Braxton CC, Lowry SF. Epinephrine inhibits tumor necrosis factor-alpha and potentiates interleukin 10 production during human endotoxemia. J Clin Invest 1996; 97(3):713–719.
232. Jilg S, Barsig J, Leist M, Kusters S, Volk HD, Wendel A. Enhanced release of interleukin-10 and soluble tumor necrosis factor receptors as novel principles of methylxanthine action in murine models of endotoxic shock. J Pharmacol Exp Ther 1996; 278(1):421–431.
233. Hopewell, PC. Adult respiratory distress syndrome. In: KM Moser, RG Spragg, eds. Respiratory Emergencies. St. Louis: Mosby-Year Book, 1982:114–131.
234. Newman JH. Sepsis and pulmonary edema. Clinics in Chest Medicine 1985; 6: 371–391.
235. Sibbald WJ, Cunningham DR, Chin DN. Non-cardiac or cardiac pulmonary edema? a practical approach to clinical differentiation in critically ill patients. Chest 1983; 84(3):452–461.

7

Pulmonary Edema Associated with Bacterial Pneumonia

JEANINE P. WIENER-KRONISH, TEIJI SAWA, KIYOYASU KURAHASHI, MARIA OHARA, and MICHAEL A. GROPPER

University of California at San Francisco
San Francisco, California

I. Introduction

Pseudomonas aeruginosa infections of the lung can lead to acute lung injury with the development of increased-permeability pulmonary edema, and cause both pulmonary and systemic complications. *Pseudomonas aeruginosa* has now become the most frequent cause of gram-negative nosocomial pneumonia and is frequently associated with sepsis and multiple organ failure in hospitalized patients (1–4). Patients who have chronic lung disease, patients who require prolonged hospitalization or prolonged intervals of mechanical ventilation are at increased risk of developing nosocomial pneumonia due to *Pseudomonas aeruginosa* (5,6). The mortality of patients who develop ventilator-associated pneumonia involving *Pseudomonas aeruginosa* is greater than that of patients with nosocomial pneumonia due to other organisms (7). Therefore, *Pseudomonas aeruginosa* is an important bacterial pathogen in patients with acute lung injury.

Bacterial infections of the lung can lead to the development of pulmonary edema via two basic mechanisms. Bacteria in the lung can disseminate into the circulation, leading to bacteremia and sepsis. As the source of sepsis, these bacteria can injure the lung endothelial and epithelial barriers either directly by release of toxins, or indirectly via mediator release (8) (see Chap. 6). In a recent study of acute lung injury, sepsis due to a pulmonary or nonpulmonary source was the most common clinical disorder associated with the development of acute lung injury (41% of the acute lung injury patients) (9). Primary pneumonia was the third most frequent disorder associated with development of acute lung injury in that investigation (20% of the acute lung injury patients) (10). When

Table 1 Organisms Recovered in 842 Episodes of Bacteremia with (n = 221) or Without (n = 621) Associated Severe Sepsis

	Bacteremic severe sepsis		Bacteremic sepsis	
Organisms[a]	No.	%	No.	%
Gram-positive, n = 473				
Staphylococcus aureus	50	19.8	130	19.3
Coagulase-negative *Staph.*	15	6.0	75	11.2
Enterococci	9	3.6	37	5.5
β-hemolytic streptococci	10	4.0	24	3.6
Streptococcus pneumoniae	22	8.7	52	7.7
Other streptococci	10	4.0	23	3.4
Other gram-positive	4	1.6	12	1.8
Gram-negative, n = 407				
Escherichia coli	57	22.6	189	28.1
Klebsiella sp.	13	5.2	23	3.4
Enterobacter, Citrobacter, Serratia spp.	11	4.4	17	2.5
Salmonella sp.	2	0.8	7	1.0
Proteus sp.	7	2.8	16	2.4
Pseudomonas aeruginosa	14	5.6	18	2.7
Acinetobacter sp.	5	2.0	4	0.6
Other gram-negative aerobes	1	0.4	4	0.6
Haemophilus, Branhamella	5	2.0	5	0.7
Neisseria meningitidis	0	—	2	0.3
Other gram-negatives	2	0.8	5	0.7
Others, n = 44				
Anaerobes	9	3.6	18	2.7
Candida, fungi	6	2.4	8	1.2
Viruses and others	0	—	3	0.4

[a]Polymicrobial bacteremia occurred in 26 (12%) episodes with severe sepsis and 46 (7%) episodes without severe sepsis syndrome ($P = .05$).

Two hundred and twenty-one episodes were associated with severe sepsis in the patients and 621 episodes were not associated with signs of severe sepsis. *P. aeruginosa* is the second most frequently isolated gram negative organism in patients with severe sepsis. *Source*: Ref. 10.

bacteria remain confined to the lung, either the bacteria or the inflammatory reaction that the bacteria induce can injure the lung epithelial and endothelial barriers. Therefore, either as a cause of sepsis or as a contained infection of the lung(s), bacterial pneumonia can lead to the form of pulmonary edema known as acute lung injury.

II. Effect of *Pseudomonas aeruginosa* Bacteremia on Lungs

In a recent prospective investigation of "all clinically significant episodes of bacteremia and severe sepsis in 85,750 adults," *P. aeruginosa* was the source of severe sepsis in approximately 6% of the patients and the cause of less severe bacteremia in about 3% of the patients (Table 1) (10). This investigation suggested that the source of the infection (i.e., the lungs *vs.* the urinary tract) influenced the severity of the sepsis as well as mortality. The microbiologic identification of the organism influenced the outcome of the patient, but did not influence the severity of the septicemia (ie: the presence of organ dysfunction or shock) (10). These results suggest several possible mechanisms: (1) that the bacteria that disseminate from the lungs or from the abdomen are more virulent than the bacteria that disseminate from the urinary tract; (2) that the lung and intestinal walls are more impenetrable to bacteria and that greater epithelial injury has to occur in these organs to allow bacteremia; or finally, (3) that larger

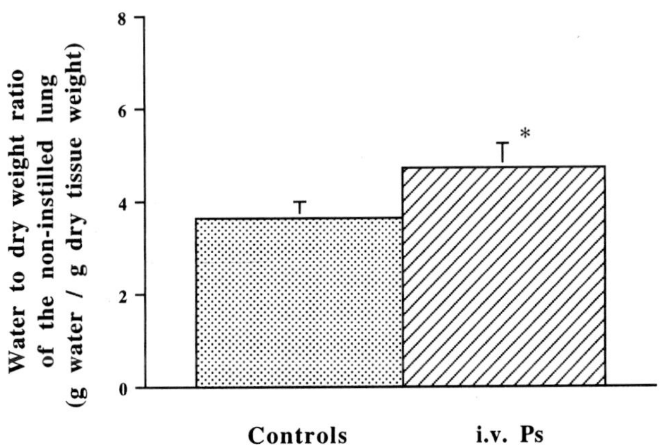

Figure 1 Rats that received intravenous *P. aeruginosa* developed significantly increased extravascular lung water content in their noninstilled lungs. These results suggest that the endothelial permeability of the lung was increased by the intravenous bacteria. (From Ref. 12.)

Table 2A Effect of Intravenous *P. aeruginosa* on Mean Systemic Arterial Pressure and Arterial pH Over 4 h in Anesthetized Rats

Experimental condition	No.	Mean systemic arterial pressure: Baseline	Mean systemic arterial pressure: Experimental	Arterial pH: Baseline	Arterial pH: Experimental
		mm Hg		units	
Controls	7	138 ± 8	123 ± 28	7.45 ± 0.04	7.44 ± 0.04
IV *P. aeruginosa*	9	122 ± 14	48 ± 30*	7.43 ± 0.03	7.12 ± 0.12*

Mean ± SD.
* $P < .05$ versus controls.

Table 2B Effect of Intravenous *P. aeruginosa* on Mean Airway Pressure, Pa_{O_2}/FI_{O_2}, and Arterial pH Over 8 h in Anesthetized Sheep[a]

Experimental condition	Mean airway pressure (mmHg)	Pa_{O_2}/FI_{O_2}	Arterial pH
Controls, n = 6			
Baseline	15 ± 3	497 ± 43	7.50 ± 0.01
Experimental	17 ± 2	281 ± 126	7.48 ± 0.08
Intravenous *P. aeruginosa*, n = 11			
Group 1, n = 8			
Baseline	15 ± 2	458 ± 71	7.51 ± 0.06
Experimental	27 ± 6[b]	196 ± 134	7.29 ± 0.10[b]
Group 2, n = 3			
Baseline	15 ± 2	455 ± 33	7.50 ± 0.04
Experimental	38 ± 7[b,c]	74 ± 49[b]	7.10 ± 0.11[b,c]

[a]Data are expressed as mean ± SD.
[b]$P < .05$ versus controls.
[c]$P < .05$ versus intravenous *P. aeruginosa*, group 1.
2A: Intravenous bolus of 10^8 cfu of PAO1. Baseline mean systemic arterial pressures and arterial pH values are similar in control and in experimental animals. Only the animals exposed to the intravenous bacteria developed hypotension and acidemia. *Source*: Ref. 12.
2B: Intravenous infusion, 3mL/h, of 3.0×10^9cfu of PAO1 for 8 hours are shown. The 11 sheep which received the iv bacteria all developed significantly increased airway pressure and acidemia. Three of these 11 sheep also developed significant hypoxemia. *Source*: Ref. 13.

quantities of bacteria enter the circulation from infected lungs or from intra-abdominal sources.

To determine the pathologic effects of bloodborne *P. aeruginosa* on the lung, experimental studies have utilized intravenous infusions of *P. aeruginosa,* and these results have then been compared to the effects of the airspace instillation of the same strain (8,11–13). The intravenous administration of live *P. aeruginosa* causes the development of severe arterial hypotension and metabolic acidosis in rats or in sheep (Table 2A, B) (12,13). In rats, the intravenous administration of *P. aeruginosa* did not lead to the development of alveolar flooding (Fig. 1); the water to dry weight ratio of the lungs was significantly increased but not to levels associated with alveolar edema (12). Furthermore, there was no evidence of increased permeability of the alveolar epithelium to protein in the rats exposed to the intravenous bacteria. In fact, the bacteremic rats were found to have accelerated alveolar liquid clearance (Fig. 2), suggesting that the alveolar epithelium had not been injured by the intravenous *P. aeruginosa* (12) and that the catecholamine release accelerated lung liquid clearance (Fig. 2).

In another investigation utilizing the same strain of *P. aeruginosa,* the intravenous administration of the bacteria led to the development of alveolar flooding in approximately 30% of sheep that received the intravenous bacteria (13). Alveolar flooding was suspected by the development of significant hypoxemia (Table 2B). Alveolar edema causes severe hypoxemia, and the resolution of the alveolar edema is associated with an improvement in arterial oxygenation (14). Since interstitial pulmonary edema should *not* cause severe hypoxemia (15), this investigation documented that significant hypoxemia and probable alveolar flooding could occur with the intravenous administration of *P. aeruginosa* in a small subset of exposed sheep (Tables 3, 4). However, the explanation for the development of alveolar edema in a fraction of the exposed animals is not clear.

Some insight into the development of the alveolar edema in the small group of sheep is provided by reviewing the physiologic data in the investigation (Tables 3, 4) (13). The alveolar epithelial injury in the three sheep that developed severe pulmonary edema was compared to the alveolar epithelial injury in the eight sheep that did not develop severe pulmonary edema; both groups of sheep had received an identical dose of intravenous *P. aeruginosa* (13). Notably the three sheep that developed alveolar flooding had lower cardiac outputs and higher mean pulmonary arterial pressures than the eight sheep that received the same intravenous dose of bacteria (Table 3). Therefore, the three sheep may have developed more cardiac failure secondary to the bacteremia, resulting in elevated pulmonary capillary pressures, although left atrial pressure was the same (Table 3).

The permeability of the alveolar epithelium to protein was also assessed in these experiments both in vivo in the bacteremic sheep and in in situ perfused

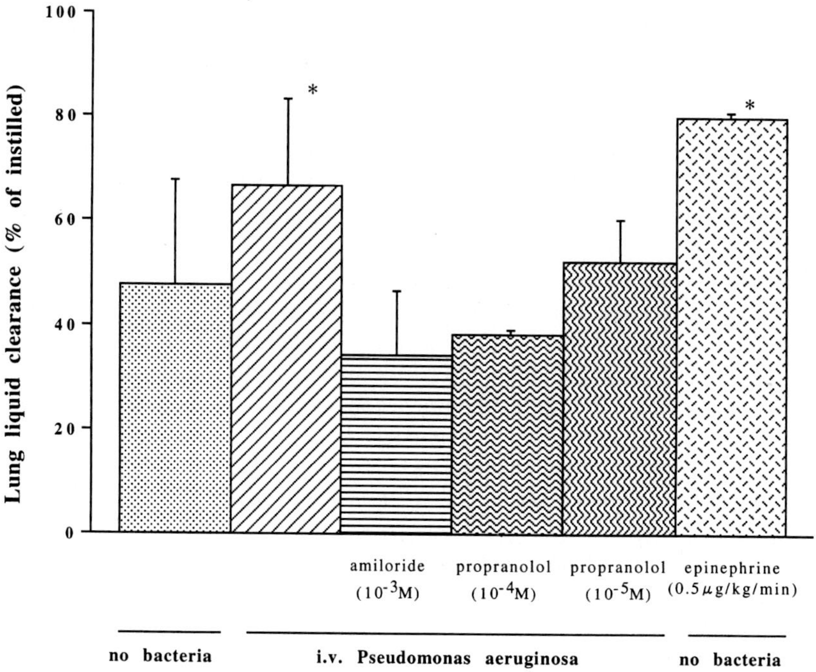

Figure 2 Lung liquid clearance in rats exposed to intravenous *P. aeruginosa.* Note that the rats that received an intravenous bolus of PA01 demonstrated significantly increased lung liquid clearance. To explore the mechanism for this increased clearance, other groups of rats that received the same dose of IV bacteria where given amiloride or different doses of propranolol. Amiloride and propranolol both were able to block the increased lung liquid clearance induced by the intravenous bacteria. Finally, the intravenous administration of 0.5 μg/kg/min of epinephrine, a dose chosen to produce comparable plasma levels of epinephrine to the levels measured in the bacteremic rats, was given to another group of rats. The epinephrine was able to increase lung liquid clearance in these rats, suggesting that catecholamines led to the increased lung liquid clearance found in the bacteremic rats. $*P<.05$ vs. controls. (From Ref. 12.)

goat lung experiments. There was no increase in the efflux of an instilled alveolar protein tracer in either experiment, suggesting that the alveolar epithelium had not been injured as measured by increased permeability to protein. However, measurements reflecting the ability of the alveolar epithelium to actively transport sodium in these three sheep suggested that either (1) the alveolar epithelium was unable to normally transport sodium so that the concentration of the instilled alveolar albumin did not increase, or (2) the influx of extravascular fluid into the airspaces was increased and could not be balanced by the normal functioning

Table 3 Effect of Intravenous *P. aeruginosa* on Systemic and Pulmonary Hemodynamics Over 8 h in Anesthetized Sheep[a]

Experimental condition	Mean systemic arterial pressure (mm Hg)	Mean pulmonary arterial pressure (mm Hg)	Left atrial pressure (mm Hg)	Cardiac output (L/min)
Controls, n = 6				
Baseline	86 ± 21	15 ± 3	4 ± 1	3.2 ± 0.6
Experimental	75 ± 14	16 ± 2	2 ± 2	2.8 ± 0.4
Intravenous *P. aeruginosa*, n = 11				
Group 1, n = 8				
Baseline	87 ± 9	15 ± 2	4 ± 2	3.6 ± 0.8
Experimental	38 ± 8[b]	33 ± 7[b]	0 ± 3	1.7 ± 0.6[b]
Group 2, n = 3				
Baseline	88 ± 29	13 ± 2	4 ± 3	3.6 ± 0.6
Experimental	45 ± 15[b]	40 ± 2[b]	1 ± 3	1.3 ± 0.5[b]

[a]Data are expressed as mean ± SD.

[b]$P < .05$ versus controls.

The mean systemic arterial pressure and central hemodynamics are shown in control sheep and in 11 sheep which received intravenous infusions of *P. aeruginosa* bacteria. Note that the 3 of the 11 sheep which developed more severe pulmonary edema also had higher pulmonary arterial pressures and lower cardiac outputs. *Source*: Ref. 13.

Table 4 Effect of Intravenous *P. aeruginosa* on Changes in Alveolar Concentration of Albumin Over 4 h in Anesthetized Sheep[a]

Experimental condition	No.	Alveolar albumin (g/100 mL) Initial	Final
Controls	6	4.2 ± 0.1	6.1 ± 0.5
Intravenous *P. aeruginosa*, group 1	8	4.6 ± 0.7	8.3 ± 1.9[b]
Intravenous *P. aeruginosa*, group 2	3	4.6 ± 0.7	4.3 ± 1.5[b,c]

[a]Data are expressed as mean ± SD.
[b]$P < .05$ versus controls.
[c]$P < .05$ versus intravenous *P. aeruginosa*, group 1.
Intravenous administration of bacteria on the ability of sheep to concentrate airspace-instilled albumin is shown. Note that 8 of the sheep were able to concentrate the albumin to levels significantly greater than the control animals. However, 3 sheep which developed more severe pulmonary edema were unable to concentrate the albumin. These results suggest that, in the 3 sheep the ability of the alveolar epithelium to transport liquid was impaired or that the influx of liquid from the interestitium was so profound that even a normally functioning alveolar epithelium could not clear the airspace liquid. *Source*: Ref. 13.

alveolar epithelium (Table 4) (13). These results confirm that the three sheep developed significantly increased quantities of pulmonary edema; however, the question remains as to why the three sheep were more susceptible than the other sheep.

III. Exoproducts Produced by Intravenous *P. aeruginosa*

Alveolar flooding and severe pulmonary edema are uncommonly produced after the short-term intravenous administration of live bacteria because of the resistance of the alveolar epithelial barrier (see above). However, the alveolar epithelial barrier may be adversely affected by the bacteremia; products produced by the bacteria or the inflammatory host response produced by the presence of the circulating bacteria could affect the lung epithelial barrier. There is in vitro evidence that suggests *P. aeruginosa* elastase injures the vascular endothelium and the basolateral surface of the alveolar epithelium (16,17). In contrast, there are in vitro and in vivo reports demonstrating that the apical surface of the alveolar epithelium is resistant to injury from *P. aeruginosa* elastase (18,19). The nebulization of 20 mg of *P. aeruginosa* elastase to the lungs of anesthetized sheep did not increase the extravascular lung water, nor did it alter the lung endothelial or epithelial permeability to protein (18). These reports suggest, therefore, that strains of *P. aeruginosa* that produce elastase would be more harmful to the alveolar epithelium if they were administered intravenously than if the strains were administered to the apical surface of the alveolar epithelium.

A recent investigation has demonstrated that the intravenous administration of a strain of *P. aeruginosa* that produces elastase (PAO1) did injure the lung endothelium and was less harmful to the alveolar epithelium (8). The intravenous administration of this strain did not increase the permeability of the alveolar epithelium to protein, nor did the administration of this strain change the ability of the epithelium to actively transport sodium. The intravenous administration of the strain did, however, increase the vulnerability of the alveolar epithelium to a second injury. When a noninjurious bacterial inoculum was instilled into the airspaces 60 min after the intravenous administration of a bolus of PAO1, there were a significant increase in the the alveolar epithelial permeability to protein, a significant increase in the severity of the pulmonary edema, and production of infected pleural effusions. In contrast, when an isogenic strain of PAO1, selectively mutated to be unable to produce elastase, was administered intravenously 60 min prior to this airspace instillation, no significant lung injury was produced. Furthermore, when a different strain of *P. aeruginosa* that does not produce elastase, PA103, was administered 60 min before the same airspace instillation of bacteria, no significant lung injury was produced. Thus, only the intravenous administration of elastase-producing strains of *P. aeruginosa* are able to increase the vulnerability of the apical surface of the alveolar epithelium to bacterial-induced injury.

Possible mechanisms for the intravenous elastase-induced vulnerability of the apical surface of the alveolar epithelium include the influence of *P. aeruginosa* elastase on epithelial cell tight junctions. *P. aeruginosa* elastase interrupts intercellular tight junctions and appears to damage the cell membranes of the type I pneumocytes (20,21). After interruption of the intercellular tight junctions of the alveolar epithelium, inflammatory mediators, bacterial products, or even the bacteria may be able to gain entry to the apical surface of the alveolar epithelium. These agents may then decrease the resistance of the apical surface of the alveolar epithelium to injury or they may interact synergistically with airspace bacteria to injure the apical surface of the alveolar epithelium.

The movement of neutrophils through intercellular tight junctions is unlikely to be an important factor in the production of secondary apical alveolar epithelial injury; after intravenous administration of the elastase-producing *P. aeruginosa,* the airspace instillation of *E. coli* endotoxin did not injure the alveolar epithelium, suggesting that the secondary apical injury required the presence of live bacteria (8). The airspace instillation of *E. coli* endotoxin has been shown to cause large quantities of neutrophils to enter the airspaces of the lung without changing the protein permeability of the alveolar epithelium (22). Therefore, it is doubtful that the entry of neutrophils via the altered intercellular junctions led to the increase in vulnerability of the apical surface of the alveolar epithelium after the intravenous administration of elastase-producing bacteria.

Several important conclusions are suggested from investigations of *P. aeruginosa* exoproducts. *P. aeruginosa* bacterial products appear to produce different degrees of injury to the exposed barriers of the lung. *P. aeruginosa* elastase is more injurious to the lung vascular endothelium and to the basolateral surface of the alveolar epithelium and is less injurious to the apical surface of the alveolar epithelium (see above). Clinical practice involves determination of the strain of a circulating bacteria in a patient to guide antibiotic therapy. In the future, it may become equally important to determine which exoproducts are produced by the strain of the circulating bacteria. Patients who become bacteremic from elastase-producing *P. aeruginosa* strains may be more vulnerable to apical alveolar epithelial injuries; airspace colonization of these elastase-exposed patients might lead to acute lung injury. More effective treatments of sepsis will probably include agents targeted against specific bacterial exoproducts, including elastase. These issues demand further investigation.

IV. Exoproducts Produced by Airspace *P. aeruginosa*

Three different strains of *P. aeruginosa* were compared for their ability to injure the alveolar epithelium when instilled into the airspaces. The three strains were chosen because they had been characterized as to which exoproducts the three strains produced, and there were isogenic, transposon-mutated strains available for the three wild-type strains. The isogenic, transposon-mutated strains do not make one or two particular exoproducts, but make most of the other exoproducts of the parental, wild-type strains. Therefore, the role of individual exoproducts in the production of alveolar epithelial injury could be established. Alveolar epithelial lung injury was determined by multiple measurements, including the efflux of an airspace radioactive protein tracer, the influx of a different circulating radioactive protein tracer, the determination of extravascular lung water, and the production of pleural effusions. Pleural effusion formation had been associated with the formation of severe interstitial and/or alveolar edema formation in other experimental models (23).

The first strain to be evaluated was PAO1 and three of its isogenic transposon mutant strains, PAO-S21, PLC-SRN, and PAO-R1, deficient in exoenzyme S, phospholipase C, and elastase and protease production, respectively (Tables 5, 6) (24). This investigation demonstrated that PAO1, an elastase-producing strain, was not injurious to the alveolar epithelium until an inoculum of 10^9 cfu was instilled into the distal airspaces of anesthetized, ventilated rabbits (24). In contrast, different *P. aeruginosa* strains producing other exoproducts

Table 5 Effects of Isogenic *P. aeruginosa* Strains on Accumulation of Alveolar and Vascular Protein Tracers in Pleural Space

Condition	n	Pleural fluid volume, ml/kg	^{125}I-albumin in pleural space, % of instilled	Pleural ^{131}I-albumin/ plasma ^{131}I-albumin
Control	6	0.16 ± 0.05	0.02 ± 0.01	0.06 ± 0.02
PAO-R1	4	0.33 ± 0.08[a]	0.15 ± 0.06[a]	0.20 ± 0.09[a]
PLC-SRN	6	0.32 ± 0.09[a]	0.20 ± 0.31	0.20 ± 0.06[a]
PAO-S21	5	0.12 ± 0.06	0.03 ± 0.03	0.10 ± 0.09

Values are means ± SD.
n, No. of animals.
[a]Significantly different ($P < .05$) from control.
Three isogenic strains of PAO1 on the formation of pleural effusions. The two isogenic strains that did not produce elastase were still able to produce alveolar epithelial injury and infected pleural effusions. Only the isogenic strain that did not produce exoenzyme S, PAO-S21, was unable to injure the alveolar epithelium nor was it able to produce infected pleural effusions. These results suggest that exoenzyme S was an important bacterial exoproduct in injuring the alveolar epithelium. *Source*: Ref. 24.

Table 6 Effect of Isogenic Strains of *P. aeruginosa* on Protein Flux Across Alveolar Epithelial Barrier

Condition	n	^{125}I-albumin in lung, % instilled	^{125}I-albumin in blood, % instilled	Alveolar ^{131}I-albumin/plasma ^{131}I-albumin	Final-to-initial instilled protein concentration ratio
Control	6	93 ± 2	3 ± 2	0.2 ± 0.1	3.0 ± 0.6
PAO-R1	4	86 ± 4[a]	11 ± 3[a]	0.5 ± 0.1[a]	2.4 ± 0.4[a]
PLC-SRN	6	90 ± 2	5 ± 2	0.5 ± 0.2[a]	2.5 ± 0.2[a]
PAO-S21	5	90 ± 2	4 ± 1	0.3 ± 0.1	2.9 ± 5.0

Values are means ± SD.
n, No. of animals.
[a]Significantly different ($P < .05$) from control.
The effects of three isogenic strains of PAO1 on the protein permeability of the alveolar epithelial barrier. Note that only the isogenic strain of PAO1 that did not produce exoenzyme S, PAO-S21, did not produce any increase in the protein permeability of the alveolar epithelial barrier. These results suggest that exoenzyme S, and not elastase, was an important bacterial exoproduct in injuring the alveolar epithelium. *Source*: Ref. 24.

Table 7 *Pseudomonas aeruginosa* Strains and Exoproducts

Strain	Toxin A		Exoenzyme S		Elastase		Phospholipase C activity
	Activity	Antigen	Activity (49 kDa)	Antigen (53 kDa)	Activity	Antigen	
PAK (parent)	+	+	++++	+	+	+	+
PAK *exsA*::Ω ($exoS^-$)	+	+	−	−	+	+	+
PA103 (parent)	++++	++++	−	++	−	−	+
PA103 *tox*Ω ($toxA^-$)	−	−	−	++	−	−	+
PA103 *exsA*Ω ($exoS^-$)	++	++	−	−	−	−	+

Presence of activity or antigen (+); lack of activity or antigen (−).
The exoproducts of two parental strains of *P. aeruginosa,* PAK and PA103, are shown, as well as their isogenic strains. The isogenic strains have been engineered not to produce selective exoproducts. *Source*: Ref. 19.

were found to cause significantly increased quantities of alveolar epithelial damage, even when 100-fold smaller inocula were instilled (19). Therefore, only modest alveolar epithelial injury over an 8-hour interval could be produced by the airspace instillation of large inocula of the elastase-producing PAO1 (24).

The role of specific exoproducts in the production of alveolar injury was determined by the instillation of 10^9 cfu of each of the isogenic stains of PAO1 (Tables 5, 6). The isogenic transposon mutant strain, PAO-R1, deficient in elastase and proteases, was as virulent as the wild-type strain, PAO1; this non-elastase-producing strain produced similar quantities of lung injury as PAO1. The instillation of 10^9 cfu of the isogenic transposon mutant strain, PAO-S21, deficient in the production of exoenzyme S and other proteins regulated by exoenzyme S, led to a significantly decreased quantitiy of alveolar epithelial injury (Table 6). These results suggested that exoenzyme S, or the proteins regulated by exoenzyme S, was important for the production of the alveolar epithelial injury associated with the parental strain, PAO1 (24). Based on these results, two strains of *P. aeruginosa* were obtained that produced increased amounts of exoenzyme S. These two strains, PAK and PA103, differ in the exoenzyme S-associated proteins they produce (Table 7). There are two or more proteins regulated by the genes for exoenzyme S (25) (Fig. 3). Preliminary

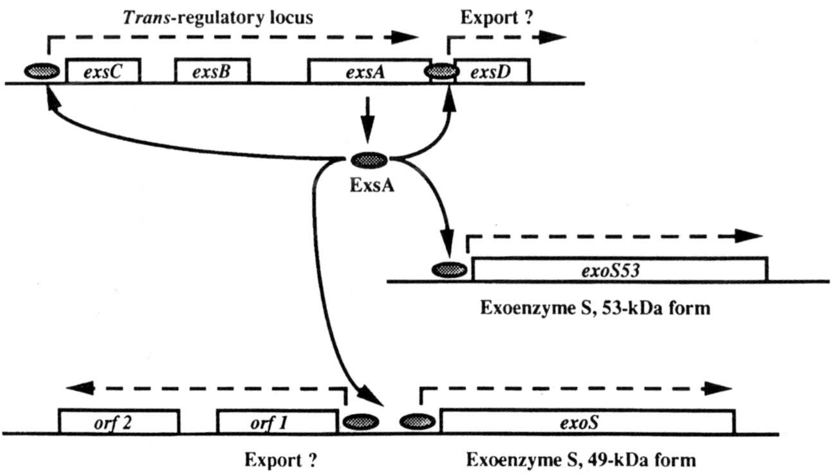

Figure 3 The exoenzyme S regulon is shown. Synthesis of exoenzyme S, encoded by two independent loci (*exoS* and *exoT*), requires a copy of the transcriptional activator, ExsA. The binding of ExsA is depicted by a filled oval in the promoter regions. The open reading frames are illustrated as open boxes with gene designation inside. The direction of transcription is indicated by dashed arrows. (From Ref. 25.)

evidence suggests that exoenzyme S and the Yop virulence determinants of *Yersinia* share significant homology between the proteins involved in their synthesis and secretion (25,26). These results and others suggests that the bacterial strains of *Pseudomonas* and *Yersinia* may have similar virulence factors and may cause similar problems for host defense (27).

The airspace instillation of 10^9 cfu of the wild-type PAK strain or of the wild-type PA103 strain led to significant alveolar epithelial injury. The instillation of the same dose of the wild-type PAO1 strain caused 8% of the instilled airspace radioactive protein tracer to leave the airspaces and enter the circulation. The instillation of PAK caused 16% of the instilled airspace tracer to leave the airspaces and enter the circulation and the instillation of the same dose of PA103 led to even greater injury, since 21% of the radioactive protein tracer entered the circulation (Table 8) (19). Significant pleural effusions were formed after the instillation of either of these strains; the pleural effusions contained the airspace bacteria and the airspace radioactive protein tracer, (Table 9) suggesting that these bacteria were able to cross the epithelium and enter the pleural space.

Table 8 Movement of Alveolar Tracer (^{125}I-Albumin) from the Lung into the Circulation Over 8 h

		Percentage of alveolar tracer	
Condition	*n*	Lung, % of instilled	Blood, % of instilled
Control	6	93 ± 2	3 ± 2
PAK (parent)	5	80 ± 4[a]	16 ± 4[a]
PAK *exsA*::Ω (exoS$^-$)	5	91 ± 2	6 ± 1
PA103 (parent)	5	56 ± 2[a,b]	21 ± 7[a]
PA103 *exsA*::Ω (exoS$^-$)	5	89 ± 3	5 ± 3
PA103 *tox*Ω (toxA$^-$)	5	54 ± 12[a,b]	27 ± 12[a]

Values are means ± SD. Control, rabbit albumin alone instilled.
[a]$P < .05$ compared with control.
[b]$P < .05$ compared with PAK parental strain.
The effect of the instillation of the two parental strains, PAK and PA103, and their isogenic strains on the permeability of the alveolar epithelium to protein. Note that the airspace instillation of either of the parental strains caused a significant increase in the permeability of the alveolar epithelium to protein. When the isogenic strains that could not produce exoenzyme S or proteins regulated by ExsA, PAK exsA::Ω, or PA103exsA::Ω were instilled, no increase in the protein permeability of the alveolar epithelium to protein was produced. These results confirmed that exoenzyme S, or a protein regulated by ExsA, was involved in the production of increased protein permeability. *Source*: Ref. 19.

Table 9 Effects on the Pleural Fluid Adjacent to the Instilled Lung Over 8 h

Condition	*n*	Pleural volume, ml	Alveolar tracer in pleural fluid
Control	6	0.6 ± 0.2	0.06 ± 0.1
PAK (parent)	5	0.9 ± 0.5[a]	0.3 ± 0.3[a]
PAK *exsA*::Ω ($exoS^-$)	5	0.6 ± 0.3	0.03 ± 0.01
PA103 (parent)	5	2.5 ± 1.1[a,b]	8.9 ± 3.2[a,b]
PA103 *exsA*::Ω ($exoS^-$)	5	0.7 ± 0.4	0.02 ± 0.02
PA103 *tox*Ω ($toxA^-$)	5	2.6 ± 1.7[a,b]	6.9 ± 4.2[a,b]

Values are means ± SD.
Control, rabbit albumin alone instilled.
Alveolar tracer, % instilled ^{125}I-albumin.
[a]$P < .05$ compared with control.
[b]$P < .05$ compared to PAK parental strain.
The effect of the instillation of the two parental strains, PAK and PA103, and their isogenic strains on the production of infected pleural effusions. The airspace instillation of either of the parental strains produced significantly increased quantities of infected pleural fluid. The airspace instillation of the two isogenic strains that could not produce exoenzyme S or proteins regulated by ExsA, PAK exsA::Ω, or PA103exsA::Ω did not increase pleural fluid volume. These results confirmed that exoenzyme S, or a protein regulated by ExsA, was involved in the production of infected pleural effusions. *Source*: Ref. 19.

When the isogenic transposon mutant strains of either PAK or PA103, unable to produce exoenzyme S or its regulated proteins, were instilled, alveolar epithelial injury was significantly decreased (Tables 8, 9). Therefore, some if not all of the proteins regulated by the genes for exoenzyme S are involved with causing the cytotoxicity of the alveolar epithelium. Investigations are underway to determine which of these proteins are necessary for the production of the cytotoxicity and the mechanisms by which they cause the epithelial cytotoxicity.

The mutant strains of *P. aeruginosa* have now been instilled into rabbits, rats, and mice (19,28,29); the results have been consistent in that the *P. aeruginosa* strains that make several of the proteins regulated by exoenzyme S are cytotoxic to the apical alveolar epithelium. To produce cytotoxicity, a minimum dose of the *P. aeruginosa* had to be instilled. (Fig. 4) A small inoculum of the "cytotoxic" strains of *P. aeruginosa* also causes the death of animals within 48 hours. Severe pulmonary edema was caused by these strains (Fig. 5); the pulmonary edema is induced because animals infected with these strains have increased permeability to protein of the epithelial and endothelial barriers. In contrast, animals exposed to intravenous injections of these cyto-

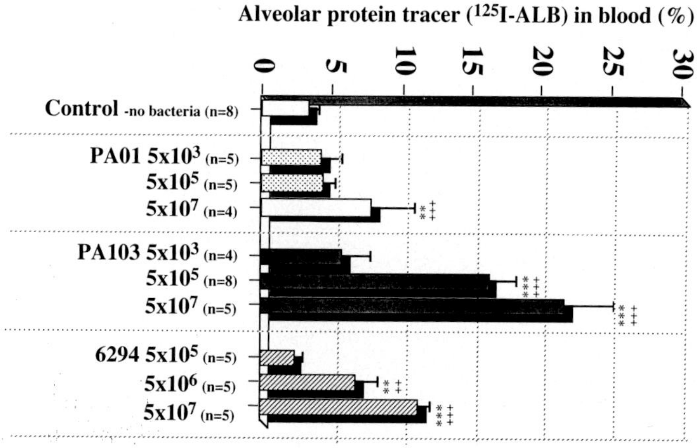

Figure 4 The effects of the airspace instillation of different doses of the parental strains, PA01, PA103, and 6294 on the protein permeability of the alveolar epithelium in mice. The instillation of PA103 caused the largest increase in protein permeability at every dose of instilled bacteria. However, when larger doses (10^7 cfu) of the "less injurious" bacteria, PA01 and 6294, were instilled, these bacteria could also significantly increase the protein permeability of the alveolar epithelium. These results suggest that although certain strains of *P. aeruginosa* produce "cytotoxic" exoproducts that injure the alveolar epithelium at low doses, all strains of *P. aeruginosa* can injure the alveolar epithelium when large quantities of the bacteria are instilled. $+++P < .01$ vs. controls; $***P < .01$ compared to other groups at same dose of bacteria. Mean $\pm$ SD.

toxic strains develop less severe pulmonary edema; alveolar epithelial permeability to protein is not increased after the intravenous administration of these strains (see above).

In vitro investigations have shown that supernatants made from PA103 or PAK are not cytotoxic to epithelial cells and that the presence of the live *P. aeruginosa* was necessary for the production of cytotoxicity (30). Interestingly, *Yersinia pseudotuberculosis* also requires physical contact with target cells for expression of its virulence factors (31). The type III secretion system coordinates the secretion of the Yersinia virulence factors with the expression of the genes for the virulence factors after the physical contact with the target cell (32). Recently, it has been established that *P. aeruginosa* secretes exoenzyme S via a type III secretion pathway (33). Furthermore, the type III secretion system appears to be an increasingly common feature of pathogenic gram negative bacteria (32). Therefore, there may be similar patterns of virulence caused by several of the gram-negative bacteria that cause lung disease.

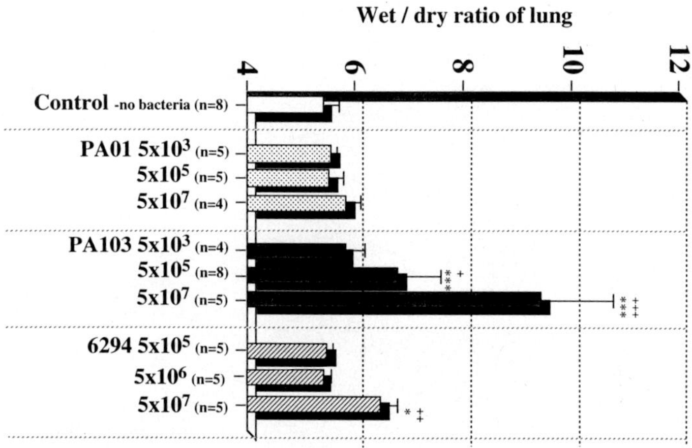

Figure 5 Airspace instillation of different doses of the parental strains, PA01, PA103 and 6294, in mice. The instillation of 10^5 and 10^7 cfu of PA103 and the instillation of 10^7 cfu of 6294 produced significant increases in extravascular lung water. Even large doses of PA01 did not significantly increase the extravascular lung waters of the exposed mice. These results suggest that the *P. aeruginosa* strain that is cytotoxic (PA103) produces more lung edema, presumably because this strain disseminates to the circulation. $+++P < .01$ vs. controls; $***P < .01$ vs. other groups at the same dose of bacteria. Mean $\pm$ SD.

V. Noncytotoxic *P. aeruginosa* Strains and the Lung

Several strains of *P. aeruginosa* that do not possess the genes for exoenzyme S were evaluated in in vitro and in vivo experiments. These strains did not cause cytotoxicity to the apical alveolar epithelium in vivo or to other epithelia in vitro (34). However, these "noncytotoxic" strains of *P. aeruginosa* invaded the epithelial cells (34) (Fig. 6) In fact, the strains of *P. aeruginosa* that possess the genes for exoenzyme S also appear to invade epithelial cells (Fig. 7). However, the cytotoxic strains cause necrosis of the epithelial cells and disseminate into the circulation of infected animals, whereas the noncytotoxic strains remain intracellular (34). These are dose-dependent phenomena; the instillation of very large doses of the noncytotoxic bacteria will cause some necrosis of the epithelium, dissemination of these bacteria, and formation of small amounts of pulmonary edema (Figs. 4, 5).

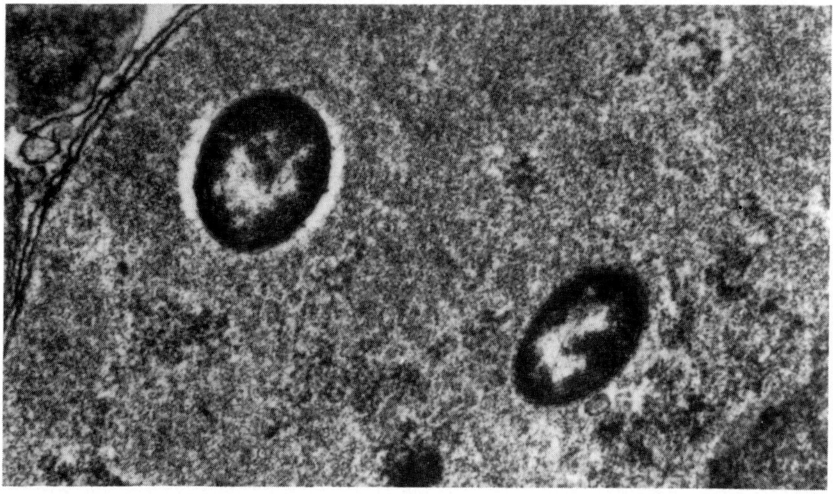

Figure 6 Electron micrograph of an infected mouse trachea. An invasive, noncytotoxic strain, 6294, was applied to the trachea of an anesthetized mouse for 4 hours. Intracellular bacteria were found inside the tracheal epithelium (magnification × 25,500). (From Ref. 34.)

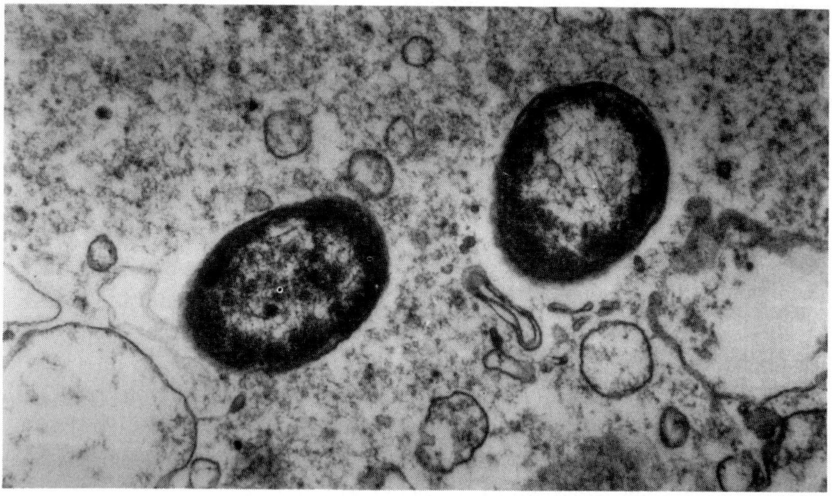

Figure 7 Electron micrograph of a trachea infected with the cytotoxic strain, PA103, applied to the trachea of an anesthetized mouse for 4 hours. Intracellular bacteria were found in epithelial cells. However, necrosis of the epithelial cells is also apparent. Therefore, the cytotoxic bacteria are invasive, but they also cause necrosis of the invaded epithelial cells. Magnification × 25,500. (From Ref. 34.)

VI. Conclusion

The mechanisms for pulmonary edema formation by *P. aeruginosa* include the production of cytotoxic exoproducts that cause alveolar epithelial necrosis; the cytotoxic bacteria are able to disseminate to the circulation and increase endothelial permeability to protein. Animals that have been given airspace instillations of the cytotoxic strains develop severe pulmonary edema. In contrast, the intravenous administration of these cytotoxic strains of *P. aeruginosa* will cause an increase in endothelial permeability that only leads to the formation of mild pulmonary edema. The intravenous administration of elastase-producing *P. aeruginosa* strains usually produces mild pulmonary edema but occasionally the intravenous administration of these strains has been associated with the formation of severe pulmonary edema. The intravenous administration of the elastase-producing strains also increases the vulnerability of the apical alveolar epithelium to subsequent injuries. Finally, the airspace instillation of noncytotoxic *P. aeruginosa* strains leads to the formation of pulmonary edema only when very large inocula are instilled.

It appears that for severe lung injury to occur, *P. aeruginosa* needs to make direct contact with the apical epithelium. This requirement for direct bacterial-to-cell contact for the production of cytotoxicity has also been demonstrated in experiments utilizing *Yersinia.* Molecular techniques are being employed to determine the mechanisms whereby these bacteria can induce cellular damage which results in increased permeability and subsequent dissemination.

Acknowledgments

Dr. Wiener-Kronish is supported by grants from the NIH-NHLI 49810 and 55980. Dr. Gropper is supported by a grant from the FAER Young Investigator Award.

References

1. Bryan CS, Reynolds KL. Bacteremic nosocomial pneumonia: analysis of 172 single episodes from one metropolitan area. Am Rev Respir Dis 1984; 129:668–671.
2. Horan TC, White WJ, Jarvis WR, Emori TG, Culver DH, Munn VP, Thornsberry C, Olson DR, Hughes JM. Nosocomial infection surveillance. CDC Surveillance Summary 1986; 32:1SS–16SS.
3. Bodey GP, Bolivar R, Fainstein V, Jadeja L. Infections caused by *Pseudomonas aeruginosa.* Rev Infect Dis 1993; 5:270–313.
4. Fabregas N, Torres A, El-Ebiary M, Ramfrez J, Hernandez C, Gonzalez J, de la Bellacasa JP, de Anta J, Rodriguez-Roisin R. Histopathologic and microbiologic aspects of ventilator-associated pneumonia. Anesthesiology 1996; 84:760–771.

5. Rouby JJ. Nosocomial infection in the critically ill: the lung as a target organ. Anesthesiology 1996; 84:757–758.
6. Torres A, Aznar R, Gatell JM, Jimenez P, Gonzalez J, Ferrer A, Celis R, Rodriguez-Roisin R. Incidence, risk, and prognosis factors of nosocomial pneumonia in mechanically ventilated patients. Am Rev Respir Dis 1990; 142:523–528.
7. Brewer SC, Wunderink RG, Jones CB, Leeper KV Jr. Ventilator-associated pneumonia due to *Pseudomonas aeruginosa.* Chest 1996; 109:1019–1029.
8. Pittet JF, Kudoh I, Wiener-Kronish JP. Experimental model of bacteremia-induced acute lung injury in rabbits. 1997. In press.
9. Doyle RL, Szaflarski N, Modin GW, Wiener-Kronish JP, Matthay MA. Early identification of patients with acute lung injury: predictors of morality. Am J Respir Crit Care Med 1995; 152:1818–1824.
10. Brun-Buisson C, Doyon F, Carlet J. Bacteremia and severe sepsis in adults: a multicenter prospective survey in ICUs and wards of 24 hospitals. Am J Respir Crit Care Med 1996; 154:617–624.
11. Pittet JF, Matthay MA, Pier G, Grady M, Wiener-Kronish JP. *Pseudomonas aeruginosa* induced lung and pleural injury in sheep: differential protective effect of circulation versus alveolar IgG antibody. J Clin Invest 1993; 92:1221–1228.
12. Pittet JF, Wiener-Kronish JP, McElroy MC, Folkesson HG, Matthay MA. Stimulation of lung epithelial liquid clearance by endogenous release of catecholamines in septic shock in anesthetized rats. J Clin Invest 1994; 94:663–671.
13. Pittet JF, Wiener-Kronish JP, Serikov V, Matthay MA. Resistance of the alveolar epithelium to injury from septic shock in sheep. Am J Respir Crit Care Med 1995; 151:1093–1100.
14. Matthay MA, Wiener-Kronish JP. Intact epithelial barrier function is critical for the resolution of alveolar edema in man. Am Rev Respir Dis 1990; 142:1250–1257.
15. Comroe JH, Forster RE, Dubois AB, Briscoe WA, Carlsen E. Arterial blood oxygen; carbon dioxide; pH. In: The Lung: Clinical Physiology and Pulmonary Function Tests. Chicago: Yearbook Medical Publishers, 1977:140–150.
16. Bejarano P, Langeveld J, Hudson B, Noelken M. Degradation of basement membranes by *Pseudomonas* elastase. Infect Immun 1989; 57:3783–3787.
17. Miller R, Britigan B. Protease-cleaved iron-transferrin augments oxidant-medicated endothelial cell injury via hydroxyl radical formation. J Clin Invest 1995; 95: 2491–2500.
18. Peterson P, Collins M, Gray L, Azghani A. Aerosolized *Pseudomonas* elastase and lung fluid balance in anesthetized sheep. J Appl Physiol 1992; 72:1927–1933.
19. Kudoh I, Wiener-Kronish JP, Pittet JF, Frank D. Exoproduct secretions of *Pseudomonas aeruginosa* strains influence severity of alveolar epithelial injury. Am J Physiol 1994; 267:L551–L556.
20. Azghani AO, Gray LD, Johnson AR. A bacterial protease perturbs the paracellular barrier function of transporting epithelial monolayers in culture. Infect Immun 1993; 61:2681–2686.
21. Azghani AO. *Pseudomonas aeruginosa* and epithelial cell permeability: role of virulence factors elastase and exotoxin A. Am J Respir Cell Mol Biol 1996; 15: 132–140.

22. Hashimoto S, Pittet JF, Hong K, Bagby G, Folkesson H, Kobzik L, Watanabe K, Tsurufuji S, Wiener-Kronish JP. Depletion of alveolar macrophages abolishes neutrophil chemotaxis to *Pseudomonas* airspace infections. Am J Physiol 1996; 270 (Lung Cell Mol Physiol 14):L819–L828.
23. Wiener-Kronish JP, Broaddus VC, Albertine KH, Gropper M, Matthay MA, Staub NC. Pleural effusions are associated with increased permeability pulmonary edema in anesthetized sheep. J Clin Invest 1988; 82:1422–1429.
24. Wiener-Kronish JP, Sakuma T, Kudoh I, Pittet JF, Frank D, Dobbs L, Matthay MA. Alveolar epithelial injury and pleural empyema in acute *P. aeruginosa* pneumonia in anesthetized rabbits. J Appl Physiol 1993; 75:1661–1669.
25. Goranson J, Frank DW. Genetic analysis of exoenzyme expression by *Pseudomonas aeruginosa.* FEMS Microbiol Lett 1996; 135:149–155.
26. Yahr TL, Hovey AK, Kulich SM, Frank DW. Transcriptional analysis of the *Pseudomonas aeruginosa* exoenzyme S structural gene. J Bacteriol 1995; 177:1169–1178.
27. Brubaker RR. Factors promoting acute and chronic diseases caused by *Yersinia.* Clin Microbiol Rev 1991; 4:309–324.
28. McElroy MC, Pittet JF, Hashimoto S, Allen L, Wiener-Kronish JP, Dobbs LG. A type I cell specific protein is a biochemical marker of epithelial injury in a rat model of pneumonia. Am J Physiol 1995; (Lung Cell Mol Biol 12):L181–L186.
29. Sawa T, Corry DB, Gropper MA, Ohara M, Kurahashi K, Wiener-Kronish JP. IL-10 improves lung injury and survival in *Pseudomonas aeruginosa* pneumonia. J Immunol 1997; 159:2858–2866.
30. Apodaca G, Bomsel M, Lindstedt R, Frank D, Mostov KE, Wiener-Kronish JP. Characterization of *Pseudomonas aeruginosa*-induced MDCK cell injury: glycosylation defective host cells are resistant to bacterial killing. Infect Immun 1995; 3:1541–1551.
31. Rosqvist R, Magnusson KE, Wolf-Watz H. Target call contact triggers expression and polarized transfer of *Yersinia* yopE cytotoxin into mammalian cells. EMBO J 1994; 13:964–972.
32. Rosqvist R, Hakansson S, Forsberg A, Wolf-Watz H. Functional conservation of the secretion and translocation machinery for virulence proteins of yersiniae, salmonellae and shigellae. EMBO J 1995; 14:4187–4195.
33. Yahr TL, Goranson J, Frank DW. Exoenzyme S of *Pseudomonas aeruginosa* is secreted by a type III pathway. Mol Microbiol 1996; 22:991–1003.
34. Fleiszig SMJ, Wiener-Kronish JP, Miyazaki H, Vallas V, Mostov KE, Kanada D, Sawa T, Yen TSB, Frank DW. *Pseudomonas aeruginosa*–mediated cytotoxicity and invasion correlate with distinct genotypes at the loci encoding exoenzyme S. Infect Immun 1997; 65:579–586.

8

Aspiration Syndromes

Acid, Salt Water, and Fresh Water

HANS G. FOLKESSON

Lund University
Lund, Sweden

RICHARD M. EFFROS

Medical College of Wisconsin
Milwaukee, Wisconsin

I. Introduction

Aspiration syndromes may be conveniently divided into two general categories. *Endogenous* aspiration usually refers to the entry of fluid from the stomach into the airways and is frequently associated with exposure of the lungs to acid solutions. *Exogenous* aspiration occurs during near-drowning incidents, and these fluids may be either hypertonic or hypotonic. Both categories of aspiration can induce lung injury and edema formation within the lung. This chapter will consider the pulmonary disorders associated with each of these fluid challenges to the integrity of the pulmonary endothelial and epithelial barriers in terms of both pathogenesis and possible future treatment strategies.

II. Acid Aspiration

Aspiration of gastric secretions represents the second or third most common cause of acute lung injury in man. Respiratory insufficiency following massive aspiration of gastric contents carries a mortality rate of between 40% and 50% (1,2). Treatment is currently limited to positive-pressure ventilation and careful management of fluid therapy. In theory, it might be possible to develop more effective treatment since the time of onset of the aspiration is frequently known with certainty when gastric aspiration is witnessed (3), whereas the time of onset is often difficult to identify in other clinical conditions which cause injury to the lungs, such as sepsis (4). Because there is a delay in onset of the acid-aspiration injury, treatment could begin before damage to the lung has become severe. These clinical considerations would justify research into the pathogenesis and potential therapy of acute lung injury caused by the aspiration of acid.

A. Neutralization of Acid in the Lungs

Mendelson was the first investigator to describe the effects of gastric aspiration that occurred during labor in 66 women (5). Further research in rabbits led him to conclude that it was the acid in gastric fluid that caused the severe lung injury in these patients. Aspiration of gastric contents and acid into the lungs causes severe pulmonary injury, which is characterized by hypoxia, increased intrapulmonary shunting, and diffuse pulmonary infiltrates (6,7). Schwartz and colleagues (8) reported that aspiration of gastric contents with a pH 2.5 or greater is relatively benign, while aspiration of fluids with lower pH cause severe pulmonary injury. In an earlier study, Wynne and colleagues (7) demonstrated that, as the pH decreased toward 1.5, the pulmonary injury increased, but lowering pH below this level appeared to cause no further injury. The dispersion of large volumes low-pH solutions in the lungs have nearly always been associated with high mortality rates (9).

Although acid is presumably the most important agent in the gastric fluid that injures the lungs, the fluid may be very alkaline if secretions from the bile and pancreas reach the gastric lumen. In addition, the stomach often contains a variety of other substances that may affect the outcome of the aspiration of gastric contents. However, the initial injury to the lung cannot be attributed to aspiration of food particles, and appears to be related to the low pH of the solution. Aspiration of food particles and bacteria may complicate the recovery phase from acid aspiration and result in the subsequent development of bacterial pneumonia (3,7).

It has been recognized that acids are rapidly neutralized in the lungs (10), but the mechanisms responsible for this process have remained largely unexplored. Studies of the cystic fibrosis transmembrane conductance regulator (CFTR) indicate that this channel permits the diffusion of both HCO_3^- and Cl^- across the apical membranes of epithelial cells (11,12). Recent studies have suggested that efficient neutralization of acids instilled into the lungs requires exchange of these anions across the membranes separating the vascular and airspace compartments of the lungs (13). It is possible that defects in CFTR in patients with cystic fibrosis may contribute to the chronic airway injury, primarily bronchiectasis, which is observed in children with this disorder. Recurrent gastric reflux has been documented in most of these children (14,15), and inefficient neutralization of aspirated acid could lead to airway damage.

B. Pathology of Acid Aspiration-Induced Acute Lung Injury

Most of our knowledge concerning the pathologic changes underlying acid aspiration-induced acute lung injury is based on results from animal experiments. Acid is dispersed throughout the lungs rapidly after aspiration, and injury to the alveolar epithelial-endothelial barrier is immediate and primarily due to chemical injury from the low-pH solution. Histological examination of the lung during the first few hours after aspiration reveals extensive epithelial degeneration of the bronchi, pulmonary edema, and hemorrhage (7). Electron microscopic evaluation demonstrates necrosis of the alveolar epithelial type I cells and free lamellated inclusion bodies derived from the type II cells in the pulmonary edema fluid. Within 4 hours after acid aspiration, an acute infiltration of polymorphonuclear leukocytes as well as accumulation of fibrin can be seen in the alveolar spaces. Further degeneration of both alveolar type I and type II cells is observed. After instillation of acid into rabbit lungs, structural changes were observed, involving dehiscence of the endothelial layer of the alveolar-capillary membranes, neutrophil accumulation, and alveolar tissue necrosis (16). Similar morphological changes have been shown to be involved in pulmonary edema formation by other investigations (17) as well.

Soon after acid aspiration, the alveolar-capillary membrane, which is normally resistant to transport of ^{51}Cr-EDTA, becomes highly permeable to this indicator (18). In another study it was shown that hydrochloric acid causes an immediate pulmonary capillary leak (19). During the following 24 to 36 hours, marked neutrophilia is associated with alveolar consolidation, and the damage to the distal airway epithelium may result in sloughing of the epithelium. Later, hyaline membranes can be observed (7), which may begin to resolve after 72 hours. This injury is associated with regeneration of bronchial epithelium, proliferation of fibroblasts, and a decrease in the acute inflammatory response (see Chap. 2). Lungs from animals obtained 2 to 3 weeks after acid aspiration are normal in appearance, with slight parenchymal scarring.

C. Role of Neutrophils in Lung Injury Induced by Acid Exposure

There is good reason to believe that acute lung injury following acid aspiration may be mediated in part by neutrophil-dependent mechanisms (20–28). The importance of neutrophils in determining vascular barrier function after acid aspiration is supported by the following observations:

1. A strong correlation exists between the number of sequestered neutrophils and the degree of pulmonary edema after acid aspiration.

2. Neutropenia protects the vascular barrier against increases in permeability induced by aspiration of acid and decreases the alveolar-arterial oxygen differences associated with this event (26,29).
3. Inhibition of neutrophil activation and H_2O_2 synthesis reduces neutrophil sequestration and limits the degree of pulmonary edema following acid aspiration.

In several studies, acid-induced lung injury was reduced either by blocking neutrophil products or by depleting neutrophils (21,24,26,28–34). Presumably, acid aspiration induces neutrophil recruitment into the lung by stimulating the release of a variety of chemotactic and inflammatory molecules, chiefly from alveolar macrophages (21,24,31,32). Once they have been recruited to the lung, neutrophils may then induce injury by binding to and migrating through the pulmonary capillary endothelium (35–37).

Mediators of Inflammation

Injury to endothelial and epithelial membranes by acidic solutions may stimulate the release of substantial quantities of cytokines, e.g., TNF-α, and a number of chemokines, including IL-8, and other pro-inflammatory molecules. These mediators are derived from a variety of cells in the lung including airway epithelial cells, alveolar epithelial cells, and alveolar macrophages (31,38–40).

Interleukin-8

Considerable evidence has been gathered implicating the importance of interleukin-8 (IL-8) as a major chemotactic factor for recruiting neutrophils to extravascular sites of inflammation, including those in the lung (41,42). Not only is IL-8 a potent chemoattractant for neutrophils, it also upregulates neutrophil β_2 adhesion receptors for endothelium (43), mediates neutrophil migration across activated endothelium (44,45), and primes neutrophils for activation (46,47). IL-8 is produced by several cell types in the lung, including alveolar macrophages, alveolar type II epithelial cells, bronchial epithelial cells, and pulmonary fibroblasts (38–40,48,49).

Measurements of IL-8 in pulmonary edema fluid and bronchoalveolar lavage fluid support an important role for IL-8 in patients with acute lung injury (37,50,51). In one study of patients with acute lung injury (37), higher IL-8 concentrations were associated with an increase in mortality, and in a study of patients at risk for acute lung injury, IL-8 concentrations were higher in those who developed ARDS than in those who did not (51). In two recent experimental studies in rats and rabbits, antibodies to human IL-8 reduced neutrophil influx and lung injury caused by IgG immune complexes (52) and ischemia reperfusion (53). Anti-IL-8 antibodies also prevented influx of neutrophils into the pleural spaces following endotoxin-induced pleurisy in rabbits (54).

A recent study suggests that IL-8 plays a key role in recruiting neutrophils into the airspaces after acid aspiration (29). Treatment with a neutralizing monoclonal anti-IL-8 antibody reduced the extent of acute lung injury by 70% (Fig. 1). Although much of the action of IL-8 may be mediated by neutrophils, other cells may also be involved since depletion of neutrophils does not afford as much protection as antibody to IL-8. Though relatively specific for neutrophils, IL-8 is also chemotactic for T lymphocytes (55) and eosinophils (56).

Folkesson and colleagues (29) investigated whether IL-8 was important for development of lung injury and neutrophil activation/sequestration following acid aspiration and whether administration of monoclonal, species-specific antibodies would attenuate the observed acute lung injury. This work was done as both a pretreatment study and a treatment study. Administration of anti-IL-8 antibodies was effective both before and 1 hour after acid aspiration. After acid was instilled into rabbit lungs, large numbers of neutrophils were recoverable from the airspaces in association with markedly elevated quantities of

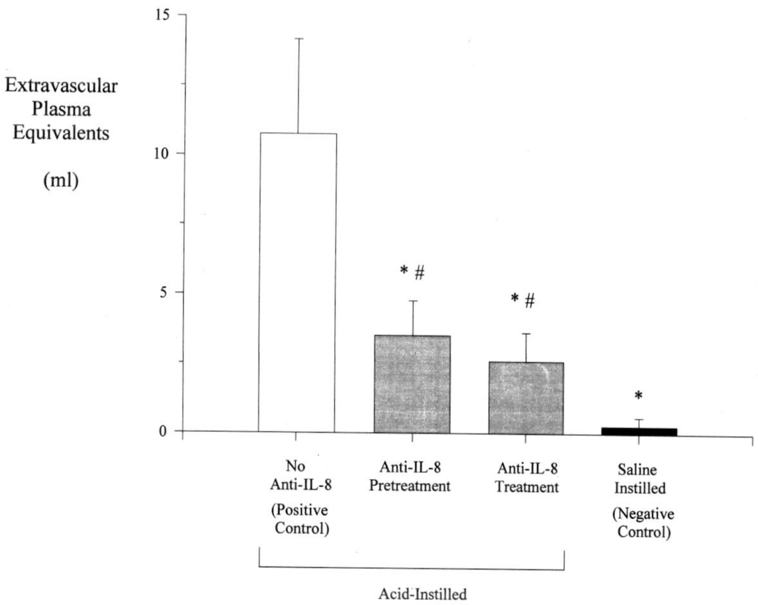

Figure 1 Endothelial permeability was significantly increased after acid aspiration in rabbit lungs. This increase was decreased by 70% after pretreatment and treatment with anti-IL-8 antibodies, but was still elevated as compared to control rabbits instilled with saline alone. $*P < .05$ relative to positive control (acid alone); $\#P < .05$ relative to negative control group (saline alone). (Reproduced from *The Journal of Clinical Investigation*, 1995, 96:107–116 by copyright permission of The American Society for Clinical Investigation.)

IL-8. The concentrations of IL-8 in the air spaces 6 hours after acid aspiration (41 ± 18 ng/mL) were biologically relevant (concentrations were 10 times greater than those needed to initiate chemotaxis and neutrophil priming in vitro assays [57]). The use of the anti-IL-8 monoclonal antibody led to a > 50% decrease in the neutrophil influx and, more importantly, to a dramatic reduction in the severity of the acute lung injury due to acid aspiration. Anti-IL-8 antibodies attenuated hypoxia, edema formation, and endothelial leak by approximately 75% and provided protection for at least 24 hours after acid aspiration (Figs. 1, 2) (29). Because IL-8 is a distal cytokine, its neutralization may have more limited effects than neutralization of a more proximal, pluripotent cytokine, such as TNF-α. Also, neutralization therapy might be required only for a short time, during the time that IL-8 is generated. Following stimulation with endotoxin, IL-8 concentrations return toward normal in < 12 hours (54,58).

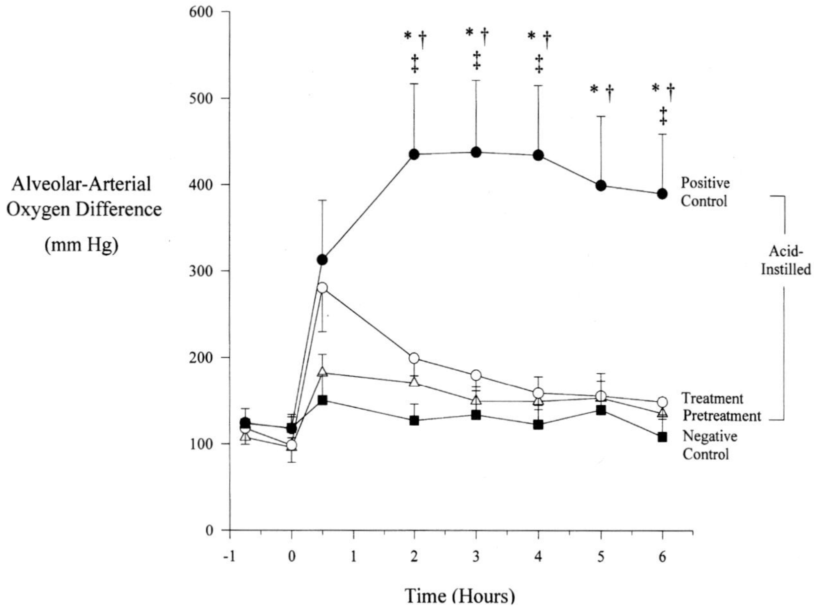

Figure 2 Alveolar-arterial oxygen tension difference increased drastically after acid instillation into the rabbit lungs. The increase in alveolar-arterial oxygen tension difference after acid instillation was attenuated by both pretreatment and treatment with anti-IL-8 antibodies and was no different from control rabbits instilled with saline only. Data are means ± SEM; $*P < .05$ relative to the negative control group (saline only); $\dagger P < .05$ relative to the pretreatment group; $\ddagger P < .05$ relative to the treatment group. (Reproduced from *The Journal of Clinical Investigation*, 1995, 96:107–116 by copyright permission of The American Society for Clinical Investigation.)

A potential limitation of anti-IL-8 therapy is that, like any anti-inflammatory therapy, it might impair host immunity and increase the risk of infection. Indeed, secondary bacterial pneumonia is a known complication of acid aspiration, occurring 2 to 10 days after aspiration (3). This issue surely deserves further experimental studies, although there are reasons to believe that anti-IL-8 therapy would not drastically increase the risk of infection. Anti-IL-8 therapy does not completely prevent the neutrophil influx into the air spaces of the lungs. In fact, the total number of neutrophils in the air spaces remained high, which may be important for host defense. Furthermore, a reduction in the underlying lung injury may reduce the risk of subsequent lung bacterial infections following acid aspiration. Finally, in mice lacking a murine homolog of an IL-8 receptor, bacterial infections have not been a problem despite an impairment in extravascular neutrophil recruitment to stimuli such as endotoxin (59).

Tumor Necrosis Factor-α (TNF-α)

Another cytokine that is probably important in the development of acid aspiration-induced acute lung injury is TNF-α. TNF-α may be produced by monocytes and/or alveolar macrophages after they have been directly stimulated by the aspirated acid. TNF-α mediates systemic and local injury by a mechanism that involves upregulation of neutrophil-endothelial adhesion receptors. Protein synthesis is necessary for this step. After septic shock, treatment with a TNF-α antibody was protective against the neutrophil-dependent systemic organ injury (60,61). TNF-α, leukotriene B_4, and thromboxane A_2 have all been shown to upregulate the neutrophil CD18-adhesion receptor complex (62). Treatment of cultured endothelium with TNF-α induces expression of two varieties of endothelial adhesion receptors—ELAM-1 and ICAM-1 (63). Expression of these adhesion receptors occurs during the course of 2 to 3 hours. This timing is consistent with the delayed occurrence of leukosequestration in the lungs following acid aspiration (20). In a study in rats, localized acid aspiration-induced injury was largely inhibited by the administration of an anti-TNF-α antiserum (Fig. 3) (31). Leukosequestration, protein leak, wet/dry weight ratios, and myeloperoxidase activities were all reduced by the anti-TNF-α treatment. The results suggested that TNF-α mediated acid aspiration-induced lung injury, in part by inducing an endothelial adhesion protein (Table 1). However, the failure of anti-TNF-α antiserum to inhibit the immediate neutropenia that follows acid aspiration argues against the involvement of TNF-α in the early neutrophil activation steps.

The failure of anti-TNF-α antiserum to fully prevent leukosequestration in the lung after acid aspiration suggests that other mechanisms may be active. Treatment of acid aspiration-induced acute lung injury with anti-TNF-α antibodies resulted in reduced edema formation in the lungs (Fig. 3), an effect also observed after inhibition of protein synthesis with cycloheximide (31). However,

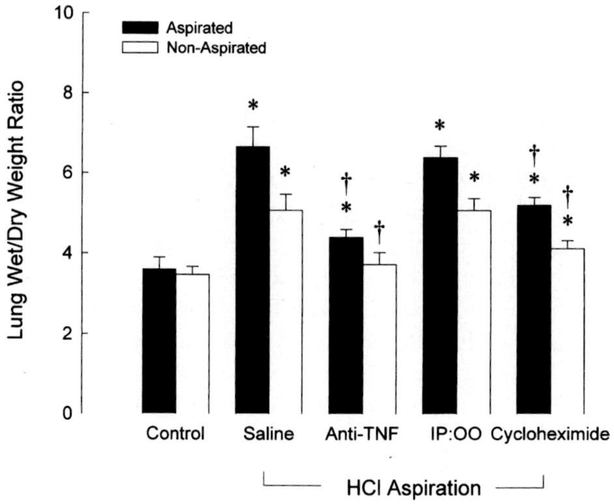

Figure 3 Localized aspiration led to increased lung wet/dry weight ratios in both aspirated and nonaspirated lungs. This increase was largely prevented by administration of anti-TNF-α antibodies and cycloheximide. * and † indicate $P < .05$ relative to control group and saline instilled group, respectively. (From Ref. 31)

treatment with the anti-TNF-α antibodies did not reduce the early leukosequestration after acid aspiration, suggesting that this part of the pathological picture might be mediated by non-TNF-α-mediated pathways.

Adhesion Molecules

Another group of inflammatory molecules that might become activated by acid aspiration-induced acute lung injury are adhesion molecules which govern migration of inflammatory cells across the endothelium. The neutrophil adhesion complex, CD11,118, (LFA-1/Mac-1/p150,95) (64), mediates stimulated neutrophil adhesion to the endothelium (65). The CD11,18 family of integrins is necessary for normal leukocyte trafficking. Patients lacking CD11,18 integrins on their circulating monocytes and neutrophils have defective functions which are specific to these cells (66,67).

Neutrophils frequently cause damage to the endothelium when they migrate through capillaries and release their granular contents (25,26). This occurs when CD11,18 integrins on the neutrophils bind to ICAM-1 receptors on the endothelium. Doerschuk and colleagues (22) studied neutrophil migration in the systemic (abdominal wall) and pulmonary circulation of rabbits following

Table 1 Factors That Have Been Demonstrated to Be Involved and Important in Mediating Acid Aspiration-Induced Acute Lung Injury

Factor	Effect	Animal species	Reference
β-Adrenergic receptors	Affecting systemic blood pressure	Rabbit	103
Leukotriene B_4	Chemotactic for neutrophils	Rabbit	21
		Rat	32
C5a	Chemotactic for neutrophils and alveolar macrophages	Rabbit	21
CD11,18	Mediating neutrophil adherence in the systemic circulation	Rabbit	22
		Cat	33
			68
CD11b,18	Mediating neutrophil activation	Rabbit	34
Atrial natriuretic peptide	Elevated in plasma after lung injury and may prevent pulmonary edema with its diuretic activity	Rat	137
Tumor necrosis factor-α	Mediates local and systemic organ injury, partly by inducing an endothelial adhesion protein	Rat	31
Thromboxane	Local thromboxane synthesis is required for neutrophil sequestration and an increased lung permeability	Rat	24
			32
Reactive oxygen species	Decrease the vascular barrier function	Rat	25
			26
Elastase	Decrease the vascular barrier function	Rat	25
Serine proteases	Decrease the vascular barrier function	Rat	26
Interleukin-8	Chemokine for neutrophils	Rabbit	29
Complement	Mediate microvascular permeability defects	Rat	27

stimulation by different inflammatory stimuli, including hydrochloric acid. They determined the role of the leukocyte adhesion complex, CD11,18, in each of these vascular beds by blocking neutrophil adhesion with a monoclonal anti-CD18 antibody (mAb 60.3). This antibody was able to block neutrophil migration into inflammatory foci in the abdominal wall produced by implantation of sponges containing either hydrochloric acid, *Streptococcus pneumoniae, Escherichia coli* endotoxin, or PMA (Table 2). In the pulmonary circulation, the effects of the antibody varied with the introduced stimulus. It inhibited neutrophil migration after PMA-induced pneumonia, partly after endotoxin-induced pneumonia, but failed to inhibit migration after *S. pneumoniae*-induced pneumonia or hydrochloric acid-induced acute lung injury (Table 3). Therefore, the investigators concluded that neutrophil adherence in the pulmonary circulation can occur by either CD18-dependent or CD18-independent mechanisms. CD18 mediates neutrophil emigration in the systemic circulation.

In a subsequent study of acid aspiration in rabbits, acute lung injury from the acid aspiration was reduced by pretreatment with a monoclonal anti-CD18 antibody (Table 1), even though the number of alveolar neutrophils, as assessed by bronchoalveolar lavage, was not decreased. The number of alveolar neutrophils after the anti-CD18 treatment was almost double the number of alveolar neutrophils observed after acid alone (28,34,68). Following neutralization of binding to CD18, acid-induced abnormalities in gas exchange, extravascular lung water, and lung vascular permeability were nearly completely prevented. It was proposed that inhibition of these adhesion molecules may have interfered with the activation of the neutrophils without affecting their migratory capacities. Therefore, less active and less injurious neutrophils may have entered the airspaces and resulted in a more modest injury to the lungs.

Table 2 PMN Migration into the Abdominal Wall of Rabbits After Pretreatment with a Monoclonal Antibody Against CD18[a]

	No. of PMN/0.10 mm^2 tissue[b]			
Pretreatment	*S. pneumoniae* 10 hours	Hydrochloric acid 4–5 hours	PMA 10 hours	Endotoxin 4 hours
mAb 60.3	4.1 ± 3.1[c] (6)	0[c] (1)	2.0 ± 1.5[c] (2)	2.2 ± 0.5[c] (4)
Saline	362 ± 27(6)	17.1 (1)	229 ± 48 (2)	152 ± 23 (4)

[a]The data demonstrate that in all cases, PMN migration is CD18-dependent.
[b]Mean ± SE and n = number of animals (shown in parentheses).
[c]Although the group size is small, the values are completely disjointed from the control values by a factor of at least 10.
Source: Doerschuk and colleagues (22). Copyright 1990, The American Association of Immunologists.

Table 3 Percent Inhibition by mAb 60.3 of PMN Emigration Induced by *E. coli* Endotoxin or *S. pneumoniae* in the Pulmonary and Systemic Circulations[a]

	% Inhibition	
Stimulus	Lung	Abdominal wall
E. coli endotoxin	72 ± 3[b]	98 ± 0.3[c]
S. pneumoniae	0.3 ± 5	99 ± 0.4[c]

[a]Inhibition of PMN migration was only partial after *E. coli* endotoxin, while no inhibition was seen after *S. pneumoniae.* Also, mAb 60.3 did not inhibit PMN migration after HCI instillation in the lung (data not shown in table), but inhibited PMN migration after PMA pneumonia. mAb 60.3 inhibited PMN migation in all cases after abdominal wall exposure. Rabbits pretreated with mAb 60.3 (n = 4) or saline (n = 4) were given *E. coli* endotoxin in the right lung and *S. pneumoniae* in the left lung, as well as sponges infiltrated with these stimuli within the abdominal wall. The number of PMN/alveolus and the number of PMN/mm^2 abdominal wall were quantitated histologically, and the percent inhibition of neutrophil emigration induced by mAb 60.3 was calculated.

[b]Statistically significant inhibition of PMN emigration ($P < .01$).

[c]Significantly more inhibition compared to the same stimulus in the lung ($P < .03$).

Source: Doerschuk et al. (22).

An alternative explanation for finding significantly elevated neutrophil numbers in the bronchoalveolar lavage fluid after anti-CD18 treatment (28) may be related to similar observations made after endotoxin injury to the liver (69). Neutrophils accumulated continuously in the livers of mice, reaching very high numbers, after exposure to galactosamine and endotoxin. Inhibition of CD11b,18 by pretreatment with monoclonal antibodies significantly attenuated the liver injury and reduced the number of neutrophils sequestered in the liver by 50%. However, treatment with a monoclonal antibody against CD11a,18 was ineffective in reducing neutrophil number and liver injury. It is therefore possible that the reduction in lung injury and higher lavage neutrophil numbers that were observed may be related to the fact that acute lung injury after acid aspiration is mediated by CD11b,18, but migration across the vascular endothelium is independent of CD11a,18.

Selectins

The selectins belong to a family of molecules that all contain an NH_2 terminal lectin-like domain, an epidermal growth factor (EGF) repeat, and a discrete number of modules (approximately 60 amino acids each), similar to those found in certain complement binding proteins. So far, three members of the selectin family have been identified, named by the cell type originally discovered on: E-selectin (endothelium), P-selectin (platelets), and L-selectin (lymphocytes).

L-selectin was the first selectin molecule to be described. It was found in studies that used a monoclonal antibody against a murine lymphoma. This antibody blocked lymphocyte adhesion to high endothelial venules of lymph nodes, and also blocked lymphocyte homing (70,71). P-selectin was discovered in studies on platelet activation in which it was found that antibodies that bound to activated platelets did not bind to resting platelets (72,73). P-selectin was also found to be part of the Weibel-Palade bodies in the vascular endothelial cells (74,75). P-selectin is rapidly shed from the platelets and endothelial cells following stimulation by thrombin and other mediators (74,75). E-selectin was discovered in studies that used an antibody strategy that combined identification of a cellular activation antigen and blocking of adhesion. A monoclonal antibody was raised that recognized a cytokine-induced glycoprotein and endothelial cells at sites of inflammation together with a second antibody that blocked neutrophil adhesion (76–79). These results suggested the existence of a new adhesion molecule that was later called E-selectin. Since their discovery, each of the selectin molecules has become a subject of substantial investigative efforts.

Leukocyte recruitment, such as that observed after acid aspiration, involves an orchestration of soluble mediators (e.g., cytokines) and cell surface molecules that results in focal adhesion of the leukocytes to the vessel walls and later extravasation. The importance of selectins in this process is widely accepted. P-selectin has been demonstrated to be of significant importance for the development of acute lung injury following cobra venom infusion (80). In that study, it was shown that administration of an antihuman P-selectin antibody to rats diminished the acute lung injury, suggesting that P-selectin was needed for the full development of the acute lung injury. Elevated levels of soluble E-selectin have been described in patients with septic shock (81). Much remains to be done before the exact roles of each of the selectins in lung injury are understood.

D. Oxygen Radicals and Granular Contents Released from Sequestered Neutrophils

Acid aspiration is followed by increased neutrophil oxidative metabolism (Table 1), an event associated with lung leukosequestration and increased alveolar endothelial-epithelial barrier permeability (25). Sepsis-induced acute lung injury is associated with increased generation of reactive oxygen species, elevated quantities of extracellular fluid, and leakage of protein (82).

Acid aspiration accelerates the synthesis of thromboxane, stimulates neutrophil activation and promotes the generation of H_2O_2. Progressive sequestration of neutrophils in the lungs is associated with acid aspiration-induced acute lung injury (31). Increased pulmonary permeability and edema are associated with neutrophil sequestration. It has been suggested that pulmonary edema formation occurs after the sequestered neutrophils release their granular contents containing vasotoxic agents, including reactive oxygen species and elastase (Table 1). Although treatment of acid aspiration-induced acute lung injury with oxygen radical scavengers, such as superoxide dismutase and catalase, did not affect neutrophil sequestration, it did reduce protein leak into the alveolar spaces and reduced accumulation of extravascular lung water (25). However, other studies suggest that reactive oxygen species may not be the sole mediators of acid aspiration-induced acute lung injury. In one study, rats made neutropenic displayed the same acute lung injury as rats having normal numbers of circulating neutrophils (26). Although neutrophils were required for the full development of lung injury, treatment with oxidant scavenging substances had no protective effects. The authors found high levels of serine proteases in the bronchoalveolar lavage fluid and concluded that these enzymes are important in the development of acid aspiration-induced acute lung injury (Table 1) (26).

E. Leukotrienes and Other Arachidonic Acid Metabolites

A wide variety of arachidonic acid metabolites may be released by activated, sequestered neutrophils, including eicosanoids, thromboxane, and leukotrienes (21,23,24,32). Leukotriene B_4 (LTB_4) and C5a have been shown to be important chemotactic factors in the airspaces of the lung (21,32,83) (Table 1). Release of these factors was associated with accumulation of inflammatory cells, primarily neutrophils, but also macrophages which were recruited by C5a. Leukotriene B_4 acted synergistically with thromboxane A_2 in mediating acid aspiration-induced acute lung injury (Table 1). Inhibition of either leukotriene B_4 or thromboxane A_2 inhibited the edema formation and leukosequestration. However, inhibition of these factors only helped after neutrophils were already sequestered. Presumably, a better approach would be to inhibit the sequestration of the neutrophils in the pulmonary microcirculation. In another study, in rats, neutrophil accumulation due to pulmonary thromboxane synthesis appeared to participate in acid aspiration-induced acute lung injury (24). In this study, inhibition of thromboxane synthesis lead to an attenuation of pulmonary edema formation associated with a decreased leukosequestration (Table 1). These data indicated that after acid aspiration, local pulmonary thromboxane synthesis is required for sequestration of neutrophils and increases in permeability.

Inhibition of the cyclo-oxygenase pathway by ibuprofen in sheep attenuated the increase in bronchial blood flow seen after acid aspiration (Table 1) (23). Moreover, lung lymph flow was also significantly reduced following cyclo-oxygenase inhibition, suggesting some protection from lung injury. The data suggested that airway blood flow may be important in the generation of pulmonary edema after acid aspiration.

F. Complement System

Complement factors play an important role in various pathological conditions that involve endothelial damage and microvascular injury (84–87). The human complement receptor-1 gene has been cloned (88), and this 200-kDa protein has been shown to inhibit human C3 and C5 convertases, thereby reducing C3a and C4a formation (88). Complement factors have been shown to play central roles in various pathologic conditions that involve endothelial damage and microvascular injury, such as sepsis (84,85) and the adult respiratory distress syndrome (ARDS) (86,87). Complement inhibition by this protein has been used to effectively inhibit pulmonary microvascular injury from immunoglobulin G or cobra venom factor-induced complement activation (89), burn injury (89), interleukin-2 infusion (90), endotoxin-induced ARDS in platelet-activating factor-primed rats (91) and in acid aspiration-induced acute lung injury in rats (Table 1) (27). Rabinovici and colleagues (27) undertook a study to investigate the role of complement after acid aspiration. They postulated that inhibition or depletion of complement attenuates acid aspiration-induced acute lung injury. The design of the study was a controlled animal trial using anesthetized rats. Aspiration was induced by intratracheal instillation of hydrochloric acid and lung injury was measured by determining lung water content, myeloperoxidase activity, protein concentration, and leukocyte count in bronchoalveolar lavage fluid. Pretreatment with soluble complement receptor type 1 (complement inhibition) or cobra venom factor (complement depletion) reduced lung edema, and protein leak, improved oxygenation, but had no effects on leukosequestration in the lung. The authors therefore concluded that acid aspiration-induced acute lung injury is partly mediated through a complement-dependent pathway and that some degree of protection may be provided by inhibiting the complement activation. However, leukocyte infiltration into the lung parenchyma was apparently complement-independent since complement inhibition did not prevent the aspiration-induced increase in serum-TNF-α.

Activation of complement by acid aspiration may be due to release of proteases from acid injured airway and alveolar epithelia. Alternatively, complement activation may be initiated by mediators produced and released by the inflammatory response to the acid. TNF-α may play a role in this process, since it has been shown that TNF-α acts synergistically with endotoxin to activate the complement system in mice (92). Whether complement itself can mediate leukocyte sequestration is not known, but the complement anaphylatoxin, C5a, is involved in neutrophil chemotaxis and aggregation (21,93).

G. Therapy of Acid Aspiration-Induced Lung Injury

As noted above, a broad effort has been made to reduce lung injury after acid aspiration by reducing either the number of neutrophils or some of the inflammatory mediators associated with these cells. A wide variety of other approaches have been used that may or may not have effects on neutrophils.

Steroids were used clinically to treat acid aspiration for many years. An initial report found that corticosteroid therapy decreased the pulmonary capillary permeability to protein (94), suggesting that this drug could be beneficial after acid aspiration. The effects of corticosteroid treatment on epithelial permeability changes, hemodynamic, and ventilatory consequences after acid aspiration were studied in dogs (95–97). In both these studies, corticosteroid therapy was of no beneficial effect acutely after the acid aspiration.

In the hope that inhibition of gastric acid secretion might protect the lungs from acid injury, patients have been treated with histamine-2 receptor inhibitors before induction of anesthesia (98–100). Unfortunately, these studies have given conflicting results.

Sznajder and colleagues (102) demonstrated that plasmapheresis was more effective than hemofiltration for reducing the extent of pulmonary edema following acid aspiration in a dog model. They suggested that the relative ineffectiveness of hemofiltration was related to the generation of neutrophil chemotactic factors or neutrophil activation factors in the blood, in the circulation, or in the hemofiltration unit. Also, removal of vasoactive substances by plasmapheresis may have had an ameliorating effect on the canine HCl-induced lung injury. In contrast, hemofiltration may have induced leukocyte lung sequestration, worsening the lung lesion and augmenting the surface area for leakage.

Broe and colleagues (101) reported that the magnitude of the acid-induced injury is to some extent a function of pulmonary arterial pressure. These investigators therefore used pulmonary vasodilators to treat acid aspiration-induced acute lung injury and found that lowering the pulmonary arterial pressure decreased the magnitude of lung injury. This suggests that intrapulmonary shunting and pulmonary arterial pressure changes may be of some importance in regulating the magnitude of injury after acid aspiration has occurred. A similar observation was made by Mizus and colleagues (103), who demonstrated that isoproterenol and aminophylline attenuated increases in pulmonary artery pressure and pulmonary vascular permeability after acid aspiration-induced acute lung injury. They proposed that a common mechanism for the protective effect of these agents may involve an increase in intracellular cAMP-levels. Similar findings have been observed after ischemia/reperfusion lung injury, in which agents that raise intracellular cAMP offered protection (104).

Kudoh and colleagues (105) used pentoxifylline to treat acid aspiration-induced acute lung injury. This agent has multiple effects on neutrophils, including inhibition of phagocytosis, degranulation, and superoxide generation (106–109). Kudoh and colleagues (105) investigated whether pretreatment with pentoxifylline protected the alveolar epithelium and pulmonary endothelium from acid-induced lung injury. They demonstrated that pretreatment with pentoxifylline attenuated the increase in endothelial permeability observed after acid aspiration of both lungs by approximately 50%, thereby restoring the Pa_{O_2}/FI_{O_2} to normal in the pretreated animals (Fig. 4). However, the epithelial permeability was not affected by the pretreatment with pentoxifylline and remained elevated after the acid aspiration-induced acute lung injury. Also, in this experimental study of acid aspiration, the injury could only be partly attenuated, suggesting that other mechanisms might be involved or that a combination of different treatments is needed.

H. Conclusions

Significant progress has been made in understanding the pathophysiology responsible for acid aspiration-induced acute lung injury. It has now clearly been

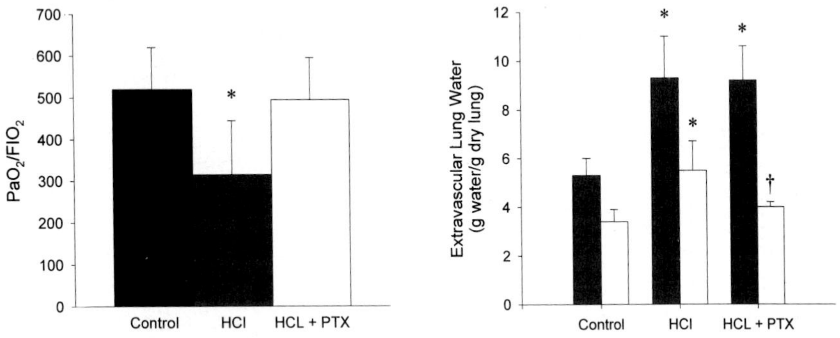

Figure 4 The measured Pa_{O_2}/FI_{O_2} 8 hours after acid instillation into rabbit lungs (a). HCI significantly decreased the Pa_{O_2}/FI_{O_2} over the 8-hour study period. Pretreatment with pentoxifylline (PTX) restored the oxygenation back to control levels. Data are means ± SD; $*P < .05$ relative to control and HCI + PTX (a). The extravascular lung water was significantly increased after acid instillation in both aspirated and nonaspirated lungs, and this increase was attenuated in the nonaspirated lung by pentoxifylline pretreatment (b). Dark-gray bars represent aspirated lung and light-gray bars represent nonaspirated lung (b). $*P < .05$ relative to control group (b); $\dagger P < .05$ relative to HCI nonaspirated lung (b); data are means ± SD. (Reproduced with permission from *Anesthesiology*.)

demonstrated that the polymorphonuclear neutrophil plays a critical role in mediating this form of lung injury. As indicated above, several approaches appear to hold promise for the future treatment of patients who either are at risk of aspiration or have already aspirated acid.

III. Aspiration of Hypotonic and Hypertonic Solutions

Drowning is the second most common cause of cardiac arrest in children and the fourth most common cause of accidental death (110). It is responsible for more than 140,000 fatalities worldwide annually (110). Death following immersion in water can be due to either laryngospasm ("dry drowning"), which occurs in 10% to 15% of drowning victims or airspace flooding with asphyxiation (111). Furthermore, occasional patients may survive an initial "near-drowning" and appear improved, only to develop adult respiratory distress syndrome some hours later ("secondary drowning") (112). Our current understanding of water transport in the lung will be reviewed, but additional information may be obtained from a variety of sources (113–121).

The sequence of events that follows aspiration of water depends on the volume and osmolality of the aspirated water. Aspiration of fresh water results in a rapid influx of water into the pulmonary circulation, which causes a significant drop in plasma osmolality and lysis of the red blood cells as well as systemic fibrinolysis (116). In contrast, aspiration of salt water results in a significant efflux of water from the circulation and surrounding tissue into the alveolar spaces, accompanied by a dramatic increase in alveolar fluid volume (121). During drowning, a subject can hold his breath until the "breaking point" is reached, which occurs at Pa_{CO_2} levels below 55 mm Hg when there is asphyxia. When the submerged victim reaches the breaking point, and an inspiration has to be made, large quantities of water are swallowed, and vomiting often occurs with aspiration of gastric contents (122). Acid aspiration, in comparison, results in a more marked endothelial injury as well as a chemical epithelial burn injury (29).

After fluid aspiration, the sequence of events can be summarized as follows:

1. Peripheral airway resistance increases.
2. Variable degrees of laryngospasm occur.
3. Reflex pulmonary vasoconstriction leads to pulmonary hypertension.
4. Lung compliance decreases.
5. Ventilation/perfusion ratios fall.
6. Fluid shifts occur across the alveolar membrane.
7. Surfactant is destroyed (salt water), or its properties are altered (fresh water or salt water).

8. Foam and froth are produced, further compromising ventilation.
9. Anatomical changes occur in alveolar epithelial cells.

The vagal effects that cause bronchoconstriction and vasoconstriction are primarily governed by the aspirated fluid's osmolality and not its volume (122). Fluids with low osmolality, such as fresh water, are especially efficient in triggering these reflexes.

Aspirated fresh water moves rapidly across the alveolar epithelium, through a basement membrane, and finally through the capillary endothelium into the capillary lumen. When the water reaches the capillary lumen, severe hemodilution occurs and the red cells lyse (122,123). This rapid water flux causes severe distortion of the pulmonary ultrastructure. Histological examination shows damage to both type 1 and type 2 alveolar epithelial cells as well as endothelial cell swelling, basement membrane detachment, and cell disruption (116).

In an experimental study on the effects from the solution's osmolality on the pulmonary injury, Orlowski and colleagues (118) demonstrated that as long as the solution contained electrolytes, injury to the alveolar epithelial-endothelial barrier was minimal. These studies, together with investigations by Kylstra (124), demonstrated that fresh water was more injurious than sea water or normal saline to the lung.

In a more recent study by Folkesson and colleagues (121), instillation of hyperosmolar seawater into rabbit lungs caused rapid translocation of large quantities of water into the distal air spaces with little injury to the alveolar epithelial-endothelial barrier. Influx of water was correlated with a significant oxygenation defect (Fig. 5), which was also observed in earlier studies (125–128). However, over time the gas exchange in the rabbit study improved significantly, suggesting that water was reabsorbed from the alveolar spaces (Fig. 5). In fact, when lung liquid clearance was measured gravimetrically on these lungs, a normal fluid clearance rate was observed (Fig. 6) (121). Therefore, the data from the experimental rabbit study (121) and the data from a case report on resolution from pulmonary edema associated with saltwater drowning (119), in which net alveolar fluid clearance was documented, provide evidence for a relatively well preserved alveolar epithelial barrier function after seawater aspiration. The situation is quite different after freshwater aspiration and acid aspiration. Both freshwater aspiration and acid aspiration result in significant destruction of the alveolar epithelial barrier functions with severe pulmonary and systemic effects (29,116,118,123,124,129).

The manner in which water crosses cell membranes remained mysterious for many years. Solomon and his colleagues (130,131) found that rate of water movement across red cell membranes induced by osmotic gradients is significantly more rapid than could be explained by diffusion. Subsequent experiments have shown that the filtration coefficient of water (P_f) is as much as 10 times

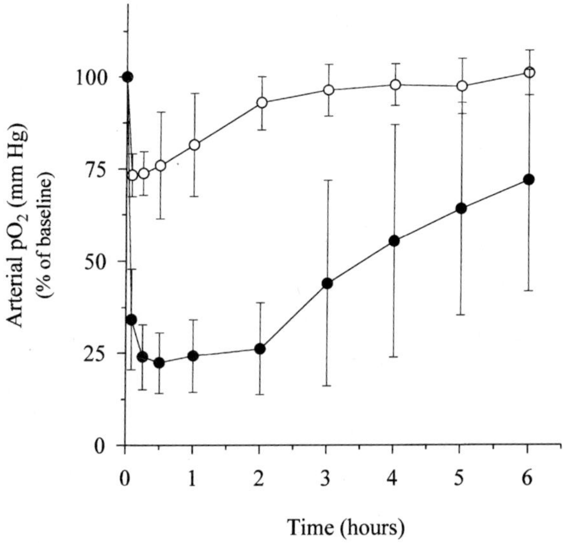

Figure 5 Changes in arterial oxygenation following instillation of seawater (closed circles) and after instillation of isosmolar saline (open circles). As water enters the air spaces to equilibrate the osmotic difference after the instillation of the hyperosmolar seawater, arterial oxygenation is severely impaired. When this fluid starts to leave the air spaces, alveolar oxygenation defect is attenuated. Values are means ± SD. (Modified from Ref. 121 with permission of *The American Journal of Respiratory and Critical Care Medicine.*)

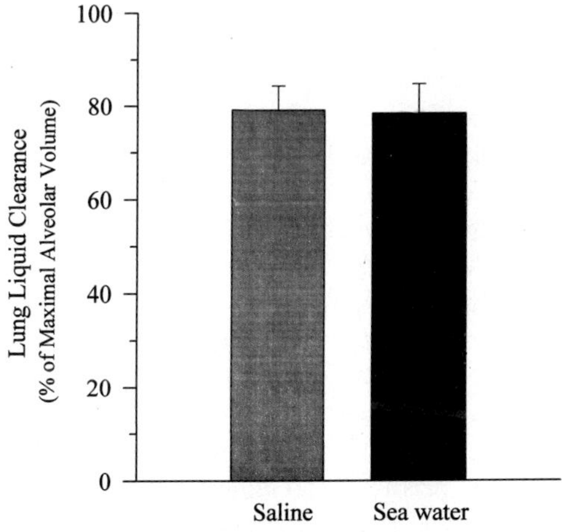

Figure 6 Lung liquid clearance in saline instilled control rabbits and in seawater instilled rabbits at 6 hours after instillation. Lung liquid clearance continued at a normal rate once isosmolar conditions had been reached after the osmotic equilibration was completed. Values are means ± SD. (Modified from Ref. 121 with permission of *The American Journal of Respiratory and Critical Care Medicine.*)

as great as the diffusion coefficient (P_d). Effros (132) and colleagues subsequently found that when lungs are perfused with hypertonic solutions of low-molecular-weight, lipophobic solutes, the fluid extracted from the pulmonary tissues is essentially devoid of solutes. In a subsequent investigation, these investigators demonstrated that when fluid-filled lungs are perfused with hypertonic solutions, the fluid lost from the airspaces is also devoid of solutes (133). Because cell membranes are relatively impermeable to lipophobic solutes, they concluded that water had crossed the endothelial-epithelial barrier through cell membranes rather than by the paracellular junctions in these experimental lungs.

The membrane channels responsible for osmotic translocation of water across cell membranes, now officially termed aquaporins, has been recently studied by several investigators (134,135). Most of these proteins are exquisitely selective for water molecules, and they have been described in many different tissues, including the lungs. Studies by Folkesson (135) indicated that the movement of water into the airspaces following instillation of hypertonic solutions into the airspaces can be inhibited by mercuric compounds, which are known to inhibit some aquaporins. Subsequent studies have indicated that most of the aquaporin-1 is located on the endothelium and some on type II epithelial cells, but none is detectable on type I cells (136). Aquaporin 5 is a water channel that is primarily located on the apical surface of alveolar type I cells (137).

Rapid water translocation through aquaporins induced by osmotic gradients presumably acts to keep the water content of the airspace gas close to saturation and prevents drying of the epithelium, which would impair gas exchange. In addition, it may enhance water movement out of the airspaces in response to active sodium transport from edematous areas of the lungs. Although water translocation from the airspaces is very rapid, it is by no means instantaneous. Recent indicator dilution studies indicate that clearance of water from the airspaces is slower than that of labeled water after instillation of water with ^{3}HOH into the tracheas of isolated rat lungs. This difference in clearance rates is readily explained by the fact that osmotic flows are induced by comparatively small differences in water concentration in the airspace and vascular compartments (55 vs. 54.7 mole/L). There is consequently considerable backdiffusion of unlabeled water from the perfusate to the airspaces in these experiments, whereas there is initially no ^{3}HOH in the perfusate and consequently no back-diffusion. It can be concluded that osmotic shifts of water in the lung tissues are limited by the permeability of the barriers to water flow rather than to the rate at which the lungs are perfused, and inhibition of aquaporins with mercurials consequently results in measurable changes in water translocation rates (see Chap. 18 for more details).

In summary, the major factors determining the injury from water aspiration and near-drowning accidents are the osmolality and presence of electrolytes in the aspirated water. Fresh water is more injurious to the alveolar epithelial-endothelial barrier than salt water since it destroys both the alveolar epithelial cells and the endothelial cells. Salt water induces a large transcellular flux of water into the distal air spaces, resulting in a significant oxygenation defect, but without significant injury to the alveolar epithelial barrier. This oxygenation defect gradually resolves over time as the water is reabsorbed into the blood circulation. Acid aspiration, in contrast, injures the barrier initially chemically by its low pH and high H^+ ion content, and in the second phase by significant influx on activated inflammatory cells, primarily neutrophils (29). Several new anti-inflammatory strategies may be useful in the clinical setting to reduce acute lung injury from aspiration of gastric contents (139).

References

1. Pepe PE, Potkin RT, Reus DH, Hudson CD, Carrico CJ. Clinical predictions of the adult respiratory distress syndrome. Am J Surg 1982; 144:124–130.
2. Fowler AA III, Hamman RF, Good JT. Adult respiratory distress syndrome: risk with common predispositions. Ann Intern Med 1983; 98:593–597.
3. Bynum LJ, Pierce AK. Pulmonary aspiration of gastric contents. Am Rev Respir Dis 1976; 114:1129–1136.
4. Rubin DB, Wiener-Kronish JP, Murray JF, Green DR, Turner J, Luce JM, Montgomery AB, Marks JD, Matthay MA. Elevated von Willebrand factor antigen is an early plasma predictor of acute lung injury in nonpulmonary sepsis syndrome. J Clin Invest 1990; 86:474–480.
5. Mendelson CL. The aspiration of stomach contents into the lungs during obstetric anesthesia. Am J Obstet Gynecol 1946; 52:191–200.
6. Stewardson RH, Nyhus LM. Pulmonary aspiration: an update. Arch Surg 1977; 112:1192–1197.
7. Wynne JW, Modell JH. Respiratory aspiration of stomach contents. Ann Intern Med 1977; 87:465–474.
8. Schwartz DJ, Wynne JW, Gibbs CP, Hood CI, Kuck EJ. The pulmonary consequences of aspiration of gastric contents at pH values greater than 2.5. Am Rev Respir Dis 1980; 121:119–126.
9. Cameron JL, Mitchell WH, Zuidema GD. Aspiration pneumonia: clinical outcome following documented aspiration. Arch Surg 1973; 106:49–52.
10. Awe WC, Fletcher WS, Jacob SW. The pathophysiology of aspiration pneumonitis. Surgery 1966; 60:232–239.
11. Smith JJ, Welsh MJ. cAMP stimulates bicarbonate secretion across normal, but not cystic fibrosis airway epithelia. J Clin Invest 1992; 89:1148–1153.
12. Poulsen JH, Fischer H, Illek B, Machen TE. Bicarbonate conductance and pH regulatory capability of cystic fibrosis transmembrane conductance regulator. Proc Natl Acad Sci USA 1994; 91:5340–5344.
13. Effros RM, Darin C. Efficient anion transport is essential for prompt neutralization of inspired acid: a possible model of acute lung injury in cystic fibrosis (abstr). Am J Respir Crit Care Med 1995; 151:A741.
14. Malfroot A, Dab I. New insights on gastro-oesophageal reflux in cystic fibrosis by longitudinal follow up. Dis Child 1991; 66:617–622.

15. Vic P, Tassin E, Turck D, Gottrand F, Launay V, Farriaux JP. Frequency of gastroesophageal reflux in infants and in young children with cystic fibrosis. Arch Pediatr 1995; 2:742–746.
16. Alexander IGS. The ultrastructure of the pulmonary alveolar vessels in Mendelson's (acid pulmonary aspiration) syndrome. Br J Anaesth 1968; 40:408–414.
17. Montaner JSB, Tsang J, Evans KG, Mullen JBM, Burns AR, Walker DC, Wiggs B, Hogg JC. Alveolar epithelial damage: a critical difference between high pressure and oleic acid induced low pressure pulmonary edema. J Clin Invest 1986; 77:1786–1796.
18. Jones JG, Grossman RF, Berry M, Slavin G, Hulands GH, Minty B. Alveolar-capillary membrane permeability. Correlation with functional, radiographic, and postmortem changes after fluid aspiration. Am Rev Respir Dis 1979; 120:399–410.
19. Grimbert FA, Parker JC, Taylor AE. Increased pulmonary vascular permeability following acid aspiration. J Appl Physiol 1981; 51:335–345.
20. Goldman G, Welbourn R, Klausner JM, Paterson IS, Kobzik L, Valeri CR, Shepro D, Hechtman HB. Localized acid aspiration leads to thromboxane dependent generalized pulmonary edema. Surg Forum 1989; 40:258–260.
21. Ishii Y, Kobayashi J, Kitamura S. Chemotactic factor generation and cell accumulation in acute lung injury induced by endotracheal acid instillation. Prostaglandins Leukot Essent Fatty Acids 1989; 37:65–70.
22. Doerschuk CM, Winn RK, Coxson HO, Harlan JM. CD18-dependent and -independent mechanisms of neutrophil emigration in the pulmonary and systemic microcirculation of rabbits. J Immunol 1990; 144:2327–2333.
23. Stothert JC Jr, Basadre JO, Gbaanador GBM, Flynn J, Traber L, Herndon DN, Traber DL. Airway aspiration of hydrochloric acid in sheep. Circ Shock 1990; 30: 237–254.
24. Goldman G, Welbourn R, Klausner JM, Kobzik L, Valeri CR, Shepro D, Hechtman HB. Neutrophil accumulations due to pulmonary thromboxane synthesis mediate acid aspiration injury. J Appl Physiol 1991; 70:1511–1517.
25. Goldman G, Welbourn R, Kobzik L, Valeri CR, Shepro D, Hechtman HB. Reactive oxygen species and elastase mediate lung permeability after acid aspiration. J Appl Physiol 1992; 73:571–575.
26. Knight PR, Druskovich G, Tait AR, Johnson KJ. The role of neutrophils, oxidants, and proteases in the pathogenesis of acid pulmonary injury. Anesthesiology 1992; 77:772–778.
27. Rabinovici R, Neville LF, Abdullah F, Phillip DR, Vernick J, Fong KL, Hillegas L, Feurstein G. Aspiration-induced lung injury: role of complement. Crit Care Med 1995; 23:1405–1411.
28. Folkesson HG, Matthay MA. Inhibition of CD11,18 attenuates acute lung injury in rabbits following HCI instillation without reducing the number of alveolar lavage neutrophils. Am J Respir Crit Care Med 1996; 153:A444. Abstract.
29. Folkesson HG, Matthay MA, Hébert CA, Broaddus VC. Acid aspiration induced lung injury in rabbits is mediated by interleukin-8 dependent mechanisms. J Clin Invest 1995; 96:107–116.
30. Kennedy TP, Johnson KJ, Kunkel RG, Ward PA, Knight PR, Finch JS. Acute acid aspiration lung injury in the rat: biphasic pathogenesis. Anesth Analg 1989; 69:87–92.

31. Goldman G, Welbourn R, Kobzik L, Valeri CR, Shepro D, Hechtman HB. Tumor necrosis factor-α mediates acid aspiration-induced systemic organ injury. Ann Surg 1990; 212:513–520.
32. Goldman G, Welbourn R, Kobzik L, Valeri CR, Shepro D, Hechtman HB. Synergism between leukotriene B_4 and thromboxane A_2 in mediating acid-aspiration injury. Surgery 1992; 111:55–61.
33. St. John RC, Mizer LA, Kindt GC, Weisbrode SE, Moore SA, Dorinsky PM. Acid aspiration-induced acute lung injury causes leukocyte-dependent systemic organ injury. J Appl Physiol 1993; 74:1994–2003.
34. Folkesson HG, Matthay MA. Inhibition of CD18 or CD11b attenuates acute lung injury after acid instillation in rabbits. J Appl Physiol. 1997; 82:1743–1750.
35. Fowler AA III, Hyers TM, Fisher BJ, Bechard DE, Centor RM, Webster RO. The adult respiratory distress syndrome: cell populations and soluble mediators in the air spaces of patients at high risk. Am Rev Respir Dis 1987; 136:1225–1231.
36. Kindt GC, Gadek JE, Weiland JE. Initial recruitment of neutrophils to alveolar structures in acute lung injury. J Appl Physiol 1991; 70:1575–1585.
37. Miller EJ, Cohen AB, Nagao S, Griffith D, Maunder RJ, Martin TR, Wiener-Kronish JP, Sticherling M, Christophers E, Matthay MA. Elevated levels of NAP-1/interleukin-8 are present in the airspaces of patients with the adult respiratory distress syndrome and are associated with increased mortality. Am Rev Respir Dis 1992; 146:427–432.
38. Standiford TJ, Kunkel SL, Basha MA, Chensue SW, Lynch JP, 3rd, Toews GB, Westwick J, Strieter RM. Interleukin-8 gene expression by a pulmonary epithelial cell line. A model for cytokine networks in the lung. J Clin Invest 1990; 86:1945–1953.
39. Nakamura H, Yoshimura K, Jaffe HA, Crystal RG. Interleukin-8 gene expression in human bronchial epithelial cells. J Biol Chem 1991; 266:19611–19617.
40. Rolfe MW, Kunkel SL, Standiford TJ, Chensue SW, Allen RM, Evanoff HL, Phan SH, Strieter RM. Pulmonary fibroblast expression of interleukin-8: a model for alveolar macrophage-derived cytokine networking. Am J Respir Cell Mol Biol 1991; 5:493–501.
41. Colditz IG, Zwahlen RD, Baggiolini M. Neutrophil accumulation and plasma leakage induced in vivo by neutrophil-activating peptide-1. J Leukoc Biol 1990; 48: 129–137.
42. Kunkel SL, Standiford T, Kasahara K, Strieter RM. Interleukin-8 (IL-8): the major neutrophil chemotactic factor in the lung. Exp Lung Res 1991; 17:17–23.
43. Detmers PA, Lo SK, Olsen-Egbert E, Walz A, Baggiolini M, Cohn ZA. Neutrophil-activating protein 1/interleukin 8 stimulates the binding activity of the leukocyte adhesion receptor CD11b/CD18 on human neutrophils. J Exp Med 1990; 171:1155–1162.
44. Huber AR, Kunkel SL, Todd RF III, Weiss SJ. Regulation of transendothelial neutrophil migration by endogenous interleukin-8. (Published errata appear in Science 1991; 254(5032):631 and 254(5037):1435.) Science 1991; 254:99–102.
45. Smith WB, Gamble JR, Clark-Lewis I, Vadas MA. Chemotactic desensitization of neutrophils demonstrates interleukin-8 (IL-8)-dependent and IL-8-independent mechanisms of transmigration through cytokine-activated endothelium. Immunology 1993; 78:491–497.

46. Yuo A, Kitagawa S, Kasahara T, Matsushima K, Saito M, Takaku F. Stimulation and priming of human neutrophils by interleukin-8: cooperation with tumor necrosis factor and colony-stimulating factors. Blood 1991; 78:2708–2714.
47. Wozniak A, Betts WH, Murphy GA, Rokicinski M. Interleukin-8 primes human neutrophils for enhanced superoxide anion production. Immunology 1993; 79: 608–615.
48. Strieter RM, Chensue SW, Basha MA, Standiford TJ, Lynch JP, Baggiolini M, Kunkel SL. Human alveolar macrophage gene expression of interleukin-8 by tumor necrosis factor-α, lipopolysaccharide, and interleukin-1β. Am J Respir Cell Mol Biol 1990; 2:321–326.
49. Boylan AM, Rüegg C, Kim KJ, Hébert CA, Hoeffel JM, Pytela R, Sheppard D, Goldstein IM, Broaddus VC. Evidence of a role for mesothelial cell-derived interleukin 8 in the pathogenesis of asbestos-induced pleurisy in rabbits. J Clin Invest 1992; 89:1257–1267.
50. Chollet-Martin S, Montravers P, Gibert C, Elbim C, Desmonts JM, Fagon JY, Gougerot-Pocidalo MA. High levels of interleukin-8 in the blood and alveolar spaces of patients with pneumonia and adult respiratory distress syndrome. Infect Immun 1993; 61:4553–4559.
51. Donnelly SC, Strieter RM, Kunkel SL, Walz A, Robertson CR, Carter DC, Grant IS, Pollok AJ, Haslett C. Interleukin-8 and development of adult respiratory distress syndrome in at-risk patient groups. Lancet 1993; 341:643–647.
52. Mulligan MS, Jones ML, Bolanowski MA, Baganoff MP, Deppeler CL, Meyers DM, Ryan US, Ward PA. Inhibition of lung inflammatory reactions in rats by an anti-human IL-8 antibody. J Immunol 1993; 150:5585–5595.
53. Sekido N, Mukaida N, Harada A, Nakanishi I, Watanabe Y, Matsushima K. Prevention of lung reperfusion injury in rabbits by a monoclonal antibody against interleukin-8. Nature 1993; 365:654–657.
54. Broaddus VC, Boylan AM, Hoeffel JM, Kim KJ, Sadick M, Chuntharapai A, Hébert CA. Neutralization of interleukin-8 inhibits neutrophil influx in a rabbit model of endotoxin-induced pleurisy. J Immunol 1994; 152:2960–2967.
55. Larsen CG, Anderson AO, Appella E, Oppenheim JJ, Matsushima K. The neutrophil-activating protein (NAP-1) is also chemotactic for T lymphocytes. Science 1989; 243:1464–1466.
56. Erger RA, Casale TB. Interleukin-8 is a potent mediator of eosinophil chemotaxis through endothelium and epithelium. Am J Physiol 1995; 268:L117–:L122.
57. Hébert CA, Luscinskas FW, Kiely J-M, Luis EA, Darbonne WC, Bennett GL, Liu CC, Obin MS, Gimbrone MA, Jr, Baker JB. Endothelial and leukocyte forms of IL-8: conversion by thrombin and interactions with neutrophils. J Immunol 1990; 145:3033–3040.
58. Harada A, Sekido N, Kuno K, Akiyama M, Kasahara T, Nakanishi I, Mukaida N, Matsushima K. Expression of recombinant rabbit IL-8 in *Escherichia coli* and establishment of the essential involvement of IL-8 in recruiting neutrophils into lipopolysaccharide-induced inflammatory site of rabbit skin. Int Immunol 1993; 5:681–690.
59. Cacalano G, Lee J, Kikly K, Ryan AM, Pitts-Meek S, Hultgren B, Wood WI, Moore MW. Neutrophil and B cell expansion in mice that lack the murine IL-8 receptor homolog. Science 1994; 265:682–684.

60. Beutler B, Milsank IW, Cerami AC. Passive immunization against cachectin/tumor necrosis factor protects mice from lethal effect of endotoxin. Science 1985; 229: 869–871.
61. Tracey KJ, Fong Y, Hesse DG. Anti-cachetin/TNF monoclonal antibodies prevent septic shock during lethal bacteraemia. Nature 1987; 330:662–664.
62. Tonnesen MG, Anderson DC, Springer TA, Knedler A, Avdi N, Henson PM. Adherence of neutrophils to cultured human microvascular endothelial cells. Stimulation by chemotactic peptides and lipid mediators and dependence upon the MAC-1, LFA-1, p150,95 glycoprotein family. J Clin Invest 1989; 83:637–646.
63. Rothlein R, Czajkowski M, O'Neill MM, Marlin SD, Mainolfi E, Merluzzi VJ. Induction of intercellular adhesion molecule-1 on primary and continuous cell lines by pro-inflammatory cytokines. Regulation by pharmacologic agents and neutralized antibodies. J Immunol 1988; 141:1665–1669.
64. Cobbold S, Hale G, Waldmann H. Non-lineage, LFA-1 family, and leukocyte common antigens: new and previously defined clusters. In: McMichael AJ, ed. Leukocyte Typing III. White Blood Cell Differentiation Antigens. Oxford, U.K.: Oxford University Press, 1987:788–803.
65. Harlan JM, Killen PO, Senecal FM, Schwartz BP, Yee EK, Taylor RF, Beatty PG, Price TH, Ochs HD. The role of neutrophil membrane glycoprotein GP-150 in neutrophil adherence to endothelium in vitro. Blood 1985; 66:167–178.
66. Harlan JM. Leukocyte adhesion deficiency syndrome: insights into the molecular basis of leukocyte emigration. Clin Immunol Immunopathol 1993; 67:S16–S24.
67. von Andrian UH, Berger EM, Ramezani L, Chambers JD, Ochs HD, Harlan JM, Paulson JC, Etzioni A, Arfors K-E. In vivo behavior of neutrophils from two patients with distinct inherited leukocyte adhesion deficiency syndromes. J Clin Invest 1993; 91:2893–2897.
68. Goldman G, Welbourn R, Kobzik L, Valeri CR, Shepro D, Hechtman HB. Neutrophil adhesion receptor CD18 mediates remote but not localized acid aspiration injury. Surgery 1995; 117:83–89.
69. Jaeschke H, Farhood A, Smith CW. Neutrophil-induced liver cell injury in endotoxin shock is a CD11b/CD18-dependent mechanism. Am J Physiol 1991; 261: G1051–G1056.
70. Gallatin WM, Weissman IL, Butcher EC. A cell-surface molecule involved in organ-specific homing of lymphocytes. Nature (Lond) 1983; 304:30–34.
71. Lewinsohn DM, Bargatze RF, Butcher EC. Leukocyte-endothelial cell recognition: evidence of a common molecular mechanism shared by neutrophils, lymphocytes, and other leukocytes. J Immunol 1987; 138:4313–4321.
72. Hsu-Lin SC, Berman CL, Furie BC, August D, Furie B. A platelet membrane protein expressed during platelet activation and secretion. Studies using a monoclonal antibody specific for thrombin-activated platelets. J Biol Chem 1984; 259:9121–9126.
73. Stenberg PE, McEver RP, Shuman MA, Jacques YV, Bainton DF. A platelet alpha-granule membrane protein (GMP-140) is expressed on the plasma membrane after activation. J Cell Biol 1985; 101:880–886.
74. Bonfanti R, Furie BC, Furie B, Wagner DD. PADGEM (GMP140) is a component of Weibel-Palade bodies of human endothelial cells. Blood 1989; 73:1109–1112.

75. McEver RP, Beckstead JH, Moore KL, Marshall-Carlson L, Bainton DF. GMP-140, a platelet alpha-granule membrane protein, is also synthesized by vascular endothelial cells and is localized in Weibel-Palade bodies. J Clin Invest 1989; 84:92–99.
76. Bevilacqua MP, Pober JS, Wheeler ME, Cotran RS, Gimbrone MA Jr. Interleukin 1 acts on cultured human vascular endothelium to increase the adhesion of polymorphonuclear leukocytes, monocytes, and related leukocyte cell lines. J Clin Invest 1985; 76:2003–2011.
77. Cotran RS, Gimbrone M Jr, Bevilacqua MP, Mendrick DL, Pober JS. Induction and detection of a human endothelial activation antigen in vivo. J Exp Med 1986; 164:661–666.
78. Pober JS, Bevilacqua MP, Mendrick DL, Lapierre LA, Fiers W, Gimbrone MA. Two distinct monokines, interleukin 1 and tumor necrosis factor, each independently induce biosynthesis and transient expression of the same antigen on the surface of cultured human vascular endothelial cells. J Immunol 1986; 136:1680–1687.
79. Bevilacqua MP, Pober JS, Mendrick DL, Cotran RS, Gimbrone MA Jr. Identification of an inducible endothelial-leukocyte adhesion molecule. Proc Natl Acad Sci USA 1987; 84:9238–9242.
80. Mulligan MS, Polley MJ, Bayer RJ, Nunn MF, Paulson JC, Ward PA. Neutrophil-dependent acute lung injury. Requirement for P-selectin (GMP-140). J Clin Invest 1992; 90:1600–1607.
81. Newman W, Beall LD, Carson CW, Hunder GG, Graben N, Randhawa ZI, Gopal TV, Wiener-Kronish J, Matthay MA. Soluble E-selectin is found in supernatants of activated endothelial cells and is elevated in the serum of patients with septic shock. J Immunol 1993; 150:644–654.
82. Carey PD, Jenkins JK, Byrne K, Schneider AM, Walsh CJ, Fowler AA III, Sugerman HJ. Neutrophil short-lived oxidant production: enhancement following onset of sepsis-induced lung injury. Circ Shock 1992; 36:256–264.
83. Martin TR, Pistorese BP, Chi EY, Goodman RB, Matthay MA. Effects of leukotriene B_4 in the human lung. Recruitment of neutrophils into the alveolar spaces without a change in protein permeability. J Clin Invest 1989; 84:1609–1619.
84. Shatney CH, Benner C. Sequential serum complement (C3) and immunoglobulin levels in shock/trauma patients developing acute fulminant systemic sepsis. Circ Shock 1985; 16:9–17.
85. Antrum RM, Solomkin JS. Monocyte dysfunction in severe trauma: evidence for the role of C5a in deactivation. Surgery 1986; 100:29–37.
86. Stevens JH, O'Hanley P, Shapiro JM, Mihm FG, Satoh PS, Collins JA, Raffin TA. Effects of anti-C5a antibodies on the adult respiratory distress syndrome in septic primates. J Clin Invest 1986; 77:1812–1816.
87. Parsons PE, Giclas PC. The terminal complement complex (sC5b-9) is not specifically associated with the development of the adult respiratory distress syndrome. Am Rev Respir Dis 1990; 141:98–103.
88. Weisman HF, Bartow T, Leppo MK, Marsh HC, Jr, Carson GR, Concino MF, Boyle MP, Roux KH, Weisfeldt ML, Fearon DT. Soluble human complement receptor

type 1: in vivo inhibitor of complement suppressing post-ischemic myocardial inflammation and necrosis. Science 1990; 249:146–151.
89. Mulligan MS, Yeh CG, Rudolph AR, Ward PA. Protective effects of soluble CR1 in complement- and neutrophil-mediated tissue injury. J Immunol 1992; 148: 1479–1485.
90. Rabinovici R, Sofronski MD, Borboroglu P, Spirig AM, Hillegas LM, Levine J, Vernick J, Scesney SM, Feuerstein N, Feuerstein G. Interleukin-2-induced lung injury. The role of complement. Circ Res 1994; 74:329–335.
91. Rabinovici R, Yeh CG, Hillegass LM, Griswold DE, DiMartino MJ, Vernick J, Fong KL, Feuerstein G. Role of complement in endotoxin/platelet-activating factor-induced lung injury. J Immunol 1992; 149:1744–1750.
92. Hsueh W, Sun X, Rioja LN, Gonzalez-Crussi F. The role of the complement system in shock and tissue injury induced by tumour necrosis factor and endotoxin. Immunology 1990; 70:309–314.
93. Gallinaro R, Cheadle WG, Applegate K, Polk HC Jr. The role of the complement system in trauma and infection. Surg Gynecol Obstet 1992; 174: 435–440.
94. Toung TJ, Bordos D, Benson DW, Carter D, Zuidema GD, Permutt S, Cameron JL. Aspiration pneumonia: experimental evaluation of albumin and steroid therapy. Ann Surg 1976; 183:179–184.
95. Glauser FL, Millen JE, Falls R. Increased alveolar epithelial permeability with acid aspiration: the effects of high-dose steroids. Am Rev Respir Dis 1979; 120: 1119–1123.
96. Glauser FL, Millen JE, Falls R. Effects of acid aspiration on pulmonary alveolar epithelial membrane permeability. Chest 1979; 76:201–205.
97. Wynne JW, DeMarco FJ, Hood CI. Physiological effects of corticosteroids in foodstuff aspiration. Arch Surg 1981; 116:46–49.
98. Toung T, Cameron JL. Inefficiency of antacid in prevention of aspiration pneumonia. Br J Anaesth 1980; 52:241–242. Letter.
99. Toung T, Cameron JL. Cimetadine as a preoperative medication to reduce the complications of aspiration of gastric contents. Surgery 1980; 87:205–208.
100. Coombs DW, Hooper DW. Cimetidine as a prophylactic against acid aspiration at tracheal extubation. Can Anaesth Soc J 1981; 28:33–38.
101. Broe PJ, Toung TJ, Permutt S, Cameron JL. Aspiration pneumonia: treatment with pulmonary vasodilators. Surgery 1983; 94:95–99.
102. Sznajder JI, Zucker AR, Wood LDH, Long GR. The effects of plasmapheresis and hemofiltration on canine acid aspiration pulmonary edema. Am Rev Respir Dis 1986; 134:222–228.
103. Mizus I, Summer W, Farrukh I, Michael JR, Gurtner GH. Isoproterenol or aminophylline attenuate pulmonary edema after acid lung injury. Am Rev Respir Dis 1985; 131:256–259.
104. Taylor AE. Pulmonary edema: ischemia reperfusion endothelial injury and its reversal by cAMP. Proc Natl Sci Counc Repub China 1991; 15:191–195.
105. Kudoh I, Ohtake M, Nishizawa H, Kurahashi K, Hattori S, Okumura F, Pittet J-F, Wiener-Kronish JP. The effect of pentoxifylline on acid-induced alveolar epithelial injury. Anesthesiology 1995; 82:531–541.

106. Bessler H, Gilgal R, Djaldetti M, Zahavi I. Effect of pentoxifylline on the phagocytic activity, cAMP levels, and superoxide anion production by monocytes and polymorphonuclear cells. J Leukoc Biol 1986; 40:747–754.
107. Currie MS, Rao KMK, Padmanabhan J, Jones A, Crawford J, Cohen HJ. Stimulus-specific effects of pentoxifylline on neutrophil CR3 expression, degranulation, and superoxide production. J Leukoc Biol 1990; 47:244–250.
108. Thiel M, Bardenheuer H, Poch G, Madel C, Peter K. Pentoxifylline does not act via adenosine receptors in the inhibition of the superoxide anion production of human polymorphonuclear leukocytes. Biochem Biophys Res Commun 1991; 180: 53–58.
109. Crouch SPM, Fletcher J. Effect of ingested pentoxifylline on neutrophil superoxide anion production. Infect Immun 1992; 60:4504–4509.
110. Karch SB. Pathology of the lung in near-drowning. Am J Emerg Med 1986; 4:4–9.
111. Modell JH, Graves SA, Ketover A. Clinical course of 91 consecutive near-drowning victims. Chest 1976; 70:231–238.
112. Fine NL, Meyerson DA, Myerson PJ, Pagliaro JJ. Near-drowning presenting as the adult respiratory distress syndrome. Chest 1974; 65:347–349.
113. Swann HG, Spafford NR. Body salt and water changes during fresh and sea water drowning. Texas Rep Biol Med 1951; 9:356–382.
114. Halmagyi DFJ, Colebatch HJH. The drowned lung. A physiological approach to its mechanism and management. Aust Ann Med 1961; 10:68–77.
115. Modell JH, Moya F, Newby EJ, Ruiz BC, Showers AV. The effects of fluid volume in seawater drowning. Ann Intern Med 1967; 67:68–80.
116. Nopanitaya W, Gambill TG, Brinkhous KM. Fresh water drowning. Pulmonary ultrastructure and systemic fibrinolysis. Arch Pathol 1974; 98:361–366.
117. Yagil Y, Stalnikowicz R, Michaeli, J, Mogle P. Near drowning in the Dead Sea. Electrolyte imbalances and therapeutic implications. Arch Intern Med 1985; 145:50–53.
118. Orlowski JP, Abulleil MM, Phillips JM. Effects of tonicities of saline solutions on pulmonary injury in drowning. Crit Care Med 1987; 15:126–130.
119. Cohen DS, Matthay MA, Cogan MG, Murray JF. Pulmonary edema associated with salt water near-drowning: new insights. Am Rev Respir Dis 1992; 146: 794–796.
120. Olshaker JS. Near drowning. Emerg Med Clin North Am 1992; 10:339–350.
121. Folkesson HG, Kheradmand F, Matthay MA. The effect of salt water on alveolar epithelial barrier function. Am J Respir Crit Care Med 1994; 150:1555–1563.
122. Pearn J. Pathophysiology of drowning. Med J Aust 1985; 142:586–588.
123. Sarnaik AP, Vohra MP. Near-drowning: fresh, salt, and cold water immersion. Clin Sports Med 1986; 5:33–46.
124. Kylstra JA. Drowning: the role of salts in the drowning fluid. A preliminary report on observations in mice. Acta Physiol Pharmacol Neerland 1962; 10:327–334.
125. Halmagyi DFJ, Colebatch HJH. Ventilation and circulation after fluid aspiration. J Appl Physiol 1961; 16:35–40.
126. Modell JH, Moya F, Williams HD, Weibley TC. Changes in blood gases and A-aDO_2 during near-drowning. Anesthesiology 1968; 29:456–465.

127. Bergquist RE, Vogelhut MM, Modell JH, Sloan SJ, Ruiz BC. Comparison of ventilatory patterns in the treatment of freshwater near-drowning in dogs. Anesthesiology 1980; 52:142–148.
128. Greenberg MI, Baskin SI, Kaplan AM, Urrichio FJ. Effects of endotracheally administered distilled water and normal saline on the arterial blood gases of dogs. Ann Emerg Med 1982; 11:600–604.
129. Orlowski JP, Abulleil MM, Phillips JM. The hemodynamic and cardiovascular effects of near-drowning in hypotonic, isotonic, or hypertonic solutions. Ann Emerg Med 1989; 18:1044–1049.
130. Paganelli CV, Solomon AK. The rate of exchange of tritiated water across the human red cell membrane. J Gen Physiol 1957; 41:259–277.
131. Sidel VW, Solomon EK. Entrance of water into human red cells under an osmotic pressure gradient. J Gen Physiol 1957; 41:243–257.
132. Effros RM. Osmotic extraction of hypotonic fluid from the lungs. J Clin Invest 1974; 5:935–947.
133. Effros RM, Mason GR, Sietsema K, Hukkanen J, Silverman P. Pulmonary epithelial sieving of small solutes in rat lungs. J Appl Physiol 1988; 65:640–648.
134. Agre P, Preston GM, Smith BL, Jung JS, Raina S, Moon C, Guggino WB, Nielsen S. Aquaporin CHIP: the archetypal molecular water channel. Am J Physiol 1993; 265:F463–F476.
135. Folkesson HG, Matthay MA, Hasegawa H, Kheradmand F, Verkman AS. Transcellular water transport in lung alveolar epithelium through mercury-sensitive water channels. Proc Natl Acad Sci USA 1994; 91:4970–4974.
136. Effros RM, Darin C, Jacobs ER, Rogers RA, Krenz G, and Schneeberger EE. Water transport and the distribution of aquaporin-1 in pulmonary air spaces. J Appl Physiol 1997; 83:1002–1016.
137. Borok Z, Lubman R, Danto SI, Zhang-X-L, Zabski S, King L, Lee DM, Agre P, Crandall ED. Keratinocyte growth factor modulates alveolar epithelial cell phenotype in vitro: expression of aquaporin 5. Am J Resp Cell Mol Biol 1998. In press.
138. Matthay MA, Rosen GD. Acid aspiration-induced lung injury: new insights and therapeutic options. Am J Resp Crit Care Med 1996; 154:277–278.

9

Increased-Permeability Edema Following Hemorrhagic and Traumatic Shock

KATHARINA MODELSKA and JEAN-FRANÇOIS PITTET

University of California at San Francisco
San Francisco, California

I. Introduction

Trauma and hemorrhagic shock are among the major causes of acute lung injury in humans. For example, a recently published clinical study reported that 25% of patients with severe trauma develop acute lung injury, and that trauma was the second most common cause of acute lung injury after sepsis (1). In the same study, the risk for developing acute lung injury was even higher after multiple transfusions for emergency resuscitation (40%). Despite major advances in supportive treatment for critically ill patients, mortality among patients with acute lung injury remains high (1). However, a significant decrease in fatality rates has been reported in one study in patients less than 60 years old and in those with sepsis syndrome, although this trend was less evident for patients with trauma (2), and not all studies have found this reduction in mortality (3).

Although trauma and hemorrhagic shock are among the major causes of acute lung injury in humans, it has been difficult to separate clinically the possible contribution of lung contusion, aspiration, fat embolization, hypoxia, hypotension, and volume resuscitation in producing acute lung damage in these patients. Therefore, several laboratory studies have been undertaken to focus on one of these individual insults to evaluate their potential for causing the development of acute lung injury. For example, there is good experimental evidence that hemorrhagic shock and fluid resuscitation can cause lung endothelial injury in animals (4–8). In contrast, although it is well established that increased permeability to protein is a hallmark of clinical acute lung injury (9–11), the critical importance of the alveolar epithelial barrier in the pathogenesis and recovery from acute lung injury after hemorrhagic shock has only recently been appreciated.

Thus, the purpose of this chapter is to discuss the mechanisms by which hemorrhagic shock causes the development of increased permeability pulmonary edema and clinically significant acute lung injury. The first objective is to review recent experimental studies on the effect of hemorrhagic shock and fluid resuscitation on the barrier function of both the lung endothelium and the alveolar epithelium. The second objective is to consider clinical characteristics and risk factors that have been associated with the development of acute lung injury in severely traumatized patients.

II. Experimental Studies

A. Hemorrhagic Shock and Lung Endothelial Injury

Hemorrhagic shock may be considered as a whole-body ischemia/reperfusion syndrome. Hemorrhagic shock increases the vascular endothelial permeability to fluid and protein in the systemic and pulmonary circulations by mechanisms that are partially understood (12). In the systemic circulation, the reduction of the rate of metabolism during the ischemic phase results in a decline in the generation of high-energy compounds associated with altered ion homeostasis and calcium influx into the cells, and may be responsible for some mitochondrial and membrane dysfunction of the endothelial cells (13). However, there is a large body of evidence indicating that the increase in vascular endothelial permeability in ischemia/reperfusion syndrome is mainly caused by the release of oxygen radicals produced by the xanthine oxidase pathway on reintroduction of oxygen during reperfusion, in association with the production of lipid mediators as platelet-activating factor, leukotriene B4, and polypeptide mediators (e.g., C5a) (14) (see Chap. 12). Oxygen radicals and platelet activating factor originate to a large extent from the endothelial cells. These mediators of inflammation cause endothelial cell dysfunction that results in a marked decrease in the release of nitric oxide (NO) and prostacyclin by endothelial cells (15). The decrease in the NO production along with the release of other chemotactic factors promotes neutrophil recruitment to the perfusion site and adherence to and diapedesis of these cells through the dysfunctional endothelium (16). Neutrophils adhering to the vascular endothelium then release pro-inflammatory mediators (cytokines, oxygen radicals, elastase) that amplify the endothelial injury. Therefore, the critical event in the early phase of reperfusion injury in the systemic circulation appears to be the endothelial dysfunction caused by the release of non-neutrophil-derived oxygen radicals that lead later to the activation of neutrophils. Also, it should be pointed out that not only regional ischemia/reperfusion, but whole-body ischemia/reperfusion results in a marked degree of endothelial dysfunction (17). Preliminary results suggest that oxygen radicals also play a major role since the pretreatment with superoxide dismutase can significantly attenuate the endothelial dysfunction associated with whole-body ischemia/reperfusion (18).

The importance of the lack of NO production in the pathogenesis of the endothelial injury after ischemia/reperfusion in the systemic circulation has been demonstrated by studies reporting that replacement of NO during the reperfusion phase of regional ischemia/reperfusion preserves the endothelium of the ischemic vasculature (19) and protects the underlying parenchymal tissue from reperfusion injury (20). Comparable results have been obtained with NO donors in experimental hemorrhagic shock, a whole-body ischemia/reperfusion syndrome (21). Also, Ma et al. (22) have reported that the diminution in the NO production observed in postischemic venules correlated closely with increased leukocyte adhesion, suggesting that diminished basal release of NO during reperfusion was a key reason for the increased neutrophil adhesion. In addition, inhibition of NO synthesis has been shown to increase microvascular permeability and edema formation in the nonischemic systemic circulation by early neutrophil-independent and late neutrophil-dependent mechanisms (23). The mechanisms by which NO donors exert their neutrophil antiadhesive properties are not known, although a recently published work suggests that this effect might be related to their ability to inactivate oxygen radical production (24).

Ischemia/reperfusion injury also occurs in the lung where increased endothelial permeability (25–27) leads to pulmonary edema (28,29). In contrast to the systemic circulation, pulmonary ischemia is not always synonymous with hypoxia if normoxic or hyperoxic ventilation is maintained. In fact, in some studies, hypoxemia during lung ischemia reduces lung injury (30), since oxygen radical generation in the lung seems to directly correlate with oxygen tension (31). These results have raised the possibility that ischemia/reperfusion-mediated endothelial injury in the ventilated lung might already occur during ischemia (32). However, there is a striking discrepancy in models of lung reperfusion injury between the relative resistance to ischemic injury of in vivo models versus the relative sensitivity of the lung ex vivo to ischemia. Data obtained from isolated perfused lung models support the existence of an oxygen radical-mediated lung vascular injury which begins during the ischemic phase (32–35) and might be continued or amplified after reperfusion (34,35). In contrast, data obtained from in vivo experimental models indicate that the pulmonary ischemia/reperfusion-mediated endothelial injury is mainly detected after reperfusion (27,36,37) (see Chap. 12).

Our own experimental data confirm this latter observation. There was a significant increase in the extravascular lung water content of rats that underwent hemorrhagic shock and fluid resuscitation with a 4% albumin solution or shed autologous blood compared with controls, a result consistent with lung endothelial injury and interstitial pulmonary edema (38). In contrast, in another group of rats that underwent hemorrhagic shock but were not resuscitated, the extravascular lung water content was not increased compared with controls (39).

The explanation for the difference observed between the data from isolated perfused lungs and in vivo experimental models is probably multifactorial. First, it has been suggested that the maintenance of the bronchial circulation and the presence of a reverse pulmonary venous blood flow may offer some protection to the lung endothelium (40,41), although this concept has been challenged (27,42,43). Second, since the pulmonary blood flow is never completely interrupted in hemorrhagic shock, the endogenous release of catecholamines accompanying the development of systemic hypotension might attenuate the oxidant-mediated lung endothelial injury during the ischemic phase of the ischemia/reperfusion syndrome by increasing the intracellular content of cAMP of the lung endothelium. It has previously been reported that the exogenous administration of drugs able to increase intracellular cAMP attenuate the increase in the microvascular permeability associated with lung ischemia/reperfusion (44–46), perhaps by inhibiting endothelial gap formation (47). Third, in vivo measurements of lung endothelial injury depend on both surface area and vascular permeability. If the pulmonary blood flow is abnormally low, the endothelial injury might not be detected until reperfusion, although it might already have developed during the ischemic phase of this syndrome. Finally, in addition to the alterations of lung endothelial permeability, the reperfusion phase of the lung ischemia/reperfusion syndrome is also characterized by an increase in pulmonary vascular resistance (26,29) caused in part by the release of thromboxane A_2, a vasoconstrictor that probably contributes to the development of pulmonary edema observed in this pathological condition by increasing lung microvascular hydrostatic pressure (48,49).

Although less well studied, the mechanisms of lung endothelial injury caused by the ischemia/reperfusion syndrome might be similar to those described for the systemic circulation. For example, in hemorrhagic shock, it has been shown that large numbers of neutrophils aggregate in pulmonary capillaries (50,51), and these cells appear to contribute to the lung endothelial injury (52). Inhibition of neutrophil adhesion to the vascular endothelium by a monoclonal antibody directed against the common beta-subunit of the leukocyte adhesion glycoprotein complex CD11/CD18 significantly attenuated the pulmonary endothelial damage associated with ischemia/reperfusion (25). As for the systemic circulation, initiation of the endothelial injury in the pulmonary circulation appears to be neutrophil-independent, although the activation of neutrophils causes an amplification of the injury (53). In fact, sequestration of neutrophils in the pulmonary microcirculation during hemorrhagic shock also appears to depend on a xanthine oxidase-related mechanism (54) and/or on the activation of cytochrome P-450 enzymes (55).

Since the injury to the lung endothelium in the ischemia-reperfusion syndrome is dependent on a nonneutrophil source of toxic oxygen metabolites, it is reasonable to hypothesize that, as for the systemic circulation, the lack of NO production by dysfunctional endothelial cells may also play a key role in the pathogenesis of the lung endothelial injury caused by the development of acute hemorrhagic shock. The results of a recently published study indicate that the manipulation of NO plasma levels in vivo alters ischemia/reperfusion lung injury (56). Elevation of plasma NO levels with sodium nitroprusside diminishes neutrophil sequestration and the associated increase in pulmonary endothelial permeability, whereas inhibition of NO synthesis with NG-nitro-L-arginine methyl ester (L-NAME) enhances neutrophil infiltration and lung injury. However, despite these preliminary results, the role of NO donors in protecting the lung vascular endothelium from the injurious effect of oxygen toxic metabolites released during the reperfusion phase of the hemorrhagic shock is largely unknown and needs to be further studied.

B. Hemorrhagic Shock and Alveolar Epithelial Injury

Although considerable progress has been made in understanding the basic transport mechanisms across the alveolar epithelium in the normal lung, the effects of severe hemorrhagic or traumatic shock on the barrier properties of the alveolar epithelium are still not completely clear. In particular, the critical importance of the alveolar epithelial barrier in the pathogenesis and recovery from acute lung injury secondary to hemorrhagic shock has not been well appreciated. Recently, two major properties of the alveolar epithelial barrier have been assessed clinically and experimentally. First, the quantity of protein that accumulates in the distal airspaces appears to be a good index of epithelial permeability, because this barrier is mostly impermeable to protein under physiological conditions. Second, changes in the protein concentration in sequential alveolar fluid samples represent a physiological index of the ability of the alveolar epithelium to remove edema fluid, because concentration of protein in alveolar fluid reflects net alveolar fluid clearance (57,58). Using these two indicators of the alveolar epithelial function, we have conducted several experimental studies on the effect of hemorrhagic shock and fluid resuscitation on the alveolar epithelial barrier function that will be discussed in the next sections.

Hemorrhagic Shock and Aveolar Epithelial Permeability to Protein

Earlier experimental studies have indicated that the alveolar epithelium is more resistant to injury than the nearby vascular endothelium. For example, the short-term intravenous administration of high doses of live *P. aeruginosa* caused a moderate increase in lung endothelial permeability but did not increase the permeability of the alveolar epithelium to protein in anesthetized rats (59). However, there was evidence of injury to the alveolar epithelium after prolonged administration of live *P. aeruginosa* in sheep that had the most severe systemic injury secondary to septic shock (60).

To study this important issue further, we have developed an experimental animal model to determine the differential effects of ischemic and reperfusion phases of hemorrhagic shock on the barrier function of the alveolar epithelium. The results of these studies indicate that during the ischemic phase of hemorrhagic shock, the alveolar epithelial barrier maintained its relative impermeability to protein despite the presence of a severe systemic hypotension and metabolic acidosis (39). Similar results were obtained during the ischemic phase of septic shock (59). Interestingly, these results are also comparable with those obtained during the ischemia/reperfusion injury in the systemic circulation. For example, during the 30-min ischemic period of perfused segments of rat jejunum, the ^{51}Cr-EDTA clearance did not change significantly from controls (61). However, within 10 min after reperfusion of these perfused segments of rat jejunum, there was a significant increase in the ^{51}Cr-EDTA clearance across the intestinal epithelium (61).

In contrast, after short-term (15 min) but severe hemorrhagic shock followed by fluid resuscitation, there was a significant unidirectional increase in the alveolar epithelial protein permeability from the lung interstitium into the alveolar space (38). This increase in the alveolar epithelial permeability to protein was associated with injury to alveolar epithelial type I cells. In fact, the bronchoalveolar lavage (BAL) fluid content of rTI40, a specific and sensitive biochemical marker of alveolar epithelial type I cell injury (62), was increased in hemorrhaged rats that were fluid resuscitated, but not in those rats that were not (Table 1) (63).

These results suggest that there is injury to alveolar epithelial type I cells during the early reperfusion phase, but not during the ischemic phase of hemorrhagic shock. However, in an earlier study, Gorin et al. (8) did not find any change in alveolar epithelial permeability to protein 24 hours after hemorrhagic shock and fluid resuscitation in sheep despite a significant increase in lung endothelial permeability to fluid and protein. The discrepancy between the results of these studies might be explained either by a difference in the sensitivity of the methods used to detect injury to the alveolar epithelium, or by the ability of this barrier to recover within a few hours from the shock-dependent injury.

Table 1 Protein and rTI40 Concentration in Bronchoalveolar Lavage (BAL) in Controls, Hemorrhaged, and Hemorrhaged and Fluid-Resuscitated Rats

Experimental condition	n	Protein (μg/mL BAL)	rTI40 (RDU/mL BAL)
Controls	3	0.15 ± 0.07	2.93 ± 0.86
Hemorrhagic shock and fluid resuscitation	4	1.20 ± 0.04*	25.00 ± 18.80*
Hemorrhagic shock without fluid resuscitation	4	0.07 ± 0.03	4.40 ± 2.43

Data as mean ± SD.
*$P < .05$ vs. controls.

However, more studies will be necessary to examine the mechanisms responsible for the increase in the epithelial permeability to protein after hemorrhagic shock and for the restoration of the integrity of the alveolar epithelial barrier after shock-mediated injury. Also, additional studies should be done to determine how shock-mediated changes in the lung endothelial permeability may affect the barrier function of the alveolar epithelium.

Fluid Transport Across Alveolar Epithelium

Recent experimental studies have provided insights into the function of the alveolar epithelial barrier under pathologic conditions such as septic shock, acid aspiration, saltwater aspiration, and hyperoxia (59,64–69) (see Chap. 14). These studies have shown that even when mild to moderate alveolar epithelial injury occurs, the capacity of alveolar epithelium to transport salt and water is often preserved (70,71). However, whether the ability of the alveolar epithelial barrier to remove fluid from the airspaces after hemorrhagic and traumatic shock is preserved, was still unknown. Therefore, we studied the differential effect of the ischemic and reperfusion phases of hemorrhagic shock on the fluid transport across the alveolar epithelium.

The results of these studies indicated that during the ischemic phase of hemorrhagic shock, the capacity of the alveolar epithelium to remove fluid transport from the airspaces was maintained (39). In fact, there was an upregulation of the sodium-dependent transport mechanism secondary to the shock-mediated release of endogenous catecholamines, since fluid transport mechanism was blocked by the addition of amiloride or propranolol to the protein solution instilled into the distal airspaces of the lung (39). These data were comparable with those obtained during the ischemic phase of septic shock (59). Therefore, the results of both studies suggest the presence of a new, previously unrecognized mechanism that may protect against alveolar flooding in the acute phase of hemorrhagic or septic shock.

A second series of experiments was conducted to determine whether this protective transport mechanism was still present 6 hours after fluid resuscitation following a brief but severe hemorrhagic shock in rats. The results of these studies indicated that the capacity of the alveolar epithelium to remove fluid from the alveolar space was also preserved despite a significant increase in the permeability to protein across this barrier (38), a finding also observed after exposure to sublethal hyperoxia (63). In fact, there was an upregulation of the fluid transport across pulmonary epithelium comparable with that found during the ischemic phase of hemorrhagic shock. This effect was sodium-dependent and catecholamine-mediated because it was reduced by administration of amiloride, a sodium transport inhibitor, propranolol, a β-adrenergic antagonist into the airspaces, or bilateral adrenelectomy prior to the hemorrhagic shock (Fig. 1).

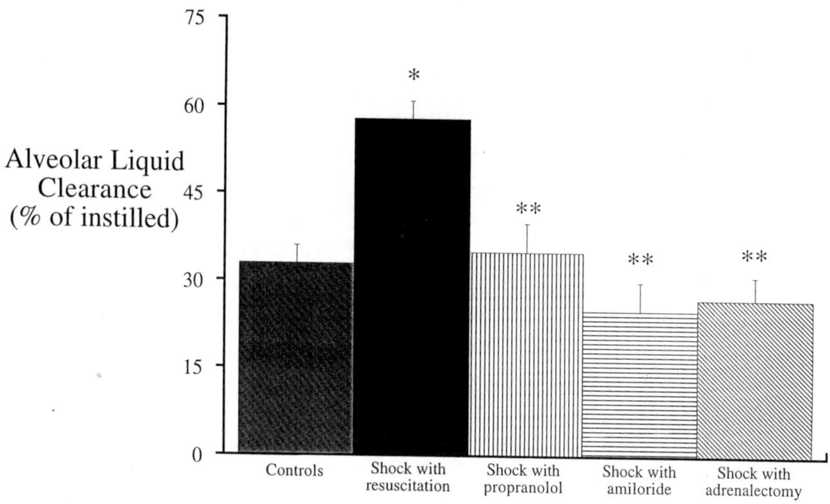

Figure 1 Alveolar liquid clearance (% of instilled liquid) (mean ± SE) is shown for control and hemorrhaged rats, as well as hemorrhaged rats instilled with and propranolol (10^{-4} M) or amiloride (10^{-4} M) and for adrenelectemized and hemorrhaged rats. Short hemorrhagic shock (15 min) and fluid resuscitation were associated with a significant increase in the alveolar liquid clearance compared with controls. This effect was prevented by the addition to the instilled solution of propranolol, a β-adrenergic antagonist or amiloride, a sodium transport inhibitor, and also by bilateral adrenelectomy prior to hemorrhagic shock and fluid resuscitation. $*P < .05$ from control rats; $**P < .05$ from hemorrhaged and resuscitated rats.

Upregulation of alveolar epithelial fluid transport has previously been reported in different pathological conditions, such as the ischemic phase of septic (59) and hemorrhagic shock (39), and after exposure to hyperoxia (68,69,72). However, these results are the first to demonstrate that this mechanism that protects against alveolar flooding in the acute phase following hemorrhagic shock is also present several hours after fluid resuscitation. The upregulation of alveolar liquid clearance after hemorrhagic shock and fluid resuscitation was associated with a significant increase in the endogenous release of epinephrine during the ischemic and resuscitative phases of hemorrhagic shock. Compared with baseline values, there was a 70-fold increase in the mean plasma epinephrine levels measured at the end of the ischemic phase of hemorrhagic shock, and a 20-fold increase in the mean plasma epinephrine levels measured 6 hours later, at the end of the study (Table 2). These data are comparable with those reported for severely injured patients in whom plasma levels of epinephrine remained significantly increased for at least 6 hours after trauma (73). Interestingly, this prolonged exposure to high levels of epinephrine did not appear to downregulate the response to β-adrenergic stimulation in the lung.

However, these results cannot completely exclude that hormones other than catecholamines, such as glucocorticoids, might be involved in the shock-induced stimulation of fluid transport across the alveolar epithelium. Glucocorticoids have an important role in the lung fluid balance of the mature fetus, although their effect on alveolar epithelial sodium transport in the adult lung is unclear. For example, cortisol, in association with tri-idothyrorine, increases lung liquid clearance in thyroidectomized fetal sheep (74), and accelerates expression of sodium channels in fetal rats (75). In addition, maternal corticosteroids

Table 2 Effect of Short-Term and Prolonged Hemorrhagic Shock and Fluid Resuscitation on Plasma Epinephrine Levels (pg/mL)

		Plasma levels of epinephrine (pg/mL)		
Experimental condition	n	Baseline	Ischemic phase of hemorrhagic shock	6 hours after hemorrhagic shock
Controls—no shock	10	< 100	< 100	< 100
Short-term hemorrhagic shock + resuscitation	7	< 100	7180 ± 1707*	2415 ± 381*,#
Prolonged hemorrhagic shock + resuscitation	6	< 100	2414 ± 381*	742 ± 203*,#

Mean ± SEM.
*$P < .05$ from baseline.
#$P < .05$ vs. shock.

increase expression of a water channel, aquaporin-1, in rat fetal lung, an effect also seen in adult rats (76). Also, tretreatment of rats with dexamethasone upregulates alveolar fluid clearance in rats (77).

A third series of experiments was conducted to determine whether the protective effect of endogenous catecholamines against alveolar flooding was also present after prolonged hemorrhagic shock and fluid resuscitation. The results from these experiments indicate that there was no upregulation of alveolar fluid clearance after a prolonged hemorrhagic shock and fluid resuscitation, despite a significant increase in plasma epinephrine levels. Morever, the intravenous or intra-alveolar administration of exogenous catecholamines did not upregulate alveolar liquid clearance in hemorrhaged and fluid-resuscitated rats. Because both prior depletion of neutrophils and pretreatment with N-acetylcysteine, an oxygen radical scavenger that increases lung tissue glutathione levels, restored the catecholamine-mediated upregulation of alveolar fluid clearance, these results suggest the presence of an oxidative injury to the alveolar epithelium after prolonged hemorrhagic shock and fluid resuscitation (78).

In summary, the alveolar epithelium is much more resistant to injury than the nearby vascular endothelium. During the ischemic and reperfusion phases of acute hemorrhagic shock endogenous release of catecholamines markedly stimulates alveolar fluid clearance by a β-adrenergic-mediated stimulation of active sodium transport. This mechanism may be clinically relevant because it may protect against alveolar flooding during the acute phase of hemorrhagic shock in humans. Interestingly, it has recently been reported that the human lung responds to exogenous catecholamines by an increase in the alveolar liquid clearance (79). In contrast, after prolonged hemorrhagic shock followed by fluid resuscitation, there is no upregulation of alveolar liquid clearance by endogenous or exogenous catecholamines, suggesting the presence of an oxidative injury of the alveolar epithelium (78). Several non-catecholamine-dependent mechanisms have been demonstrated to increase the rate of alveolar epithelial fluid clearance under different pathological conditions (71). However, the importance of these mechanisms after hemorrhagic or traumatic shock is still unknown.

III. Clinical Studies

Acute lung injury is a syndrome of respiratory failure that usually develops within 72 hours of clinical risk factors. Among these clinical predispositions, severe trauma has been identified in several studies as the second most important cause of acute lung injury after sepsis (1,80–82). The victims of major trauma constitute a heterogeneous population of patients who are at risk for acute lung injury with an incidence that ranges from 2% to 40%. In a study including more than 3000 trauma patients studied prospectively, pulmonary complications accounted for a 30% of all disease complications (83). Pneumonia was the most common pulmonary complication in this population of trauma patients, but only 1.2% of the patients developed acute lung injury. The low incidence of acute lung injury in this large population of trauma patients may be explained by the fact that all trauma patients who were hospitalized for more than 3 days were included in the study. In a retrospective study including patients with multiple trauma who had an injury severity score (ISS) > 20, the incidence of acute lung injury was 12% for the period 1982 to 1991 and 18% for the period 1972 to 1981 (84). In another study, which included 271 trauma patients with well-defined risk conditions for acute lung injury (pulmonary contusion, multiple transfusions, or multiple fractures), the incidence of acute lung injury was 25% in the presence of one of the defined risk conditions. The incidence of acute lung injury increased to 40% if a combination of any of two of the three trauma risks was present (1). Only 12% of the trauma patients who developed acute lung injury during the study period were missed. These data were comparable to those of an earlier study conducted by the same investigators, although more than half of the patients who developed acute lung injury were missed in their original study (80).

Each of these studies defined the incidence of acute lung injury in a high-risk hospitalized cohort. However, while all studies employed adequate definitions of acute lung injury, there were sufficient differences to make comparison between them difficult. Thus, several meetings of North American and European investigators resulted in a consensus statement that proposed a more precise definition for acute lung injury, in part so that investigators can study patients early in the course of their respiratory failure, using uniform criteria (85). Early identification of patients with risk factors for developing acute lung injury, including sepsis, aspiration, or pneumonia, did not appear to alter the hospital mortality or the clinical characteristics associated with more traditional definitions of acute lung injury that have used stricter oxygenation criteria (3). Since this study did not include trauma patients, we conducted a clinical study to determine whether the use of recently proposed criteria for acute lung injury results in a significant change in the incidence, clinical characteristics, and risk factors for acute lung injury in severely traumatized patients at high risk for the development of this syndrome.

There were 916 trauma patients who met the trauma team activation criteria over a period of 17 months and were included in the study. From these 916 trauma patients, 102 patients were retained in the study because they had an ISS ≥ 16, were aged between 18 and 75, and were mechanically ventilated for at least 48 hours. From these 102 severely traumatized patients, 42 patients (41.2%) developed acute lung injury, and 60 patients did not. Of the 42 patients, seven met the criteria for acute lung injury (ALI) ($PaO_2/FIO_2 < 300$) but did not progress to ARDS; 35 patients met the criteria for acute respiratory distress syndrome (ARDS) ($PaO_2/FIO_2 < 200$) (85). All patients had bilateral pulmonary infiltrates on the chest radiograph. From the 814 trauma patients who were not retained in the study because they had an ISS < 16 or because they were mechanically ventilated for less than 48 hours, only three patients subsequently met the criteria for acute lung injury. These data indicate that 93% of the trauma patients who developed acute lung injury over the 17-month study period were included in the study (86). Thus, this study identified a homogeneous subset of trauma patients with a high risk (40%) for developing acute lung injury. The data also suggest that early identification of trauma patients with risk factors for developing acute lung injury did not appear to alter the incidence of this syndrome in this patient population at risk when compared with more traditional definitions of acute lung injury that have used stricter oxygenation criteria. Indeed, in this study, most of the trauma patients (83%) who developed acute respiratory failure met the criteria for ARDS.

While the association between trauma with acute lung injury has been consistent, it is difficult to explain its precise etiologic role. Therefore, prospective cohort studies have been designed to identify risk factors associated with the development of acute lung injury in trauma patients. For example, in a previously mentioned study including more than 3000 trauma patients studied prospectively, the authors employed a nested case-case control design, in which patients with subsequent cases of acute lung injury were compared with members of the cohort who did not develop the syndrome. These groups were compared and analyzed to identify potential risk factors using logistic regression analysis. Multiply adjusted odd ratios showed that patients who developed acute lung injury were most likely to have blunt trauma, to have an ISS of > 16, and to undergo head surgery (83). In another prospective cohort study, several factors were independently associated with an increased risk for development of acute lung injury in trauma patients: older age (> 70 years old), female gender, APACHE II > 20, ISS > 40, massive transfusion (defined as > 15 units of blood in 24 hours), and the development of sepsis between the admission of the patient to the hospital and the onset of acute lung injury (1).

Although well designed, there are several limitations in the interpretation of the results of this study. First, the data were collected > 10 years ago. Second, the design of this study did not permit to determine whether the clinical risks used were causally associated with the development of acute lung injury or whether they were simply markers of systemic endothelial injury rather than true etiologic risks. Data from animal and human studies indicate that endothelial activation and injury occurs early in endotoxemia and bacteremia (87–92). Moreover, the severity of systemic injury, as indicated by the presence of systemic hypotension and metabolic acidosis, and endothelial cell activation measured by plasma levels of Von Willebrand factor antigen (vWfAg), were significantly correlated with the risk of developing acute lung injury in an homogenous group of patients with nonpulmonary sepsis (91). When patients at risk of acute lung injury from etiologies other than sepsis, such as severe trauma, were studied, the correlation between prior systemic injury, endothelial cell activation and development of acute lung injury was less evident (89,90,93). For example, two of three indicators of endothelial cell activation (soluble ICAM-1 and soluble E-selectin) were not increased over control values in severely traumatized patients studied 8 hours after trauma despite a 25% incidence of acute lung injury in this patient population (90). Interestingly, mean plasma levels vWfAg from severely traumatized patients measured 8 hours after trauma were significantly increased above controls (2.5-fold), but significantly lower than the values measured in septic patients despite an incidence of acute lung injury comparable in the two groups of patients studied (25%) (90). To explain this apparent discrepancy between data obtained from septic and trauma patients at high risk for developing acute lung injury, we hypothesized that systemic endothelial cell activation might occur immediately after injury, and might be of shorter duration in trauma patients than in septic patients.

Thus, the objective of our study was to determine whether the early severity of systemic endothelial injury is a primary determinant for the development of acute lung injury in a homogeneous group of severely traumatized patients. Our results indicate that trauma patients who later developed acute lung injury had a significantly more severe initial metabolic acidosis than those who did not (arterial pH: 7.23 ± 0.02 vs. 7.30 ± 0.01; base deficit: -8.8 ± 0.7 vs. -5.6 ± 0.7). In a subset of patients in this study, there was also a more pronounced systemic endothelial cell activation, as indicated by the significantly greater mean initial plasma vWfAg concentration measured in those patients than in trauma patients who did not develop acute lung injury (418 ± 55 vs. $320 \pm 23\%$, $P < .05$). This was associated with the presence of an early hematological dysfunction in 36% of trauma patients who later develop acute lung injury, but only in 15% of trauma patients who did not develop this syndrome ($P < .05$).

To further evaluate the early predictors of acute lung injury in this subset of severely traumatized patients, a stepwise multiple logistic-regression analysis was then carried out. Two variables were independently associated with the development of ALI in this population of severely traumatized patients: (1) ISS ($P < .05$); (2) initial arterial pH measured in the emergency room at the arrival of the patient to the hospital ($P < .01$). When the initial arterial pH was excluded from the stepwise multiple logistic-regression analysis, then the calculated base deficit from the initial arterial blood gas measurement also became an independent predictor of ALI in this population of severely traumatized patients ($P < .05$) (86). Comparable results were reported in a large retrospective study including 3000 trauma patients. Admission base deficit identified trauma patients likely to require early blood transfusion and to develop acute lung injury (94).

In summary, the results of these studies support the conclusion that the initial severity of systemic endothelial injury, as reflected physiologically by the metabolic acidosis, is a primary determinant for the development of acute lung injury in patients who have sustained severe trauma.

Although there is no doubt that the presence of acute lung injury increases the morbidity of trauma patients, the association between development of this syndrome and mortality rate of this patient population is less evident. Data from a large prospective study conducted $>$ 10 years ago indicate that mortality rate of trauma patients increased by 4.3-fold if they developed acute lung injury (1). However, during the past 10 years, there has been a reduction in the mortality rate of patients of acute lung injury, although this trend was stronger in septic than in trauma patients after adjustment for age and ISS 2. The mortality rate of trauma patients with acute lung injury may also have been affected by the cause of acute lung injury secondary to trauma. For example, trauma patients who develop fat embolism syndrome after long-bone fractures have a much better prognosis than patients with acute lung injury secondary to major trauma, arterial hypotension, and surgical treatment. Finally, the presence of severe head injury is an important cause of mortality in severely traumatized patients who survive the initial phase of trauma (95). In our recent study in severely traumatized patients, the mortality rate of this patient population was not influenced by the development of acute lung injury, but was strongly dependent on the presence of severe head injury (86).

IV. Conclusions

The overall objective of this chapter was to review the mechanisms of increased permeability pulmonary edema following hemorrhagic or traumatic shock. Recent experimental studies have showed that the shock-dependent release of catecholamines stimulates active fluid removal from the airspaces by the alveolar epithelium, indicating the presence of a new, previously unrecognized mechanism that may protect against alveolar flooding in the acute phase of hemorrhagic shock. Neutrophil-mediated oxidative injury appears to be one of the important mechanisms responsible for the alteration of the barrier function of both the lung endothelium and the alveolar epithelium after severe hemorrhagic shock. Finally, the shock-mediated oxidant injury to the alveolar epithelium may predispose to alveolar edema by blunting the capacity of this barrier to upregulate fluid removal from the airspaces in response to the release of endogenous catecholamines.

Clinical studies have identified risk factors associated with the development of acute lung injury in severely traumatized patients. However, whether these clinical risks are causally associated with the development of acute lung injury or they are simply markers of systemic endothelial injury rather than true etiologic risks, is still unclear. In fact, the results of recent clinical studies indicate that the initial severity of systemic endothelial injury appears to be a major determinant in the development of acute lung injury in trauma patients. However, available measurable soluble markers of endothelial cell activation are neither sensitive nor specific enough to easily identify trauma patients at high risk for developing acute lung injury. Therefore, more studies are necessary to define a pattern of physiological and biochemical markers that will identify a subset of trauma patients at high risk for acute lung injury in whom early therapeutic intervention may be achieved, thus reducing the morbidity and perhaps the mortality rate of this population of patients.

References

1. Hudson LD, Milberg JA, Anardi D, Maunder RJ. Clinical risks for development of the acute respiratory distress syndrome. Am J Respir Crit Care Med 1995; 151: 293–301.
2. Milberg JA, Davis DR, Steinberg KP, Hudson LD. Improved survival of patients with acute respiratory distress syndrome (ARDS). JAMA 1995; 273:306–309.
3. Doyle RL, Szaflarski N, Modin GW, Wiener-Kronish JP, Matthay MA. Identification of patients with acute lung injury: predictors of mortality. Am J Respir Crit Care Med 1995; 152:1818–1824.
4. Todd TR, Baile JE, Hogg JC. Pulmonary capillary permeability during hemorrhagic shock. J Appl Physiol 1978; 45:298–306.
5. Pretorius JP, Schlag G, Redl H, et al. The lung in shock as a result of hypovolemic-traumatic shock in baboons. J Trauma 1987; 27:1344–1353.
6. Michel RP, Laforte M, Hogg JC. Physiology and morphology of pulmonary microvascular injury with shock and reinfusion. J Appl Physiol 1981; 50:1227–1235.
7. Holcroft JW, Trunkey DD. Pulmonary extravasation of albumin during and after hemorrhagic shock in baboons. J Surg Res 1975; 18:91–97.
8. Gorin AB, Mendiondo G. Permeability of barriers to albumin flux in lungs of sheep resuscitated from hemorrhagic shock. J Appl Physiol 1986; 61:2156–2161.
9. Matthay MA, Eschenbacher WL, Goetzl EJ. Elevated concentrations of leukotrienes D_4 in pulmonary edema fluid of patients with the adult respiratory distress syndrome. J Clin Immunol 1984; 4:479–483.
10. Fein A, Grossman RF, Jones JG, Overland E, Pitts L, Murray JF, Staub NC. The value of edema fluid protein measurement in patients with pulmonary edema. Am J Med 1979; 67:32–38.
11. Clark JG, Milberg JA, Steinberg KP, Hudson LD. Type III procollagen peptide in the adult respiratory distress syndrome: association of increased peptide levels in bronchoalveolar lavage fluid with increased risk for death. Ann Intern Med 1995; 122:17–23.
12. Lefer AM, Lefer DJ. Pharmacology of the endothelium in ischemia-reperfusion and circulatory shock. Annu Rev Pharmacol Toxicol 1993; 33:71–90.

13. Cheung JY, Bonventre JV, Malis CD, Leaf A. Calcium and ischemic injury. N Engl J Med 1986; 314:752–756.
14. McCord JM. Oxygen-derived free radicals in postischemic tissue injury. N Engl J Med 1985; 312:159–163.
15. Lefer AM, Tsao PS, Lefer DJ, Ma XL. Role of endothelial dysfunction in the pathogenesis of reperfusion injury after myocardial ischemia. FASEB J 1991; 5: 2029–2034.
16. Lorant DE, Patel KD, McIntyre TM, McEver RP, Prescott SM, Zimmerman GA. Coexpression of GMP-140 and PAF by endothelium stimulated by histamine or thrombin: a juxtacrine system for adhesion and activation of neutrophils. J Cell Biol 1991; 115:2233–2234.
17. Kovach AGB, Szabo C, Benyo Z, Csaki C, Greenberg JH, Reivich M. Effects of NG-nitro-L-arginine and L-arginine on regional cerebral blood flow in the cat. J Physiol 1992; 449:183–196.
18. Lefer AM, Ma XL. Endothelial dysfunction as an early critical event in ischemia and shock. Host Defense Dysfunction in Trauma, Shock, and Sepsis 1992:107–112.
19. Siegfried MR, Erhardt J, Rider T, Ma XL, Lefer AM. Cardioprotection and attenuation of endothelial dysfunction by organic nitric oxide donors in myocardial ischemia-reperfusion. J Pharmacol Exp Ther 1992; 260:668–675.
20. Siegfried MR, Carey C, Ma XL, Lefer AM. Beneficial effects of SPM-5185, a novel NO donor, in myocardial ischemia reperfusion. Am J Physiol 1992; 263: H771–H777.
21. Symington PA, Ma XL, Lefer AM. Protective actions of S-nitroso-N-acetyl penicillamine in a rat model of hemorrhagic shock. Meth Find Exp Clin Pharmacol 1992; 14:789–797.
22. Ma XL, Weyrich AS, Lefer DJ, Lefer AM. Diminished basal nitric oxide release after myocardial ischemia and reperfusion promotes neutrophil adherence to coronary endothelium. Circ Res 1993; 72:403–412.
23. Kurose I, Kubes P, Wolf R, Anderson DC, Paulson J, Miyasaka M, Granger DN. Inhibition of nitric oxide production: mechanisms of vascular albumin leakage. Circ Res 1993; 73:164–171.
24. Payne D, Kubes P. Nitric oxide donors reduce the rise in reperfusion-induced intestinal mucosal permeability. Am J Physiol 1993; 265:G189–G195.
25. Adkins WK, Taylor A. Role of xanthine oxidase and neutrophils in ischemia-reperfusion injury in rabbit lung. J Appl Physiol 1990; 69:2012–2018.
26. Allison RC, Kyle J, Adkins WK, Prasad VR, McCord JM, Taylor AE. Effect of ischemia-reperfusion or hypoxia reoxygenation on lung vascular permeability and resistance. J Appl Physiol 1990; 69:597–603.
27. Bishop MJ, Lamm W, Guidotti SM, Albert RK. Pulmonary artery occlusion is sufficient to increase pulmonary vascular permeability in rabbits. J Appl Physiol 1992; 73:272–275.
28. Bishop MJ, Boatman ES, Ivey TD, Jordan JP, Cheney FW. Reperfusion of ischemic dog lung results in fever, leukopenia, and lung edema. Am Rev Respir Dis 1986; 134:752–756.
29. Kennedy TP, Rao NV, Hopkins C, Pennington L, Tolley E, Hoidal JR. Role of reactive oxygen species in reperfusion injury to the rabbit lung. J Clin Invest 1989; 83:1326–1335.

30. Freeman BA, Crapo JD. Hyperoxia increases oxygen radical production in rat lungs and lung mitochrondria. J Biol Chem 1981; 256:674–679.
31. Koyama I, Toung TJK, Rogers MC, Gurtner GH, Traystman RJ. O_2 radicals mediate reperfusion lung injury in ischemic O_2-ventilated canine pulmonary lobe. J Appl Physiol 1987; 63:111–115.
32. Becker PM, Pearse DB, Permutt S, Sylvester JT. Separate effects of ischemia and reperfusion on vascular permeability in ventilated ferret lungs. J Appl Physiol 1992; 73:2616–2622.
33. Qiao RL, Sadurski R, Bhattacharya J. Hydraulic conductivity of ischemic pulmonary venules. Am J Physiol 1993; 264:L382–L386.
34. Eckenhoff RG, Dodia C, Tan Z, Fisher AB. Oxygen-dependent reperfusion injury in the isolated lung. J Appl Physiol 1992; 72:1454–1460.
35. Fisher PW, Huang YCT, Kennedy TP, Piantadosi CA. PO_2-dependent hydroxyl radical production during ischemia-reperfusion lung injury. Am J Physiol 1993; 265: L279–L285.
36. Hamvas A, Palazzo R, Kaiser L, Cooper J, Shuman TL, Velazquez M, Freeman B. Inflammation and oxygen free radical formation during pulmonary ischemia-reperfusion injury. J Appl Physiol 1992; 72:621–628.
37. Gilroy RJ, Batte MJ, Wickersham NE, Pou NA, Loyd JE, Overholser KA. Postischemic hypoperfusion during unilateral lung reperfusion in vivo. Am Rev Respir Dis 1993; 147:276–282.
38. Modelska K, Matthay MA, McElroy MC, Pittet JF. Upregulation of alveolar liquid after hemorrhagic shock and fluid resuscitation in rats. Am J Physiol 273 (Lung Cell Mol Physiol 17) 1997:L305–L314.
39. Pittet JF, Brenner T, Modelska K, Matthay MA. Alveolar liquid clearance is increased by endogenous catecholamines in hemorrhagic shock in rats. J Appl Physiol 1996; 81:830–837.
40. Hamvas A, Schuster DP. Bronchial and reverse pulmonary venous blood flow protects the lung from ischemia-reperfusion injury. J Appl Physiol 1994; 77:731–736.
41. Obermiller T, Lakshminarayan S, Willoughby S, Mendenhall J, Butler J. Influence of lung volume and left atrial pressure on reverse pulmonary venous blood flow. J Appl Physiol 1991; 70:447–453.
42. Agostoni PG, Deffebach M, Kirk W, Mendenhall JM, Albert RK, Butler J. Temperature alters bronchial blood flow response to pulmonary arterial obstruction. J Appl Physiol 1987; 62:1907–1911.
43. Kowalski TF, Guidotti S, Deffebach M, Kubilis P, Bishop MJ. The bronchial circulation in pulmonary artery occlusion and reperfusion. J Appl Physiol 1990; 68: 125–129.
44. Seibert AF, Thompson J, Taylor AE, Wilborn WH, Barnard J, Haynes J. Reversal of increased microvascular permeability associated with ischemia-reperfusion: role of cAMP. J Appl Physiol 1992; 72:389–395.
45. Adkins WK, Barnard JW, Seibert AF, Haynes J, Taylor AE. Compounds that increase cAMP prevent ischemia-reperfusion pulmonary capillary injury. J Appl Physiol 1992; 72:492–497.
46. Barnard JW, Seibert AF, Prasad VR, Smart DA, Strada SJ, Taylor AE, Thompson WJ. Reversal of pulmonary capillary ischemia-reperfusion injury by rolipram, a cAMP phosphodiesterase inhibitor. J Appl Physiol 1994; 77:774–781.

47. Baluk P, McDonald DM. The β_2-adrenergic receptor agonist formoterol reduces microvascular leakage by inhibiting endothelial gap formation. Am J Physiol 1994; 266:L461–L468.
48. Ljungman AG, Grum CM, Deeb GM, Bolling SF, Morganroth ML. Inhibition of cyclooxygenase metabolite production attenuates ischemia-reperfusion lung injury. Am Rev Respir Dis 1991; 143:610–617.
49. Zamore CA, Baron DA, Heffner JE. Thromboxane contributes to pulmonary hypertension in ischemia-reperfusion lung injury. J Appl Physiol 1993; 74:224–229.
50. Ratliff NB, Wilson JW, Mikat E, Hackel DB, Graham TC. The lung in hemorrhagic shock. IV. The role of neutrophil polymorphonuclear leukocytes. Am J Pathol 1971; 65:325–334.
51. Redl H, Schlag G, Hammerschmidt DE. Quantitative assessment of leukostasis in experimental hypovolemic-traumatic shock. Acta Chir Scand 1984; 150:113–117.
52. Barroso-Aranda J, Schmid-Schonbein GW, Zwerfach BW, Engler RL. Granulocytes and no-reflow phenomenon irreversible hemorrhagic shock. Circ Res 1988; 63: 437–447.
53. Deeb GM, Grum CM, Lynch MJ, Guynn TP, Gallagher KP, Ljungman AG, Bolling SP, Morganroth ML. Neutrophils are not necessary for induction of ischemia-reperfusion injury. J Appl Physiol 1990; 68:374–381.
54. Anderson BO, Moore EE, Moore FA, Left JA, Terada LS, Harken AH, Repine JE. Hypovolemic shock promotes neutrophil sequestration in lungs by a xanthine-oxidase-related mechanism. J Appl Physiol 1991; 71:1862–1865.
55. Bysani GK, Kennedy TP, Ky N, Rao NV, Blaze CA, Hoidal JR. Role of cytochrome P-450 in reperfusion injury of the rabbit lung. J Clin Invest 1990; 86:1434–1441.
56. Abdih H, Kelly CJ, Bouchier-Hayes D, William R, Watson G, Redmond HP, Burke P, Bouchier-Hayes DJ. Nitric oxide endothelium-derived relaxing factor attenuates revascularization-induces lung injury. J Surg Res 1994; 57:39–43.
57. Matthay MA, Landolt C, Staub NC. Differential liquid and protein clearance from the alveoli of anesthetized sheep. J Appl Physiol 1982; 53:96–104.
58. Matthay MA, Berthiaume Y, Staub NC. Long term clearance of liquid and protein from the lungs of unanesthetized sheep. J Appl Physiol 1985; 59:928–934.
59. Pittet JF, Wiener-Kronish JP, McElroy MC, Folkesson HF, Matthay MA. Stimulation of lung epithelial liquid clearance by endogenous release of catecholamines in septic shock in anesthetized rats. J Clin Invest 1994; 94:663–671.
60. Pittet JF, Wiener-Kronish JP, Serikov V, Matthay MA. Resistance of the alveolar epithelium to injury from septic shock in sheep. Am J Respir Crit Care Med 1995; 151:1093–1100.
61. Kanwar S, Kubes P. Mast cells contribute to ischemia-reperfusion-induced granulocyte infiltration and intestinal dysfunction. Am J Physiol 1994; 267:G316–G321.
62. McElroy MC, Pittet JF, Hashimoto S, Allen L, Wiener-Kronish JP, Dobbs LG. A type I cell-type specific protein is a biochemical marker of epithelial injury in a rat mode of pneumonia. Am J Physiol 1995; 268:L181–L186.
63. McElroy MC, Modelska K, Matthay MA, Dobbs LG, Pittet JF. Increased BAL concentrations of an alveolar epithelial type I cell-specific antigen after hemorrhagic and fluid resuscitation in rats. Am J Respir Crit Care Med 1997; 155:A581.
64. Folkesson HG, Kheradmand F, Matthay MA. The effect of salt water on alveolar epithelial barrier function. Am J Respir Crit Care Med 1994; 150.

65. Folkesson HG, Matthay MA, Hebert C, Broaddus CV. Acid aspiration-induced lung injury in rabbits is mediated by IL-8 dependent mechanisms. J Clin Invest 1995; 96:107–116.
66. Nici L, Dowin R, M. Gilmore-Heber, Jamieson JD, Ingbar DH. Upregulation of rat lung Na-K-ATPase during hyperoxic injury. Am J Physiol 1991; 261: L307–L314.
67. Olivera W, Ridge LDW, Sznajder JI. Active sodium transport and alveolar epithelial Na-K-ATPase increase during subacute hyperoxia in rats. Am J Physiol 1994; 266: L577–L584.
68. Sznajder JI, Olivera WG, Ridge KM, Rutschman DH. Mechanism of lung liquid clearance during hyperoxia in isolated rat lungs. Am J Respir Crit Care Med 1995; 151:1519–1525.
69. Yue G, Russel WJ, Bensos DJ, Jackson RM, Olman MA, Matalon S. Increased expression and activity of sodium channels in alveolar type II cells of hyperoxic rats. Proc Natl Acad Sci USA 1992; 92:8418–8422.
70. Pittet JF, Hashimoto S, Pian M, McElroy MC, Nitenberg G, Wiener-Kronish JP. Exotoxin A stimulates fluid reabsorption from distal airspaces of lung in anesthetized rats. Am J Physiol 1996; 270:L232–L241.
71. Matthay MA, Folkesson HG, Verkman AS. Salt and water transport across alveolar and distal airway epithelia in the adult lung. Am J Physiol 1996; 270:L487–L503.
72. McElroy MC, Wiener-Kronish JP, Miyazaki H, Sawa T, Modelska K, Dobbs LG, Pittet JF. Nitric oxide attenuates lung endothelial injury caused by sublethal hyperoxia in rats. Am J Physiol 1997; 272:L631–L638.
73. Jaattela A, Alho A, Avikainen V, Karaharju E, Kataja J, Lahdensuu M, Lepisto P, Rokkanen P, Tervo T. Plasma catecholamines in severely injured patients: a prospective study on 45 patients with multiple injuries. Br J Surg 1975; 62: 177–181.
74. Barker PM, Markiewicz KAP, Walters DV, Strang LB. Synergistic action of triiodothyronine and hydrocortisone on epinephrine-induced reabsorption of fetal lung liquid. Pediatr Res 1991; 27:588–591.
75. O'Brodovich H, Canessa C, Ueda J, Rafii B, Rossier BC, Edelson J. Expression of the epithelial Na^+ channel in the developing rat lung. Am J Physiol 1993; 265: C491–C496.
76. King LS, Nielsen S, Agre P. Aquaporin-1 water channel protein in lung: ontogeny, steroid-induced expression, and distribution in rat. J Clin Invest 1996; 97:2183–2191.
77. Folkesson HG, Norlin A, Siller M, Knutsson RM, Matthay MA. Dexamethasone upregulates alveolar epithelial liquid clearance in anesthetized ventilated rats. FASEB J 1997; 11:A561.
78. Modelska K, Matthay MA, Pittet JF. Catecholamine-dependent upregulation of alveolar epithelial liquid clearance is reduced after prolonged hemorrhagic shock in rats. Am J Respir Crit Care Med 1997; 155:A858.
79. Sakuma T, Okaniwa G, Nakada T, Nishimura T, Fujimura S, Matthay MA. Alveolar fluid clearance in the resected human lung. Am J Respir Crit Care Med 1994; 150: 305–310.
80. Pepe PE, Potkin RT, Reus DH, Hudson LD, Carrico CJ. Clinical predictors of the adult respiratory distress syndrome. Am J Surg 1982; 144:124–131.

81. Sloane PJ, Gee M, Gottlieb JE, et al. A multicenter registry of patients with acute respiratory distress syndrome. Physiology and outcome. Am Rev Respir Dis 1992; 146:419–426.
82. Lewandowski K, Metz J, Deutschmann C, et al. Incidence, severity, and mortality of acute respiratory failure in Berlin, Germany. Am J Respir Crit Care Med 1995; 151:1121–1125.
83. Hoyt DB, Simons RK, WInchell RJ, et al. A risk analysis of pulmonary complications following major trauma. J Trauma 1993; 35:524–531.
84. Regel G, Lobenhoffer P, Grotz M, Pape HC, Lehmann U, Tscherne H. Treatment results of patients with multiple trauma: an analysis of 3406 cases treated between 1972 and 1991 at German level I trauma center. J Trauma 1995; 38:70–78.
85. Bernard GR, Artigas A, Brigham KL, et al. The American-European consensus conference on ARDS. Definitions, mechanisms, relevant outcomes, clinical trial coordination. Am J Respir Crit Care Med 1994; 149:818–824.
86. Pittet JF, Campbell AR, Morabito DJ, et al. Both the initial severity of metabolic acidosis and systemic endothelial injury are primary determinants for the development of acute lung injury in trauma patients. Am J Respir Crit Care Med 1997; 155:A91.
87. Brigham KL, Woolvertson WC, Blake LH, Staub NC. Increased sheep lung vascular permeability caused by *Pseudomonas* bacteremia. J Clin Invest 1974; 54:792–804.
88. Brigham KL, Bowers RE, Haynes J. Increased lung vascular permeability caused by *E. coli* endotoxin. Circ Res 1979; 45:292–297.
89. Moss M, Ackerson L, Gillespie MK, Moore FA, Moore EE, Parsons PE. Von Willebrand factor antigen levels are not predictive for the adult respiratory distress syndrome. Am J Respir Crit Care Med 1995; 151:15–20.
90. Moss M, Gillespie MK, Ackerson L, Moore FA, Moore EE, Parsons PE. Endothelial cell activity varies in patients at risk for the adult respiratory distress syndrome. Crit Care Med 1996; 24:1782–1786.
91. Rubin DB, Wiener-Kronish JP, Murray J, et al. Elevated von Willebrand factor antigen is an early plasma predictor of acute lung injury in nonpulmonary sepsis syndrome. J Clin Invest 1990; 86:474–480.
92. Suffredini AF, Harpel PC, Parillo JE. Promotion and subsequent inhibition of plasminogen activation after administration of intravenous endotoxin to normal subjects. N Engl J Med 1989; 320:1165–1172.
93. Sabharwal AK, Bajaj SP, Ameri A, et al. Tissue factor pathway inhibitor and von Willebrand factor antigen levels in adult respiratory distress syndrome and in a primate model of sepsis. Am J Respir Crit Care Med 1995; 151:758–767.
94. Davis JD, Parks SN, Kaups KL, Gladen HE, O'Donnell-Nicol S. Admission base deficit predicts transfusion requirements and risk of complications. J Trauma 1996; 41:769–774.
95. Schonfeld SA, Ploysongsang Y, DiLisio R, et al. Fat embolism prophylaxis with corticosteroids. Ann Intern Med 1983; 99:438–443.

10

Neurogenic Pulmonary Edema

MICHAEL B. MARON and CHARLES F. PILATI

Northeastern Ohio Universities College of Medicine
Rootstown, Ohio

I. Introduction

Neurogenic pulmonary edema (NPE) is a form of edema that may develop after injury or other disorders of the central nervous system (CNS), and can occur in the absence of preexisting left ventricular dysfunction. Although the focus of this review will be on the mechanisms responsible for the development of the edema, it should be noted that CNS injury can result in a broad spectrum of pulmonary abnormalities that include hypoxemia, abnormal ventilatory patterns, hypermetabolism, and, in the extreme, pulmonary edema (1). Despite much investigation, the mechanisms responsible for the development of NPE remain controversial. Cameron and De (2) originally proposed that an increase in vascular permeability was responsible for the development of NPE. This hypothesis was soon challenged by Sarnoff and Sarnoff (3), who concluded that the edema resulted from extreme pulmonary capillary hypertension produced by the translocation of blood from the systemic to the pulmonary circuit. These disparate views set the stage for a continuing argument that has yet to be completely resolved. Complicating the basic question of increased permeability versus increased pressure is evidence of the involvement of a variety of hydrostatic and increased permeability mechanisms. For example, decreases in left ventricular compliance, mitral valve regurgitation, pulmonary venoconstriction, and catecholamine-induced left ventricular dysfunction have been proposed as contributing or additional mechanisms. Additionally, increased permeability has been variously considered either to occur independently of changes in vascular pressure (pressure-independent) or to be a direct result of extremely high pressures (pressure-dependent).

II. NPE in Humans: Insight from Case and Clinical Studies

NPE has been reported to develop after a wide variety of CNS injuries and disorders. These include head trauma (4–20), intracranial hemorrhage (5,6, 8,18,21–24), subarachnoid hemorrhage (6,13,18,25–32), brainstem hemorrhage or tumors (33,34), cerebrovascular thrombosis (35), acute hydrocephalus (36), spinal cord injuries (37,38), epileptic seizures (13,18,39–55), bulbar poliomyelitis (56), medulla oblongata injury or edema (57–59), intrathecal hypertonic saline injection (60), cerebral air embolism (61), trigeminal nerve blockade (62), vertebral artery ligation (63), cerebral hypoxia and edema due to drug-induced ventilatory insufficiency (64), potential complications resulting from surgical removal of intracranial tumors (65), missile embolization of the cerebral circulation (66), Guillain-Barré syndrome (67), and Reye syndrome (68). These disorders are often associated with either an increase in intracranial pressure or the development of cerebral ischemia, both of which can result in an increase in sympathetic nervous system (SNS) activity. The incidence of NPE has been determined from postmortem studies of individuals with intracranial hemorrhage (5,21), intracranial lesions (69), subarachnoid hemorrhage (27), cerebral infarction (70), and isolated head injuries (5,20) and has been found to range from 33% to 71%, with most studies reporting an incidence of > 50% in individuals dying from these causes.

NPE may develop very rapidly. In this regard, pulmonary edema fluid has been observed almost immediately after seizures (18,40,47,52), subarachnoid hemorrhage (13,18,26), gunshot wounds to the head (7,18), and the injection of bupivacaine into the trigeminal space (62). Additionally, the lungs of individuals who have died immediately or soon after head injuries (7,20,21), subarachnoid hemorrhage (8), or the development of seizures (8,40,48,51) have been found to be edematous at necropsy. The increase in extravascular lung water (EVLW) may be substantial, and the appearance of pink frothy edema fluid has frequently been reported (6,8,12,18,19,23,24,26,29,31,36,38,55,57,58,61,63,65). Since the pulmonary interstitium can accommodate an increase in EVLW of approximately 25–35% before alveolar flooding occurs (71), the appearance of edema fluid indicates that EVLW must have increased by at least this amount. Far greater degrees of edema have been reported in some case studies. For example, Carlson et al. (23) suctioned approximately 300 ml of fluid from the endotracheal tube of a patient with an intracranial hemorrhage. Measurements of lung weight at necropsy also indicate that the degree of pulmonary edema may be substantial (6–8,20,21,40,48,57). Finally, measurements of EVLW (determined from thermal dye dilution) have been obtained in some patients with NPE and have been found to be increased from 50% to 70% above control values (15,72–74). It is important to note, however, that the increase in lung water may be variable and can range from interstitial edema to alveolar flooding. Consequently, not all individuals have an increase in EVLW that results in alveolar edema.

Sarnoff and Sarnoff (3) and Theodore and Robin (75) hypothesized that the sequence of events leading to the development of NPE was initiated by a CNS trauma-induced massive discharge of the SNS. The resultant systemic vasoconstriction in turn was considered to translocate blood from the systemic to the pulmonary circuit, thus producing marked increases in pulmonary blood volume and vascular pressures that favor the development of edema. The time course of the above events can be extremely rapid, often occurring within minutes of the initiating event. The following observations in humans support this hypothesis. First, elevations in both plasma catecholamine and urinary catecholamine metabolite concentrations have been observed in patients with a variety of CNS injuries and disorders (76–81), indicating an increase in SNS activity. More interestingly, three case reports (22,23,66) documenting the sudden development of severe increases in pulmonary arterial (P_{pa}) and wedge (P_w) and/or arterial (P_a) pressures in patients (Table 1) suggest that the sequence of events discussed above may occur in humans. In all three patients, the hypertensive episodes developed suddenly. The hypertensive period appears to be transient, however. In the patient studied by Wray and Nicotra (22), P_a, P_{pa}, and

Table 1 Systemic and Pulmonary Hypertensive Crises in Three CNS-Injured Patients Who Developed NPE

Study	Disorder	Peak pressure (torr)		
		P_a	P_{pa}	P_w
Wray and Nicotra (22)	Intracranial hemorrhage	410/200	110/60	48
Carlson et al. (23)	Intracranial hemorrhage	260/155	77/44	40
Reines et al. (66)	Missle embolization of cerebral circulation	230/120	nm	nm

P_a, arterial pressure; P_{pa}, pulmonary arterial pressure; P_w, pulmonary arterial wedge pressure; nm, not measured. P_a and P_{pa} are shown as systolic and diastolic pressures.

P_w returned to baseline values within 5 min, and a marked reduction in P_a was observed within 10 min in the patient observed by Reines et al. (66). Two of the studies (22,66) indicated that pulmonary edema either developed soon after the hypertensive episode or worsened after subsequent episodes. Finally, there may be multiple periods of pulmonary hypertension and edema development (22,35). A similar pattern of massive SNS activation has been observed in patients with seizures (82). The above observations indicate that severe but transient increases in pulmonary microvascular pressure can produce NPE in humans.

Theodore and Robin (75) also suggested that if the pulmonary hypertension was of sufficient magnitude, damage to the alveolar-capillary barrier could result, which could allow EVLW to continue to increase even after normal vascular pressures were reattained. It is thus conceivable that an increased permeability might contribute to the edema development in some patients who develop increases in pulmonary vascular pressure large enough to disrupt the integrity of the vessels. This possibility might explain the relatively high edema fluid protein concentrations (29,33,65,73,83–86) and the development of intrapulmonary hemorrhages (7,48,51,56,84) observed in some patients.

A number of investigators have compared the protein concentrations of edema fluid and plasma in patients with NPE to determine whether the edema was due to increased pressure or permeability (23,29,33,65,73,83–86). Low edema-fluid/plasma-protein concentration ratios (E/P) indicate that microvascular protein sieving has been maintained and are consistent with a hydrostatic mechanism, whereas high E/P ratios suggest that there has been an increase in vascular protein permeability. It is commonly stated in the literature that the edema fluid in NPE is protein-rich. This statement appears to be based, in part, on observations of patients with NPE who produced edema fluid having E/P ratios approaching unity (33,73,84,85) and has led many to conclude that NPE is permeability-based. Recent observations, however, question this generalization. First, care is required in the interpretation of the E/P ratio, because recent studies have shown that alveolar fluid protein concentration increases over time as edema fluid is reabsorbed from the airspaces (87). It is thus difficult to determine (particularly in cases where the airway fluid is collected later in the illness) if the protein concentration is high because of increased permeability or fluid reabsorption. Secondly, in a recent study of 12 patients with NPE, Smith and Matthay (86) found that the E/P ratio ranged between low values (typical of those observed in hemodynamic pulmonary edema) and high values, with many of the patients having ratios below 0.65. In their analysis, they accounted for the potential confounding effects of time. These data suggest that hydrostatic mechanisms play a more predominant role in the development of NPE than had been previously realized, but also indicate that there appears to be an increase in vascular protein permeability in some patients.

The commonly made observation that the edema fluid is pink suggests that some erythrocytes must be present. The fact that the color is pink rather than red indicates that the hematocrit is low; in one case report it was found to average only 1.6% (23). There are occasional reports, however, of the appearance of bloody edema fluid or hemoptysis (7,10,40,41,45,47,52,56,62), and some necropsy reports have documented the presence of intrapulmonary hemorrhages (48,56,65,84). However, these cases tend to be less frequent, and in general, the observations suggest that vascular permeability is not increased globally to the point where erythrocytes readily leave the blood, but are more consistent with the development of focal areas of injury.

Based on the disappearance of pulmonary infiltrates in follow-up roentgenograms and the reestablishment of normal blood gas values, the edema appears to resolve within 24 to 72 hours in many patients (13,17,18,24, 30,31,35–37,39,42–47,49,50,52,54,60,62,64). This seems to be particularly the case in NPE associated with seizures, a situation in which there is no ongoing CNS injury to potentially interfere with the recovery process. In some instances, however, the edema may persist and even worsen. In this regard, Mackersie et al. (72) found elevations in thermal lung water over a 4-day study period in head-injured patients, with the mean value increasing during the first 2 postinjury days. Similarly, Singbartl (73) observed that nonsurviving patients with cerebral lesions had elevated thermal lung water values at the initial measurement and that these continued to increase substantially during the next several days. The reason(s) why lung water remains elevated and/or continues to increase in some patients is unknown, but could relate to either a progressive fall in plasma protein osmotic pressure observed in some patients (73), an increased vascular permeability due to either a pressure-dependent or pressure-independent mechanism, or catecholamine-induced cardiac dysfunction.

Although NPE frequently develops rapidly, it may not develop for some time after the original insult in some individuals. Delays ranging from 12 hours to several days have been observed (28,29,53,58,61,63,65), leading some investigators to conclude that there may be two forms of NPE (53). The delayed development in itself is not what makes these cases of interest, because it is conceivable that the intense SNS discharge could have occurred sometime after the initial injury. Rather, many of these cases appear to develop in the absence of evidence for hemodynamic changes, and the edema often develops slowly rather than suddenly. Some of these patients exhibit very high A/P ratios, suggestive of an increase in protein permeability. This has led some investigators to conclude that under these circumstances, NPE results from an increase in vascular permeability that was not related to the development of pulmonary hypertension.

It has recently become clear that depressed cardiac contractility is also one of the consequences of massive SNS activation (30,32,88–98). The relationship between this type of neurogenic cardiac dysfunction and NPE has not been clearly elucidated, but recent observations from clinical studies suggest that cardiac dysfunction can play a major role in the development of NPE (25,30,32).

For example, Schell et al. (30) observed NPE and depressed left ventricular (LV) contractility in a patient with subarachnoid hemorrhage. Pulmonary vascular wedge pressure was elevated, and hypokinesis was observed in the septum and basolateral wall of the left ventricle. Because the pulmonary edema began to resolve as LV function improved over the next 2 days, they concluded that the edema was cardiogenic. Although depressed cardiac contractility may underlie some forms of NPE, it may not be a significant factor in all cases of NPE, particularly those in which the edema develops almost immediately after the CNS injury. In this regard, Mayer et al. (32) described five patients who developed pulmonary edema rapidly after subarachnoid hemorrhage, and none had evidence of LV dysfunction at the time of edema formation. However, wedge pressure, monitored in four of the patients, became significantly elevated in each beyond 15 hours of the initial hemorrhage. LV wall motion abnormalities and reduced ejection fraction were also observed at this time, and pulmonary edema persisted for more than 1 week in three of the four individuals. Thus, the above cases suggest that depressed cardiac contractility can be a significant factor contributing to the development of NPE. It would seem, however, to play a greater role in situations in which the edema development is delayed or is persistent in nature.

In summary, the available clinical data indicates that NPE can develop rapidly after the initiating CNS disturbance and support Sarnoff and Sarnoff's (3) and Theodore and Robin's (75) hypothesis that NPE can develop due to severe pulmonary hypertension resulting from the translocation of blood from the systemic to the pulmonary circuit. In some cases, the edema may persist, possibly due either to an increase in lung vascular permeability or to cardiac dysfunction. These mechanisms might also be involved in explaining the delayed form of NPE that occurs in some patients.

III. Insight from Animal Models

Further insight into the mechanisms responsible for the development of NPE has been derived from the study of animal models in which the SNS can be centrally activated by either increasing intracranial pressure or by administering substances that massively activate the SNS (e.g., veratrine, sodium citrate, mixtures of thrombin and fibrinogen, tityustoxin, aconitine) to the intracranial cerebrospinal fluid. These stimuli produce a severe but transient episode of systemic and pulmonary hypertension and increases in lung water that mimic the events observed in humans who rapidly develop NPE after CNS injury. In particular, the veratrine model has been extensively studied, with the results suggesting that multiple mechanisms may be involved in the development of NPE.

A. Evidence for Hemodynamic Mechanisms

Systemic Arterial and Venous Vasoconstriction

Within minutes after intense SNS activation, severe systemic and pulmonary hypertension develops in most animals (3,99–110). A representative set of pressure tracings depicting these events in the dog after the intracisternal administration of veratrine is shown in Figure 1. The arterial hypertension results from arterial vasoconstriction, is accompanied by extreme increases in plasma catecholamine concentrations (92,111–114) (Fig. 2), and can be prevented or attenuated by α-adrenoceptor blockade (103,115), sympathetic ganglionic blockade (3), or spinal cord transection (100,101,115,116).

The pulmonary hypertension is characterized by extreme increases in both P_{pa} and P_{la}, with the pulmonary arteriovenous pressure gradient frequently becoming very small (Fig. 1). The pulmonary capillaries are thus exposed to very

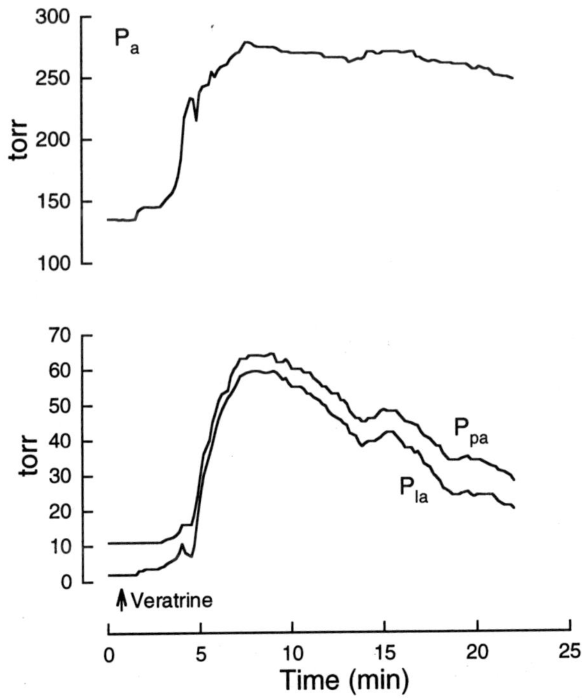

Figure 1 Rapid development of systemic and pulmonary hypertension after intracisternal veratrine administration in the dog. P_a, arterial pressure; P_{pa}, pulmonary arterial pressure; P_{la}, left atrial pressure.

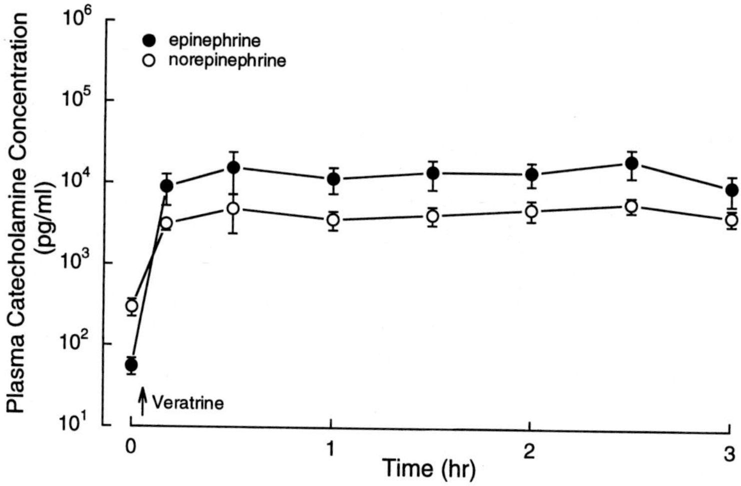

Figure 2 Plasma epinephrine and norepinephrine concentrations in dogs administered veratrine. (From Ref. 111.)

high pressures under these conditions, and edema can develop if the lungs' safety factors that normally prevent EVLW from increasing are overwhelmed. There appears to be general agreement that the increase in pulmonary capillary pressure results from a transient imbalance in right ventricular (RV) and LV outputs with the resultant translocation of a large quantity of blood from the systemic to the pulmonary circulation (3,102,106,117–121). The translocation hypothesis is supported by observations of increased in situ lung weight (120,122), central blood volume (103,104), and pulmonary blood volume (PBV) (105) during the episode of pulmonary hypertension. For example, Maron et al. (105) measured PBV by indicator dilution in dogs administered veratrine at a time when P_{pa} had started its recovery (39.2 torr) after having reached its peak value of 57.5 torr. At this time, PBV was increased an average 2.5 times above baseline values. Some animals exhibited much larger increases in PBV (Fig. 3), and it is possible that even larger increases might have been observed if the measurements could have been made earlier, when P_{pa} was at its peak value. This hemodynamic basis for the pulmonary edema prompted Sarnoff and Sarnoff (3) to suggest that the term "neurohemodynamic pulmonary edema" would be more appropriate than "neurogenic pulmonary edema" because it was more descriptive of the mechanism.

The possible component mechanisms that have been proposed to play a role in producing the transient imbalance in ventricular outputs are (1) an afterload-related decrease in LV output due to the development of intense arterial

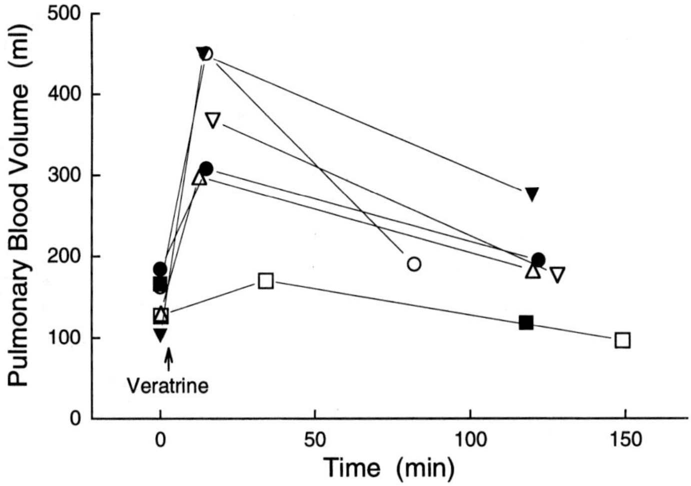

Figure 3 Pulmonary blood volume before and after veratrine administration. Different symbols represent different dogs. Symbols not connected by lines are from experiments with missing data points. (From Ref. 105.)

vasoconstriction, and (2) a transient augmentation of RV output due to constriction of systemic capacitance vessels which increases blood flow back to the right heart (3,106,117–119). A reduction in left ventricular output is considered to play a prominent role, and in this regard, a decrease in left ventricular function has been observed within minutes after the development of arterial hypertension (92). The relative contributions of the two pump outputs in producing the imbalance are not clear, however. Sarnoff and Berglund (118) considered both elements to be necessary for the development of severe pulmonary hypertension produced by thrombin and fibrinogen in the dog, and Novitsky et al. (106) found that the pulmonary vascular-left heart volume increased in baboons with acutely raised intracranial pressure due to a concurrent fall in aortic flow and an increase in pulmonary arterial flow. On the other hand, Chen et al. (102,120), in making the same flow measurements as Novitsky et al., concluded that only an increased LV afterload was critical in rats subjected to intense cerebral compression. Complicating this issue is that several other factors that may contribute to the ventricular imbalance have been identified. These include relative mitral valve insufficiency (due to extreme dilation of the left ventricle) (123), pulmonary venoconstriction (117), and a decrease in left ventricular diastolic compliance (100).

When the degree of pulmonary hypertension is severe, EVLW can increase dramatically within minutes, and edema fluid may suddenly appear in the airways (104,105,120,124). The time course and the magnitude of the increase in EVLW have been quantified by Maron et al. (105) in dogs administered veratrine. In their studies, EVLW was initially measured an average 5.6 to 11.2 min after P_{pa} had reached its highest value. Increases in EVLW were observed during this interval, but only in dogs in which P_{pa} had increased to levels >60 torr (Fig. 4). These results are noteworthy not only for the rapidity of the edema development, but also because they indicate that there is a threshold pressure that must be reached before edema is produced. At extreme pressures, EVLW increased by 200% in some animals in this short time period. Consistent with the rapid time course are earlier observations indicating that arterial hypoxemia, hypercapnia, and acidosis can develop within minutes after veratrine administration when severe edema is produced (99).

In general, the degree of edema has been found to be related to the magnitude of the hypertensive episode. For example, Maron (99) observed that the

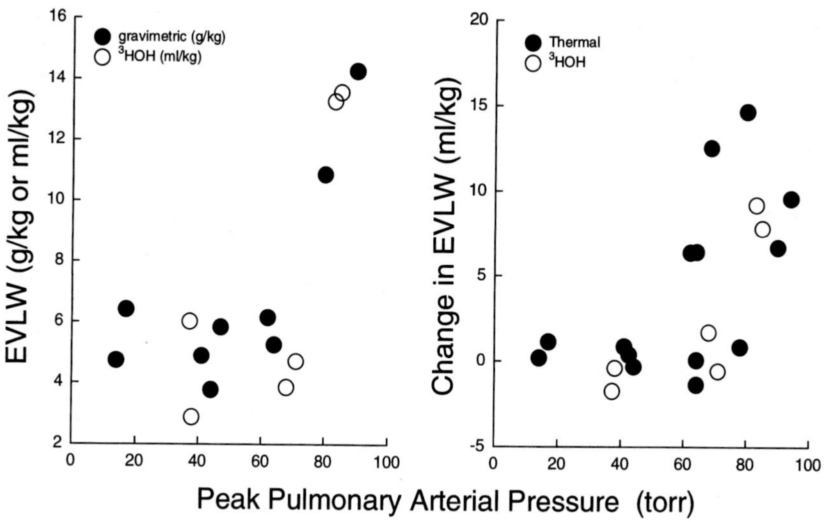

Figure 4 Relationship between EVLW and peak P_{pa} observed in dogs 5.6 to 11.2 min after P_{pa} had reached its highest value after veratrine administration. *Left*: EVLW determined gravimetrically or by indicator dilution using ^{125}I-human serum albumin (^{125}I-HSA) and ^{3}HOH as vascular and extravascular indicators. *Right*: Change in EVLW determined using thermal dye technique and by indicator dilution using ^{125}I-HSA and ^{3}HOH. EVLW is expressed as a change from baseline value for this analysis, because the absolute thermal dye EVLW value includes extravascular water from nonpulmonary sources. ^{125}I-HSA and ^{3}HOH data in both panels are from the same measurements. (From Ref. 105.)

edema was more severe in dogs that exhibited larger increases in P_{pa} (74.5 torr) and left ventricular end-diastolic pressure (P_{LVED}, 42.8 torr) than in animals that developed less hypertension (P_{pa}, 52.5 torr; P_{LVED} = 24.8 torr) (Table 2). Lung water was increased (over that observed in a group of control dogs) an average 122.8 g in the former animals, but only 14.7 g in the later group. Nevertheless, there appears to be considerable variability in the magnitude of the increase in EVLW that may occur even at high pressures. Whereas many dogs exhibit substantial increases in EVLW when P_{pa} rises to 60 to 80 torr, others exhibit little or no increase in EVLW (105) (Fig. 4). The reason for this variability is unknown but the degree to which the high pulmonary microvascular pressure increases protein permeability could contribute to some of the variability. In this regard, very large increases in pulmonary microvascular pressure (~ 80 torr) are required to produce decreases in the osmotic reflection coefficient (σ_d) of the canine lung, but not all lungs exhibit decreases in σ_d when pressures reach these levels (125,126). Lungs having an impaired ability to sustain a transcapillary oncotic pressure gradient would be expected to develop more edema during continued exposure to elevated pressures than uninjured lungs. Differences in the duration of the pulmonary hypertensive episode between animals and the ability to remove filtered fluid from the lung by lymphatic flow and other fluid clearance mechanisms may also contribute to the variability in EVLW accumulation.

In the two groups of animals discussed above that developed different degrees of pulmonary hypertension and edema, the increase in systemic arterial pressure was virtually identical (Table 2). Thus, an important question is, why

Table 2 Hemodynamic Responses of Dogs That Developed Alveolar or Interstitial Edema After Veratrine Administration

	Alveolar edema group		Interstitial edema group	
	Control	Veratrine	Control	Veratrine
EVLW	3.75 ± 0.09	7.30 ± 0.46	3.75 ± 0.09	4.45 ± 0.24
P_a	147 ± 5	273 ± 9	147 ± 7	268 ± 15
P_{cv}	1.2 ± 0.4	9.0 ± 1.7	0.7 ± 0.5	7.7 ± 1.6
P_{pa}	12.6 ± 1.3	74.5 ± 4.9	12.8 ± 1.2	52.5 ± 6.7
P_{lved}	4.2 ± 0.6	42.8 ± 4.5	3.2 ± 1.2	24.8 ± 4.0

EVLW, extravascular lung water content (g H_2O/g dry wt); P_a, P_{cv}, P_{pa}, P_{lved}, arterial, central venous, pulmonary arterial, and left ventricular end-diastolic pressures (torr). Values are means ± SE. Control and veratrine determinations are from the same animal, except in the case of EVLW where a separate control group was used. Alveolar edema group, n = 11; interstitial edema group, n = 6. *Source*: Ref. 99.

do some animals develop greater degrees of pulmonary hypertension (and consequently edema) than others when the increases in systemic arterial pressure are similar? The answer to this question is not known but presumably relates to differences in the degree to which the right and left ventricular outputs become imbalanced. Another unanswered question is how the increased pulmonary vascular pressures revert back to baseline values. To unload the lung of excess blood and restore normal pressure, LV output must transiently exceed RV output. This might occur during the time that the arterial pressure (and LV afterload) is returning to normal values.

In contrast to the explosive form of NPE discussed above, a more slowly developing variant has been found to occur in rats with lesions of the rostral hypothalamus or nucleus of the tractus solitarius (127,128). These lesions produce persistent arterial hypertension, and edema may eventually develop hours later due to heart failure. It is not clear, however, if this sequence of events can explain the delayed development of edema observed in some patients, because severe hypertension does not seem to develop in these individuals.

Catecholamine-Induced Left Ventricular Dysfunction

The ability of catecholamines to damage the heart was first reported nearly 100 years ago (129) and has since been confirmed numerous times. The damage is similar in many respects to that of myocardial infarction except that the injury is diffuse rather than localized. Typically, small areas of necrosis, interspersed between normal myocardium, are scattered throughout the left ventricle, especially in the subendocardium (130–136). The precise mechanism is still unresolved, but there is general agreement that the damage is due to excessive exposure to catecholamines. Myocardial damage identical to that produced by catecholamine administration has also been observed after injuries to the CNS that cause intense SNS activation (137–141). The question whether this degree of SNS activation might also diminish myocardial contractility has been addressed by Pilati et al. (92,94–96). They observed depressed LV contractility in rabbits after massive SNS activation with veratrine which did not occur if the animals were pretreated with α- or β-adrenoceptor antagonists (Fig. 5) (95). The latter observation suggests that SNS-induced cardiac dysfunction is also due to high concentrations of catecholamines. Findings consistent with those of Pilati et al. have also been observed in experimental brain death models in which the onset of brain death produces a massive SNS discharge that is soon followed by a marked depression in LV contractility (88,89,93,98,142).

Despite considerable effort, the mechanism by which catecholamines or intense SNS activation injure the heart has not been determined. Fleckenstein et al. (143) observed a sixfold increase in myocardial calcium uptake after administering isoproterenol to rats, and proposed that the histologic damage re-

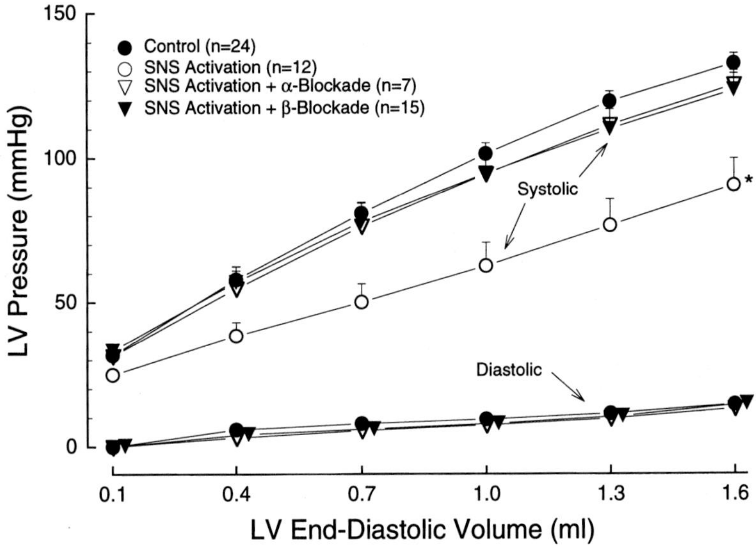

Figure 5 LV function of hearts isolated from rabbits 2.5 hours after massive SNS activation. LV function was significantly diminished by the intense SNS activity, but pretreatment with phentolamine or propranolol prevented the dysfunction. *Curve significantly different from control. (From Ref. 95.)

sulted from adrenoceptor-mediated calcium overload. However, the results from other laboratories indicate that myocardial ischemia might be the underlying mechanism (144–146). In this regard, Pilati and co-workers (95,147) reported that normal LV contractility was preserved if the hypertension or the tachycardia that normally accompanies massive SNS activation was not allowed to develop. Because both of these variables have pronounced effects on myocardial energy demand, myocardial O_2 supply/demand imbalance would seem to be at least partly responsible for SNS-induced depression of cardiac function.

Lang et al. (92) evaluated LV performance sequentially in intact anesthetized dogs after massively activating the SNS with veratrine, and found that cardiac function was diminished within 5 min after activating the SNS and remained depressed over a 3-hour period (Fig. 6). The extreme degree of hypertension that was present during the first 30 to 60 min probably played a major role in reducing function at this time, but the persistent impairment after this time could not be explained by a change in either preload or afterload and thus most likely resulted from a decrease in contractility. The impaired function was accompanied by elevated pulmonary vascular and LV filling pressures. These observations raise the possibility that a longlasting impairment in

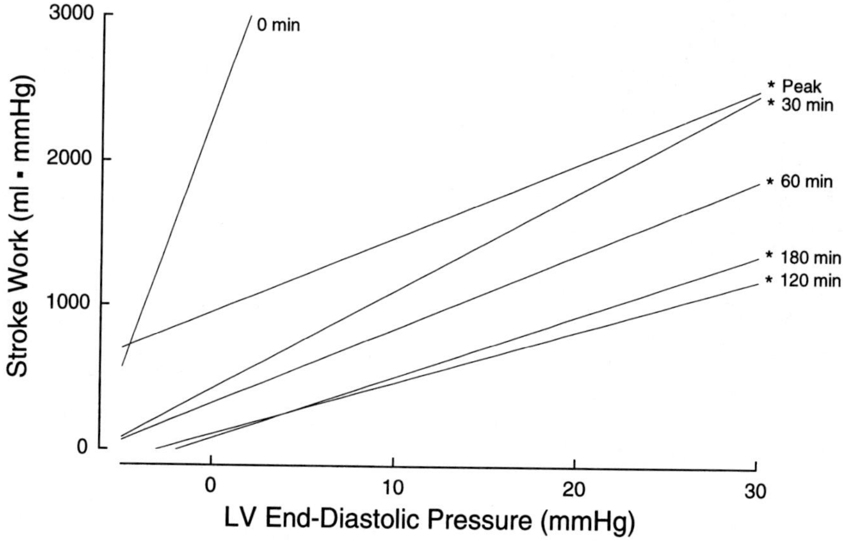

Figure 6 Temporal changes in LV function after massive SNS activation in intact dogs. Baseline LV function is labeled "0 min." "Peak" is the time when systemic and pulmonary vascular pressures had attained their highest values (~5 min after veratrine administration). *Curve significantly different from curve at 0 min. (From Ref. 92.)

myocardial contractility might allow edema to continue to develop over a prolonged period or play a role in producing the delayed edema observed in some patients.

Pulmonary Venoconstriction

The possibility that the centrally mediated massive SNS discharge is also directed to the pulmonary vasculature has been of considerable interest, but remains problematic. Controversy exists concerning both the nature of the vascular response (e.g., no response [148]), vascular resistance changes of varying magnitude and direction [121,149–156], and decreased vascular compliance [121,157] have all been reported for various central stimuli) and the possibility that circulating agents can account for some of the observed changes in vascular tone (149,150,153,156). In the dog, varying degrees of pulmonary vasoconstriction have been observed after massive central SNS activation (117,149–151,153,155) under conditions where the potential confounding effects of changes in cardiac output and left atrial pressure are eliminated. Both pulmonary arterial and venous resistances increase, with the preponderant effect being on the venous side of the circulation (117,150,153).

The increase in capillary pressure produced under these conditions, however, is generally small. It thus seems unlikely that this degree of increased pulmonary venous tone could contribute significantly to the development of NPE acutely when the pulmonary vasculature may be exposed to a far greater degree of passively induced hypertension. In fact, the increase in vascular resistance produced by pulmonary vasoconstriction after SNS activation is attenuated or abolished when vascular pressure is mechanically raised to levels observed during the development of NPE (121,149,153). Similarly, structures suggestive of sphincters in the pulmonary vein of the rat can be observed to appear to contract after head injury when the translocation of blood to the pulmonary circulation is prevented (158,159), but passive factors appear to play the predominant role in producing the pulmonary hypertension and edema observed in this species after head injury (120). These observations suggest that passive factors probably outweigh any actively mediated changes in pulmonary hemodynamics during the development of NPE. It is possible, however, that pulmonary venoconstriction might be significant over a longer time course if it is maintained and vascular permeability is increased. Finally, some investigators have suggested that a decrease in compliance of the pulmonary vasculature might increase the degree of hypertension that develops by passive mechanisms (120).

Is it possible that pulmonary venoconstriction might produce pulmonary edema under conditions where the degree of sympathetic activation is not of sufficient intensity to produce passive changes in pulmonary hemodynamics? If so, such a mechanism might explain the slow development of NPE that occurs in some patients with stable arterial blood pressures. Insight into this question has been provided by Simon and Bayne (160). They found that the elevation of intracranial pressure in sheep to levels equaling baseline arterial pressure (75 to 120 torr) produced only a modest increase in arterial pressure, but caused pulmonary arterial pressure to increase by 67% with no significant change in left atrial pressure. Pulmonary vascular resistance was thus increased, and pulmonary lymph flow doubled. These observations are compatible with the development of pulmonary venoconstriction. The critical question, however, whether such an increase in venous tone is sufficient to produce pulmonary edema, remains to be answered because EVLW was not measured.

Recent observations suggest that the lung may actively reduce its vascular resistance by the production of nitric oxide (NO) during massive SNS activation. In this regard, Pilati et al. (110) observed that rabbits pretreated with the NO inhibitor, N^{ω}-nitro-L-arginine (L-NNA), exhibited a significant increase in pulmonary vascular resistance after SNS activation, whereas this did not occur in nontreated animals. The L-NNA-treated animals also exhibited a greater reduction in cardiac output during this period and, interestingly, a lower frequency of pulmonary edema development. A possible explanation for these observations is that NO inhibition allowed pulmonary arteriolar resistance to markedly increase, diminishing output from the right ventricle, and thus reducing both the volume of blood translocated into the pulmonary circulation and the increase in capillary presssure.

B. Evidence for Increased Permeability Mechanisms

Pressure-Dependent Increases in Vascular Permeability

Theodore and Robin (75) proposed that the extreme increases in pulmonary capillary pressure that develop after massive SNS activation might damage the vasculature, thus leaving it with an increased protein permeability and an impaired ability to sustain a transvascular oncotic pressure gradient. The latter could allow edema to continue to accumulate at lower pressures after normal pulmonary vascular pressures are reattained, and might explain the prolonged or continued development of edema observed in some patients. This possibility has recently received considerable attention but remains an enigmatic problem, given experimental results suggesting that increased pressure might affect vascular permeability in different ways, with the exact result likely dependent on the degree of hypertension. In this regard, the results of several studies suggest that elevated vascular pressures might increase permeability by a reversible process ("stretched-pore" hypothesis), with normal permeability returning soon after pressure is normalized (161–163). West, Mathieu-Costello, and colleagues (164–169) have recently described what may be a more extreme state of pore stretching. They observed that capillary endothelial and alveolar epithelial layer disruptions developed at high capillary transmural pressures (Fig. 7) and that a substantial number of these breaks closed within 3 to 6 min after lowering capillary pressure. Some of the observed breaks were large enough to permit the egress of erythrocytes. This phenomenon has been termed "stress failure," because the calculated stresses on the capillary walls are very large. Finally, still higher pressures might damage the vasculature (170), with repair taking some longer period of time. It is thus conceivable that permeability might be increased by one or more of these mechanisms in a given patient, with the exact mechanism being dependent on the degree of pulmonary hypertension that develops. In the following paragraphs, we discuss the evidence supporting the hypothesis that pulmonary vascular pressures may rise to levels that increase vascular permeability in animals with NPE.

Studies of rat, rabbit, guinea pig, and cat models of NPE indicate that pulmonary vascular pressure may commonly rise to levels sufficient to disrupt the integrity of the alveolarcapillary barrier. In this regard, the production of airway fluid having a high protein concentration (2,107), lung hemorrhages (2,124,171–178), erythrocytes within alveoli or in edema fluid (2,107,108, 124,173,176,177,179–181), and discontinuities in the capillary endothelial

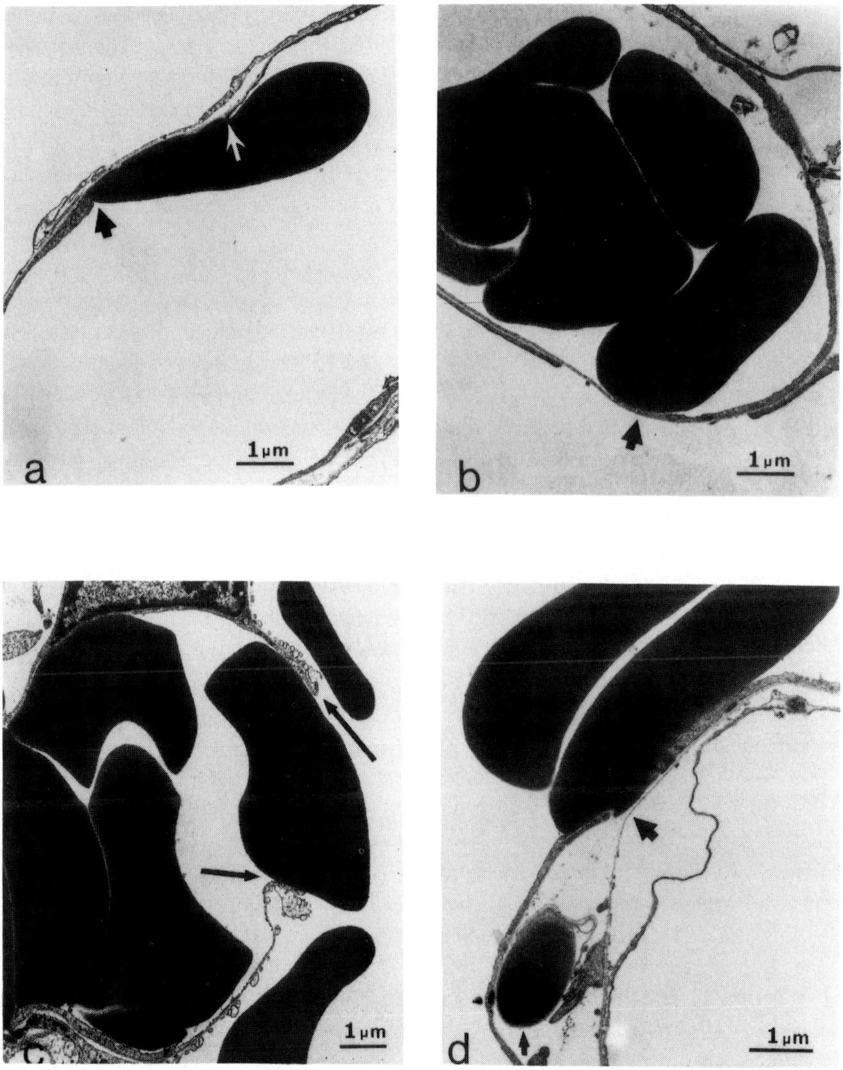

Figure 7 Electron micrographs showing ultrastructure of blood-gas barrier in rabbit lungs perfused at 52.5 (b and d) and 72.5 cm H_2O capillary transmural pressure (a and c). (a) Endothelial discontinuity (arrows) with an intact basement membrane and an adjacent erythrocyte (RBC). (b) Epithelial discontinuity. (c) Complete dislocation of blood-gas barrier with epithelial "blebbing" and with the RBC passing through the opening. (d) Endothelial discontinuity with RBC in close proximity, distension of epithelial layer, and increased interstitial space. Note the RBC in interstitium (small arrow). (From Ref. 165.)

(107,124,171,173,174,177) and alveolar epithelial lining (171,173,174,177) have been observed soon after the development of NPE in these species. The severity of these events appears to depend on the degree of pulmonary hypertension (108). There appear to be species differences, however. For example, Beckman (182) found that the rat is more susceptible to developing NPE after head injury than other species. In contrast, Ducker et al. (104) saw few erythrocytes in the edema fluid of chimpanzees that developed severe edema after intracranial pressure elevation.

Measurement of edema fluid protein concentration in dogs with veratrine-induced NPE (99,183) suggests that vascular protein permeability is increased in some, but not all, animals. In these experiments, edema fluid was collected soon after the development of edema, and the E/P ratios ranged from 0.48 to 0.93. This range is similar to that observed in humans with NPE (86). Since all of the animals developed severe pulmonary hypertension, the edema had at least a hydrostatic basis. Values in the upper end of the range suggest, however, that protein permeability had increased. In dogs in which the total protein E/P ratio was high, the E/P ratio was increased for each of four endogenous protein fractions having molecular radii ranging from 31 to 114 Å, with the smallest protein (albumin) becoming almost freely permeable (E/P = 0.93). In addition to these changes in protein permeability, the lungs removed from dogs with NPE may exhibit numerous petechiae (99), and eythrocytes may be present in the airway fluid (183). The hematocrit, however, has been found to be very small (average 2.6%), suggesting that the permeability defect was generally not large enough to allow significant numbers of erythrocytes to leave the blood (183).

Another approach used to address the question of increased permeability has been to mechanically elevate pulmonary vascular pressure to determine at what pressure macromolecules leave the vasculature and changes in membrane permeability coefficients or ultrastructure occur. In the dog lung, elevation of left atrial pressure to levels > 55 cm H_2O (40.5 torr) produces an increase in the microvascular filtration coefficient (K_f) (162,184,185) that may revert to normal after pressure is decreased (162,185). Additionally, hemoglobin has been observed to escape the canine pulmonary vasculature at pulmonary arterial pressures of > 50 torr with no apparent ultrastructural alterations (186). In the above studies, permeability was evaluated while the pressure was elevated. To determine if a transient episode of pulmonary hypertension (similar to that occurring during the development of NPE) leaves the vasculature with an impaired ability to sieve proteins, Maron (125) and Bosso et al. (126) measured the osmotic reflection coefficient for total proteins (σ_d) in both canine isolated perfused lung lobes and in situ lung lobes under baseline conditions and after pressure had been restored to normal after microvascular pressure had been transiently raised to values ranging from 9.8 to 103 torr. No reductions in σ_d were observed in lobes in which the peak microvascular pressure was < 80

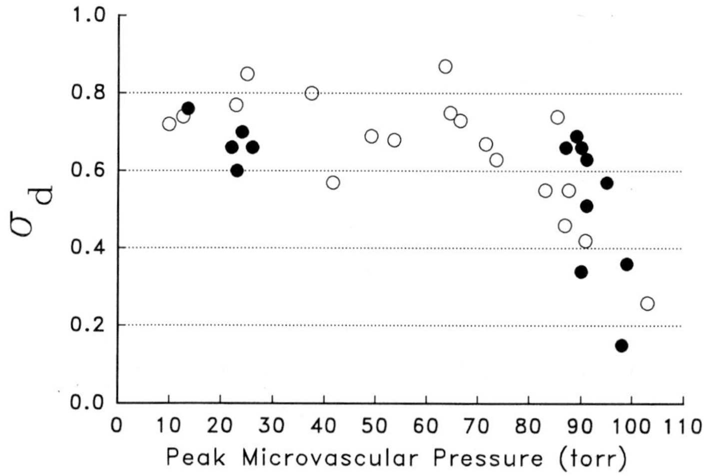

Figure 8 Effect of elevated microvascular pressure on osmotic reflection coefficient (σ_d). Open circles, σ_d determined by hematocrit-protein double indicator technique; closed circles, σ_d determined by lymph washdown. (From Ref. 126.)

torr (Fig. 8). At higher pressures, σ_d fell in relation to the magnitude of the pressure transient. The pressure interval between 80 and 90 torr appeared to be a critical level, however, because some lobes exhibited decreases in σ_d whereas others did not. In a subsequent study (187), transient elevation of capillary pressure to an average 86 torr left the lung lobes with significant decreases in σ_d and increases in K_f, but with no evidence for an increased incidence of capillary endothelial or alveolar epithelial breaks when the lung lobes were fixed for ultrastructural analysis at the same pressure that σ_d and K_f were determined. These data suggest that the increased water and protein leakage occurred through sites smaller than that which can be resolved by electron microscopy.

The above observations in dog lungs suggest that large increments in vascular pressure are required to increase permeability in this species and are also consistent with studies indicating that the sheep lung can be exposed to pulmonary microvascular or left atrial pressures of at least 40 torr with no evidence for an increased permeability (188–192). In contrast, Nicolaysen et al. (163) observed that abrupt increases in fluid filtration were observed at lower pressures (25 to 30 torr) in isolated rabbit lungs, with the increases sometimes being reversible when pressure was lowered. Additionally, Bachofen et al. (193) observed that the elevation of capillary transmural pressure to moderate levels

(~14 torr) for a period sufficient to produce edema in the isolated rabbit lung, resulted in the appearance of alveolar epithelial blebs when the lungs were fixed after pressure had been returned to normal. After exposure to higher capillary transmural pressures (~29 torr), frank disruptions of the epithelial barrier were observed. Taken together, these observations suggest that there may be species differences in susceptibility to pressure-induced increases in permeability. This issue has recently been clarified by studies of West, Mathieu-Costello, and colleagues (164,165,167–169), who found that the capillary pressure at which capillary stress failure develops is species-dependent. In this regard, the threshold for stress failure was found to be ~52 cm H_2O (39 torr) in the rabbit, 90 cm H_2O (67 torr) in the dog, and 130 cm H_20 (96 torr) in the horse. These differences have been found to correlate primarily with the thickness of the blood gas barrier.

In conclusion, the results of recent investigations have indicated that there are species differences in the strength of the blood gas barrier. The critical determinant for the development of an increased permeability in NPE is thus not the absolute increase in pulmonary capillary pressure that occurs, but rather the degree to which the developed pressure exceeds the threshold required to increase permeability. For example, pulmonary vascular pressures can rise during the development of NPE to levels that cause stress failure in the rabbit (107,109), but pressures of this magnitude (e.g., 40 torr) would be well tolerated in the horse. With respect to humans, critical questions relate to where in the continuum between the rabbit and horse does the strength of the human blood gas barrier lie, and does pulmonary capillary pressure rise during the development of NPE to levels that disrupt vascular integrity? Case study observations of pink edema fluid suggest that at least a mild degree of stress failure commonly occurs in humans with NPE, but the severity of the permeability defect generally does not seem to be as severe as that which develops in other species, such as the rat.

Finally, at this time, it is not possible to provide an unequivocal answer to Theodore and Robin's hypothesis that pulmonary capillary pressure might rise during the development of NPE to levels that damage the vasculature. A fundamental problem is that the ultrastructural appearance of the disrupted blood gas barrier caused by reversible stress failure looks like what one would expect to see if outright damage had occurred. A possible key to resolving this dilemma may be the condition of the basement membrane. In this regard, Elliot et al. (166) suggested that capillary endothelial and alveolar epithelial breaks produced by elevated pressure were more likely to close upon reduction of vascular pressure if the underlying basement membranes remained intact. It is thus possible that the integrity of the basement membrane might be a differentiating factor between a reversible increase in permeability and one that requires time to repair.

Pressure-Independent Increases in Permeability

The hypothesis that pulmonary vascular permeability might be increased in NPE by a mechanism unrelated to the development of pulmonary hypertension has been suggested by clinical observations of patients who appeared to develop edema without exhibiting significant changes in pulmonary vascular pressures. This remains a controversial question and is complicated in that in some cases, alternative mechanisms have been subsequently proposed to explain observations originally interpreted as due to an increased permeability. For example, Cameron and De (2) originally concluded that the edema produced by the intracisternal injection of a mixture of thrombin and fibrinogen in rabbits resulted from a pressure-independent increase in permeability even though no measurements of pulmonary vascular pressure were made. Bosso et al. (109) subsequently repeated Cameron and De's study, with the additional measurement of pulmonary arterial pressure, and observed that edema developed only if severe pulmonary hypertension occurred. The protein-rich edema fluid observed in some rabbits by both Cameron and De and Bosso et al. thus most likely resulted from a pressure-induced increase in permeability. Similarly, observations of increased lung lymph flow and lymphatic protein clearance in the absence of significant increases in pulmonary microvascular pressure in sheep with increased intracranial pressure (194,195) were also originally interpreted as due to an increase in permeability. Subsequent studies have suggested, however, that an increase in the vascular surface area available for the exchange of water and solutes might explain or contribute to the increased lymph flow and solute clearance (189,196,197). If, for the sake of argument, however, one does consider that the two- to threefold increase in lymph flow typically observed after intracranial pressure elevation in sheep did result from an increased permeability, the magnitude of the permeability defect had to be small, because either no increases (195) or only modest (24%) increases in EVLW (197) were found. The fact that EVLW does not increase substantially indicates that an increase in permeability of this magnitude, if it were to occur, is unlikely by itself to cause severe NPE. Finally, the induction of seizures in sheep produced a transient episode of severe pulmonary hypertension but an increase in lung lymph flow that was maintained for hours after normal pressures were reattained (116). The sustained increases in lymph flow in the presence of normal pulmonary vascular pressures could reflect either an increased permeability or surface area. Subsequent studies found, however, that the increased lymph flow was not due to a neurally or neurohumorally induced increase in vascular permeability, because prevention of the pulmonary hypertension eliminated the increase in lymph flow (198), and a similar pattern of increased lymph flow was observed after transient mechanical elevation of left atrial pressure (199).

There are observations, however, where increased permeability might explain increases in EVLW. For example, cats exposed to either low-level concussive brain trauma (200) or increased intracranial pressure (201) have been found to develop small increases (~14%) in EVLW even when pulmonary capillary pressure did not rise. Since a hemodynamic basis for the edema was not apparent, the increased lung water was considered to result from an increase in permeability. Additionally, McClellan et al. (202) found that the rate of extravasation of radiolabeled proteins increased threefold in dogs after a mild elevation of intracranial pressure, and that EVLW was elevated 36%. Since the increased protein leakage could not be duplicated by elevation of left atrial pressure, they interpreted the increased rate of protein extravasation and edema as being due to an increased protein permeability. These observations are intriguing, but further studies of these particular models would be helpful to more fully understand the mechanism of the edema formation.

If pulmonary vascular permeability can be increased by autonomic activation, what is the mechanism? Both neural (i.e., "permeability nerves") and humoral mechanisms have been postulated. With respect to the former, several investigators have examined the possibility that the sympathetic and parasympathetic innervation to the lungs might modulate permeability. In the sheep, stellate ganglion stimulation causes an increased lymph flow and protein clearance that resembles that which occurs after intracranial pressure elevation (203). These results were interpreted as being due to an increase in permeability, but as discussed above, increases in surface area might have also caused the observed changes (204). Ishikawa and colleagues (205) have reported evidence of increased vascular permeability after the sympathetic nerves of an isolated perfused rat lung preparation were stimulated. Further studies (206,207) suggested that the increased permeability may have been mediated by neuropeptide Y (NPY). It is not clear, however, whether the site of leakage is the pulmonary or the bronchial vasculature (205). In any event, the data suggest that the increase in permeability is most likely small. In this regard, sympathetic stimulation did not increase lung weight at physiological pressures (205), and NPY receptor blockade, although decreasing the airway/serum protein concentration ratio, did not decrease the amount of edema in rats in which NPE was produced by the intracisternal administration of thrombin and fibrinogen (207).

Bilateral vagus nerve stimulation in the guinea pig produces an increase in the rate of extravasation of labeled albumin from the pulmonary vasculature that is not mediated by adrenergic neural pathways, acetylcholine-mediated cholinergic pathways, or sensory peptides (208). The rate of leakage, however, was potentiated by β-adrenoceptor blockade and by nitric oxide synthase inhibition, suggesting that endogenous catecholamines and nitric oxide attenuate this response. Further study of this model would be interesting to completely rule out the possibility that pulmonary hemodyanamic changes do not contribute to the increased albumin extravasation and to determine if vagal stimulation also increases EVLW. These results are consistent with Cameron and De's (2) original observations that bilateral vagotomy prevented the development of NPE in rabbits produced by the intracisternal administration of thrombin and fibrinogen, but are difficult to reconcile with the results of more recent studies using the same means to massively activate the SNS in which vagotomy was found to either increase the degree or incidence of NPE (109,209).

Several investigators have examined the possibility that humoral mediators might increase vascular permeability in NPE, but at this time there is little definitive evidence to support this hypothesis. In this regard, neither epinephrine nor norepinephrine has been found to increase vascular protein permeability of the sheep lung by a mechanism independent of their hemodynamic effects (210). Moreover, changes in vascular protein permeability in the dog lung are no different after vascular pressure has been increased by massive SNS activation or by mechanical means (211), and the administration of oxidant scavengers to rats prior to cerebral compression does not alter the observed pattern of arterial hypertension and edema (212). These observations suggest that in the early stages of pulmonary edema any increase in vascular permeability that may occur after massive SNS activation can be explained by stress failure. On the other hand, Tsukimoto et al (213) found elevated leukotriene B_4 (LTB_4) concentrations in bronchioalveolar lavage fluid in isolated rabbit lungs exposed to large elevations in vascular pressure. No increase in LTB_4 was observed after exposure to smaller pressures. These observations indicated that inflammatory mediators may be produced when pressure rises sufficiently to produce stress failure, and suggest that the initial pressure-dependent increase in permeability might set the stage for the development of further increases in permeability mediated by other mechanisms.

In summary, although there has been considerable interest in the possibility that a pressure-independent increase in permeability contributes to the development of NPE, the significance of this mechanism remains unclear. The issue is complicated by more recent work suggesting that hemodynamic mechanisms, rather than an increase in permeability, may account for some of the earlier observations. In any event, the increases in EVLW that have been observed in these studies generally appear to be modest, suggesting that such an increase in permeability is unlikely to play the primary role in the initial rapid development of NPE. The identification of inflamatory mediators in pulmonary edema fluid after the development of severe hypertension, however, raises the possibility that these substances might play a role in the delayed form of edema or in its prolongation in some individuals.

C. Recovery from NPE

In patients who survive, the pulmonary edema appears to resolve relatively quickly. Recent studies have suggested that the rate of recovery may be accelerated by endogenous epinephrine. In this regard, excess water has been shown to be cleared from the alveolar spaces by a mechanism involving sodium transport across the alveolar epithelium (214). This process can be accelerated by the administration of β-adrenergic agonists, such as terbutaline and epinephrine (214,215) (see Chaps. 14 and 20). In the dog, extreme and prolonged increases in plasma epinephrine concentration develop in NPE produced by veratrine administration (92,111,112), and indicator dilution lung water measurements suggest that the pulmonary edema resolves relatively quickly (105). Recently, the rate of alveolar liquid reabsorption in this model of massive SNS activation has been found to be increased substantially over baseline rates (216,217). The increased fluid reabsorption could be reduced by pretreatment with either ICI 118,551 (a highly selective β_2-adrenoceptor antagonist) or amiloride (a sodium channel inhibitor) (217). Additionally, increases in alveolar liquid reabsorption of a similar magnitude can be produced by the infusion of epinephrine in doses calculated to reproduce the pattern of elevated plasma epinephrine concentrations that occurs after veratrine activation, and the increases can be reduced by the administration of ICI 118,551 (217). These observations suggest that the increased plasma catecholamine concentrations that may be in part responsible for the development of NPE may also play a role in its resolution.

Acknowledgments

Supported by National Heart, Lung and Blood Institute grant HL-56366, a grant from the American Heart Association Ohio Affiliate, and the Northeastern Ohio Universities College of Medicine. The authors thank Dr. Odile Mathieu-Costello for kindly providing Figure 7.

References

1. Demling R, Riessen R. Pulmonary dysfunction after cerebral injury. Crit Care Med 1990; 18:768–774.
2. Cameron GR, De SE. Experimental pulmonary oedema of nervous origin. J Pathol Bacteriol 1949; 61:375–387.
3. Sarnoff SJ, Sarnoff LC. Neurohemodynamics of pulmonary edema. II. The role of sympathetic pathways in the elevation of pulmonary and systemic vascular pressures following the intracisternal injection of fibrin. Circulation 1952; 6: 51–62.
4. Moutier F. Hypertension et mort par oedème pulmonaire aigu chez les blessés cranio-encéphalique (relation de ces faits aux recherches recentes sur les fonctions des capsules surrénales). Presse Med 1918; 26:108–109.
5. Cameron GR. Pulmonary oedema. Br Med J 1948; 1:965–972.

6. Ducker TB. Increased intracranial pressure and pulmonary edema. Part 1. Clinical study of 11 patients. J Neurosurg 1968; 28:112–117.
7. Simmons RL, Martin AM Jr, Heisterkamp CA III, Ducker TB. Respiratory insufficiency in combat casualties. II. Pulmonary edema following head injury. Ann Surg 1969; 170:39–44.
8. Ducker TB, Simmons RL, Martin AM Jr. Pulmonary edema as a complication of intracranial disease. Am J Dis Child 1969; 118:638–664.
9. Felman AH. Neurogenic pulmonary edema. Observations in 6 patients. Am J Roentgenol Radiat Ther Nucl Med 1971; 112:393–396.
10. James HE, Tsueda K, Wright B, Young AB, McClosky J. The effect of positive end-expiratory pressure (PEEP) ventilation in neurogenic pulmonary oedema. Report of a case. Acta Neurochir 1978; 43:275–280.
11. Milley JR, Nugent SY, Rogers MC. Neurogenic pulmonary edema in childhood. J Pediatr 1979; 94:706–709.
12. Loughan PM, Brown TCK, Edis E, Klug GL. Neurogenic pulmonary oedema in man: aetiology and management with vasodilators based on haemodynamic studies. Anaes Intens Care 1980; 8:65–71.
13. Lagerkranser M, Pehrsson K, Sylvén C. Neurogenic pulmonary oedema. A review of the pathophysiology with clinical and therapeutic implications. Acta Med Scand 1982; 212:267–271.
14. Kushner J, Holschub K. Insidious development of neurogenic pulmonary edema in a child. Md State Med J 1982; 31:58–60.
15. Eggleston CA. Clinical correlation of neurogenic pulmonary edema to increased intracranial pressure. J Neurosurg Nurs 1982; 14:245–254.
16. Casey WF. Neurogenic pulmonary oedema. Anaesthesia 1983; 38:985–988.
17. Wohns RN, Tamas L, Pierce KR, Howe JF. Chlorpromazine treatment for neurogenic pulmonary edema. Crit Care Med 1985; 13:210–211.
18. Pender ES, Pollack CV Jr. Neurogenic pulmonary edema: case reports and review. J Emerg Med 1992; 10:45–51.
19. Locke CF, Sing RF, Sing RF. Neurogenic pulmonary edema. JAOA 1993; 93: 382–384.
20. Rogers FB, Shackford SR, Trevisani GT, Davis JW, Mackersie RC, Hoyt DB. Neurogenic pulmonary edema in fatal and nonfatal head injuries. J Trauma: Injury Infect Crit Care 1995; 39:860–866.
21. Weisman SJ. Edema and congestion of the lungs resulting from intracranial hemorrhage. Surgery 1939; 6:722–729.
22. Wray NP, Nicotra MB. Pathogenesis of neurogenic pulmonary edema. Am Rev Respir Dis 1978; 118:783–786.
23. Carlson RW, Schaeffer RC Jr, Michaels SG, Weil MH. Pulmonary edema following intracranial hemorrhage. Chest 1979; 75:731–734.
24. Yabumoto M, Kuriyama T, Iwamoto M, Kinoshita T. Neurogenic pulmonary edema associated with ruptured intracranial aneurysm: case report. Neurosurgery 1986; 19:300–304.
25. Hammermeister KE, Reichenbach DD. QRS changes, pulmonary edema, and myocardial necrosis associated with subarachnoid hemorrhage. Am Heart J 1969; 78:94–100.

26. Ciongoli AK, Poser CM. Pulmonary edema secondary to subarachnoid hemorrhage. Neurology 1972; 22:867–870.
27. Weir BK. Pulmonary edema following fatal aneurysm rupture. J Neurosurg 1978; 49:502–507.
28. Fisher A, Aboul-Nasr HT. Delayed nonfatal pulmonary edema following subarachnoid hemorrhage. J Neurosurg 1979; 51:856–859.
29. Fein IA, Racknow EC. Neurogenic pulmonary edema. Chest 1982; 81:318–320.
30. Schell AR, Shenoy MM, Friedman SA, Patel AR. Pulmonary edema associated with subarachnoid hemorrhage. Evidence for a cardiogenic mechanism. Ann Intern Med 1987; 147:591–592.
31. Knudsen F, Jensen HP, Peterson PL. Neurogenic pulmonary edema: treatment with dobutamine. Neurosurgery 1991; 29:269–270.
32. Mayer SA, Fink ME, Homma S, Sherman D, LiMandri G, Lennihan L, Solomon RA, Klebanoff LM, Beckford A, Raps EC. Cardiac injury associated with neurogenic pulmonary edema following subarachnoid hemorrhage. Neurology 1994; 44:815–820.
33. Harari AS, Rapin M, Regnier B, Comoy J, Caron JP. Normal pulmonary-capillary pressures in the late phase of neurogenic pulmonary oedema. Lancet 1976; 1:494. Letter.
34. Yamour BJ, Sridharan MR, Rice JF, Flowers NC. Electrocardiographic changes in cerebrovascular hemorrhage. Am Heart J 1980; 99:294–300.
35. Cohen JA, Abraham E. Neurogenic pulmonary edema: a sequella of nonhemorrhagic cerebrovascular accidents. Angiology 1976; 27:280–292.
36. Findler G, Cotev S. Neurogenic pulmonary edema associated with a colloid cyst in the third ventricle. J Neurosurg 1980; 52:395–398.
37. Poe RH, Reisman JL, Rodenhouse TG. Pulmonary edema in cervical spinal cord injury. J Trauma 1978; 18:71–73.
38. Lee DS, Kobrine A. Neurogenic pulmonary edema associated with ruptured spinal cord arteriovenous malformation. Neurosurgery 1983; 12:691–693.
39. Shanahan WI. Acute pulmonary edema as a complication of epileptic seizures. NY State J Med 1908; 87:54–56.
40. Ohlmacher AP. Acute pulmonary oedema as a terminal event in certain forms of epilepsy. Am J Med Sci 1910; 139:417–422.
41. Bonbrest HC. Pulmonary edema following an epileptic seizure. Am Rev Respir Dis 1965; 91:97–100.
42. Huff RW, Fred HL. Postictal pulmonary edema. Arch Intern Med 1966; 117: 824–828.
43. Chang CH, Smith CA. Postictal pulmonary edema. Radiology 1967; 89:1087–1089.
44. Bloom S. Pulmonary edema following a grand mal epileptic seizure. Am Rev Respir Dis 1968; 97:292–294.
45. Greene R, Platt R, Matz R. Postictal pulmonary edema. NY State J Med 1975; 75:1257–1261.
46. Sarkar TK, Munshi AT. Postictal pulmonary edema. Postgrad Med 1977; 61: 281–285.

47. Archibald RB, Armstrong JD Jr. Recurrent postictal pulmonary edema. Postgrad Med 1978; 63:210–213.
48. Terrence CF, Rao GR, Perper JA. Neurogenic pulmonary edema in unexpected, unexplained death of epileptic patients. Ann Neurol 1981; 9:458–464.
49. Buisseret P. Acute pulmonary oedema following grand mal epilepsy and as a complication of electric shock therapy. Br J Dis Chest 1982; 76:194–198.
50. Darnell JC, Jay SJ. Recurrent postictal pulmonary edema: a case report and review of the literature. Epilepsia 1982; 23:71–83.
51. Mandel S, Paschall R. Anticonvulsants and neurogenic pulmonary edema. Am Fam Physician 1983; 28:167–169.
52. Mulroy JJ, Mickell JJ, Tong TK, Pellock JM. Postictal pulmonary edema in children. Neurology 1985; 35:403–405.
53. Colice GL. Neurogenic pulmonary edema. Clin Chest Med 1985; 6:473–489.
54. Fredberg U, Bøtker HE, Rømer FK. Acute neurogenic pulmonary oedema following generalized tonic clonic seizure. A case report and a review of the literature. Eur Heart J 1988; 9:933–936.
55. Bekemeyer WB, Pinstein ML. Neurogenic pulmonary edema: new concepts of an old disorder. South Med J 1989; 82:380–383.
56. Baker AB. Poliomyelitis. A study of pulmonary edema. Neurology 1957; 7: 743–751.
57. Schlesinger B. Neurogenic pulmonary edema, due to puncture wound of medulla oblongata. J Nerv Ment Dis 1945; 102:247–255.
58. Brown RH, Beyerl BD, Iseke R, Lavyne MH. Medulla oblongata edema associated with neurogenic pulmonary edema. Case report. J Neurosurg 1986; 64:494–500.
59. Simon RP, Gean-Marton AD, Sander JE. Medullary lesion inducing pulmonary edema: a magnetic resonance imaging study. Ann Neurol 1991; 30:727–730.
60. Thompson GE. Pulmonary edema complicating intrathecal hypertonic saline injection for intractable pain. Anesthesiology 1971; 35:425–427.
61. Rittenhouse EA, Merendino KA. Acute pulmonary edema in the absence of left ventricular failure. Circulation 1969; 40:823–827.
62. Wright RS, Feuerman T, Brown J. Neurogenic pulmonary edema after trigeminal nerve blockade. Chest 1989; 96:436–438.
63. Waters HR, Gooding MR. Pulmonary oedema following vertebral artery ligation. Anaesthesia 1972; 27:450–453.
64. Pollack CV Jr, Pollack ES. Neurogenic pulmonary edema. J Emerg Med 1993; 11:207–210.
65. Melon E, Bonnet F, Lepresele E, Ferrier MJ, Djindjian M, François Y, Gray F, Debras C. Altered capillary permeability in neurogenic pulmonary edema. Intens Care Med 1985; 11:323–325.
66. Reines HD, Dill L, Saad S, Hungerford GD. Neurogenic pulmonary edema and missle emboli. J Trauma 1980; 20:698–701.
67. Bredin CP. Speculations on neurogenic pulmonary edema (NPE). Am Rev Resp Dis 1976; 114:814–815. Letter.
68. Lansky LL, Linn R, Mathewson HS, Morantz RA, Brachett CE, Bone RC. Neurogenic pulmonary edema and intracranial pressure monitoring in severe Reyes syndrome. Ann Neurol 1978; 4:191. Abstract.

69. Richards P. Pulmonary oedema and intracranial lesions. Br Med J 1963; 2:83–86.
70. Crompton MR. The pathogenesis of cerebral infarction following rupture of cerebral berry aneurysms. Brain 1964; 87:491–510.
71. Iliff LD. Extra-alveolar vessels and edema development in excised dog lungs. Circ Res 1971; 28:524–532.
72. Mackersie RC, Christensen JM, Pitts LH, Lewis FR. Pulmonary extravascular fluid accumulation following intracranial injury. J Trauma 1983; 23:968–975.
73. Singbartl G. Kardio-zirkulatorische und pulmonale Veränderungen bei Patienten mit isolierter zerebraler Läsion. Anaesthesist 1989; 38:360–374.
74. Touho H, Karasawa J, Shishido H, Yamada K, Yamazaki Y. Neurogenic pulmonary edema in the acute stage of hemorrhagic cerebrovascular disease. Neurosurg 1989; 25:762–768.
75. Theodore J, Robin ED. Speculations on neurogenic pulmonary edema (NPE). Am Rev Respir Dis 1976; 113:405–411.
76. Cruickshank JM, Neil-Dwyer G, Stott AW. Possible role of catecholamines, corticosteroids, and potassium in production of electrocardiographic abnormalities associated with subarachnoid haemorrhage. Br Heart J 1974; 36:697–706.
77. Myers MG, Norris JW, Hachinski VC, Sole MJ. Plasma norepinephrine in stroke. Stroke 1981; 12:200–204.
78. Benedict CR, Loach AB. Sympathetic nervous system activity in patients with subarachnoid hemorrhage. Stroke 1978; 9:237–244.
79. Clifton GL, Ziegler MG, Grossman RG. Circulating catecholamines and sympathetic activity after head injury. Neurosurg 1981; 8:10–13.
80. Benedict CR, Loach AB. Clinical significance of plasma adrenaline and noradrenaline concentrations in patients with subarachnoid haemorrhage. J Neurol Neurosurg Psych 1978; 41:113–117.
81. Simon RP, Aminoff MJ, Benowitz NL. Changes in plasma catecholamines after tonic-clonic seizures. Neurology 1984; 34:255–257.
82. White PT, Grant P, Mosier J, Craig A. Changes in cerebral dynamics associated with seizures. Neurology 1961; 11:354–361.
83. Harari A, Rapin M, Comoy J, Caron JP. Etude hémodynamique de trois cas d'oedèmes aigus pulmonaires après interventions neurochirurgicales. Rev Neurol 1974; 130:349–356.
84. Fein A, Grossman RF, Jones JG, Overland E, Pitts L, Murray JF, Staub NC. The value of edema fluid protein measurement in patients with pulmonary edema. Am J Med 1979; 67:32–38.
85. Sprung CL, Rackow EC, Fein IA, Jacob AI, Isikoff SK. The spectrum of pulmonary edema: differentiation of cardiogenic, intermediate, and noncardiogenic forms of pulmonary edema. Am Rev Respir Dis 1981; 124:718–722.
86. Smith WS, Matthay MA. Evidence for a hydrostatic mechanism in human neurogenic pulmonary edema. Chest 1997; 111:1326–1333.
87. Matthay MA. Resolution of pulmonary edema—new insights. West J Med 1991; 154:315–321.
88. Bittner HB, Chen EB, Milano CA, Kendell SWH, Jennings RB, Sabiston DC, Van Trigt P. Myocardial β-adrenergic receptor function and high-energy phosphates in brain death-related cardiac dysfunction. Circulation 1995; 92(suppl II): II472–II478.

89. D'Amico TA, Buchanan SA, Lucke JC, Koutlas TC, Soto PF, Gall SA, Van Trigt P. The preservation of cardiac function after brain death: a myocardial pressure-dimension analysis. Surg Forum 1990; 41:277–279.
90. Handlin LR, Kindred LH, Beauchamp GD, Vacek JL, Rowe SK. Reversible left ventricular dysfunction after subarachnoid hemorrhage. Am Heart J 1993; 126: 235–240.
91. Kono T, Morita H, Kuroiwa T, Onaka H, Takatsuka H, Fujiwara A. Left ventricular wall motion abnormalities in patients with subarachnoid hemorrhage: neurogenic stunned myocardium. J Am Coll Cardiol 1994; 24:636–640.
92. Lang SA, Maron MB, Bosso FJ, Pilati CF. Temporal changes in left ventricular function after massive sympathetic nervous system activation. Can J Physiol Pharmacol 1994; 72:693–700.
93. Meyers CH, D'Amico TA, Peterseim DS, Jayawant AM, Steenbergen C, Sabiston DC, Van Trigt P. Effects of triiodothyronine and vasopressin on cardiac function and myocardial blood flow after brain death. J Heart Lung Transplant 1993; 12: 68–80.
94. Pilati CF, Clark RS, Gilloteaux J, Bosso FJ, Holcomb P, Maron MB. Excessive sympathetic nervous system activity decreases myocardial contractility. Proc Soc Exp Biol Med 1990; 193:225–231.
95. Pilati CF, Bosso FJ, Maron MB. Factors involved in left ventricular dysfunction after massive sympathetic activation. Am J Physiol 1992; 263:H784–H791.
96. Pilati CF, Maron MB, Bosso FJ. Role of EDRF in the cardiopulmonary dysfunction produced by massive sympathetic activation. J Appl Physiol 1995; 78: 1642–1650.
97. Pollick C, Cujec B, Parker S, Tator C. Left ventricular wall motion abnormalities in subarachnoid hemorrhage: an echocardiographic study. J Am Coll Cardiol 1988; 12:600–605.
98. Shivalkar B, Van Loon J, Wieland W, Tjandra-Maga TB, Borgers M, Plets C, Flameng W. Variable effects of explosive or gradual increase in intracranial pressure on myocardial structure and function. Circulation 1993; 87:230–239.
99. Maron MB. A canine model of neurogenic pulmonary edema. J Appl Physiol 1985; 59:1019–1025.
100. Luisada AA. Mechanisms of intracisternal vertatrine pulmonary edema. Dis Chest 1969; 55:45–48.
101. Ducker TB, Simmons RL. Increased intracranial pressure and pulmonary edema. Part 2. The hemodynamic responses of dogs and monkeys to increased intracranial pressure. J Neurosurg 1968; 28:118–123.
102. Chen HI, Lin JD, Liao JF. Participation of regional sympathetic outflows in the centrogenic pulmonary pathology. Am J Physiol 1981; 240:H109–H115.
103. Brashear RE, Ross JC. Hemodynamic effects of elevated cerebrospinal fluid pressure: alterations with adrenergic blockade. J Clin Invest 1970; 49:1324–1333.
104. Ducker TB, Simmons RL, Anderson RW. Increased intracranial pressure and pulmonary edema. Part 3. The effect of increased intracranial pressure on the cardiovascular hemodynamics of chimpanzees. 1968; 29:475–483.
105. Maron MB, Holcomb PH, Dawson CA, Rickaby DA, Clough AV, Linehan JH. Edema development and recovery in neurogenic pulmonary edema. J Appl Physiol 1994; 77:1155–1163.

106. Novitsky D, Wicomb WN, Rose AG, Cooper DKC, Reichart B. Pathophysiology of pulmonary edema following experimental brain death in the Chacma baboon. Ann Thorac Surg 1987; 43:288–294.
107. Minnear FL, Kite C, Hill LA, van der Zee H. Endothelial injury and pulmonary congestion characterize neurogenic pulmonary edema in rabbits. J Appl Physiol 1987; 63:335–341.
108. Chen HI, Chai CY. Pulmonary edema and hemorrhage as a consequence of systemic vasoconstriction. Am J Physiol 1974; 227:144–151.
109. Bosso FJ, Lang SA, Maron MB. Role of hemodynamics and vagus nerves in development of fibrin-induced pulmonary edema. J Appl Physiol 1990; 69: 2227–2232.
110. Pilati CF, Maron MB, Bosso FJ. Role of EDRF in the cardiopulmonary dysfunction produced by massive sympathetic activation. J Appl Physiol 1995; 78: 1642–1650.
111. Lang SA, Maron MB, Signs SA. Oxygen consumption after massive sympathetic nervous system discharge. Am J Physiol 1989; 256:E345–E351.
112. Maron MB. Pulmonary vasoconstriction in a canine model of neurogenic pulmonary edema. J Appl Physiol 1990; 68:912–918.
113. Graf CJ, Rossi NP. Catecholamine response to intracranial hypertension. J Neurosurg 1978; 49:862–868.
114. Benowitz NL, Simon RP, Copeland JR. Status epilepticus: Divergence of sympathetic activity and cardiovascular response. Ann Neurol 1986; 19:197–199.
115. Cicardo VH. Arterial hypertension by veratrum derivates injected into the nervous centres. Arch Int Pharmacodyn Ther 1953; 94:65–74.
116. Simon RP, Bayne LL, Tranbaugh RF, Lewis FR. Elevated pulmonary lymph flow and protein content during status epilepticus in sheep. J Appl Physiol 1982; 52: 91–95.
117. Aravanis C, Libretti A, Jona E, Liu, CK, Luisada AA. Pulmonary reflexes in pulmonary edema? Am J Physiol 1957; 189:132–136.
118. Sarnoff SJ, Berglund E. Neurohemodynamics of pulmonary edema. IV. Effect of systemic vasoconstriction and subsequent vasodilation on flow and pressures in systemic and pulmonary vascular beds. Am J Physiol 1952; 170:588–600.
119. Stein P, MacAnespie CL, Rothe CF. Total body vascular capacitance changes during high intracranial pressure in dogs. Am J Physiol 1983; 245:H947–H956.
120. Chen HI, Liao JF, Kuo L, Ho ST. Centrogenic pulmonary hemorrhagic edema induced by cerebral compression in rats. Mechanism of volume and pressure loading in the pulmonary circulation. Circ Res 1980; 47:366–373.
121. Chen HI, Wang DJ. Systemic and pulmonary hemodynamic responses to intracranial hypertension. Am J Physiol 1984; 247:H715–H721.
122. Sarnoff SJ, Berglund E, Sarnoff LC. Neurohemodynamics of pulmonary edema. III. Estimated changes in pulmonary blood volume accompanying systemic vasoconstriction and vasodilation. J Appl Physiol 1953; 5:367–374.
123. Jacono A, Kaplan M, Luisada AA. Relative mitral insufficiency as a factor of paroxysmal pulmonary edema. Cardiologica 1961; 39:1–11.
124. Chen HI, Sun SC, Chai CY. Pulmonary edema and hemorrhage resulting from cerebral compression. Am J Physiol 1973; 224:223–229.

125. Maron MB. Effect of elevated vascular pressure transients on protein permeability in the lung. J Appl Physiol 1989; 67:305–310.
126. Bosso FJ, Maron MB, Pilati CF, Jarjoura DG. Pulmonary vascular protein sieving capability after exposure to high vascular pressures. J Appl Physiol 1992; 73: 50–58.
127. Doba N, Reis DJ. Acute fulminating neurogenic hypertension produced by brainstem lesions in the rat. Circ Res 1973; 32:584–593.
128. Nathan MA, Reis DJ. Fulminating arterial hypertension with pulmonary edema from release of adrenalmedullary catecholamines after lesions of the anterior hypothalamus in the rat. Circ Res 1975; 37:226–235.
129. Ziegler K. Uber die Wirkung intervenoser Adrenalininjektion auf das Gefasssystem und ihre Beziehung zur Arteriosklerose. Ziegler's Beitrage 1905; 38:229–254.
130. Szakacs JE, Cannon A. L-Norepinephrine myocarditis. Am J Clin Pathol 1958; 30:425–434.
131. Rona G, Chappel CI, Balazs T, Gaudry R. An infarct-like myocardial lesion and other toxic manifestations produced by isoproterenol in the rat. AMA Arch Pathol 1959; 67:443–455.
132. Haft JI. Cardiovascular injury induced by sympathetic catecholamines. Prog Cardiovasc Dis 1974; 17:73–86.
133. Milei J, Nunez RG, Rapaport M. Pathogenesis of isoproterenol-induced lesions: its relation to human 'coagulative myocytolysis'. Cardiol 1978; 63:139–151.
134. Todd GL, Baroldi G, Pieper GM, Clayton FC, Eliot RS. Experimental catecholamine-induced myocardial necrosis. II. Temporal development of isoproterenol-induced contraction band lesions correlated with ECG, hemodynamic, and biochemical changes. J Mol Cell Cardiol 1985; 17:647–656.
135. Khullar M, Datta BN, Wahi PL, Chakravarti RN. Catecholamine-induced experimental cardiomyopathy—a histopathological, histochemical and ultrastructural study. Ind Heart J 1989; 41:307–313.
136. Veprek P, Batra S, Korecky B, Raklusan K. Isoproterenol induced rat endomyocardial damage in relationship to local capillary geometry. Basic Res Cardiol 1991; 86:434–440.
137. Hunt D, Gore I. Myocardial lesions following experimental intracranial hemorrhage: prevention with propranolol. Am Heart J 1972; 83:232–236.
138. Neil-Dwyer G, Walter P, Cruickshank JM, Doshi B, O'Gorman P. Effect of propranolol and phentolamine on myocardial necrosis after subarachnoid haemorrhage. Br Med J 1978; 2:990–992.
139. Kolin A, Norris JW. Myocardial damage from acute cerebral lesions. Stroke 1984; 15:990–993.
140. Hachinski VC, Smith KE, Silver MD, Gibson CJ, Ciriello J. Acute myocardial and plasma catecholamine changes in experimental stroke. Stroke 1986; 17:387–390.
141. Shanlin RJ, Sole MJ, Rahimifar M, Tator CH, Factor SM. Increased intracranial pressure elicits hypertension, increased sympathetic activity, electrocardiographic abnormalities and myocardial damage in rats. J Am Coll Cardiol 1988; 12: 727–736.

142. Bittner HB, Kendall SWH, Campbell KA, Montine TJ, Van Trigt P. A valid experimental brain death organ donor model. J Heart Lung Transplant 1995; 14: 308–317.
143. Fleckenstein A, Janke J, Doring HJ, Pachinger O. Ca overload as the determinant factor in the production of catecholamine-induced myocardial lesions. In: Bajusz E, Rona G, Brink AJ, Lochner A, eds. Recent Advances in Studies on Cardiac Structure and Metabolism. Baltimore: University Park Press, 1973:455–466.
144. Lehr D. Studies on the cardiotoxicity of α- and β-adrenergic amines. In: Balazs T, ed. Cardiac Toxicology. Boca Raton: CRC Press, 1981:75–112.
145. Rona G, Kahn DS, Chappel CI. Studies on infarct-like myocardial necrosis produced by isoproterenol: a review. Rev Can Biol 1963; 22:241–255.
146. Rona G, Boutet M, Huttner I, Peters H. Pathogenesis of isoproterenol-induced myocardial alterations: functional and morphological correlates. In: Dhalla NS, ed. Recent Advances in Studies on Cardiac Structure and Metabolism. Baltimore: University Park Press, 1972:507–525.
147. Bosso FJ, Allman FD, Pilati CF. Myocardial work load is a major determinant of norepinephrine-induced left ventricular dysfunction. Am J Physiol 1994; 266: H531–H539.
148. Maron MB, Hakim TS, Dawson CA. Pulmonary hemodynamic responses to elevated cerebral spinal fluid pressure in the dog. J Appl Physiol 1979; 46:84–88.
149. Maron MB, Dawson CA. Adrenal component to pulmonary hypertension induced by elevated cerebrospinal fluid pressure. J Appl Physiol 1979; 47:153–160.
150. Maron MB, Dawson CA. Pulmonary venoconstriction caused by elevated cerebrospinal fluid pressure in the dog. J Appl Physiol 1980; 49:73–78.
151. Lloyd TC Jr. Effect of increased intracranial pressure on pulmonary vascular resistance. J Appl Physiol 1973; 35:332–335.
152. Hessler JR, Cassin S. Effects of increased intracranial pressure on pulmonary vascular resistance of fetal and neonatal goats. Am J Physiol 1977; 232:H671–H675.
153. Maron MB. Pulmonary vasoconstriction in a canine model of neurogenic pulmonary edema. J Appl Physiol 1990; 68:912–918.
154. Anderson FL, Brown AM. Pulmonary vasoconstriction elicited by stimulation of the hypothalamic integrative area for the defense reaction. Circ Res 1967; 21: 747–756.
155. Chen HI, Wang YC, Chai CY. The Cushing responses in the systemic and pulmonary circulation: the role of adrenal glands, bronchial circulation and pulmonary innervation. Chin J Physiol 1987; 30:29–43.
156. Hyman AL, Dempsey CW, Fontana C, Richardson DE, Rieck RW, Kadowitz PJ. Pulmonary vascular responses to forebrain stimulation in the cat. Circ Res 1988; 63:492–501.
157. Szidon JP, Fishman AP. Participation of pulmonary circulation in the defense reaction. Am J Physiol 1971; 220:364–370.
158. Schraufnagel DE, Patel KR. Sphincters in pulmonary veins. An anatomic study in rats. Am Rev Respir Dis 1990; 141:721–726.
159. Schraufnagel DE, Thakkar MB. Pulmonary venous sphincter constriction is attenuated by alpha-adrenergic antagonism. Am Rev Respir Dis. 1993; 148:477–482.

160. Simon RP, Bayne LL. Pulmonary lymphatic flow alterations during intracranial hypertension in sheep. Ann Neurol 1984; 15:188–194.
161. Shirley HH Jr, Wolfram CC, Wasserman K, Mayerson HS. Capillary permeability to macromolecules: stretched pore phenomenon. Am J Physiol 1957; 190: 189–193.
162. Rippe B, Townsley M, Thigpen J, Parker JC, Korthuis RJ, Taylor AE. Effects of vascular pressure on the pulmonary microvasculature in isolated dog lungs. J Appl Physiol 1984; 57:233–239.
163. Nicolaysen G, Waaler BA, Aarseth P. On the existence of stretchable pores in the exchange vessels of the isolated rabbit lung preparation. Lymphology 1979; 12: 201–207.
164. West JB, Tsukimoto K, Mathieu-Costello O, Prediletto R. Stress failure in pulmonary capillaries. J Appl Physiol 1991; 70:1731–1742.
165. Tsukimoto K, Mathieu-Costello O, Prediletto R, Elliott AR, West JB. Ultrastructural appearances of pulmonary capillaries at high transmural pressures. J Appl Physiol 1991; 71:573–582.
166. Elliot AR, Fu Z, Tsukimoto K, Prediletto R, Mathieu-Costello O, West JB. Short-term reversibility of ultrastructural changes in pulmonary capillaries caused by stress failure. J Appl Physiol 1992; 73:1150–1158.
167. West JB, Mathieu-Costello O, Jones JH, et al. Stress failure of pulmonary capillaries in racehorses with exercise induced pulmonary hemorrhage. J Appl Physiol 1993; 75:1097–1109.
168. Birks ER, Mathieu-Costello O, Fu Z, Tyler WS, West JB. Comparative aspects of the strength of pulmonary capillaries in rabbit, dog, and horse. Respir Physiol 1994; 97:235–246.
169. Mathieu-Costello O, Willford DC, Fu X, Garden RM, West JB. Pulmonary capillaries are more resistant to stress failure in dogs than in rabbits. J Appl Physiol 1995; 79:908–917.
170. Cassen B, Kistler K. Development of acute pulmonary edema in mice and rats and an interpretation. Am J Physiol 1954; 178:49–52.
171. Minnear FL, Connell RS. Increased permeability of the capillary-alveolar barriers in neurogenic pulmonary edema (NPE). Microvasc Res 1981; 22:345–366.
172. Campbell GS, Visscher MB. Pulmonary lesions in guinea pigs with increased intracranial pressure, and the effect of bilateral cervical vagotomy. Am J Physiol 1949; 157:130–134.
173. Almeida HO, Lima EG, Freire-Maia L. Mechanism of the acute pulmonary edema induced by intracerebroventricular injection of scorpion toxin (tityustoxin) in the unanesthetized rat. Toxican 1976; 14:435–440.
174. Minnear FL, Connell RS. Prevention of aconitine-induced neurogenic pulmonary edema (NPE) with hypovolemia or methylprednisone. J Trauma 1982; 22:121–128.
175. Cruchaud S, Vermeil G. Etude expérimentale de l'œdème aigu du poumon (O.A.P.) provoqué par une irritation du système nerveux central. Helvet Med Acta 1950; 17:525–527.
176. Chan SHH, Chong APY, Ong BT, Chong OK, Lim HC. Pulmonary edema as a cause for fulminant death following microinjection of kainic acid into the rat medulla oblongata. Neurosci Lett 1985; 62:341–346.

177. Hücker H, Schäfer U, Meinen K. Early morphological alterations of the rat lung with increased intracranial pressure. I. A light and electron microscopic study. Virchows Arch A Path Anat Histol 1974; 362:331–342.
178. Bean JW, Beckman DL. Centrogenic pulmonary pathology in mechanical head injury. J Appl Physiol 1968; 27:807–812.
179. Jarisch A, Richter H, Thoma H. Zentrogenes Lungenödem. Klin Wochenschr 1939; 18:1440–1443.
180. Schäfer U, Hücker H, Meinen K. Early morphological alterations of the rat lung with increased intracranial pressure. II. A scanning electron microscope study using different fixation procedures. Res Exp Med 1975; 165:1–8.
181. Hoff JT, Nishimura M. Experimental neurogenic pulmonary edema in cats. J Neurosurg 1978; 48:383–389.
182. Beckman DL. Rat hyper-reactivity to stress. Aviat Space Environ Med 1978; 49:70–72.
183. Maron MB. Analysis of airway fluid protein concentration in neurogenic pulmonary edema. J Appl Physiol 1987; 62:470–476.
184. Ehrhart IC, Hofman WF. Pressure-dependent increase in lung vascular permeability to water but not protein. J Appl Physiol 1992; 72:211–218.
185. Townsley MI, Lim EH, Sahawneh TM, Song W. Interaction of chemical and high vascular pressure injury in isolated canine lung. J Appl Physiol 1990; 69:1657–1664.
186. Pietra GG, Szidon JP, Leventhal MM, Fishman AP. Hemoglobin as a tracer in hemodynamic pulmonary edema. Science 1969; 166:1643–1646.
187. Maron MB, Fu Z, Mathieu-Costello O, West JB. Effect of extreme transient increases in pulmonary capillary pressure (Pc) on functional and ultrastructural measures of vascular permeability in the dog lung (abstr). FASEB J 1996; 10:A351.
188. Erdmann AJ III, Vaughan TR, Brigham KL, Woolverton WC, Staub NC. Effect of increased vascular pressure on lung fluid balance in unanesthetized sheep. Circ Res 1975; 37:271–284.
189. Jones TA, Townsley MI, Weidner WJ. Effects of intracranial and left atrial hypertension on lung fluid balance in sheep. J Appl Physiol 1982; 52:1324–1329.
190. Minnear FL, Barie PS, Malik AB. Effects of transient pulmonary hypertension on pulmonary vascular permeability. J Appl Physiol 1983; 55:983–989.
191. Parker, RE, Roselli RJ, Harris TR, Brigham KL. Effect of graded increases in pulmonary vascular pressures on lung fluid balance in unanesthetized sheep. Circ Res 1981; 49:1164–1172.
192. Weidner WJ, Jones TA, Townsley MI, DeFouw DO. Ultrastructural analysis of sheep lungs after increased intracranial pressure and development of pulmonary edema. Microcirc Endoth Lymphatics 1987; 3:397–410.
193. Bachofen H, Schürch S, Weibel ER. Experimental hydrostatic pulmonary edema in rabbit lungs. Barrier lesions. Am Rev Respir Dis 1993; 147:997–1004.
194. Bowers RE, McKeen CR, Park BE, Brigham KL. Increased pulmonary vascular permeability follows intracranial hypertension in sheep. Am Rev Respir Dis 1979; 119:637–641.

195. van der Zee H, Malik AB, Lee BC, Hakim TS. Lung fluid and protein exchange during intracranial hypertension and role of sympathetic mechanisms. J Appl Physiol 1980; 48:273–280.
196. van der Zee H, Neumann PH, Minnear FL, Malik AB. Effects of transient intracranial hypertension on lung fluid and protein exchange. J Appl Physiol 1983; 54: 178–184.
197. Peterson BT, Ross JC, Brigham KL. Effect of naloxone on the pulmonary vascular responses to graded levels of intracranial hypertension in anethetized sheep. Am Rev Respir Dis 1983; 128:1024–1029.
198. Johnston SC, Darragh TM, Simon RP. Postictal pulmonary edema requires pulmonary vascular pressure increases. Epilepsia 1996; 37:428–432.
199. Simon RP, Bayne LL, Naughton MP. Left atrial pressure elevation recreates the altered lung lymph flow of seizures. J Appl Physiol 1982; 53:432–435.
200. Millen JE, Glauser FL. Low levels of concussive brain trauma and pulmonary edema. J Appl Physiol 1983; 54:666–670.
201. Beckman DL, Ginty DD, Gaither AC. Neurogenic pulmonary edema in a pulmonary hypertensive model. Proc Soc Exp Biol Med 1987; 186:170–173.
202. McClellan MD, Dauber IM, Weil JV. Elevated intracranial pressure increases pulmonary vascular permeability to protein. J Appl Physiol 1989; 67:1185–1191.
203. Hakim TS, van der Zee H, Malik AB. Effects of sympathetic nerve stimulation on lung fluid and protein exchange. J Appl Physiol 1979; 47:1025–1030.
204. Malik AB. Mechanisms of neurogenic pulmonary edema. Circ Res 1985; 57: 1–18.
205. Sakakibara H, Hashiba Y, Taki K, Kawanishi M, Shimada Y, Ishikawa N. Effect of sympathetic nerve stimulation on lung vascular permeability in the rat. Am Rev Respir Dis 1992; 145:685–692.
206. Hirabayashi A, Nishiwaki K, Taki K, Shimada Y, Ishikawa N. Effect of neuropeptide Y on lung vascular permeability in the pulmonary circulation of rats. Eur J Pharmacol 1994; 256:227–230.
207. Hirabayashi A, Nishiwaki K, Shimada Y, Ishikawa N. Role of neuropeptide Y and its receptor subtypes in neurogenic pulmonary edema. Eur J Pharmacol 1996; 296: 297–305.
208. Liu S, Kuo H-P, Sheppard MN, Barnes PJ, Evans TW. Vagal stimulation induces increased pulmonary vascular permeability in guinea pig. Am Rev Respir Crit Care Med 1994; 149:744–750.
209. Hashiba Y, Ishikawa N, Sumita T, Takagi K, Hikada H, Satake T. Capsaicin-sensitive nerves exert an inhibitory effect on the development of fibrin-induced pulmonary edema in rats. Am Rev Respir Dis 1989; 140:652–658.
210. Minnear FL, Barie PS, Malik AB. Effects of epinephrine and norepinephrine infusion on lung fluid balance in sheep. J Appl Physiol 1981; 50:1353–1357.
211. Lang SA, Maron MB. Effect of severe pulmonary hypertension on pulmonary vascular permeability to proteins (abstr). Proceedings 5th World Congress for Microcirculation 1991:56.

212. Chen HI, Huang H-S, Yang J-G, Wang D. Vasodilator and oxidant scavenger in the neurogenic pulmonary edema produced by cerebral compression. Chin J Physiol 1992; 35:121–131.
213. Tsukimoto K, Yoshimura N, Ichioka M, Tojo N, Mizazoto I, Marumo F, Mathieu-Costello O, West JB. Protein, cell, and LTB4 concentrations of lung edema fluid produced by high capillary pressures in the rabbit. J Appl Physiol 1994; 76: 321–327.
214. Saumon G, Basset G. Electrolyte and fluid transport across the mature alveolar epithelium. J Appl Physiol 1993; 74:1–15.
215. Sakuma T, Okaniwa G, Nakada T, Nishimura T, Fujimura S, Matthay MA. Alveolar fluid clearance in the resected human lung. Am Rev Resp Dis 1994; 150: 305–310.
216. Lane SA, Grimme JD, Maron MB. Alveolar fluid reabsorption is increased during recovery from neurogenic pulmonary edema (abstr). FASEB J 1995; 9:A569.
217. Lane SM, Maron MB. An endogenous β_2-adrenergic receptor agonist increases alveolar liquid reabsorption (ALR) in a canine model of neurogenic pulmonary edema (NPE) (abstr). FASEB J 1997; 11:A559.

11

High-Altitude Pulmonary Edema

HERBERT N. HULTGREN[†]

Stanford University School of Medicine
Stanford, California

I. Introduction

High-altitude pulmonary edema (HAPE) is a unique form of lung edema which occurs in susceptible persons who visit altitudes in excess of 2500 m. Symptoms typically appear on the second or third day after arrival and are usually preceded by heavy physical activity such as climbing or skiing. Dyspnea, cough, chest congestion associated with weakness, and marked limitation of physical activity are common. Cyanosis, rales, and a pulmonary infiltrate by chest x-ray are usually present as well as tachycardia, tachypnea, and a reduced arterial oxygen saturation.

Recovery occurs with descent, oxygen, or bed rest. In mountaineers at very high altitudes where descent is not possible and oxygen is not available, several deaths continue to occur annually. Fatal cases in trekkers are less common due to educational efforts and the ready accessibility of prompt descent or oxygen therapy. In the United States, most instances of HAPE occur in skiers. The incidence is low, but due to the several million visitors per year to ski resorts in the Rocky Mountains, a substantial number of cases occur annually. Deaths in this setting are extremely rare due to the small number of severe cases, the ease of rapid descent, and the availability of prompt medical care.

[†]Deceased.

The unique physiologic features of HAPE include the absence of the usual causes of lung edema such as left ventricular failure, infection, or hypersensitivity. Left ventricular function is normal. Individual susceptibility is common, and repeat episodes in the same individual occur frequently. Many of the basic mechanisms responsible for the edema are poorly understood and represent an opportunity for continued research. These aspects make a review of the clinical and physiologic features of HAPE appropriate.

II. Historical Aspects

Mosso in 1898 described a case of probable HAPE that occurred in 1891 in a physician climber who descended from a summit climb on Mount Blanc to the Vallot Hut at 4300 m (1). Here he developed severe dyspnea, progressive mental confusion, and coma. Prior to death his companion noted a respiratory rate of 50 to 70 breaths per minute. An autopsy was performed and the cause of death was ascribed to "suffocative catarrh accompanied by acute edema of the lungs due to pneumonitis." Mosso also noted cases of "pneumonia or inflammation of the lungs" in some recent arrivals at high altitude in the Alps. He was struck by the presence of a high heart rate, a rapid respiratory rate, and severe symptoms in the presence of only slight elevation of temperature. In one instance the heart rate was 125/min, the respiratory rate was 32/min, and rales were present at the right posterior base of the lung. The temperature was 39.5°C. These findings are typical of HAPE.

In 1913 Ravenhill, a British physician who was working as a medical officer in the mines in the Andes of northern Chile published accurate clinical descriptions of acute mountain sickness, high-altitude cerebral edema, and HAPE. His report of the clinical features of HAPE is very accurate and consistent with present-day observations including rapid recovery with descent by train (2). Ravenhill's publication received little attention since it was published in the Journal of Tropical Medicine and Hygiene. In the late 1930s and 1940s physicians at the Chulec General Hospital in the Peruvian Andes (3782 m) were aware of persons who, after arrival by train from sea level, developed a cough, dyspnea, and weakness and who recovered completely upon descent (3). The condition was recognized as pulmonary edema (soroche agudo edema de pulmon).

In 1955 Lizarraga published his medical thesis describing 14 cases of HAPE seen at the Chulec Hospital between 1950 and 1954 (4). Subsequently several similar reports were published by Peruvian physicians (5,6). These publications in Spanish attracted little attention in the United States despite a brief letter in the Journal of the American Medical Association by Bardales in 1956 (7). In May 1960 a brief report of 41 cases of HAPE seen at the Chulec

Hospital was published by Hultgren (8). In September 1960 a report of a case of HAPE in a skier was published by Houston (9). Subsequently a more detailed report of cases of HAPE in Peru as well as probable cases in mountaineers was published by Hultgren and Houston (10). Prior to that time cases of HAPE in mountaineers were thought to be due to pneumonia (10,11). Reports of cases seen in India among troops rapidly deployed to high altitude were published by Singh (12) and Menon (13). The basic etiologic mechanisms involved in HAPE were not understood at that time, and the most common concept was that left ventricular (LV) failure due to hypoxia was the cause.

III. Definition

In 1991 a consensus committee at the International Hypoxia Symposium proposed the following criteria for the diagnosis of HAPE: the presence of at least two of the following symptoms in the setting of a recent gain in altitude, dyspnea at rest, cough, weakness, decreased exercise performance, chest tightness or congestion, and at least two of the following signs—rales or wheezing, central cyanosis, tachycardia, or tachypnea (14). The use of these criteria will increase the accuracy of case reports of HAPE, differentiate it from other conditions such as acute mountain sickness or pneumonia, and facilitate communication. Where clinical facilities are available I would suggest as additional criteria the presence of a pulmonary infiltrate or abnormal vascular congestion in the chest radiograph as well as a decrease in arterial oxygen saturation below the accepted normal value for the altitude of occurrence.

A. Severity Classification

A functional grading of disability has been proposed (14), and a modification of this system has been made by the author as follows:

1. Strenuous or heavy activity limited by symptoms.
2. Symptoms on normal activity, cannot perform heavy activity but the patient is ambulatory.
3. Severe symptoms requiring bed rest. The patient may be able to carry out bodily functions.
4. Life-threatening symptoms–disturbance of consciousness, mental confusion, obtundation. The patient cannot stand or walk.

B. Clinical Features

Since HAPE in the United States most commonly occurs in skiers and climbers in the Rocky Mountains, the clinical features of HAPE in skiers will be described in 150 patients seen at a ski resort medical clinic (2928 m) over a 27-month period. All patients satisfied the diagnostic criteria proposed above including the presence of rales or an abnormal chest radiograph (15).

The mean age of the patients was 34 ± 16 years. Males constituted 84% of all patients. The mean time from arrival to the day of onset of symptoms of sufficient severity to seek medical attention was 3 ± 1.3 days (range 1 to 9). The most common symptoms were dyspnea, cough, chest congestion, nausea or vomiting, and headache. A total of 126 patients (84%) had three or more symptoms.

C. Physical Signs

Tachycardia was common. The mean heart rate was 104 beats/min. In 40 patients (27%), the rate was 120 beats/min or more. The mean respiratory rate was 23 ± 6 min. A mild temperature elevation was common (16). In 30 patients (20%) a temperature exceeding 100°F was present. Seventeen patients (12%)

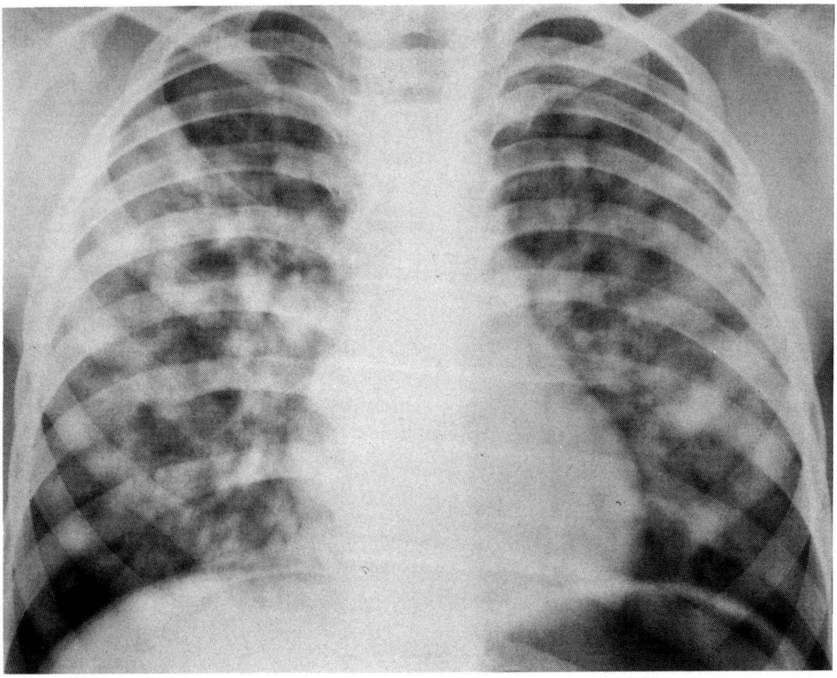

Figure 1 Chest film of a 14-year-old boy who developed HAPE after an ascent to 3750 m from sea level. After 48 hours of bed rest and oxygen, complete recovery occurred.

had a blood pressure of 150/90 mm Hg or more. This was more common in elderly patients. Rales were present in 127 patients (85%), usually bilateral (55%) or only over the right lung field (24%).

D. Radiologic Features

A pulmonary infiltrate was present in 132 patients (88%). Most of the infiltrates were bilateral and involved the central portion of both lung fields in 80 patients (53%). The right lung field was involved in only 51 patients (34%). One patient had an infiltrate only in the left lung. Only seven patients (4.7%) had all four lung fields involved. Typical chest films are shown in Figures 1 and 2.

E. Pulse Oximetry

Arterial oxygen saturation was determined in 43 patients using a fingertip oximeter. The mean saturation was 74% (range 38% to 93%). The mean normal value for healthy recent arrivals at 2500 m is 92% ± 1% (17).

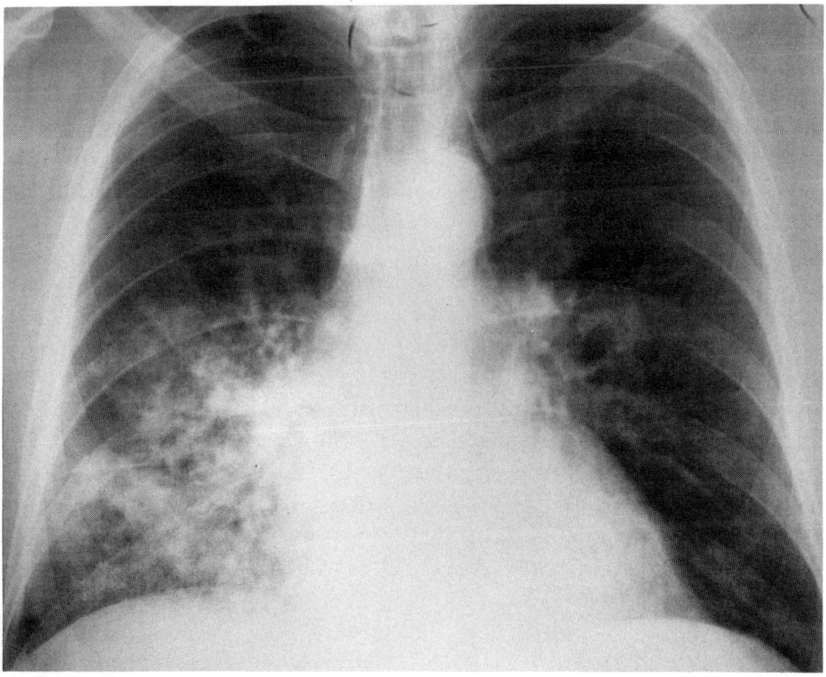

Figure 2 Chest film of a 42-year-old skier who developed HAPE after skiing from 2600 m to 3500 m over a 4-day period.

IV. Management and Treatment

The following management methods were employed: On entry to the clinic a history and physical examination were performed followed by vital signs, a chest x-ray, and pulse oximetry. Oxygen at a flow rate of 4 L/min was administered via a plastic face mask. Ten milligrams of nifedipine was given sublingually and followed by 30 mg every 6 hours. When the patient was stabilized, several options were employed depending on the severity of the condition. Very mild cases elected to return to Denver. Others returned to their quarters to rest and receive low-flow oxygen via nasal cannula. If recovery was complete the following day, a day of rest or light activity was permitted before returning to ski. More severe cases were admitted to a local hospital or sent to a Denver hospital for observation and oxygen therapy.

There were no deaths in the series of cases studied. This was due to the fact that most cases were mild and prompt medical therapy was instituted.

Similar reports of HAPE in a ski resort have been published by Sophocles (18,19).

A. Incidence

The incidence of HAPE is dependent upon several variables including the altitude attained, speed and mode of ascent, physical activity after arrival, age, gender, and individual susceptibility. Adults ascending to 3782 m in Peru experience an incidence of 3% (20). In Swiss climbers at 4559 m, the incidence was 5.2% (21). The incidence in Indian troops transported by air to 3500 m was 5.7% (12). At lower altitudes, 2500 to 2750 m, the incidence is about one in 10,000 (20). Subclinical cases are common, Hackett and Rennie observed rales in 23% of trekkers in Nepal, of whom only 4.5% had clinical HAPE (22).

B. Altitude of Occurrence

HAPE rarely occurs below 2450 m. The Lake Tahoe area, at 1922 m in California, is visited by several million skiers and vacationers annually, yet HAPE is practically never seen at this altitude. At 2450 m and higher in the Colorado Rockies, HAPE is a well-recognized problem, largely among skiers. Of 56 patients with HAPE evacuated from the Swiss Alps over a 4-year period, no cases had occurred below 2500 m (23). The sleeping altitude is probably more important in the genesis of HAPE than the altitude attained during the day.

C. Age and Gender

Studies in Peru have shown that HAPE is about six times as common in children as in adults, and it also appears to be more serious. In a study of 97 individuals who experienced a total of 1157 rapid ascents to 3730 m, 90% of the episodes occurred in those under 19 years. The highest incidence, accounting for 46.7% of all cases was in the 5- to 9-year age group (24).

In adults, HAPE appears to occur more frequently in men. In visitors to Vail, Colorado, at 2500 m the incidence of HAPE was 0.74/100,000 women compared to 10.0/100,000 men (18,19). In a nearby ski resort at 2928 m, 84% of the cases of HAPE occurred in men (15). The higher incidence of HAPE in men is probably related to the observations that men respond to the hypoxia of high altitude with a lower pulmonary ventilation than women (25). The higher ventilation in women may be due to the effect of estrogen and progesterone (26). Subjects with a history of HAPE have a blunted hypoxic ventilatory drive (27). Sleep apnea is more common in men (28). Men have a lower arterial PO_2 and thus a greater degree of pulmonary vasoconstriction and pulmonary hypertension.

D. Reentry HAPE

Early observations in Peru indicated that a substantial number of cases of HAPE occurred in high-altitude dwellers who descended to a lower altitude and returned to high altitude. The time spent at a lower altitude was usually 10 days or longer. In 113 cases of reentry HAPE, only 10.5% had a stay of < 7 days (29). Children living in Leadville, Colorado, may develop HAPE upon reascent after 3 to 5 days at a lower altitude (30). Reascent pulmonary edema does not appear to differ clinically or physiologically from first-ascent HAPE.

E. Mortality

In cases of HAPE seen at ski resorts, mortality is extremely low due to the fact that most cases are mild and access to descent or medical care is readily available (15). Most fatal cases occur at higher altitudes, where oxygen or medical care may not be available and descent is difficult. Many early deaths occurred because the diagnosis was not made and pneumonia was thought to be present (10). An analysis of 166 cases of HAPE collected worldwide revealed 19 deaths (11.4%). Of 61 patients who descended or were treated with oxygen, four died (6%); in 23 patients who neither descended nor received oxygen, 10 deaths (49%) occurred (31).

F. Physiologic Studies

Only a few hemodynamic studies of HAPE have been performed at high altitude during the acute stage and before treatment has been started (32–38). The results have been consistent in demonstrating the following abnormalities: (1) an elevated mean pulmonary artery pressure (mean = 46 mm Hg); (2) a normal or low pulmonary artery wedge pressure (mean 3.6 mm Hg); (3) a moderately

Table 1 Mean Hemodynamic Values from 21 Cases of HAPE Studied at High Altitude (variable-mean; range)

	Hultgren	Antezana	Kobayashi	Normal
Number studied	13	5	5	26
Heart rate	103[a]	117	—	72
Altitude	3750 m	3650 m	2935 m	3750 m
Arterial O_2 sat.	71% (55–87)	74% (72–86)	(41)[a]	85% (70–91)
PA mean mm Hg	46 mm (22–117)	62 mm (54–70)	26 mm (15–36)	22 mm (14–28)
PA wedge mm Hg	4 mm (1–9)	5 mm (1–9)	6 mm (3–7)	8 mm (2–13)
BA mean mm Hg	79	87	ND	110
Cardiac index L/min/m^2 (range)	3.0 (2.3–4.5)	2.1 (1.3–2.9)	3.8 (3.0–4.9)	3.4 (1.8–4.5)
Arterial P_{CO_2} mm Hg	28 (24–35)	29 (24–36)	30.6 (27–34)	32 (26–36)

Note. Values in column 3 (Kobayashi) are more normal than the others because the altitude of occurrence was lower and studies were done within 4.5 hours after hospital entry and after descent to 2000 feet (610 m).

Abbreviations: PA, pulmonary artery; BA, brachial artery; ND, not done.

[a]Arterial P_{O_2}.

Sources. Data from Hultgren, Ref. 45; Antezana, Ref. 34; Kobayashi, Ref. 32. (Normal data from Ref. 45.)

reduced cardiac index (mean 3.0 $L/min/m^2$); (4) a decreased mean systemic blood pressure (mean = 79 mm Hg); and (5) an increased pulmonary vascular resistance (mean = 1040 $dynes\text{-}sec\text{-}cm^{-5}$). The results of 21 cases are shown in Table 1. The pulmonary artery wedge pressure is probably an accurate reflection of the left atrial pressure, since in one patient the catheter fortuitously entered the left atrium via a foramen ovale and recorded a normal pressure (36). The administration of 100% oxygen rapidly lowers pulmonary artery pressure, but normal values are not always attained. Exercise and induced hypoxia will result in a marked rise in pulmonary artery pressure but without a change in pulmonary artery wedge pressure (35). The hemodynamic data clearly indicate that HAPE is not due to left ventricular failure and that the abnormality resulting in edema must reside in the lung.

A common feature of severe cases of HAPE is a markedly reduced arterial oxygen saturation in the presence of a moderate decrease in arterial pCO_2. In some cases it is possible that a right-to-left shunt across a patent foramen ovale may accentuate the hypoxemia (39).

V. Pathology

Knowledge of the pathology of HAPE is limited by the paucity of well-conducted autopsy studies (40–45). Twenty-six autopsy reports were evaluated by the author. The mean age was 31 years (range 9 to 62 years). All were males. The mean duration of symptoms before death was 2 days (range 1 to 3 days). The following gross findings were present:

1. All lungs showed diffuse pulmonary edema with bloody, foamy fluid being readily expressed from the cut surfaces and usually filling the airways. Mean total lung weight was 1960 g (range 1200 to 3000 g). Normal combined weight of normal lungs is between 750 and 800 g. Grossly evident pulmonary emboli or thrombosis was present in two cases, one of which had pulmonary infarcts. There were no areas of substantial purulent consolidation indicating extensive pneumonia.
2. There was no evidence of LV failure. Neither hypertrophy nor dilatation of the left ventricle or left atrium was present. There was no myocardial infarction or coronary occlusion. The right ventricle, right atrium, and proximal pulmonary arteries were often distended.
3. Cerebral edema was present in three of eight cases in which the brain was examined, and petechial hemorrhages were present in three. No thrombotic cerebral lesions were seen. Two brains were weighed, with values of 1750 and 1610 g (normal value, 1350).

Histologic studies in 24 cases revealed thrombi in small pulmonary arteries and capillaries (46%), focal areas of pneumonitis (21%), infiltration with leukocytes (75%), alveolar hyaline membranes (37%), and alveolar hemorrhages (58%). These changes indicated the presence of capillary injury and a capillary leak syndrome with a high protein content of edema fluid. The cellular infiltrate indicates an inflammatory response to cellular or tissue damage. Pneumonia in some instances may be associated with HAPE and may in some cases facilitate the development of pulmonary edema (41).

Nayak and co-workers reported the autopsy findings in 13 patients with HAPE with similar results (42). Seven cases had hyaline membranes, and six had microscopic evidence of thrombi in small pulmonary arteries and capillaries. Focal pneumonitis was found in six cases.

The above autopsy studies excluded patients who exhibited gross evidence of pneumonia or pulmonary embolism. Both these conditions can be fatal at high altitude, and both can be accompanied by pulmonary edema (44). Acute myocarditis and myocardial infarction may also result in fatal pulmonary edema in persons who were well and fit at the beginning of a trip.

Certain conclusions can be derived from these data:

1. There is no evidence of LV failure or underlying cardiac disease.
2. The degree of pulmonary edema is severe and widespread, and can result in death by hypoxia.
3. Although small foci of pneumonitis may be demonstrated histologically, in about one-third to one-half of cases lung infection appears to be coincidental and not a causative factor.
4. The protein-rich alveolar exudate with numerous areas of alveolar hemorrhage and the presence of alveolar hyaline membranes indicate that the edema fluid has a high protein content, compatible with capillary injury.
5. Thrombotic lesions in small pulmonary arteries and capillaries in half the cases suggest that in some patients thrombotic vascular obstruction may play a role in elevating the pulmonary artery pressure.
6. Cerebral edema is not universally present and therefore can be excluded as a causative factor.

An important question regarding pathogenesis is whether the initial initiating factor is a rise in pulmonary artery pressure or an increase in capillary permeability. These possibilities were examined in the following study: In five men with a history of prior episodes of HAPE, hemodynamics and pulmonary gas exchange were measured at sea level and again 24 hours after ascent to 3100 m. A 3-hour period of altitude hill walking preceded the altitude study. At sea level all findings were essentially normal, except for a mean pulmonary artery pressure of 33 mm Hg during supine exercise in one subject. At altitude mean pulmonary artery pressure increased abnormally in all subjects being 30 $\pm$ 10 mm Hg at rest and 53 $\pm$ 12 mm Hg during moderate exercise (mean oxygen consumption of 1196 ml/min). A respiratory alkalosis was present (pH 7.49). Oxygen breathing only partially relieved the pulmonary hypertension. Arterial blood gases were normal at sea level. At altitude, in spite of hyperventilation, arterial P_{O_2} was only 51 ± 6 mm Hg at rest and fell to 41 ± 3 mm Hg during exercise with a widened alveolar arterial oxygen difference of 28 ± 7 mm Hg. None of the subjects developed clinically detectable HAPE. Therefore these men developed excessive pulmonary hypertension and impaired oxygen exchange without pulmonary edema following ascent to high altitude (24). These results indicate that the initial abnormality in HAPE is an increase in pulmonary artery pressure due to the hypoxia of high altitude. An important question is, how does hypoxic pulmonary hypertension lead to in pulmonary edema in HAPE?

In 1966, the author suggested the following concept of the etiology of HAPE, which was later studied in an animal model (46–48). It was proposed that the primary cause of HAPE was nonhomogeneous obstruction of the pulmonary vascular bed by hypoxic vasoconstriction and possibly intravascular thromboses. During periods of exercise with increased cardiac output, unobstructed areas of the pulmonary circulation would be subjected to high pressure and flow and the precapillary arterioles would be dilated, permitting the pressure to be transmitted directly to the capillary bed, with resulting interstitial and alveolar edema. With dilatation of arterioles and capillaries, the pulmonary veins would then become the site of resistance to flow, which would also facilitate a high capillary pressure. Small pulmonary arteries and arterioles have relatively thin muscular walls and are easily dilated by small pressure elevations. Thus, an important mechanism of HAPE may be regional failure of hypoxic vasoconstriction and dilatation of nonconstricted vessels in local areas of the lung with high pressure being transmitted to the pulmonary capillaries. Johansson and coworkers have proposed a similar concept for the pathogenesis of hypertensive encephalopathy (49).

There is considerable evidence that hypoxic pulmonary vasoconstriction is not uniform throughout the lung.

Lehr injected India ink into the veins of rabbits before and after acute hypoxia and examined the distribution of the ink particles in the lungs. With normoxia, most particles had traversed the lung. With hypoxia, irregular areas of the lung had trapped ink particles, suggesting local areas of vasoconstriction and blockage of blood flow, while other areas were free of particles, suggesting the absence of vasoconstriction (50). Lung scans in persons with a history of HAPE show areas of increased and decreased flow when subjected to hypoxia that are not observed in normal subjects (51).

Dawson showed that alveolar hypoxia nearly doubled the dispersion of transit times through the circulation of a lobe of a dog lung, strongly suggesting that vasoconstriction was uneven (52). Scherrer and his associates provided further evidence of the uneven blood flow in HAPE. They showed that inhaled nitric oxide in patients with HAPE lowered pulmonary artery pressure, improved oxygenation, and shifted blood flow in the lung away from the edematous regions toward nonedematous areas, thereby improving the matching of ventilation and perfusion with a decrease in the alveolar-arterial oxygen difference (53). Nitric oxide is an endothelium-derived relaxing factor synthesized locally in the pulmonary circulation.

The overperfusion concept of the mechanism of HAPE has been evaluated in the following experimental model. Anesthetized 16-kg dogs with controlled mechanical ventilation had a left thoracotomy, incision of the pericardium, and a right ventricular bypass from the right atrium to the main pulmonary artery using a roller pump. Measurements were made of cardiac output, pulmonary artery pressure, and left atrial pressure. Slow ligation of the right pulmonary artery was performed. After control measurements, gradual ligation of the branches of the pulmonary artery branches to the left lower and left middle lobes was performed. While maintaining blood flows of 0.5, 1.1, and 1.5 L/min into the perfused left upper lobe, repeat measurements were made. When perfusion of the isolated left upper lobe was continued, the lobe became engorged with blood and a continuous thrill and murmur was present over the lobe's surface. After 10 to 20 min of perfusion the lobe became cyanotic and stiff, and blood-tinged edema fluid filled the alveoli. Arterial oxygen saturation rapidly decreased. The excised, perfused lobe was firm and exuded edema fluid upon pressure, and the weight was 66% heavier than the nonperfused lobe corrected for volume. The protein content of the edema fluid was elevated to 4.3 to 5.3 g/100 mL. Histologic studies revealed marked capillary dilatation and engorgement and a diffuse hemorrhagic alveolar edema. The left atrial and pulmonary artery wedge pressures remained normal throughout the study. Just prior to the onset of pulmonary edema the mean pulmonary artery pressure was 48 mm Hg (range 23 to 68 mm Hg). The cardiac output and the total pulmonary artery flow were within normal limits. The estimated pulmonary vascular resistance was 800 dynes-sec-cm^{-5} (normal = 100 to 150 dynes-sec-cm^{-5}. From measurements of the weights of normal pulmonary lobes it was estimated that the blood flow through the perfused lobe was increased by approximately five- to sixfold (48). These studies indicate that a marked increase in blood flow in a portion of a canine lung is accompanied by pulmonary edema with a high protein content while the left atrial pressure remains normal. The pulmonary capillary pressure is probably increased. The high pulmonary artery pressure is similar to that found in humans with HAPE (35,37). These studies support the author's concept of the mechanism of HAPE in man (Fig. 3).

Younes studied a similar model of pulmonary edema in a dog preparation by pneumonectomy and removal of lung tissue so that 33% to 55% of the lung was perfused by a blood flow estimated to be four to five times normal (54). Pulmonary artery mean pressure was 35 mm Hg. Pulmonary capillary pressure

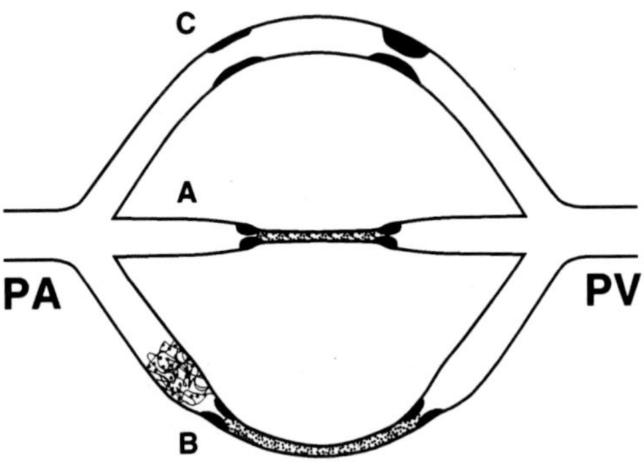

Figure 3 Diagram of the pulmonary circulation in HAPE according to the author's overperfusion concept. (A) Hypoxic arteriolar constriction closes off part of the pulmonary circulation. (B) Arteriolar constriction and obstruction of precapillary vessels by thrombus obstructs the pulmonary circulation. (C) Remaining nonobstructed circulatory bed is subjected to high pressure and flow with a resulting increase in capillary pressure. Capillary wall injury increases capillary permeability. Pulmonary veins may now be the site of pressure drop due to high flow and/or venous constriction.

was elevated, but not left atrial pressure. Younes speculated that the pulmonary venules and veins were relatively indistensible and thus acted as loci of resistance to flow with a resulting increase in capillary pressure and edema. Pulmonary edema fluid protein was not determined. Landolt and associates evaluated the effect of increased pulmonary flow (by partial lung resection), hypoxia, and elevation of left atrial pressure upon lymph flow and lymph protein concentration in sheep with a maintained cardiac output. While lymph flow increased moderately, there was no increase in lymph protein concentration, indicating a maintained microvascular permeability. The overperfused lobe showed interstitial edema with a 24% increase in extravascular water. The pulmonary artery pressure increased to 30 mm Hg (55). One can only speculate that a higher flow and pressure might have increased lymph protein concentration and perhaps caused more edema.

A. Pulmonary Venous Obstruction

It is possible that under conditions of hypoxia and high flow, pulmonary venules and veins may act as the site of some of the resistance to flow. Studies of perfused intact dog lungs have shown that when blood flow to a pulmonary lobe is increased more than fourfold, the pressure drop in the precapillary vessels is diminished, capillary pressure rises, and the site of resistance is shifted to the pulmonary veins with an increase in small vein pressure (56). While acute hypoxia is accompanied by an increase in pulmonary precapillary resistance, prolonged hypoxia results in pulmonary vein constriction (57). Nagasaka and colleagues have shown that the lung microvascular pressure profile during hypoxia in cats is associated with constriction of pulmonary venules (58).

B. Pulmonary Vascular Obstruction by Thrombi

The finding of thrombi in pulmonary arterioles and capillaries in many cases of HAPE raises the possibility that thrombi may obstruct flow, increase pulmonary artery pressure, and cause regional differences in blood flow. Some studies have suggested that a coagulopathy may be present in HAPE since in some patients clotting factors have been abnormal (59). In 27 patients with HAPE studied in Japan by Kobayashi and associates, platelet counts were decreased and the prothrombin time was slightly prolonged upon hospital admission compared with recovery values (32).

Further studies by Bärtsch and associates revealed that in mild cases no coagulation abnormalities were observed but in severe cases several abnormalities occurred including increases in fibrinopeptide A and other factors. It was concluded that since coagulation abnormalities were not present in mild cases but only in severe cases, an initial causative role could not be ascribed to thrombi which appears to be a late manifestation of HAPE (60).

C. Sympathetic Nervous System

The role of sympathetic stimulation in the geneses of HAPE remains largely unknown. Ascent to high altitude is associated with a transient increase in epinephrine blood levels and a more sustained increase in norepinephrine levels (61).

Hackett and colleagues studied the effect of alpha-adrenergic blockage by phentolamine mesylate in patients with HAPE. Phentolamine increased heart rate and cardiac index, reduced pulmonary artery pressure and pulmonary vascular resistance, and increased arterial oxygen saturation. The effect was greater than oxygen, nifedipine, and hydralazine. Beta blockade had no significant effect on pulmonary hemodynamics (62). The results of the study suggested that part of the pulmonary vasoconstriction in HAPE might be mediated via the sympathetic nervous system. In addition it provided additional support for the concept of treating HAPE by pulmonary vasodilators such as nifedipine. Nitroglycerin will lower pulmonary vascular resistance and may be a simple addition to the use of nifedipine (63).

VI. Sea Level Analogs to HAPE

Several sea level conditions illustrate that pulmonary edema may occur if portions of the pulmonary vascular bed are occluded while remaining portions of the lung are subjected to an increased blood flow.

1. In most cases of pulmonary embolism the amount of the pulmonary vascular bed that is obstructed is not sufficient to result in a significant rise in pulmonary artery pressure. In severe pulmonary embolism, pulmonary edema has been observed in regions of the lung where the circulation was not obstructed. An example of pulmonary edema associated with pulmonary embolism was reported by Combret (64). A young woman developed an embolus obstructing a large portion of the main pulmonary trunk. Angiography indicated that perfusion was present only in the upper and middle lobes of the left lung. Pulmonary edema was present only in these areas. Hemodynamic studies revealed a pulmonary artery pressure of 45/19 mm Hg, a pulmonary artery wedge pressure of 9 mm Hg, and a cardiac index of 1.9 L/min/m^2. This case represents the human analogy to the overperfusion canine studies reported in this paper and indicates that at least 50% to 75% of the pulmonary vascular bed must be obstructed to permit overperfusion pulmonary edema.

2. Successful balloon dilatation of peripheral pulmonary artery stenosis has been followed by pulmonary edema in the portion of the lung supplied by the stenotic artery. Mean pressures in the artery after dilatation varied from 22 to 28 mm Hg. Four patients with pulmonary edema had systemic pressures in the right ventricle, three had Fallot's tetralogy, and one had transposition of the great arteries. In 15 patients who had dilatations without pulmonary edema, mean pulmonary artery pressure after dilatations was $<$ 20 mm Hg in all but one patient, who had a mean pressure of 22 mm Hg (65).

3. In thromboembolic pulmonary hypertension surgical removal of occluding thrombi from branches of the pulmonary arteries has been accompanied by pulmonary edema in the reperfused segments (66,67).

4. Congenital absence of the right pulmonary artery is a risk factor for HAPE (68). The anomaly results in an increased flow to the left lung with a moderate degree of pulmonary hypertension (69). The pulmonary edema is confined to the left lung. Other conditions that restrict blood flow to a portion of the lung and increase susceptibility to HAPE include severe spinal scoliosis (15), proximal interruption of the left pulmonary artery (70), hypoplasia of the right pulmonary artery (71), and anomalous pulmonary venous connection of drainage with intact atrial septum (72).

VII. Capillary Permeability

Autopsy studies in HAPE indicate that capillary injury and increased permeability are probably present by the frequent occurrence of alveolar hemorrhages, hyaline membranes, and leucocyte infiltrates (41–43). In the dog lung perfusion studies described earlier in this review, the edema fluid protein concentration was increased, suggesting an increase in permeability. The high flow through the perfused lobe was associated with a palpable thrill and a continuous bruit compatible with considerable turbulence. Increased permeability was therefore considered to be due not only to the increased capillary pressure but capillary wall injury due to increased flow and high shear forces.

Schoene and colleagues obtained lung lavage fluid from three patients with HAPE on Mount McKinley and from three controls. The fluid exhibited a marked increase in high-molecular-weight proteins, erythrocytes, and leucocytes, most of which were alveolar macrophages (73,74). Similar observations were made by Kobayashi and colleagues (32). These results in humans indicated that HAPE is clearly associated with an increased capillary permeability, or a "large pore" leak. The role of increased permeability due to high shear forces was challenged by the work of West and associates, who demonstrated that, in the rabbit, elevation of capillary pressure without an increase in flow resulted in edema fluid with an increased protein content as well as electron microscopic evidence of disruption of the capillary endothelial layer, alveolar epithelial layer, and sometimes all layers of the wall. In the rabbit model pulmonary venous pressure and capillary pressure were raised by elevating the pulmonary venous reservoir to approximately 40 to 56 mm Hg. The flow through the system was low (75,76). This pressure was higher than produced in sheep by Landolt and associates in which lymph protein was not increased (55).

An increase in capillary pressure and possibly shear forces due to the high flow may injure capillary walls and result in the release of cell-derived factors from platelets, leucocytes, alveolar macrophage, and other cells. Thromboxane, a mediator of pulmonary hypertension, and leukotriene B_4, a potent chemotatic factor for leucocytes, are also present in pulmonary edema fluid (73,74). These factors probably play an important role in the increase in permeability. For example, Flick and associates have shown that leucocytes are required for increased microvascular permeability after microembolization in sleep (77). Richalet has reviewed the evidence for the importance of pulmonary vascular leakage of fluid in the pathogenesis of HAPE (78). Further studies are clearly indicated to differentiate the role of high flow versus high pressure in increasing capillary permeability.

VIII. Treatment

Several treatment options are now available, depending on the location availability of medical facilities (Table 2).

1. Bed rest. Mild cases of HAPE may be safely treated by bed rest alone if frequent observations are made to ascertain that clinical improvement is occurring. Recovery is slower than that observed with oxygen therapy (79).

2. Descent. Rapid descent of even a few thousand feet may result in rapid improvement and may be lifesaving. Rapid descent is the most important, usually most easily available method of treatment. Other methods of therapy

Table 2 Treatment Methods Employed in HAPE

Method	Comment
Physical	
1. Bed rest (79)	Useful in mild cases. Continued observation necessary.
2. Descent (80)	Most simple, effective measure if terrain is suitable or methods of descent available.
3. Oxygen (79)	Effective when given at an optimal flow rate. At very high altitudes higher flow rates needed. Limited by the supply available.
4. Hyperbaric bag (81,82)	Useful for expeditions. Used for temporary improvement prior to descent.
5. Positive expiratory pressure grunt breathing (83,84)	Of doubtful value. May result in pneumothorax or mediastinal emphysema. Hyperventilation may provide a similar increase in oxygen saturation.
6. Chest compression to remove airway fluid (85)	Of temporary use when excessive fluid is present in airways.
Pharmacological agents	
7. Nifedipine (86,87)	For temporary benefit and relief of symptoms. Lowers pulmonary artery pressure and increases arterial oxygen saturation. May prevent HAPE in susceptible persons.
8. Acetazolamide (89)	No controlled studies. May prevent HAPE in susceptible subjects during ascent.
9. Morphine (80,90)	Of doubtful value. May be tried in very anxious patients.
10. Furosemide (10,91)	Of no proven value. May be dangerous due to volume depletion.

should be considered, not as substitutes for descent, but to provide sufficient clinical improvement so that descent is facilitated (80).

3. Oxygen. High-flow oxygen by plastic face mask or nasal cannulae will result in rapid improvement of symptoms and physical signs (79).

4. Hyperbaric bag. The use of a hyperbaric bag (Gamow bag) is now widespread and has been used successfully in the treatment of HAPE,

high-altitude cerebral edema, and acute mountain sickness. At 4246 m, inflation to a pressure of 2 lb/in.^{2} reduces the altitude to an equivalent of 2662 m. The bag weighs less than an oxygen cylinder, can be used several times, and can be dropped from an aircraft. The pressure is maintained by a foot pump. Continual pumping is necessary but can be tiring, so a relay of persons is needed to maintain a continuous pressure. It is best used to improve symptoms so that descent can be facilitated (81). Kasic and associates have shown that the bag compares favorably with oxygen in improving symptoms and increasing arterial oxygen saturation (82).

5. Expiratory Positive Airway Pressure (EPAP). This method commonly employs a Downs mask or a variation thereof consisting of a tightly fitting plastic mask providing positive expiratory pressure by a spring-loaded exhalation valve. Studies in four climbers with HAPE and 13 healthy volunteers at rest and during exercise revealed a modest increase in oxygen saturation of about 7% at 10 cm water expiratory pressure. The authors suggested that voluntary hyperventilation would be a better and safer method of increasing arterial oxygen saturaiton (83). Another method of increasing expiratory pressure is by "grunt breathing," where forced expiration is performed through pursed lips. These methods are not without complications including pneumothorax and mediastinal emphysema (84). Another method of increasing intrathoracic pressure to expel airway fluid consists of forcible compression of the chest in a head-down position. This may expel enough fluid to result in a temporary respite from severe dyspnea and near suffocation (85).

6. Nifedipine. Nifedipine has proven to be a useful adjunct to the treatment of HAPE. Oelz et al. gave nifedipine to six patients with HAPE with good results (86). The subjects were able to continue exercise at the same altitude, with continued improvement in symptoms. Bärtsch and associates (87) gave 20 mg of slow-release nifedipine every 8 hours for 4 days, starting the day of ascent to 4590 m, to subjects with a prior history of HAPE. HAPE was prevented in nine of 10 subjects, although it occurred in seven of 11 subjects given a placebo. Subjects given nifedipine had a lower pulmonary artery pressure, a lower alveolar arterial pressure gradient, and a lower symptom score. No significant side effects were observed. Nifedipine probably acts by reversing hypoxic pulmonary vasoconstriction (88). One would expect nitroglycerin to have a similar effect (63).

Other medications have been used in the treatment of HAPE without clear evidence of benefit or with serious side effects. Acetazolamide may provide some benefit, but controlled trials have not been done. It may prevent HAPE in susceptible subjects during ascent (89). Morphine may be of benefit in patients who are very anxious, dyspneic, and tachypneic (80). One anecdotal report by a physician with HAPE described a worsening of symptoms following the self-administration of morphine (90). Digitalis preparations have no significant benefit in HAPE, which is understandable because heart failure is absent. Glucocorticoids have no effect on the symptoms of HAPE, but may be useful if cerebral edema is present. Glucocorticoids have no objective physiologic effects that would favorably affect HAPE for either prevention or treatment (79). Furosemide was originally used in the treatment of HAPE by Singh and his associates (10). However, a careful review of his report does not show a significant benefit of furosemide compared to a placebo. Gray has reported adverse effects of furosemide in subjects brought to 5340 m on Mt. Logan (91). The major problem is the occasional severe fall in blood pressure, especially with intravenous administration. In some instances shock has resulted, with the need for intravenous fluids and a prolongation of the recovery time.

A. Emergency Room Management

Most instances of HAPE occur at mountain resorts where emergency rooms and hospital facilities are nearby and available. Management methods will therefore be different than in an isolated mountain environment. General guidelines in one medical clinic emergency room at a Rocky Mountain ski resort can be summarized as follows. A medical history, physical examination, vital signs, and pulse oximetry are obtained upon entry. Oxygen is administered via a plastic face mask at a flow rate of 4 to 6 L/min. A posterior-anterior and lateral chest roentgenogram is done. Other studies, if available, include a blood count, urinalysis, serum enzymes, and electrocardiogram. Sustained-release nifedipine, 30 mg twice daily, is started after an initial 10-mg sublingual dose of regular nifedipine. Medication for headache is provided. If dehydration due to vomiting or prolonged dyspnea is present, intravenous fluids are given. After 2 to 3 hours of oxygen therapy, improvement is usually rapid and a decision for future management is made. In mild cases, the patient may be allowed to return to the hotel room, condominium, or house for 24 hours of bed rest alone or with oxygen therapy. In most areas, hospital supply companies will provide the patient with oxygen via a tank or concentrator and instruct the patient in its use via nasal cannulae. If the patient is symptom-free the following day, another day or 2 of light activity without oxygen is usually advised before returning to more strenuous activities, such as skiing. Severe cases not responding promptly to initial therapy are admitted to a local hospital or clinic for 1 or 2 nights of more intensive therapy. Most cases of HAPE can usually be treated in this manner, without the necessity of canceling a family vacation by descending to a larger medical facility.

B. Prevention

It is prudent for anyone with a prior history of HAPE to observe preventive measures. Acclimatization for several days at an intermediate altitude and a slow ascent to over 2450 m are effective measures. Awareness of the early symptoms of HAPE will facilitate the early institution of therapy. Extended-release nifedipine given the day before ascent and continued for 5 to 7 days after ascent may be used. Although there are no systematic studies of acetazolamide in the prevention of HAPE, a report from Bolivia (89) and Peru indicates that its use in children ascending to high altitude after a sojourn at sea level has greatly reduced the previously high incidence of HAPE.

References

1. Mosso A. In: Landon A, Fisher T, eds. Life of Man on the High Alps, London: Unwin, 1898:179, 323.
2. Ravenhill T. Some experiences of mountain sickness in the Andes. J Trop Med Hygiene 1913; 20:313–320.
3. Crane H. Soroche. Mountain sickness. Anoxemia. An Fac Med 1927; 11:306–312.
4. Lizarraga L. Soroche, agudo, edema agudo de pulmón. An Facul Med, Lima 1955; 38:244–276.
5. Bardales A. Algunos casos de edema pulmonar agudo por soroche grave. An Facul Med, Lima 1955; 38:233–240.
6. Bardales A. Edema pulmonar agudo por soroche grave. Rev Peru Cardiol 1957; 6:115–139.
7. Bardales A. Edema of the lung in mountain sickness. JAMA 1956; 160:698. Foreign letters.
8. Hultgren H, Spickard W. Medical experiences in Peru. Stanford Med Bull 1960; 18:76–95.
9. Houston C. Acute pulmonary edema of high altitude. N Engl J Med 1960; 263: 478–480.
10. Hultgren H, Spickard W, Hellriegel K, Houston C. High altitude pulmonary edema. Medicine 1961; 40:289–313.
11. Siri W. Cordillera Blanca. Sierra Club Bull 1953; 38:1–12.
12. Singh I, Kapila C, Khanna P, Nanda R, Rao B. High altitude pulmonary edema. Lancet 1965; 30:229–234.
13. Menon N. High altitude pulmonary edema. N Engl J Med 1965; 273:66–74.
14. Hackett P, Oelz O. The Lake Louise Consensus of the Definition and Quantification of Altitude Illness. In: Sutton J, Coates G, Houston C, eds. Hypoxia and Mountain Medicine. Burlington, VT: Queen City Printers, 1992:327–330.
15. Nicholas R, Theis K, Honigman B, Hultgren H. High altitude pulmonary edema in a ski resort. West J Med 1996; 164:222–227.
16. Roach R, Houston C, Honigman B, et al. How well do older persons tolerate moderate altitude. West J Med 1995; 162:32–36.
17. Maggiorini M, Bärtsch P, Oelz O. Elevated body temperature in severe mountain sickness (AMS). In: Sutton J, Coates G, Houston C (eds): Hypoxia and Mountain Medicine, Burlington, VT: Queen City Printers, 1992:311. Abstract.
18. Sophocles A, Bachman J. High altitude pulmonary edema among visitors to Summit County, Colorado. J Fam Pract 1983; 17:1015–1017.

19. Sophocles A. High altitude pulmonary edema in Vail, Colorado 1972–1982. West J Med 1986; 144:569–573.
20. Hultgren Y, Marticorena E. High altitude pulmonary edema: epidemiologic observations in Peru. Chest 1978; 74:372–376.
21. Maggiorini M, Buhler M, Waiter M, Oelz O. Prevalence of acute mountain sickness in the Swiss Alps. Br Med J 1990; 301:853–855.
22. Hackett P, Rennie D. The incidence, importance and prophylaxis of acute mountain sickness. Lancet 1976; 2:1149–1154.
23. Hochstrasser J, Mazer A, Oelz O. Altitude edema in the Swiss Alps: observations on the incidence and clinical course in 50 patients. Schweiz Med Wochenschr 1986; 116:866–873.
24. Marticorena E. Edema agudo pulmonar de altura. Doctoral thesis. Universidad Peruana Cayetano Heridia, Lima, Peru. 1971.
25. Hannon J. Comparative adaptability of young men and women. In: Folinsbee L, Wagner J, Borgia J, Drinkwater B, Gliner J, Bedi J, eds. Environmental Stress: Individual Human Adaptation. New York: Academic Press, 1978:335–350.
26. Regensteiner J, Woodard W, Hagerman D, et al. Combined effects of female hormones and metabolic rate on ventilatory drives in women. J Appl Physiol 1989; 66:808–813.
27. Matsuzawa Y, Fujimoto K, Kobayashki T, et al. Blunted hypoxic ventilatory drive in subjects susceptible to high altitude pulmonary edema. J Appl Physiol 1989; 66: 1152–1157.
28. Block A, Boysen P, Wynne J, Hunt L. Sleep apnea, hypopnea and oxygen desaturation in normal subjects. A strong male predominance. N Engl J Med 1979; 3300:513–517.
29. Lopez C. Edema agudo pulmónbar de altura in niños. Doctoral thesis. Universidad Peruana Cayetano Heridia, Lima, Peru. 1971.
30. Scoggin C, Hyers T, Reeves J, Grover R. High altitude pulmonary edema in the children and young adults of Leadville, Colorado. N Engl J Med 1977; 297: 1269–1272.
31. Lobenhoffer H, Zink R, Brendel W. High altitude pulmonary edema: analysis of 166 cases. In: Brendel W, Zink R, eds. High Altitude Physiology and Medicine, New York: Springer-Verlag, 1982.
32. Kobayshi T, Koyama S, Lubo K, Fukushima M, Kusama S. Clinical features of patients with high altitude pulmonary edema in Japan. Chest 1987; 92:814–821.
33. Fukushima M, Yochimura I, Kubol K, Kobayashi T, Handa K, Kusama S. A case of high altitude pulmonary edema. Jpn J Thorac Dis 1980; 18:753–757.
34. Antezana G, Leguia G, Guzman A, et al. Hemodynamic study of high altitude pulmonary edema (12,200 ft). In: Brendel W, Zink R, eds. High Altitude Physiology and Medicine. New York: Springer-Verlag, 1982:232–241.
35. Hultgren H, Lopez C, Lundberg E. Physiologic studies of pulmonary edema at high altitude. Circulation 1964; 29:393–408.
36. Fred H, Schmidt A, Bates T, Hecht H. Acute pulmonary edema of high altitude: clinical and physiologic observations. Circulation 1962; 25:929.
37. Penaloza D, Sime D. Circulatory dynamics during high altitude pulmonary edema. Am J Cardiol 1969; 23:369.

38. Roy S, Guleria J, Khana P. Hemodynamic studies in high altitude pulmonary edema. Br Heart J 1969; 31:52–58.
39. Levine B, Trayburn P, Voyles W, Greene R, Roach R, Hackett P. Intracardiac shunting across a patent foramen ovale may exacerbate hypoxemia in high altitude pulmonary edema. Ann Intern Med 1991; 114:569–570.
40. Dickinson J, Heath D, Gasney I, Williams D. Altitude-related deaths in seven trekkers in the Himalayas. Thorax 1983; 38:646–656.
41. Hultgren H, Spickard W, and Lopez D. Further studies of high altitude pulmonary edema. Br Heart H 1962; 24:95–102.
42. Arias-Stella J, Kruger H. Pathology of high altitude pulmonary edema. Arch Pathol 1963; 76:147–157.
43. Nayak N, Roy S, Narayanan T. Pathologic features of altitude sickness. Am J Pathol 1964; 45:381–391.
44. Nakagawa S, Kubo K, Koizumi T, et al. High altitude pulmonary edema with pulmonary thromboembolism. Chest 1993; 103:948–950.
45. Hultgren H, Kelly J, Miller H. Effect of oxygen upon pulmonary circulation in acclimatized men at high altitude. J Appl Physiol 1965; 20:239–243.
46. Hultgren H., Robinson M., Wuerflein R. Overperfusion pulmonary edema. (abstr) Circulation 1966; 33:132.
47. Hultgren H. High altitude pulmonary edema. In: Staub N, ed. Water and Solute Exchange, New York: Marcel Dekker, 1978:437–464.
48. Hultgren H. High altitude pulmonary edema—current concepts. Annu Rev Med 1995; 47:267–284.
49. Johansson B, Strandgaard S, Lassen N. On the pathogenesis of hypertensive encephalopathy: the hypertensive "breakthrough" of autoregulation of cerebral blood flow with forced vasodilatation, flow increase, and blood-brain-barrier damage. Circ Res 1974; 34–35(suppl 1):167–171.
50. Lehr D, Triller M, Fisher L, Ellis K, Fishman A. Induced changes in the pattern of pulmonary blood flow in the rabbit. Circ Res 1963; 13:119–131.
51. Viswanathan R, Subramanian S, Radha T. Effect of hypoxia on regional lung perfusion by scanning. Resp 1979; 37:142–144.
52. Dawson C, Bronikowski T, Linehan J, Hakim T. Influence of pulmonary vasoconstriction on lung water and perfusion heterogeneity. J Appl Physiol 1983; 54: 654–660.
53. Scherrer U, Vollenweider L, DeLabays A, et al. Inhaled nitric oxide for high altitude pulmonary edema. N Engl J Med 1996; 334:624–629.
54. Younes M., Bshouty Z. Effect of high blood flow, ventilation, breathing pattern, and alveolar hypoxia on lung fluid flux, In: Sutton J, Coates G, Remmers J, eds. Hypoxia: The Adaptations. Toronto; Decker, 1990:155–162.
55. Landolt C, Matthay M, Albertine K, Roos P, Wiener-Kronish J, Staub N. Overperfusion, hypoxia, and increased pressure cause only hydrostatic pulmonary edema in anesthetized sheep. Circ Res 1983; 52:335–341.
56. Hyman A. Effects of large increases in pulmonary blood flow on pulmonary venous pressure. J Appl Physiol 1961; 217:1177–1178.
57. Welling K, Sanchez R, Raven J, Larsen B, Amtorp O. Effect of prolonged alveolar hypoxia on pulmonary artery pressure and segmental vascular resistance. J Appl Physiol 1993; 75:1194–1200.

58. Nagaaka Y, Battacharya Y, Nanjo S, Gropper M, Staub N. Micropuncture measurement of lung microvascular pressure profile during hypoxia in cats. Circ Res 1984; 54:90–95.
59. Bärtsch P, Waber U, Haeberli A, et al. Enhanced fibrin formation in high altitude pulmonary edema. J Appl Physiol 1987; 63:752–757.
60. Bärtsch P, Haeberli N, Nanzer A, et al. High altitude pulmonary edema: blood coagulation. In: Sutton J, Coates G, Houston C, eds. Hypoxia and Molecular Medicine. Burlington, VT, Queen City Printers, 1993:252–258.
61. Wolfel E, Selland M, Mazzeo R, Reeves J. Systemic hypertension at 4,300 m is related to sympathoadrenal activity. J Appl Physiol 1994; 76:1643–1650.
62. Hackett P, Roach R, Hartig G, Green E, Levine B. The effect of vasodilators on pulmonary hemodynamics in high altitude pulmonary edema. A comparison. Int J Sports Med 1992; 13:568–571.
63. Pearl R, Rosenthal M, Schroeder J, Ashton J. Acute hemodynamic effects of nitroglycerine in pulmonary hypertension. Ann Intern Med 1983; 99:9–13.
64. Combret M, Rouby J, Smiegan J, Brun P, Saroux J, Marmuse J. Pulmonary edema during pulmonary embolism. Br J Dis Chest 1987; 81:407–414.
65. Arnold L, Keane J, Kan J, Fellows K, Lock J. Transient unilateral pulmonary edema after successful balloon dilatation of peripheral pulmonary artery stenosis. Am J Cardiol 1988; 62:327–330.
66. Moser K, Daily P, Peterson K, et al. Thromboendarterectomy for chronic, major-vessel thromboembolic pulmonary hypertension: immediate and long-term results in 42 patients. Ann Intern Med 1987; 107:560–565.
67. Levinson R, Shure D, Moser K. Reperfusion pulmonary edema after pulmonary artery thromboendarterectomy. Am Rev Respir Dis 1986; 139:1291–1245.
68. Hackett P, Creagh C, Grover R, Honigman B, Houston C. High altitude pulmonary edema in persons without the right pulmonary artery. N Engl J Med 1980; 302: 1070–1073.
69. Pool P, Vogel J, Blount G, Jr. Congenital unilateral absence of a pulmonary artery. Am J Cardiol 1962; 10:706–732.
70. Levine S, White D, Fels A. An abnormal chest radiograph in a patient with recurring high altitude pulmonary edema. Chest 1988; 94:627–628.
71. Fiorenzano G, Restelli V, Greco V. Unilateral high altitude pulmonary edema in a subject with right pulmonary artery hypoplasia. Resp 1994; 61:52–54.
72. Derks A, Basch F. High altitude pulmonary edema in anomalous pulmonary venous connection of drainage with intact atrial septum. Newslett Int Soc Mt Med 1995; 5:3.
73. Schoene R, Hackett P, Henderson W, et al. High altitude pulmonary edema: characteristics of lung lavage fluid. JAMA 1986; 256:63–69.
74. Schoene R, Swenson E, Pizzo C, et al. The lung at high altitude: bronchopulmonary lavage in acute mountain sickness and pulmonary edema. J Appl Physiol 1988; 64: 2605–2613.
75. West J, Tsukimoto K, Mathieu-Costello O, Prediletto R. Stress failure in pulmonary capillaries. J Appl Physiol 1991; 70:1731–1742.
76. Tsukimoto K, Yoshimure N, Ichioka M, et al. Protein, cell and LTB_4 concentrations of lung edema fluid produced by high capillary pressures in rabbit. J Appl Physiol 1994; 76:321–327.

77. Flick M, Pereel A, Staub N. Leucocytes are required for increased lung microvascular permeability after microembolization in sheep. Circ Res 1981; 48:344–351.
78. Richalet J. High altitude pulmonary edema: still a place for controversy? Thorax 1995; 50:923–929.
79. Marticorena E, Hultgren H. Evaluation of therapeutic methods in high altitude pulmonary edema. Am J Cardiol 1979; 43:307–312.
80. Hackett P. Mountain Sickness. Prevention, Recognition and Treatment. Golden, CO: American Alpine Club, 1980.
81. Taber R. A portable hyperbaric chamber for the treatment of high altitude disorders. J Wilderness Med 1990; 1:181–192.
82. Kasic J, Yaron M, Nicholas R, et al. Treatment of acute mountain sickness: hyperbaric versus oxygen therapy. Ann Emerg Med 1991; 20:1109–1112.
83. Schoene R, Roach R, Hackett P, Harrison G, Mills W. High altitude pulmonary edema and exercise at 4,400 meters: effect of expiratory positive pressure. Chest 1985; 87:330–333.
84. Vosk A, Houston C. Mediastinal emphysema in mountain climbers. Report of two cases and review. Heart Lung 1972; 6:799–805.
85. Hultgren H. Emergency maneuver in high altitude pulmonary edema. JAMA 1986; 255:3245–3246.
86. Oelz O, Maggiorini M, Ritter M, Jeni R, Waber U, Vock P. Nifedipine for high altitude pulmonary edema. Lancet 1989; 2:1241–1244.
87. Bärtsch P, Maggiorini M, Ritter M, Noti C, Vock P, Oelz O. Prevention of high altitude pulmonary edema by nifedipine. N Engl J Med 1991; 325:1284–1289.
88. McMurty I, Davidson A, Reeves J, Grover R. Inhibition of hypoxic pulmonary vasoconstriction by calcium antagonists in isolated rat lungs. Circ Res 1976; 38: 99–104.
89. Smith L. High altitude illness. JAMA 1977; 237:1199. Letter to the Editor.
90. Bates T. Pulmonary edema of mountains. Br Med J 1972; 3:829. Letter to the Editor.
91. Gray G, Bryan A, Frayser R, Houston C. Control of acute mountain sickness. Aero Med 1971; 42:81–84.

12

Mechanisms Underlying Ischemia/Reperfusion Injury of the Lung

JOHN E. HEFFNER

University of Arizona Health Sciences Center
and St. Joseph's Hospital and Medical Center
Phoenix, Arizona

I. Introduction

Extensive investigations during the past two decades have established the importance of ischemia/reperfusion (IR) injury in the pathogenesis of numerous pulmonary conditions. It has been recognized since 1979 that temporary ischemia followed by reperfusion can initiate tissue inflammation and microvascular dysfunction through oxidant-mediated mechanisms (1). Histopathologic evidence of intrapulmonary leukosequestration supports a contributory role for neutrophil activation with overabundant release of neutrophilic toxic products for the full expression of endothelial cell injury in this condition (2). More recently, recognition that secondary organ dysfunction can occur in vascular beds distant from the primary site of IR injury indicates that bloodborne mediators can generate widespread endothelial cell dysfunction. These mediators may underlie the pathogenesis of multiorgan dysfunction in various critical illnesses.

In the past several years, intensive investigations into the pathophysiology of IR injury have focused on the generation of reactive oxygen species (ROS), mechanisms of leukosequestration, the role of adhesion molecules, the nature of proinflammatory mediators, and strategies for preventing or attenuating tissue injury in this condition. This chapter will review these investigations to develop a unifying theory of the pathophysiology of IR injury as it affects the pulmonary circulation and lung function.

II. Evidence That IR Can Alter Lung Function

The lung has three potential sources of tissue oxygenation that include the pulmonary arteries, bronchial arteries, and direct diffusion of oxygen from the alveolar space. This redundant oxygen supply system initially suggested that the lung would be relatively resistant compared to other organs to injury from IR (3,4). More recent investigations in multiple experimental models and observations made in several clinical conditions, however, indicate that the lung is uniquely subject to IR-related histopathologic changes and functional abnormalities.

In experimental models, warm ischemia followed by reperfusion increases microvasculature membrane permeability as measured by abnormal filtration coefficients (5,6). This alteration in membrane permeability is accompanied by an inflammatory response characterized by leukosequestration and release of proinflammatory mediators from multiple sources (7). These findings are accompanied by abnormalities of lung function that include increased pulmonary vascular resistance, compromised gas exchange, and impaired metabolic functions of the lung, such as synthesis and release of angiotensin-converting enzyme (ACE) (8).

Several clinical conditions appear to be analogous to experimental models of IR injury. Patients treated for pneumothorax or large pleural effusions may develop pulmonary edema after lung reexpansion. In the initial generation of this condition, termed "reexpansion pulmonary edema," atelectatic lungs experience a prolonged ischemic and hypoxic state. Lung reexpansion promotes reperfusion and initiates events that result in IR injury, characterized by increased microvascular permeability in the reexpanded lung. Experimental models of atelectatic rabbit lungs reperfused after lung reexpansion simulate the clinical events of reexpansion pulmonary edema and demonstrate regional and diffuse permeability abnormalities (9,10). These models have established IR as the mechanism for edema formation in this condition.

Ischemia/reperfusion injury also appears to be a central etiologic factor in the "reimplantation response." In this condition, transplanted human lungs develop edematous lung injury related to the duration and nature of ischemia prior to reimplantation (11). The reimplantation response has emerged as a major challenge to transplantation programs because the increasing shortage of donor lungs often requires their acquisition from greater distances resulting in prolonged delays before reimplantation (12).

Several other conditions have pathophysiologic features that may depend, at least to a degree, on the presence of IR-related stress. The acute respiratory distress syndrome (ARDS) occurs in patients who experience IR in distant organs, such as muscle crush injuries in trauma patients. In this setting, ARDS may result from the release of vasoactive mediators from injured tissue that alter function in the pulmonary microcirculation either directly or through the activation and recruitment of neutrophils (7). Patients with ARDS also develop obliteration of small pulmonary vessels and may experience alveolar overdistension during mechanical ventilation, both of which can establish regional lung ischemia. Relief of vascular obstruction or attenuation of alveolar distending volumes may then initiate reperfusion injury that has the potential for augmenting the underlying lung injury. Ischemia/reperfusion stress may also contribute to lung dysfunction after pulmonary thromboembolectomy (13,14) and cardiopulmonary bypass in patients who experience postpump pulmonary edema (15).

Regardless of the clinical setting, it now appears clear that IR stress causes microvascular endothelial damage and promotes protein leakage in the pulmonary microcirculation. Resulting pulmonary dysfunction is characterized by pulmonary edema with normal capillary hydrostatic pressures, hypoxemia, ventilation-perfusion mismatch, and reduced lung compliance (16,17).

III. Mechanisms of Lung Injury

A. Reactive Oxygen Species

Demonstration of lung protection in the presence of exogenous antioxidants provides evidence for oxidant-mediated mechanisms of IR-related lung injury in experimental models. The ability of exogenous antioxidants to attenuate lung injury induced by IR was first examined in the isolated perfused lung. This ex vivo model simplifies experimental systems allowing isolation of oxidant-antioxidant interactions without the introduction of organ interactions or, in some experimental designs, the complicating effects of circulating blood elements. Exogenous antioxidants used in these models have included superoxide dismutase (SOD, a superoxide anion scavenger), dimethylthiourea (DMTU, a scavenger of hydroxyl radical), and catalase (a scavenger of hydrogen peroxide). These investigations demonstrated in the isolated perfused rabbit lung pretreated with SOD, DMTU, or catalase (6,12,18) and isolated canine lungs pretreated with SOD or catalase (19,20) that antioxidants infused before initiation of ischemia prevented or attenuated some of the features of IR injury.

Similar results have been observed in endothelial cell monolayers exposed to hypoxia and reoxygenation, which is an analogous process to IR that occurs in organs with vascular structures. Exposure of bovine endothelial cell monolayers to hypoxia and reoxygenation causes a measurable increase in albumin flux that is blocked by the preinstillation of SOD (21,22) or catalase (22) into the monolayer nutrient solution.

Whole-animal models have provided variable results regarding the capacity of exogenous antioxidants to attenuate IR lung injury. DMTU is an attractive antioxidant for these studies because its small molecular size allows it to enter endothelial cells, a putative site for oxidant generation from IR. Jackson and co-workers infused DMTU into a rabbit pneumothorax model and attenuated the severity of reexpansion pulmonary edema (23). These investigators observed that catalase did not alter lung edema formation but decreased the degree of leukosequestration in the microcirculation of the reexpanded lungs (23). The protective effects of DMTU appeared to result from scavenging of ROS rather than inhibition of PMN function because previous investigations demonstrated that DMTU does not alter PMN migration or activation (24). Bishop and co-workers were unable to demonstrate a protective effect of DMTU in a rabbit or canine whole-animal model of IR injury (25). These negative results, however, may be a consequence of the dose of DMTU used or the degree of IR stress generated, as discussed below.

SOD has been infused conjugated to polyethylene glycol (PEG) into the whole-rabbit model of reexpansion pulmonary edema (26). PEG-conjugated SOD did not attenuate the resultant permeability edema but decreased the number of neutrophils in alveolar lavage samples. Pretreatment of rabbits with SOD before occlusion of the pulmonary arteries attenuates measured alterations in function in endothelial cells harvested from large pulmonary arteries (27).

Whole-animal studies present considerable challenges in interpreting conflicting results between laboratories because of the complexity of the systems studied. For instance, lungs perfused with blood in whole-animal studies introduce the confounding effects of circulating antioxidants that may obscure contributions from exogenous agents. Additionally, exogenous antioxidants may have differing physiological effects that depend on availability of certain substrates. For instance, SOD produces hydrogen peroxide from the dismutation of superoxide. In the presence of iron, generated hydrogen peroxide can react with residual superoxide to form hydroxyl radical by Haber-Weiss chemistry (28). SOD production of hydroxyl radical, an extremely potent ROS, would initiate rather than attenuate IR tissue injury. This dual capacity of SOD to prevent or promote oxidant injury has been emphasized by McCord (29) and demonstrated in a model of myocardial IR injury (30). In this model, SOD lost its protective capacity and promoted cell injury when infused in higher concentrations. And lastly, the ischemia and reperfusion phases of IR injury may each individually make variable contributions to the final degree of lung injury observed in a specific model (31). The protective effects of exogenous antioxidants may vary depending on whether the injurious stress is primarily generated in the ischemic or reperfusion phase.

The combined results from the in vitro, ex vivo, and whole-animal investigations, however, support the concept that exogenous antioxidants prevent or attenuate the lung edema or leukosequestration observed after exposure to ischemia (hypoxemia)/reperfusion (reoxygenation) injury. It is notable that exogenous SOD and catalase can attenuate features of IR stress in some models considering the large molecular weight of these antioxidants that prevents their penetration into cells. Extracellular concentrations of these antioxidants may consume ROS immediately adjacent to the external cell membrane. The resulting lowered concentrations of ROS in the pericellular matrix may promote diffusion of oxidants out of the intracellular compartment through anion channels down a concentration gradient (18).

Direct or indirect methods for detecting generated ROS are additional approaches for determining the importance of oxidant-induced mechanisms in IR lung injury. In cultured endothelial cells, Zweier and co-workers detected by EPR spectroscopy the presence of superoxide and superoxide-derived hydroxyl radicals after cell culture reoxygenation (32). In a whole-rabbit model of reexpansion pulmonary edema, Jackson and co-workers demonstrated the presence of cyanide-insensitive respiration, which correlates with the generation of free radicals (10). In isolated perfused rabbit lungs, IR induces a threefold increase in superoxide anion concentration in the circulating perfusate (18) and exposure to hypoxic and normoxic conditions generates reaction products of hydroxyl radical (33). Superoxide anion has also been detected in bovine endothelial cell monolayers exposed to hypoxia-reoxygenation injury (22). Studies in rat IR-exposed lungs using fluorescence microtopography demonstrate that oxidants are predominately generated in the endothelial cell, type II pneumatocytes, Clara cells, ciliated cells, and macrophages (34).

A final method for establishing the existence of oxidant-mediated mechanisms of cell injury is to measure biochemical byproducts of oxidative events. In an isolated perfused lung model of IR injury, markers of lipid peroxidation and soluble products of protein oxidation have been found to correlate directly with the presence or absence of changes in lung permeability (35–37). Exposure of isolated rat or rabbit lungs to hypoxia and reoxygenation increases the ratio of oxidized (GSSG) to reduced (GSH) glutathione in the lung perfusate (38,39) thereby supporting the presence of excess generation of hydrogen peroxide that consumes GSH. Culturing cells in hypoxic conditions results in a rapid fall in mitochondrial SOD (40). Reduced mitochondrial manganese (Mn) SOD has also been demonstrated in rabbit lungs that are maintained collapsed for 7 days (10).

Cumulative investigative findings support the role of ROS in the generation of IR lung injury. Although much of the empiric evidence is indirect, the existence of metabolic byproducts of oxidant injury and the protective effects of antioxidants in the majority of experimental models support the production of ROS as a central factor. Greater confirmation of this role, however, will depend on the development of more sensitive and reliable methods for directly measuring and characterizing generated oxidants in tissues exposed to IR stress.

It should be noted that in some experimental conditions, generated oxidants may protect rather than promote tissue injury. In the presence of excess SOD, the protective effects of the enzyme can be reversed and IR tissue injury occurs (30,41). Some basal concentration of superoxide anion may be necessary to terminate lipid peroxidation in oxidant-injured tissue; high concentrations of SOD in the system eliminate the small amount of oxidant required for protection (30).

B. Sources and Mechanisms of ROS Production

Although circulating PMN recruited to the pulmonary microcirculation and resident macrophages are potent generators of ROS, pulmonary vascular endothelial cells are capable of producing and releasing to the extracellular matrix toxic oxygen metabolites under conditions of IR stress (Fig. 1) (32). Teleologically, endothelial cells may have developed the ability to generate oxidants in order to regulate their intracellular concentration of nitric oxide (NO·) (32,42). Endothelial cell production of superoxide anion inactivates excess NO· in the following reaction:

$$NO\cdot + O_2 \rightarrow NO_3^-$$

In pathological conditions, endothelial cells can activate additional systems for generating ROS. The initial interest in IR injury developed when Fridovich suggested that ischemia alters the balance between endothelial cell xanthine dehydrogenase (XDH) and xanthine oxidase (XO), thereby priming cells to produce toxic oxygen metabolites during the reoxygenation phase (1,43). XDH and XO are isoenzymes that oxidize both various purine and pteridine substrates. Xanthine oxidase, however, reduces NAD^+ in its reactions while XO univalently and divalently donates electrons to oxygen, thereby generating superoxide anion and hydrogen peroxide as toxic metabolic byproducts.

During ischemia, XDH, which normally accounts for 80% of the isoenzymes' activity in cells (44), undergoes sulfhydryl oxidation or limited proteolysis and converts to XO (45). Ischemia also causes degradation of ATP stores, thereby increasing the intracellular concentrations of hypoxanthine and xanthine. These purine substrates promote the generation of ROS by XO when reperfusion provides oxygen as the necessary cofactor. Ischemia also produces tissue acidification, which causes enhanced hemoglobin unloading of oxygen during the reperfusion phase by the Bohr effect (46). The resulting tissue hyperoxia favors XO-mediated production of superoxide anion through the univalent reduction

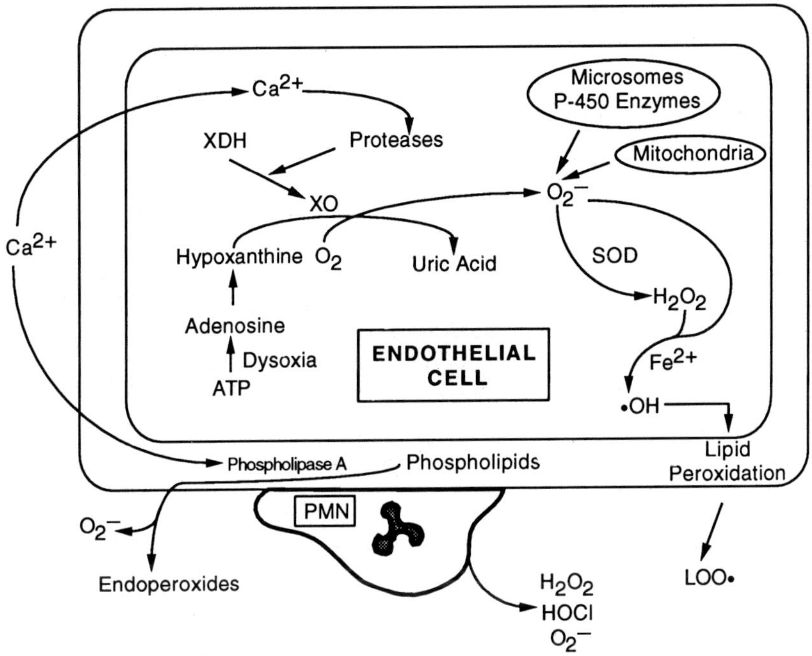

Figure 1 Potential sources of reactive oxygen metabolites during ischemia reperfusion injury of the lung. Abbreviations used: XDH = xanthine dehydrogenase; XO = xanthine oxidase; O_2^- = superoxide anion; H_2O_2 = hydrogen peroxide; SOD = superoxide dismutase; ·OH = hydroxyl radical; ATP = adenosine triphosphate; HOCL = hypochlorous acid; LOO· = lipid hydroperoxides.

of oxygen over the divalent reduction of oxygen, which produces hydrogen peroxide (47).

A role for XO-induced production of ROS in the generation of IR lung injury would seem to depend on whether the XDH/XO isoenzymes exist in sufficiently high concentrations in pulmonary vascular tissue. Pulmonary vascular endothelial cells in several species, including man, however, have been reported to be poorly endowed with XO activity compared to other organ systems (23,48,49). Adkins and co-workers reported that IR pulmonary edema occurs similarly in the lungs of rats, which have high XO activity, compared to sheep and rabbits, which hardly demonstrate any XO activity in whole-lung homogenate assays (6).

It has been argued, however, that even low concentrations of XO may produce vascular injury during IR if the enzyme is concentrated in the endothelium of the microvasculature where fluid conductance occurs (50,51). It has been suggested that XO located at this juncture on the luminal surfaces of endothelial cells may serve teleologically as a signal to activate the reticuloendothelial system to kill circulating microbes (51). Moreover, sensitive immunohistoaffinity and histochemical techniques have identified high XO enzyme levels in microvascular endothelium from organs, such as the lung and heart of some species, that were previously determined to have negligible concentrations by more standard assay techniques (31,50,52).

Experimental evidence supports a role for XO in the production of IR lung injury. Instillation of allopurinol, an inhibitor of XO, attenuates lung edema formation in isolated perfused rabbit (6,53), canine (54), and rat (55) lungs exposed to IR. Tungsten-rich diets, which depress XO activity, similarly decrease measured vascular permeability in isolated rabbit lungs (6). Allopurinol does not attenuate lung edema formation, however, in whole-animal models of reexpansion pulmonary edema (23).

In bovine endothelial cell monolayers, instillation of XO alters endothelial structure and enhances the permeability for albumin across the membrane (56). Cell structure appears to be altered through XO-induced changes on the endothelial cell cytoskeleton (57,58). Endothelial cells exposed to hypoxia followed by reoxygenation generate superoxide anion and superoxide-derived hydroxyl radical primarily from a XO source as demonstrated by EPR (32). Associated membrane permeability changes in these cell cultures exposed to hypoxia-reoxygenation are prevented by instillation of the XO inhibitors allopurinol and oxypurinol (21).

Additional studies using human cell lines demonstrate a contribution of XO to cell injury. Human umbilical vein endothelial cells grown in culture and exposed to hypoxia-reoxygenation demonstrate cell injury that is prevented by pretreatment with allopurinol (59). These investigators also detected XO activity in the injured cells (59).

Michiels and co-workers demonstrated in a human umbilical vein endothelial cell culture model that hypoxia-reoxygenation injury was prevented by allopurinol (59). They further detected XO activity in the cells exposed to hypoxia (59). Other investigators using EPR have demonstrated that suspensions of human umbilical vein endothelial cells incubated in substrate-free anoxic conditions before exposure to oxygenation are potent producers of ROS unless allopurinol is added to the solution (60). Increased XO activity has been detected in human microvascular endothelial cell cultures exposed to hypoxia-reoxygenation (61).

The above studies support a role for XO-induced generation of ROS in the pathophysiology of IR lung injury. It has been suggested that allopurinol may prevent cell injury by acting as a scavenger of superoxide anion and hydroxyl radical rather than by inhibiting XO (62). It does not appear, however, that allopurinol scavenges oxygen radicals at the concentrations used in experimental models (62,63).

In addition to the conversion of XDH to XO during ischemia and the reduction of oxygen by XO during reperfusion, other potential sources of ROS generation with endothelial cells exist. Aerobic mitochondrial metabolism normally produces a small amount of superoxide anion as a physiologic byproduct at the NADH dehydrogenase step and from auto-oxidation of ubiquinone. The mitochondrial electron transport system becomes reduced during ischemia and may generate large amounts of ROS during reperfusion (64). Evidence of this enhanced ability of mitochondria to produce toxic oxygen metabolites has been indirectly demonstrated by detecting decreased Mn SOD activity and Mn SOD content in animals after exposure to prolonged hypoxia and reperfusion (64). Myocardial cell preparations have a demonstrated capacity to produce hydrogen peroxide from mitochondrial sources during conditions of hypoxia and reoxygenation (65). Enhanced mitochondrial generation of ROS may also result from ischemia-induced cellular energy depletion that results in influxes of calcium into the cell (66) by way of a calcium channel mechanism (67).

The microsomal electron transport system is an additional, potentially important source of ROS during IR. Reactions involving NADPH cytochrome reductase and cytochrome P-450 mixed-function oxidases contribute the most to microsomal superoxide anion production (68,69). Considering that lung tissue is especially rich in cytochrome P-450 (70), microsomes may be more important in adding to IR injury affecting the lungs compared to other tissues.

Endothelial cells may also produce ROS during the metabolism of arachadonic acid. Enzyme activity at the PGH synthase and lipoxygenase steps generates superoxide anion (71). Arachidonic acid metabolism can possibly represent a positive feedback proinflammatory mechanism during IR because phospholipase A_2 is activated during IR (72) and promotes increased generation of endoperoxides by endothelial cell cyclo-oxygenase (73).

It has been suggested that the auto-oxidation of catecholamines during IR lung injury can result in superoxide anion production (74). Others have argued, however, that the autooxidation of catecholamines procedes too slowly to be of in vivo significance in pathological states (75).

C. Timing of IR Lung Injury

Because the lung has three potential sources of oxygen from the pulmonary arteries, bronchial arteries, and alveoli (3), hypoxic or anoxic conditions may not necessarily exist during the ischemia phase of IR injury. Consequently, sufficient tissue oxygen may be available during ischemia to generate ROS and produce cell injury in contrast to nonpulmonary tissue wherein ROS are formed with the reperfusion of oxygen. It is possible, therefore, that lung tissue has a unique property to become injured during ischemia as well as reperfusion. Investigations in different models have conflicted as to whether lung IR injury primarily occurs during ischemia or reperfusion (15,19,27,36,37,76–82).

Differences in investigations that attempt to isolate the relative importance of ischemia and reperfusion in IR lung injury may result from differences in the vascular site studied. For instance, tissue in the lung periphery may be exposed to hyperoxia from alveolar sources during ischemia in contrast to proximal tissue, which is distant from gas exchanging units and may therefore be relatively hypoxic during ischemia (19,73). Also, isolated perfused lung models tend to support reperfusion dependency of IR injury compared to investigations using whole animals. Conflicting findings made in these different models may result from the difficulty in whole animals of completely stopping all blood flow to ischemic regions and the confounding effects of circulating antioxidants. As a final explanation of differences in experimental models, Fisher and co-workers recently demonstrated that different types of oxidants may be generated in different experimental conditions (33). In their isolated perfused rabbit lung model, hydroxyl radical and hydrogen peroxide were generated after ischemic lungs were reperfused and reoxygenated. In ischemic lungs reperfused but not reoxygenated (ventilated with nitrogen), only hydrogen peroxide increased. Oxidant generation in lungs exposed to IR may therefore have oxygen-dependent and oxygen-independent mechanisms. Different experimental models, therefore, may observe a varying importance of the ischemia and reperfusion phases for the generation of lung injury depending on the existence of factors that initiate one or more of the mechanisms for producing ROS. It remains, however, that the multiple sources of oxygen available to lung tissue underlie more complicated processes for the production of IR injury than other organ systems. Fisher and co-workers have suggested that in the absence of hypoxia during the ischemic phase, changes in cell membranes due to alterations of normal mechanical forces may initiate injury rather than decreased tissue ATP (83).

D. Participation of Neutrophils in IR Lung Injury

In nearly all experimental models of IR injury, neutrophils can be observed adhering to endothelial surfaces (84–90). In pulmonary IR injury, attraction and adherence of neutrophils to the microcirculation occur in a parallel time course to the onset and progression of the observed lung dysfunction (91,92). Furthermore, neutrophils isolated from the pulmonary microvasculature of rats exposed to hepatic IR are highly activated, and the degree of activation correlates with the severity of lung injury (90).

Adherence of neutrophils to endothelial surfaces would seem to be a likely event for the promotion and augmentation of lung injury because of the neutrophil's tremendous capacity to release a variety of toxic compounds. Activated neutrophils release elastase, which can hydrolyze a variety of biological substrates. Neutrophil elastase has been demonstrated to augment cell damage observed in endothelial cell cultures exposed to hypoxia and reoxygenation (93).

Moreover, activated neutrophils produce toxic oxygen metabolites through myeloperoxidase and lactoferrin pathways in addition to membrane-associated NADPH oxidase (94). And finally, neutrophils can release arachidonate products that can directly affect the pulmonary microvasculature. As outlined below, extensive investigations have examined the mechanisms for recruitment of neutrophils to the pulmonary vasculature during IR and the ability of recruited neutrophils to initiate and amplify IR lung injury (95).

The generation of ROS may initiate the recruitment of neutrophils to the pulmonary vascular bed, as shown by the attenuation of leukosequestration by the instillation of exogenous antioxidants in some IR models (26). Generated ROS may stimulate endothelial cells to release pro-inflammatory mediators that attract, initiate adherence, and activate neutrophils (96,97).

Experimental models have demonstrated the release of chemotactic agents during IR stress that may serve to attract neutrophils to the pulmonary microcirculation. In a unilateral sheep lung ischemia model, mixed venous blood contains increased neutrophil chemotactic activity that is immunoreactive with interleukin-8 (IL-8), a neutrophil chemoattractant (98). A neutrophil chemoattractant has also been detected in cell cultures of human umbilical vein endothelial cells exposed to hypoxia (99). High concentrations of IL-8 and leukotriene B_4 have been measured in pulmonary edema fluid collected from a patient with reexpansion pulmonary edema (100). Moreover, oxidation of phospholipase A_2 during ischemia can generate endoperoxides that can be metabolized by neutrophils to chemoattractant leukotrienes (101).

Recent data indicate that enhanced neutrophil adherence to endothelial surfaces is a central mechanism for promoting neutrophil sequestration in the lung during IR. Specific aspects of adherence mechanisms as they relate to IR tissue injury have been reviewed (7,102). Cell culture studies demonstrate that endothelial cells exposed to hypoxia-reoxygenation alter their surfaces in a manner that enhances neutrophil adherence (88). Upregulation of endothelial cell ligand intracellular adhesion molecule 1 (ICAM-1) (55,103) and expression of neutrophil CD11/CD18 adhesion glycoprotein complexes (55,104) are critical events in promoting neutrophil adherence. Immunoneutralization of CD18 and ICAM-1 in an isolated rat lung model decreases intrapulmonary neutrophil sequestration (55). Moreover, infusion of monoclonal anti-ICAM-1 antibodies into an isolated perfused rabbit lung transplantation model preserved oxygenation capacity and attenuated leukocyte infiltration (105).

Generation of nitric oxide by endothelial cells is a potential protective mechanism against IR injury in that NO· can inhibit neutrophil adhesion (106), possibly through inactivation of superoxide anion and reduction of the superoxide-induced stimulus for adhesion (107). This protective effect of NO· has been demonstrated in an in vivo rat model of IR wherein NO· inhibits pulmonary leukosequestration and lung injury (108). As will be discussed below, the generation of NO· by endothelial cells may provide other protective mechanisms in IR injury.

Neutrophils may also become entrapped in the pulmonary microcirculation due to a decreased capacity for deformation during IR conditions (7). Neutrophils are relatively large, viscoelastic cells that must de-form substantially during their transit through capillary beds. Tissue conditions related to IR may activate neutrophils and thereby decrease their de-formability and ability to pass through pulmonary capillaries narrowed by tissue edema. Some investigators consider that decreased de-formability initiates leukosequestration, which is followed by adhesion to endothelial surfaces with the expression of adhesion molecules (109).

Additional investigative data suggest that neutrophils sequestered in the pulmonary circulation contribute to lung injury initiated by IR. These investigations have employed techniques that deplete experimental models of neutrophils, block neutrophil chemotaxis and neutrophil adhesion, and reintroduce neutrophils back into neutrophil-depleted systems.

Neutrophil depletion models have provided conflicting data regarding a necessary role for neutrophils in the pathogenesis of IR lung injury (6,22, 26,86,91,110,111). In neutrophil depletion studies of Jackson and co-workers (26), neutrophil content was decreased in alveolar lavagates from rabbits exposed to reexpansion lung injury but the severity of permeability lung edema was unaffected. Pretreatment of rabbits with nitrogen mustard to deplete circulating neutrophils similarly did not attenuate IR-induced lung injury (91). Rats made neutropenic with the infusion of antineutrophil antibodies did not have decreased sensitivity to reperfusion lung injury (110). Neutrophils have not been demonstrated to be necessary factors for the generation of IR injury in the isolated perfused rat lung (111) or hypoxia-reoxygenation injury in endothelial cell cultures (22). In models of cardiopulmonary bypass lung injury, however, pulmonary edema can be prevented by reperfusion with leukocyte-depleted blood (15). Also, neutrophils are required for lung injury to occur in a model of intestinal IR (86) and in a rabbit model of IR lung injury (6).

In contrast to the above neutrophil depletion studies, investigations that block neutrophil chemotaxis or adherence support a role for neutrophils in IR lung injury. Lodoxamide is an agent that causes a dose-dependent inhibition of neutrophil-directed migration. Instillation of this agent into animal models of IR lung injury decrease leukosequestration and attenuate the measured alterations in alveolar-capillary permeability (112). Lodoxamide, however, also inhibits XO activity (113). Other studies using monoclonal antibodies directed at neutrophil or endothelial adhesion molecules decrease neutrophil recruitment to the lung and attenuate the severity of IR lung injury (6,55,103,104,114–116). Immunoneutralization of CD18 and ICAM-1 in an isolated rat lung model decreases intrapulmonary neutrophil sequestration and attenuates the degree of pulmonary edema by 50% after IR (55). Inhibition of P-selectin has been shown to attenuate lung injury in rat models of intestinal IR (92) and isolated perfused rat lung models of IR (55), although the degree of leukosequestration appears not to be affected. Immunoneutralization of P-selectin may attenuate lung injury without decreasing intrapulmonary neutrophil sequestration possibly because (1) expression of P-selectin primes endothelial cells for injury prior to leukocyte adhesion (117), (2) P-selectin interactions with neutrophils may promote the neutrophil respiratory burst (118), or (3) IR results in decreased neutrophil deformability and promotes neutrophil entrapment but P-selectin is required for adhesion and initiation of endothelial injury (109). Immunoneutralization of L-selectin does not prevent permeability increases or neutrophil entrapment in isolated perfused rat lungs exposed to IR (55). Recent data in bovine aortic endothelial cell models indicate that hypoxia serves as a physiological signal in combination with TNF-α to promote the expression of endothelial E-selectin (119).

Introduction of neutrophils into neutrophil-free models has been demonstrated to augment IR-related injury. Addition of neutrophils to hypoxic endothelial cells in culture increases the degree of observed endothelial cell dysfunction (93).

Several considerations assist in interpreting the conflicting investigations that examine the role of neutrophils in the pathogenesis of IR lung injury. The adherence of neutrophils and the ability to demonstrate a neutrophil effect on endothelial surfaces may vary greatly depending on experimental conditions. For instance, shear forces within microvasculature and the kinetic energy of circulating neutrophils determine the degree to which neutrophils can adhere to the luminal surfaces of vessels and initiate endothelial cell injury (120). This impact of flow state on IR-induced lung injury has been examined in a rat isolated perfused lung model (121). In this model, neutrophils were instilled into the perfusate at different perfusate flow rates. Greater adherence of neutrophils to the pulmonary vasculature was observed at the lower compared to the higher perfusate flow rates. Furthermore, intravital miscroscopic studies demonstrate in mesenteric venules that the number of adherent neutrophils progressively increase as shear stresses are reduced from normal values of 18 dyn/cm^2 to 6 dyn/cm^2 (122).

It has also been demonstrated that the hemocytometer methods used in neutropenic models of IR lung injury overestimate the degree of neutropenia (121). Preparations deemed to be neutrophil-free may actually have as many as $10^3/\mu l$ circulating neutrophils. This concentration of neutrophils may be sufficient in models of IR to produce adherence of residual neutrophils and neutrophil-dependent lung injury in conditions of low flow where neutrophil adherence to endothelial surfaces is promoted.

Additionally, experimental conditions may vary depending on the relative duration and severity of the exposure to the ischemia versus the reperfusion phases of IR injury (6). Models wherein injury primarily occurs during the ischemic phase may differ in pathogenesis from models wherein injury occurs primarily during reperfusion. Fisher and co-workers demonstrated in a rabbit isolated lung model that different metabolic pathways exist for the generation of ROS when the relative "doses" of ischemia and reperfusion are altered (33). Neutrophils, therefore, may appear to have more or less of a pathogenetic effect in different experimental models.

On the basis of the reviewed data, activation of neutrophils and their sequestration in the pulmonary microcirculation appear to be central events in the pathogenesis of IR-related lung injury. Direct IR injury to the lungs initiates endothelial cell injury that can progress to pulmonary edema without the presence of neutrophils if the degreee of ischemia- or reperfusion-related events are sufficiently severe. Ischemia/reperfusion injury in tissues distant from the lungs most likely depends to a large degree on activation of circulating neutrophils and adhesion molecules to promote intrapulmonary leukosequestration and lung injury. Because neutrophils can also release inflammatory mediators that promote the conversion of endothelial cell XDH to XO (123), leukosequestration in IR injury may initiate a positive feedback loop that amplifies the severity of lung inflammation (6). Other types of leukocytes may participate in IR-induced injury, but the neutrophil is believed to the the major mediator.

E. Additional Contributory Factors

Other factors that support the generation of intracellular oxidants and promote tissue inflammation most likely participate in the pathogenesis of IR lung injury (Table 1). These contributory elements include alterations in intracellular concentrations of calcium, the status of tissue iron stores, availability of energy substrates, complement, cytokines, and enzymes of the cytochrome P-450 system. The importance of some of these noncellular mediators of tissue injury are supported by observations in models of unilateral lung IR injury. Contralateral lungs in animals exposed to unilateral lung IR demonstrate intravascular entrapment of neutrophils (81,124,125), altered membrane permeability (126), decreased antioxidant content (39), and abnormal protein flux as measured by positron emission tomography (127,128). Because activated phagocytic cells in the venous circulation of the ischemic lung would not readily cross the systemic capillary bed and sequester in the contralateral nonischemic lung, circulating factors, such as TNF-α (129), IL-8, and LTB_4 (100), would seem to participate in the generation of IR lung injury.

Ischemia results in the exhaustion of intracellular ATP energy stores (130), which may trigger the initial events of IR-related lung injury. The lung has a minimal capacity to store glycogen even though glucose is the primary energy substrate for pulmonary cells. Exhaustion of lung cell glucose stores, therefore,

Table 1 Factors That May Contribute to the Generation of Pulmonary Ischemia/Reperfusion Injury

- Cellular energy depletion with influx of calcium
- Calcium activation of proteolytic enzymes
- Proteolytic conversion of XDH to XO
- Degradation of energy stores during ischemia with conversion of ATP to hypoxanthine and xanthine
- Tissue acidosis promotion of hemoglobin unloading of oxygen (Bohr effect) with promotion of superoxide anion generation by xanthine oxidase
- Mitochondrial electron transport system production of oxygen metabolites
- Microsomal production of oxygen metabolites
- Generation of oxygen metabolites through arachidonate metabolism
- Auto-oxidation of catecholamines
- Mechanical alterations of cell membranes
- Adherence and activation of neutrophils with release of cytotoxic compounds
- Release of free iron with hydroxyl radical production through Haber-Weiss chemistry
- Complement activation
- Cytokine release
- Impairment of normal vascular vasoregulation
  —Alterations in eicosanoid metabolism
  —Impairment of nitric oxide synthesis

may underlie ATP depletion during ischemia. The importance of retaining adequate cellular concentrations of glucose is supported by observations that ischemic injury to the lungs correlates with both oxygen tension and glucose levels (77). Depletion of glucose and glucose-dependent enzyme systems can also result in decreased intracellular concentrations of reduced glutathione, thereby diminishing pulmonary antioxidant defenses (130).

Depleted energy stores can also affect calcium homeostasis. Cells require a constant source of energy in the form of ATP to remove intracellular calcium by the endoplasmic reticulum in order to maintain the normal 10,000:1 balance of extracellular to intracellular calcium (130). Depletion of ATP during ischemia allows an influx of calcium that activates proteases resulting in the irreversible transformation of XDH to XO (131). Increased intracellular concentrations of calcium can also activate thromboxane and leukotrienes, which increase vasoreactivity and activate platelets (132), and inhibit mitochondrial electron transport, which can promote the generation of hydrogen peroxide (66). An important role for calcium in IR-related lung injury is supported by observations that calcium channel blocking agents can improve oxygen transfer and pulmonary hemodynamics in lungs exposed to ischemia (133). Low ATP stores can promote an influx of calcium into the cell with subsequent dysfunction of cell mitochondria and membranes. These events have been observed within 48 hours of unilateral pulmonary arterial occlusion in dogs in a manner that correlates with depletion of ATP stores (134).

The ability of superoxide anion generated during IR to cause tissue injury is markedly amplified in the presence of free iron. Superoxide anion can reduce ferritin-bound iron to the ferrous state and thereby promote the release of iron from ferritin (35,135–137) in the following reaction:

$$O_2^- + \text{Ferritin-FE}^{3+} \rightarrow O_2 + \text{Ferritin} + Fe^{2+}$$

Free iron can then initiate lipid peroxidation by causing reductive lysis of oxygen-oxygen bonds in lipid hydroperoxide molecules (29). The major effect of free iron, however, on oxidant-induced tissue injury is through its promotion of the iron-catalyzed reaction called Haber-Weiss chemistry (28), which forms highly reactive hydroxyl radicals:

$$O_2^- + Fe^{3+} \rightarrow O_2 + Fe^{2+}$$

$$Fe^{2+} + H_2O_2 \rightarrow Fe^{3+} + \cdot OH + OH^-$$

Hydroxyl radical is an extraordinarily potent oxidant that can cause severe tissue injury. Experiments using deferoxamine, an iron-chelating agent, support a role for iron catalyzed reactions in IR-related lung injury. Rabbit isolated perfused lungs exposed to warm IR fail to develop lung edema when pretreated with deferoxamine (18). Instillation of deferoxamine into a dense suspension of human umbilical vein endothelial cells exposed to anoxia decreases the generation of ROS as measured by EPR (60). Instillation of iron chelating agents also prevent cell injury in human umbilical vein endothelial cell cultures exposed to hypoxia-reoxygenation (59).

Studies employing deferoxamine to chelate iron may be confounded by the capacity of deferoxamine to also scavenge hydroxyl radical (138). Further investigation is required to firmly establish that iron redox cycling and Haber-Weiss chemistry contribute significantly to IR lung injury.

A role for complement in IR lung injury has not been clearly established. Although some studies indicate that IR lung injury can develop despite the depletion of complement by pretreatment with cobra venom factor (139), other investigations suggest that complement may contribute to lung injury through complex interactions. In the rat model of intestinal IR injury, infusion of soluble complement receptor type 1 (sCR1) ameliorates injury in distant organs including the lung but does not prevent intrapulmonary leukosequestration (140,141). These observations suggest that endothelial cells exposed to IR injury lose their autoprotective proteins and become complement activators (142). Activation of endothelium-fixed iC3b may then promote the activation of adhered neutrophils recruited to the lung through non-complement-related mechanisms. It is also possible—although not well demonstrated—that IR in organs distant from the lung results in systemic complement activation, which in turn activates circulating neutrophils and increases the expression of adhesion molecules, resulting in leukosequestration within the lung.

Several cytokines that may be expressed by ischemic tissue appear to have a capacity for initiating or augmenting IR-related lung injury. TNFα is cytotoxic itself but also upregulates neutrophil and endothelial cell adhesion molecules (143) and activates circulating neutrophils (90). The interleukins IL-1 and IL-8 upregulate endothelial cell adhesion molecules and act as chemotaxins (144). A role for these cytokines in IR lung injury is supported by observations that hindlimb IR in rats increases plasma levels of TNFα, IL-1, and IL-8 (145). Infusion of cytokine-blocking agents prevents the observed lung injury in this model. TNFα is also released after transient occlusion of the pulmonary artery (146). Moreover, chemotactic activity for neutrophils in mixed venous blood increases and appears related to a substance that is immunoreactive to IL-8 antibody (98). Additional studies indicate that TNFα contributes to pulmonary capillary injury due to hepatic ischemia (85) and lower torso ischemia (147). It appears likely that lung injury related to TNFα is mediated through enhanced endothelial adhesion of neutrophils (148). However, direct killing of TNF-sensitive cells by TNFα is enhanced by the generation of reactive oxygen species as occurs in IR and may serve as an additional TNF-mediated mechanism (149).

Mechanisms mediated through enzymes of the P-450 system may also promote IR lung injury. In an isolated rabbit lung model of IR injury, P-450 enzyme inhibitors prevented lung edema formation and lipid peroxidation but did not alter the generation of superoxide anion (35). These inhibitors did decrease, however, the formation of non-protein-bound, low-molecular-weight chelates of iron after the establishment of reperfusion. These observations suggest that the P-450 enzyme system releases iron from intracellular stores and promotes its participation in the generation of free radicals in ischemic tissue (35).

The widely diverse effects on vascular membranes that are mediated through arachidonate metabolites suggest that these agents may participate in IR lung injury. Moreover, the generation of ROS in microvasculature and an increase in intracellular calcium content as observed in IR injury can activate thromboxane and leukotriene synthesis (150).

Arachidonate metabolites have been found to increase in concentration in several isolated perfused lung models of IR injury (73,151–153). Also, pulmonary artery occlusion and reperfusion in the canine model causes mast cells to degranulate and release LTB_4 (154). Cultures of microvascular endothelial cells exposed to hypoxia and reoxygenation have increased XO activity that parallels an enhanced synthesis of thromboxane (61).

The capacity of arachidonate metabolites to initiate or augment IR lung injury, however, is not clearly established. Inhibition of thromboxane generation in isolated perfused lung models attenuates IR lung edema (151,152). The protective mechanisms, however, may depend on the prevention of thromboxane-induced increases in capillary hydrostatic pressures, as discussed below. Fisher and co-workers attributed a significant proportion of the lipid peroxidation in an isolated perfused lung model of IR to the generation of arachidonic acid metabolites (73). Other investigators, however, observed in ischemic isolated rat lungs that inhibition of cyclo-oxygenase and lipoxygenase enzymes with eicosatetraynoic acid (ETYA) did not alter the oxidation of soluble protein (37). Moreover, treating suspensions of human umbilical endothelial cells exposed to anoxia-reoxygenation with blockers of cyclo-oxygenase does not alter the degree of oxygen radical generation as measured by EPR (60).

IV. Relationship of IR Injury to Vascular Reactivity

Most models of IR lung injury demonstrate that pulmonary vessels vasoconstrict during the reperfusion period (6,18,54,152,155). This vasoconstriction may augment edema formation because pulmonary vascular resistance shifts more toward the postcapillary venules, which increases capillary hydrostatic pressures (6,54). Inhibition of this pressor response to IR results in attenuation of edema formation in isolated perfused lung models (151,152).

Mechanisms underlying the pressor response appear to be at least partly mediated through the release of arachidonate metabolites. Instillation of indomethacin, a cyclo-oxygenase inhibitor, prevents pulmonary vasoconstriction during reperfusion (18). Treatment of a rabbit isolated lung model with a specific thromboxane/prostaglandin H_2 receptor antagonist also attenuates the pressor response to IR (152).

Other investigations suggest that nitric oxide-related mechanisms may participate in the pressor response of IR. Superoxide anion and SOD-derived reactive oxygen species generated during IR have the capacity to react with NO· and accelerate its degradation (156,157). Diminished concentrations of NO·, a vasodilator, would be expected to produce vasoconstriction. Recent investigations have further outlined mechanisms wherein oxidant stress may limit endothelial cell production of NO· through calcium-dependent mechanisms (158). Moreover, animal models indicate that NO· production is rapidly suppressed after the induction of ischemia/reperfusion injury (159,160).

V. Therapeutic Strategies and Preventive Measures

Insights into the putative mechanisms of IR-related lung injury suggest therapeutic and preventive strategies, some of which already have demonstrated clinical utility (Table 2). Calcium channel blockers have been used in lung preser-

Table 2 Potential Therapeutic Interventions to Prevent or Attenuate Ischemia/Reperfusion Lung Injury

- Calcium channel blockers
- Iron chelation
- Supplementation of intracellular energy stores
    - ATP (ATP-$MgCl_2$)
    - Hydroxybutyrate
    - Pyruvate
- Adenosine supplementation
    - Increases cAMP
    - Inhibits neutrophil activation
    - Inhibits calcium influx
    - Increases glucose transport
    - Promotes SOD activity
- Supplement intracellular cAMP
    - Adenosine
    - Hydroxybutyrate
    - Pyruvate
    - 2-Chloroadenosine
    - Rolipram
- Supplement nitric oxide
    - Nitric oxide inhalation
    - L-arginine
- Exogenous eicosanoids
    - PGE_1
- Maintain platelet function
- Therapy with licensed drugs
    - Cimetidine
    - Pentoxifylline

vation solutions to prevent the reimplantation response (161). Strategies for enhancing cellular antioxidant reserves and chelating free iron are undergoing clinical investigation for various pulmonary and nonpulmonary conditions (101,162).

Other interventions remain investigational. In vitro studies demonstrate that ATP supplementation inhibits neutrophil chemotaxis and the production of superoxide anion (163,164). In a rat model of IR injury, infusion of ATP-$MgCl_2$ results in decreased injury through mechanisms that depend on the preservation of normal activity of neutrophil *ecto*-adenosinetriphosphatase (165), which is thought to generate adenosine from ATP. It is uncertain whether ATP-$MgCl_2$ preserves lung function by supplying energy substrates or through its effects of delivering adenosine to the cell.

Factors that increase endothelial cell cAMP inhibit IR injury in isolated perfused lung models (155,166). Adenosine, which is produced by ischemic tissue, increases cAMP levels in cells through its effects on adenosine A_2 receptors and adenyl cyclase (155,167). Adenosine may also be beneficial in IR lung injury because it inhibits neutrophil activation and release of oxidants and proteases (168,169). More recently, putative cytoprotective mechanisms of adenosine in various tissues have been extended to inhibition of calcium influx into ischemic cells, increase in glucose transport and energy production, and enhancement of superoxide dismutase activity (170).

The addition of adenosine into models of neutrophil-induced injury has been shown to attenuate endothelial permeability changes (171). Moreover, inactivation of adenosine by adenosine deaminase increases neutrophil-induced endothelial injury (168). Other compounds may prevent IR lung injury through their ability to increase cAMP levels. A stable adenosine analogue, 2-chloroadenosine, has been shown to reduce lung edema in rabbits exposed to IR (8). Rolipram, an agent that inhibits phosphodiesterase-mediated cAMP breakdown, can reverse pulmonary capillary IR injury (172). Enhancement of cellular energy stores by the infusion of b-hydroxybutyrate and pyruvate have also been shown to attenuate IR lung injury (59). These agents are quickly incorporated into the Kreb's cycle as energy substrates.

Interventions to promote endogenous production of NO· or exogenous supplementation of inhaled NO· may attenuate IR injury. NO· regulates platelet aggregation, vascular tone, and neutrophil adhesion, all of which participate in IR-induced pulmonary membrane injury (106). More importantly, recent data indicate that NO· may also directly preserve endothelial membranes. Inhalation of NO· attenuates pulmonary vascular permeability after induction of hydrogen peroxide-induced injury by the infusion of purine and xanthine oxidase (173) or glucose and glucose oxidase (174). Exogenous NO· has been shown to reduce oxidant injury in the intestine or heart after exposure to IR (175,176). Also, infusion of L-arginine, a precursor of NO·, in an isolated rabbit lung model of IR results in preservation of endothelial membrane function (177). Experiments in an isolated heart IR model indicate that coinfusion of L-arginine with N^G-nitro-L-arginine, a specific inhibitor of the formation of NO· from L-arginine, prevent tissue protection (178). These findings indicate that L-arginine protects membranes exposed to IR through the generation of NO·. Recently, infusion of glyceryl trinitrate, a NO· donor, has been shown to attenuate reperfusion-induced lung injury in an animal model of aortic occlusion (179). Other NO· donors, such as S-nitroso-N-acetyl-D-penicillamine, are undergoing evaluation in models of oxidant-induced lung injury (180).

Although the protective mechanisms of NO· are unknown, several known effects of NO· have been proposed to participate in maintenance of normal membrane permeability in IR (174). As previously mentioned, NO· decreases neutrophil adhesion, emigration, and activation (107,181); suppresses mast cell degranulation (182); and inhibits the release of various cytotoxic factors (175). NO· also has the capacity to suppress oxidant-induced membrane injury by binding with free iron and other transition metal ion complexes, thereby decreasing their reactivity and ability to generate hydroxyl radicals in the Fenton reaction (183,184). By binding with iron, NO· can also inhibit lipid peroxidation initiated by myoglobin, hemoglobin, lipoxygenase, and cyclooxygenase (183, 185,186). And finally, NO· can scavenge hydroxyl radical directly (183). It should be cautioned, however, that NO· can conversely promote oxidant injury by interacting with superoxide to form peroxynitrite (187) (see Chap. 15).

Exogenous eicosanoids have been examined in IR injury. The infusion of PGE_1 has beneficial effects in an in situ rabbit model of lung IR that does not appear to occur as a result of its vasodilating, antiplatelet, neutrophil inhibitory, or TNF suppressive effects (188).

Modulation of neutrophil function by interfering with neutrophil-endothelium interactions is a promising approach to limiting IR injury. Ongoing studies suggest that inhibition of adhesion molecules (ICAM-1 and E-selectin) or leukocyte adhesion molecules (L-selectin, CD11a/CD18, CD11b/CD18) may attenuate IR-mediated lung injury (102,105). This approach may be especially valuable in lung transplantation wherein the transplanted organ can be pretreated with blocking antibodies to prevent the reimplantation response.

Interventions that modulate platelet function may reduce the severity of IR lung injury. Platelets contribute to endothelial cell viability and normal integrity of vascular membranes (189–191). In a rabbit isolated lung model of IR injury, infused human platelets attenuated the severity of lung edema formation through mechanisms that appear dependent on normal functioning of the platelet glutathione redox cycle (192). Platelets may protect membranes by delivering adenosine to endothelial cells (193).

Several licensed drugs have been investigated in IR lung injury. Cimetidine, an inhibitor of P-450 enzymes, attenuates IR lung injury (35). Pentoxifylline (PTX) reduces capillary injury and attenuates edema formation in animal models exposed to intestinal ischemia (194). PTX also attenuates lung injury in rat lungs undergoing IR stress, possibly through inhibition of intrapulmonary leukosequestration (195,196). PTX may prevent entrapment of neutrophils in the lung microcirculation by inhibiting expression of CD11/CD18 on neutrophils (197) or by decreasing cytokine production (198). PTX also inhibits neutrophil release of ROS and proteases (199), scavenges ROS (200), and directly preserves endothelial cell membrane permeability characteristics (201). A PTX analog, Procysteine, is currently in a clinical trial for the treatment of early clinical lung injury (see Chap. 20).

VI. Unifying Description of Pathophysiologic Events

It is clear that the lung is subject to IR injury on the basis of pathological changes and functional abnormalities. It is also clear that extrapulmonary tissue injured during IR can release mediators that can initiate a series of events that cause leukosequestration and alter the permeability characteristics of pulmonary microvascular membranes.

Cells directly exposed to IR experience an influx of calcium, depletion of energy substrates, generation of free iron from protein-bound iron stores, and alteration of intracellular enzyme systems. Sufficient evidence supports the hypothesis that a modest but functionally important concentration of superoxide anion is generated during reperfusion by XO that is converted from XDH during the ischemia phase. Additional sources exist, however, for endothelial cell production of oxidants from microsomes, mitochondria, and arachidonate metabolism. Combined with free iron, toxic concentrations of hydroxyl radical can be generated from superoxide anion and hydrogen peroxide by Haber-Weiss chemistry.

The initial oxidant-induced cellular injury triggers the release or activation of pro-inflammatory mediators such as TNFα, interleukins, complement, and arachidonate metabolites. In instances wherein extrapulmonary tissue is the primary target of IR injury, noncellular pro-inflammatory mediators released into the circulation can directly damage pulmonary endothelial cells and activate circulating neutrophils, which express adhesion molecules and promote leukosequestration. When IR stress directly affects the lungs, altered pulmonary microvasculature activate neutrophils during their transit through the lung.

Once entrapped in the pulmonary circulation, neutrophils can amplify lung injury through the release of oxidants and cytotoxic enzymes. Activated neutrophils can also accelerate the conversion of XDH to XO and recruit additional neutrophils to the lung by releasing chemoattractants. These cellular interactions between neutrophils and endothelial cells can perpetuate IR injury through amplification of a pro-inflammatory cascade.

References

1. Fridovich I. Hypoxia and oxygen toxicity. Adv Neurol 1979; 26:255–259.
2. Ward Pa, Till GO, Warren JS. Pathophysiology of leukocyte-mediated tissue injury. J Crit Care 1992; 6:112–116.
3. Deffebach M, Charan N, Lakshminarayan S, Butler J. The bronchial circulation: small, but a vital attribute of the lung. Am Rev Respir Dis 1987; 135:463–481.
4. Fisher A, Dodia C. The lung as a model for evaluation of critical intracellular PO_2 and PCO_2. Am J Physiol 1981; 241:E47–E50.

5. Pavlin J, Cheney F. Unilateral pulmonary edema in rabbits after re-expansion of collapsed lung. J Appl Physiol 1979; 46:31–35.
6. Adkins W, Taylor A. Role of xanthine oxidase and neutrophils in ischemia-reperfusion injury in rabbit lung. J Appl Physiol 1990; 69:2012–2018.
7. Korthuis RJ, Anderson DC, Granger DN. Role of neutrophil-endothelial cell adhesion in inflammatory disorders. J Crit Care 1994; 9:47–71.
8. Marts B, Baudendistel L, Naunheim K, Dahms T. Protective effect of 2-chloroadenosine on lung ischemia reperfusion injury. J Surg Res 1993; 54:523–529.
9. Pavlin J, Nessly M, Cheney F. Hemodynamic effects of rapidly evacuating prolonged pneumothorax in rabbits. J Appl Physiol 1987; 62:477–484.
10. Jackson R, Brannen A, Veal C, Fulmer J. Superoxide dismutase and cytochrome oxidase in collapsed lungs: possible role in reexpansion edema. J Appl Physiol 1988; 65:235–241.
11. Parquin F, Le Roy Ladurie F, Cerrina J, et al. Outcome of immediate pulmonary edema after lung transplantation (abstr). Am J Respir Crit Care Med 1993; 149:A733.
12. Stuart R, Baumgartner W, Borkon A, et al. Five-hour hypothermic lung preservation with oxygen free-radical scavengers. Transplant Proc 1985; 17:1454–1456.
13. Levinson R, Shure D, Moser K. Reperfusion pulmonary edema after pulmonary artery thromboendarterectomy. Am Rev Respir Dis 1986; 134:1241–1245.
14. Moser K, Spragg R, Utley J, Daily P. Chronic thrombotic obstruction of major pulmonary arteries. Ann Intern Med 1988; 99:299–305.
15. Kuratani T, Matsuda H, Sawa Y, Kaneko M, Nakano S, Kawashima Y. Experimental study in a rabbit model of ischemia-reperfusion lung injury during cardiopulmonary bypass. J Thorac Cardiovasc Surg 1992; 103:564–568.
16. Fantini GA, Conte MS. Pulmonary failure following lower torso ischemia: clinical evidence for a remote effect of reperfusion injury. Am Surg 1995; 61:316–319.
17. Paterson IS, Klausner JM, Pugatch R. Noncardiogenic pulmonary edema after abdominal aortic aneurysm surgery. Ann Surg 1989; 209:231–236.
18. Kennedy T, Rao N, Hopkins C, Pennington L, Tolley E, Holdal J. Role of reactive oxygen species in reperfusion injury of the rabbit lung. J Clin Invest 1989; 83: 1326–1335.
19. Koyama I, Toung J, Rogers M, Gurtner G, Traystman R. O_2 radicals mediate reperfusion lung injury in ischemic O_2-ventilated canine pulmonary lobe. J Appl Physiol 1987; 63:111–115.
20. Paull D, Keagy B, Kron E, Wilcox B. Reperfusion injury in the lung preserved for 24 hours. Ann Thorac Surg 1989; 47:187–192.
21. Inauen W, Payne D, Kvietys P, Granger D. Hypoxia/reoxygenation increases the premeability of endothelial cell monolayers: role of oxygen radicals. Free Rad Biol Med 1990; 9:219–223.
22. Lum H, Barr D, Shaffer J, Gordon R, Ezrin A, Malik A. Reoxygenation of endothelial cells increases permeability by oxidant-dependent mechanisms. Circ Res 1992; 70:991–998.
23. Jackson R, Veal C, Alexander C, Brannen A, Fulmer J. Re-expansion pulmonary edema. A potential role for free radicals in its pathogenesis. Am Rev Respir Dis 1988; 137:1165–1171.

24. Jackson J, White C, Parker N, McMurtry I, Berger E, Repine J. Dimethylthiourea decreases acute lung edema in phorbol myristate acetate-treated rabbits. J Appl Physiol 1986; 61:353–360.
25. Bishop M, Chi E, Su M, Cheney F. Dimethylthiourea does not ameliorate reperfusion lung injury in dogs or rabbits. J Appl Physiol 1988; 65:2051–2056.
26. Jackson R, Veal C, Beckman J, Brannen A. Polyethylene glycol-conjugated superoxide dismutase in unilateral lung injury due to re-expansion (re-oxygenation). Am J Med Sci 1990; 299:22–28.
27. Davenpeck K, Guo J-P, Lefer A. Pulmonary artery endothelial dysfunction following ischemia and reperfusion of the rabbit lung. J Vasc Res 1993; 30: 145–153.
28. Beauchamp C, Fridovich I. A mechanism for the production of ethylene from methional. The generation of the hydroxyl radical by xanthine oxidase. J Biol Chem 1970; 245:4641–4646.
29. McCord J. Human disease, free radicals, and the oxidant/antioxidant balance. Clin Biochem 1993; 26:351–357.
30. Omar B, Gad N, Jordan M, et al. Cardioprotection by Cu,Zn-superoxide dismutase is lost at high doses in the reoxygenated heart. Free Rad Biol Med 1990; 9: 465–471.
31. Bulkley G. Free radicals and other reactive oxygen metabolities: clinical relevance and the therapeutic efficacy of antioxidant therapy. Surgery 1993; 113: 479–483.
32. Zweier J, Kuppusamy P, Lutty G. Measurement of endothelial cell free radical generation: evidence for a central mechanism of free radical injury in postischemic tissues. Proc Natl Acad Sci USA 1988; 85:4046–4050.
33. Fisher P, Huang Y-C, Kennedy T, Piantadosi C. PO_2-dependent hydroxyl radical production during ischemia-reperfusion lung injury. Am J Physiol 1993; 265: L279–L285.
34. Al-Mehdi A, Shuman H, Fisher A. Fluorescence microtopography of oxidative stress in lung ischemia-reperfusion. Lab Invest 1994; 70:579–587.
35. Bysani G, Kennedy T, Ky N, Rao N, Blaze C, Hoidal J. Role of cytochrome P-450 in reperfusion injury of the rabbit lung. J Clin Invest 1990; 86:1434–1441.
36. Eckenhoff R, Dodia C, Tan Z, Fisher A. Oxygen-dependent reperfusion injury in the isolated rat lung. J Appl Physiol 1992; 72:1454–1460.
37. Ayene I, Dodia C, Fisher A. Role of oxygen in oxidation of lipid and protein during ischemia/reperfusion in isolated perfused rat lung. Arch Biochem Biophys 1992; 296:183–189.
38. Jenkinson S, Marcum R, Pickard J, Orzechowski Z, Lawrence R, Jordan J. Glutathione disulfide formation occurring during hypoxia and reoxygenation of rat lung. J Lab Clin Med 1988; 112:471–480.
39. Jackson R, Veal C. Effects of hypoxia and reoxygenation on lung glutathione system. Am J Physiol 1990; 259:H518–H524.
40. Liu J, Simon L, Phillips J, Robin E. Superoxide dismutase (SOD) activity in hypoxic mammalian systems. J Appl Physiol 1988; 42:107–110.
41. Bernier M, Manning A, Hearse D. Reperfusion arrhythmias: dose-related protection by anti-free radical interventions. Am J Physiol 1989; 256:H1344–H1352.

42. Moncada S, Radomski M, Palmer R. Endothelium-derived ralaxing factor. Identification as nitric oxide and role in the control of vascular tone and platelet function. Biochem Pharmacol 1988; 37:223–233.
43. McCord J. Oxygen-derived free radicals in postischemic tissue injury. N Engl J Med 1985; 312:159–163.
44. Parks D, Williams T, Beckman J. Conversion of xanthine dehydrogenase to oxidase in ischemic rat intestine: a reevaluation. Am J Physiol 1988; 254:G768–G774.
45. Engerson T, McKelvey T, Rhyne D, et al. Conversion of xanthine dehydrogenase to oxidase in ischemic rat tissues. J Clin Invest 1987; 79:1564–1570.
46. Wolbarsht M, Fridovich I. Hyperoxia during reperfusion is a factor in reperfusion injury. Free Rad Biol Med 1989; 6:61–62.
47. Fridovich I. Quantitative aspects of the production of superoxide anion radical by xanthine oxidase. J Biol Chem 1970; 245:4053–4057.
48. Eddy L, Stewart J, Jones H, Engerson T, McCord J, Downey J. Free radical producing enzyme, xanthine oxidase, is undetectable in human hearts. Am J Physiol 1987; 253:H709–H711.
49. Zweier J, Kuppusamy P, Williams R, et al. Measurement and characterization of postischemic free radical generation in the isolated perfused heart. J Biol Chem 1989; 264:18890–18895.
50. Jarasch E, Bruder G, Heid H. Significance of xanthine oxidase in capillary endothelial cells. Acta Physiol Scand 1986; 548:39–46.
51. Bulkley G. Endothelial xanthine oxidase: a radical transducer of inflammatory signals for reticuloendothelial activation. Br J Surg 1993; 80:684–686.
52. Terada L, Leff J, Repine J. Measurement of xanthine oxidase in biological tissues. Methods Enzymol 1990; 186:651–656.
53. Horgan M, Lum H, Balik A. Pulmonary edema after pulmonary artery occlusion and reperfusion. Am Rev Respir Dis 1989; 140:1421–1428.
54. Allison R, Kyle J, Adkins W, Prasad V, McCord J, Taylor A. Effect of ischemia reperfusion or hypoxia reoxygenation on lung vascular permeability and resistance. J Appl Physiol 1990; 69:597–603.
55. Moore TM, Khimenko P, Adkins WK, Miyasaka M, Taylore AE. Adhesion molecules contribute to ischemia and reperfusion-induced injury in the isolated rat lung. J Appl Physiol 1995; 78:2245–2252.
56. Shasby D, Lind S, Shasby S, Goldsmith J, Hunninghake G. Reversible oxidant-induced increases in albumin transfer across cultured endothelium: alterations in cell shape and calcium homeostasis. Blood 1985; 65:605–614.
57. Alexander J, Hechtman H, Shepro D. Phalloidin enhances endothelial barrier function and reduces inflammatory permeability in vitro. Microvasc Res 1988; 35: 308–315.
58. Rasio E, Bendayan M, Goresky C, Alexander J, Shepro D. Effect of Phalloidin on structure and permeability of rete capillaries in the normal and hypoxic state. Circ Res 1989; 65:591–599.
59. Michiels C, Arnould T, Houbion A, Remacle J. Human umbilical vein endothelial cells submitted to hypoxia-reoxygenation in vitro: implication of free radicals, xanthine oxidase, and energy deficiency. J Cell Physiol 1992; 153:53–61.

60. Zweier J, Kuppusamy P, Thompson-Gorman S, Klunk D, Lutty G. Measurement and characterization of free radical generation in reoxygenated human endothelial cells. Am J Physiol 1994; 266:C700–C708.
61. Wiles M, Hectman H, Morel N, Shepro D. Hypoxia reoxygenation induces injury of cultured pulmonary microvessel endothelial cells. J Leukocyte Biol 1993; 53: 490–497.
62. Moorhouse P, Grootveld M, Halliwel B, Quinlan J, Gutteridge J. Allopurinol and oxypurionol are hydroxyl radical scavengers. FEBS Lett 1987; 213:23–28.
63. Zimmerman B, Parks D, Grisham M, Granger D. Allopurinol does not enhance antioxidant properties of extracellular fluid. Am J Physiol 1988; 255:H202–H206.
64. Russell W, Jackson R. MnSOD protein content changes in hypoxic/hypoperfused lung tissue. Am J Respir Cell Molec Biol 1993; 9:610–616.
65. Shlafer M, Myers C, Adkins S. Mitochondrial hydrogen peroxide generation and activities of glutathione peroxidase and superoxide dismutase following global ischemia. J Molec Cell Cardiol 1987; 19:1195–1206.
66. Turrens J, Beconi M, Barilla J. Mitochondrial generation of oxygen radicals during reoxygenation of ischemic tissues. Free Rad Biol Med 1991; 12:681–684.
67. Vaca L, Kunze DL. Depletion of intracellular Ca^{2+} stores activates a Ca^{2+} selective channel in vascular endothelium. Am J Physiol 1994; 267:C920–C925.
68. White R, Coon M. Oxygen activation by cytochrome P-450. Annu Rev Biochem 1980; 49:315–356.
69. Aust S, Roerig D, Pederson T. Evidence for superoxide generation by NADPH-cytochrome C reductase of rat liver microsomes. Biochem Biophys Res Commun 1972; 47:1133–1137.
70. Schwab G, Johnson E. Enzymology of rabbit cytochromes P-450. In: Guengerich P, ed. Mammalian Cytochromes P-450. Vol. 1. Boca Raton, FL: CRC Press, 1987: 55–105.
71. Kukreja R, Kontos H, Hess M, Ellis E. PGH synthase and lipoxygenase generate superoxide in the presence of NADH or NADPH. Circ Res 1986; 59:612–619.
72. Karmazyn M, Moffat M. Toxic properties of arachidonic acid on normal, ischemic, and reperfused hearts. Indirect evidence for free radical involvement. Prostaglandins Leukotrienes Med 1985; 17:251–264.
73. Fisher A, Dodia C, Tan Z, Ayene I, Echenhoff R. Oxygen-dependent lipid peroxidation during lung ischemia. J Clin Invest 1991; 88:674–679.
74. Cohen G. Oxy-radical toxicity in catecholamine neurons. Neurotoxicol 1984; 5: 77–82.
75. Jewett S, Eddy L, Hochstein P. Is the autoxidation of catecholamines involved in ischemia-reperfusion injury? Free Rad Biol Med 1989; 6:185–188.
76. Barie P, Malik A. Effect of pulmonary arterial occlusion on lung fluid and protein exchange. J Appl Physiol 1982; 53:543–548.
77. Becker P, Pearse D, Sylvester J. Effects of oxygen tension and glucose concentration on ischemic injury in ventilated ferret lungs. J Appl Physiol 1993; 75: 1233–1237.
78. Badellino M, Morganroth M, Grum C, Lynch M, Bolling S, Deeb G. Hypothermia or continuous ventilation decreases ischemia reperfusion injury in an ex vivo rat lung. Surgery 1989; 105:752–760.

79. Overand P, Bishop M, Eistenstein B, Chi E, Menglung S, Cheney F. Lack of alveolar O_2 during lung reperfusion does not decrease edema formation. J Appl Physiol 1989; 67:528–533.
80. Bishop M, Holman R, Guidotti S, Alberts M, Chi E. Pulmonary artery occlusion and lung collapse depletes rabbit lung adenosine triphosphate. Anesthesiology 1994; 80:611–617.
81. Wickersham N, Johnson J, Meyrick B, Gilroy R, Loyd J. Lung ischemia-reperfusion injury in awake sheep: protection with verapamil. J Appl Physiol 1991; 71:1554–1562.
82. Imai T, Fujita T. Unilateral lung injury caused by ischemia without hypoxia in isolated rat lungs perfused with buffer solution. J Lab Clin Med 1994; 123: 830–836.
83. Fisher AB, Al-Mehdi A. Lipid and protein oxidation in ischemia/reperfusion of the lung. In: Weir EK, Archer SL, Reeves JT, eds. Nitric Oxide and Radicals in the Pulmonary Vasculature. Armonk, NY: Futura Publishing Co., 1996:45–61.
84. Jaeschke H, Farhood H. Neutrophil and Kupffer cell-induced oxidant stress and ischemia-reperfusion injury in rat liver in vivo. Am J Physiol 1991; 260:G355–G362.
85. Colletti LM, Burtch GD, Remick DG, et al. The production of tumor necrosis factor-α development of a pulmonary capillary injury following hepatic ischemia-reperfusion. Transplantation 1990; 49:268–272.
86. Simpson R, Alon R, Kobzik L, Valeri R, Shepro D. Neutrophil and nonneutrophil-mediated injury in intestinal ischemia-reperfusion. Ann Surg 1993; 218:444–454.
87. Terada LS, Dormish JJ, Shanley PF, et al. Circulating xanthine oxidase mediates lung neutrophil sequestration after intestinal ischemia-reperfusion. Am J Physiol 1992; 263:L394–L401.
88. Suzuki M, Inauen W, Kvietys P, et al. Superoxide mediates reperfusion-induced leukocyte-endothelial cell interactions. Am J Physiol 1989; 257:H1740–H1745.
89. Schmeling DJ, Caty MG, Oldham KT, Guice KS, Hinshaw DB. Evidence for a neutrophil-related acute lung injury following intestinal ischemia-reperfusion. Surgery 1989; 106:195–202.
90. McGuire GM, Liu P, Jaeschke H. Neutrophil-induced lung damage after hepatic ischemia and endotoxemia. Free Rad Biol Med 1996; 20:189–197.
91. Jackson R, Veal C, Alexander C, Brannen A, Fulmer J. Neutrophils in reexpansion pulmonary edema. J Appl Physiol 1988; 65:228–234.
92. Carden D, Young J, Granger D. Pulmonary microvascular injury after intestinal ischemia-reperfusion: role of P-selectin. J Appl Physiol 1993; 75:2529–2534.
93. Inauen W, Granger D, Meininger C, Schelling M, Granger H, Kvietys P. Anoxia-reoxygenation-induced, neutrophil-mediated endothelial cell injury: role of elastase. Am J Physiol 1990; 259:H925–H931.
94. Rossi F. The superoxide forming NADPH oxidase of phagocytes: nature, mechanisms of activation and function. Biochim Biophys Acta 1986; 853:65–89.
95. Seekamp A, Mulligan M, Till G, Ward P. Requirements for neutrophil products and L-arginine in ischemia-reperfusion injury. Am J Pathol 1993; 142:1217–1226.
96. Granger D, Benoit J, Suzuki M, Grisham M. Leukocyte adherence to venular endothelium during ischemia-reperfusion. Am J Physiol 1989; 257:G683–G688.

97. Granger D. Role of xanthine oxidase and granulocytes in ischemia-reperfusion injury. Am J Physiol 1988; 255:H1269–H1275.
98. Wickersham N, Loyd J, Johnson J, McCain R, Christman J. Acute inflammation in a sheep model of unilateral lung ischemia: the role of interleukin-8 recruitment of polymorphonuclear leukocytes. Am J Respir Cell Molec Biol 1993; 9:199–204.
99. Fletcher D, Osinga D, Hand K, et al. A comparison of alpha-proteinase inhibitor methoxysuccinyl-ala-ala-pro-val-chloromethylketone and specific beta-lactam inhibitors in an acute model of human polymorphonuclear leukocyte elastase-induced lung hemoorhage in the hamster. Am Rev Respir Dis 1990; 141:672–677.
100. Nakamura H, Ishizaka A, Sawafuji M, et al. Elevated levels of interleukin-8 and leukotriene B4 in pulmonary edema fluid of a patient with reexpansion pulmonary edema. Am J Respir Crit Care Med 1994; 149:1037–1040.
101. Cohen M. Free radicals in ischemic and reperfusion myocardial injury: is this the time for clinical trials? Ann Intern Med 1989; 111:918–931.
102. Lukacs NW, Ward PA. Inflammatory mediators, cytokines, and adhesion molecules in pulmonary inflammation and injury. Adv Immunol 1996; 62:257–304.
103. Horgan M, Ge M, Gu J, Rothlein R, Malik A. Role of ICAM-1 in neutrophil-mediated lung vascular injury after occlusion and reperfusion. Am J Physiol 1991; 261:H1578–H1584.
104. Horgan M, Wright S, Malik A. Antibody against leukocyte integrin (CD18) prevents reperfusion-induced lung vascular injury. Am J Physiol 1990; 259:L315–L319.
105. Buchanan SA, Mauney MC, deLima NF, et al. Enhanced isolated lung function after ischemia with anti-intercellular adhesion molecule antibody. J Thorac Cardiovasc Surg 1996; 111:941–947.
106. McCall T, Boughton-Smith N, Palmer R, Whittle B, Moncada S. Synthesis of nitric oxide from L-arginine by neutrophils: release and interaction with superoxide anion. Biochem J 1989; 261:293–296.
107. Gaboury J, Woodman R, Granger D, Reinhardt P, Kubes P. Nitric oxide prevents leukocyte adherence: role of superoxide. Am J Physiol 1993; 265:H862–H867.
108. Abdih H, Kelly C, Bouchier-Hayes D, et al. Nitric oxide (endothelium-derived relaxing factor) attenuates revascularization-induced lung injury. J Surg Res 1994; 57:39–43.
109. Doershuck CM. The role of CD-18-mediated adhesion in neutrophil sequestration induced by infusion of activated plasma in rabbits. Am J Respir Cell Molec Biol 1992; 7:140–148.
110. Steimle C, Guyunn T, Morganroth M, Bolling S, Carr K, Deeb G. Neutrophils are not necessary for ischemia-reperfusion lung injury. Ann Thorac Surg 1992; 53: 64–73.
111. Deeb G, Grum C, Lynch M, et al. Neutrophils are not necessary for induction of ischemia-reperfusion lung injury. J Appl Physiol 1990; 68:374–381.
112. Veal C, Jackson R, Brannen A, Fulmer J. Lodoxamide tromethamine prevents neutrophil accumulation in reexpansion pulmonary edema. J Cardiovasc Pharmacol 1989; 14:227–232.
113. White G. Inhibition of oxidative enzymes by anti-allergy drugs. Agents Actions 1981; 11:503–509.

114. Goldman G, Welbourn R, Rothlein R, et al. Adherent neutrophils mediate permeability after atelectasis. Ann Surg 1992; 216:372–380.
115. Kapelanski DP, Iguchi A, Niles SD, Mao HZ. Lung reperfusion injury is reduced by inhibiting a CD18-dependent mechanism. J Heart Lung Transplant 1993; 12: 294–307.
116. Seekamp A, Mulligan MS, Till GO, et al. Role of beta 2 integrins and ICAM-1 in lung injury following ischemia-reperfusion of rat hind limbs. Am J Pathol 1993; 143:464–472.
117. Harris NR, Granger DN. Leukocytes contribute to increased capillary filtration induced by inflammatory mediators. FASEB J 1993; 7:A887.
118. Kishimoto TK, Jutila MA, Berg EL, Butcher EC. Neutrophil Mac-1 and Mel-1 adhesion proteins inversely regulated by chemotactic factors. Science 1989; 245: 1238–1241.
119. Zünd G, Nelson DP, Neufeld EJ, et al. Hypoxia enhances stimulus-dependent induction of E-selectin on aortic endothelial cells. Proc Natl Acad Sci USA 1996; 93:7075–7080.
120. Hogg J. Neutrophil kinetics and lung injury. Physiol Rev 1987; 67:1249–1295.
121. Seibert A, Haynes J, Taylor A. Ischemia-reperfusion injury in the isolated rat lung. Am Rev Respir Dis 1993; 147:270–275.
122. Perry MA, Granger DN. Role of CD11/CD18 in shear rate-dependent leukocyte-endothelial cell interactions in cat mesenteric venules. J Clin Invest 1991; 87: 1798–1804.
123. Phan S, Gannon D, Varani J, Ryan V, Ward P. Xanthine oxidase activity in rat pulmonary artery endothelial cells and its alteration by activated neutrophils. Am J Pathol 1989; 134:1201–1211.
124. Bishop M, Boatmen E, Ivey T, Jordan J, Cheney F. Reperfusion in ischemic dog lung results in fever, leukopenia, and lung edema. Am Rev Respir Dis 1986; 134: 752–756.
125. Bishop M, Kowalski T, Guidotti S, Harlan J. Antibody against PMN adhesion improves reperfusion and limits alveolar infiltrate following unilateral pulmonary artery occlusion. J Surg Res 1992; 52:199–204.
126. Bishop M, Chi E, Cheney F. Lung reperfusion in dogs causes bilateral lung injury. J Appl Physiol 1987; 63:942–950.
127. Palazzo R, Hamvas A, Shuman T, Kaiser L, Cooper J, Schuster D. Injury in nonischemic lung after unilateral pulmonary ischemia with reperfusion. J Appl Physiol 1992; 72:612–620.
128. Hamvas A, Palazzo R, Kaiser L, et al. Inflammation and oxygen free radical formation during pulmonary ischemia-reperfusion injury. J Appl Physiol 1992; 72:621–628.
129. Tutor J, Mason C, Dobard E, Beckerman R, Summer W, Nelson S. Loss of compartmentalization of alveolar tumor necrosis factor after lung injury. Am J Respir Crit Care Med 1994; 149:1107–1111.
130. Cheung J, Bonventre J, Malis C, Leaf A. Calcium and ischemic injury. N Engl J Med 1986; 314:1670–1676.
131. Melgren R. Calcium-dependent proteases: an enzyme system active at cellular membranes. FASEB J 1987 Aug; 1(2):110–115.

132. Fuller B, Gower J, Green C. Free radical damage and organ preservation: fact or fiction? A review of the interrelationship between oxidative stress and physiological ion disbalance. Cryobiology 1988; 25:377–393.
133. Hachida M, Morton D. The protection of ischemic lung with verapamil and hydralazine. J Thorac Cardiovasc Surg 1988; 95:178–183.
134. Modry D, Chiu R. Pulmonary reperfusion syndrome. Ann Thorac Surg 1979; 27: 206–215.
135. Biemond P, Swaak A, Beindorff C, Koster J. Superoxide-dependent and -independent mechanisms of iron mobilization from ferritin by xanthine oxidase. Implications for oxygen-free-radical-induced tissue destruction during ischaemia and inflammation. Biochem J 1986; 239:169–173.
136. Nayini N, White B, Aust S, et al. Post resuscitation iron delocalization and malondialdehyde production in the brain following prolonged cardiac arrest. J Free Rad Biol Med 1985; 1:111–116.
137. Halliwell B, Gutteridge J. Oxygen free radicals and iron in relation to biology and medicine: some problems and concepts. Arch Biochem Biophys 1986; 246: 501–514.
138. Halliwell B. Use of desferrioxamine as a "probe" for iron-dependent formation of hydroxyl radicals. Evidence for a direct reaction between desferal and the superoxide radical. Biochem Pharmacol 1985; 34:229–233.
139. Bishop M, Giclas P, Guidotti S, Su M, Chi E. Complement activation is a secondary rather than a causative factor in rabbit pulmonary artery ischemia/ reperfusion injury. Am Rev Respir Dis 1991; 143:386–390.
140. Hill J, Lindsay TF, Ortiz F, Yeh CG, Hechtman HB, Moore FD. Soluble complement receptor type 1 ameliorates the local and remote organ injury after intestinal ischemia-reperfusion in the rat. J Immunol 1992; 149:1723–1728.
141. Lindsay TF, Hill J, Ortiz F, et al. Blockade of complement activation prevents local and pulmonary albumin leak after lower torso ischemia-reperfusion. Ann Surg 1992; 216:677–683.
142. Moore FD Jr. Therapeutic regulation of the complement system in acute injury states. Adv Immunol 1994; 56:267–299.
143. Gamble J, Harlan J, Klebanoff S, Vadas M. Stimulation of the adherence of neutrophils to umbilical vein endothelium by human recombinant tumor necrosis factor. Proc Natl Acad Sci USA 1985; 82:8667–8671.
144. Youker K, Smith C, Anderson D, et al. Neutrophil adherence to isolated adult cardiac myocytes. J Clin Invest 1992; 89:602–609.
145. Seekamp A, Warren J, Remick D, Till G, Ward P. Requirements for tumor necrosis factor-α and interleukin-1 in limb ischemia/reperfusion injury and associated lung injury. Am J Pathol 1993; 143:453–463.
146. Palace G, Del Vecchio P, Horgan M, Malik A. Release of tumor necrosis factor after pulmonary artery occlusion and reperfusion. Am Rev Respir Dis 1993; 147: 143–147.
147. Welbourn R, Goldman G, O'Riordain M, et al. Role of tumor necrosis factor as mediator of lung injury follwoing lower torso ischemia. J Appl Physiol 1991; 70: 2645–2649.

148. Lo S, Everitt J, Gu J, Malik A. Tumor necrosis factor mediates experimental pulmonary edema by ICAM-1 and CD-18-dependent mechanisms. J Clin Invest 1992; 89:981–988.
149. Pogrebniak H, Matthews W, Mitchell J, Russo A, Samuni A, Pass H. Spin trap protection from tumor necrosis factor cytotoxcity. J Surg Res 1991; 50: 469–474.
150. Allen B, Okamoto F, Buckberg G, et al. Reperfusate composition: benefits of marked hypocalcemia and diltiazem on regional recovery. J Thorac Cardiovasc Surg 1986; 92:564–572.
151. Ljungman A, Grum C, Deeb G, Bolling S, Morganroth M. Inhibition of cyclo-oxygenase metabolite production attenuates ischemia-reperfusion lung injury. Am Rev Respir Dis 1991; 143:610–617.
152. Zamora C, Baron D, Heffner J. Thromboxane contributes to pulmonary hypertension in ischemia-reperfusion lung injury. J Appl Physiol 1993; 74:224–229.
153. Palace G, Horgan M, Malik A. Generation of 5-lipoxygenase metabolites following pulmonary reperfusion in isolated rabbit lungs. Prostaglandins 1992; 43: 339–349.
154. Su M, Chi E, Bishop M, Hebderson W. Lung MAST cells increase in number and degranulate during pulmonary artery occlusion/reperfusion injury in dogs. Am Rev Respir Dis 1993; 147:448–456.
155. Adkins W, Barnard J, May S, Seibert A, Haynes J, Taylor A. Compounds that increase cAMP prevent ischemia-reperfusion pulmonary capillary injury. J Appl Physiol 1992; 72:492–497.
156. Gryglewski R, Palmer R, Moncada S. Superoxide anion is involved in the breakdown of endothelium-derived vascular relaxing factor. Nature (Lond) 1986; 320: 454–456.
157. Beckman J, Beckman T, Chen J, Marshall P, Freeman B. Apparent hydroxyl radical production by peroxynitrate: implications for endothelial injury from nitric oxide and superoxide. Proc Natl Acad Sci USA 1990; 87:1620–1624.
158. Elliott SJ, Koliwad SK. Oxidant stress and endothelial membrane transport. Free Rad Biol Med 1995; 19:649–658.
159. Summers ST, Zinner MJ, Freischlag JA. Production of endothelium-derived relaxing factor (EDRF) is compromised after ischemia reperfusion. Am J Surg 1993; 166:216–220.
160. Tao, P. S., Aoki N, Lefer DJ, Johnson G, Lefer AM. Time course of endothelial dysfunction and myocardial injury during myocardial ischemia and reperfusion in the cat. Circulation 1990; 82:1402–1412.
161. Karck M, Schmid C, Siclari F, Dammenhayn L, Haverick A. Effects of calcium channel blockage in postischemic lung reperfusion. Transplant Proc 1990; 22: 2237.
162. Hall ED, McCall JM, Means ED. Theraeputic potential of the lazaroids (21-aminosteroids) in acute central nervious system trauma, ischemia and subarachnoid hemorrhage. Adv Pharmacol 1994; 28:221–268.
163. McGarrity S, Stephenson A, Webster R. Regulation of human neutrophil functions by adenine nucleotides. J Immunol 1989; 142:1986–1994.

164. McCord J, Petrone W, Jones H. ecto-ATPase-mediated inhibition of human neutrophil functions by adenine nucleotides. Adv Inflammat Res 1985; 10: 21–29.
165. Hsu K, Wang D, Wu S-Y, Shen C-Y, Chen H. Ischemia-reperfusion lung injury attenuated by ATP-$MgCl_2$ in rats. J Appl Physiol 1994; 76(2):545–552.
166. Seibert A, Thompson W, Taylor A, Wilborn W, Barnard J, Haynes J. Reversal of increased microvascular permeability associated with ischemia-reperfusion: role of cAMP. J Appl Physiol 1992; 72:389–395.
167. Cronstein B, Kramer S, Rosenstein E, Korchak H, Weissmann G, Hirschhorn R. Occupancy of adenosine receptors raises cAMP alone and in synergy with occupancy of chemoattractant receptors and inhibits membrane depolarization. Biochem J 1988; 252:709–715.
168. Cronstein B, Levin R, Belanoff J, Weissmann G, Hirschhorn R. Adenosine: an endogenous inhibitor of neutrophil-mediated injury to endothelial cells. J Clin Invest 1986; 78:760–770.
169. Cronstein B, Kubersky S, Weissmann G, Hirschhorn R. Engagement of adenosine receptors inhibits hydrogen peroxide (H_2O_2) release by activated human neutrophils. Clin Immunol Immunopathol 1987; 42:76–85.
170. Ramkumar V, Nie Z, Rybak LP, Maggirwar SB. Adenosine, antioxidant enzymes and cytoprotection. Trends Pharmacol Sci 1995; 16:283–285.
171. Bradley J, Zanaboni P, Dahms T, Webster R. Vascular resistance and Kf in normal and PMA-injured rabbit lungs: effects of adenosine. J Appl Physiol 1991; 72: 417–424.
172. Barnard J, Seibert A, Prasad V, et al. Reversal of pulmonary capillary ischemia-reperfusion injury by rolipram, a cAMP phosphodiesterase inhibitor. J Appl Physiol 1994; 77:774–781.
173. Kavanagh BP, Mouchawar A, Goldsmith J, Pearl RG. Effects of inhaled NO and inhibition of endogenous NO synthesis in oxidant-induced acute lung injury. J Appl Physiol 1994; 76:1324–1329.
174. Poss WB, Timmons OD, Farrukh IS, Hoidal JR. Inhaled nitric oxide prevents the increase in pulmonary vascular permeability caused by hydrogen peroxide. J Appl Physiol 1995; 79:886–891.
175. Aoki N, Johnson G III, Lefer AM. Beneficial effects of two forms of NO administration in feline splanchnic artery occlusion shock. Am J Physiol 1990; 258: G275–G281.
176. Masini E, Bianchi S, Mugnai L, et al. The effect of nitric oxide generators on ischemia-reperfusion injury and histamine release in isolated perfused guinea-pig heart. Agents Actions 1991; 33:53–56.
177. Normandin L, Mazmanian M, Brink C, Chapelier A, Dartevelle P, Herve P. L-arginine and pentoxifylline attenuate pulmonary vascular dysfunction in vessels after reperfusion in blood perfused rabbit lung (abstr). Am J Respir Crit Care Med 1993; 149:A737.
178. Li XS, Uriuda Y, Wang QD, Nordlander R, Sjöquist PO, Pernow J. Role of L-arginine in preventing myocardial and endothelial injury following ischaemia/reperfusion in the rat isolated heart. Acta Physiol Scand 1996; 156:37–44.

179. Barry MC, Kelly CJ, Stokes K, et al. Glyceryl trinitrate prevents neutrophil activation but not thromboxame release following ischaemia-reperfusion injury. Br J Surg 1996; 83:1095–1100.
180. Chang J, Rao NV, Markewitz BA, Hoidal JR, Michael JR. Nitric oxide donor prevents hydrogen peroxide-mediated endothelial cell injury. Am J Physiol 1996; 270:L931–L940.
181. Pinsky DJ, Oz MC, Koga S, et al. Cardiac preservation is enhanced in a heterotropic rat transplant model by supplementing the nitric oxide pathway. J Clin Invest 1994; 93:2291–2297.
182. Kurose I, Wolf R, Grishham MB, Granger DN. Modulation of ischemia/reperfusion-induced microvascular dysfunction by nitric oxide. Circ Res 1994; 74: 376–382.
183. Kanner J, Harel S, Granit R. Nitric oxide as an antioxidant. Arch Biochem Biophys 1991; 289:130–136.
184. Stamler JS, Osborne JA, Jaraki O, et al. Adverse vascular effects of homocysteine are modulated by endothelium-derived relaxing factor and related oxides of nitrogen. J Clin Invest 1993; 91:308–318.
185. Bruckdorfer KR, Dee G, Jacobs M, Rice-Evans CA. The protective action of nitric oxide against membrane damage induced by myoglobin radicals. Biochem Soc Trans 1990; 18:285–286.
186. Kanner J, Harel S, Granit R. Nitric oxide, an inhibitor of lipid oxidation by liposygenase, cyclooxygenase and hemoglobin. Lipids 1992; 27:46–49.
187. Radi R, Beckman JS, Bush KM, Freeman BA. Peroxynitrite oxidation of sulfhydryls. The cytotoxic potential of superoxide and nitric oxide. J Biol Chem 1991; 266:4244–4250.
188. Matsuzaki Y, Waddell T, Puskas J, et al. Amelioration of post-ischemic lung reperfusion injury by prostaglandin E_1. Am Rev Respir Dis 1993; 148: 882–889.
189. Heffner JE, Sahn SA, Repine JE. State of the art: the role of platelets in the adult respiratory distress syndrome. Am Rev Respir Dis 1987; 135:482–489.
190. Heffner J, Katz S, Halushka P, Cook J. Human platelets attenuate oxidant injury in isolated rabbit lungs. J Appl Physiol 1988; 65:1258–1266.
191. Heffner JE, Cook JA, Halushka PV. Human platelets modulate edema formation in isolated rabbit lungs. J Clin Invest 1989; 84:757–764.
192. Zamora C, Baron D, Heffner J. Washed human platelets prevent ischemia-reperfusion edema in isolated rabbit lungs. J Appl Physiol 1991; 70:1075–1084.
193. Paty P, Sherman P, Shepard J, Malik A, Kaplan J. Role of adenosine in platelet-mediated reduction in pulmonary vascular permeability. Am J Physiol 1992; 262: H771–H777.
194. Carter MB, Wilson MA, Wead WB, Garrison RN. Pentoxifylline attenuates pulmonary macromolecular leakage after intestinal ischemia-reperfusion. Arch Surg 1995; 130:1337–1344.
195. Chapelier A, Reignier J, Mazmanian M, et al. Pentoxifylline and lung ischemia-reperfusion injury: application to lung transplantation. J Cardiovasc Pharmacol 1995; 25(suppl 2):S130–S133.

196. Reigner J, Mazmanian M, Detruit H, et al. Reduction of ischemia-reperfusion injury by pentoxifylline in the isolated rat lung. Am J Respi Crit Care Med 1994; 150:342–347.
197. Sullivan GW, Carpenter HT, Mandell GL. Pentoxifylline modulates activation of human neutrophils by amphotericin B in vitro. Antimicrob Agents Chemother 1992; 36:408–416.
198. Lilly CM, Sandhu JS, Ishizaka A, et al. Pentoxifylline prevents tumor necrosis factor-induced acute lung injury in guinea pigs. Am Rev Respir Dis 1989; 139: 1361–1368.
199. Mandell GL. ARDS, neutrophils, and pentoxyphylline. Am Rev Respir Dis 1988; 138:1103–1105.
200. Pasquier C, Franzini E, Abedinzadea Z, Kaouadjii MN, Hakim J. Gamma and pulse radiolysis study of pentoxifylline, a methylxanthine. Int J Radiat Biol 1991; 60:433–447.
201. Sato K, Stelzner TJ, O'Brien RF, Weil JV, Welsh CH. Pentoxifylline lessens the endotoxin-induced increase in albumin clearance across pulmonary artery endothelial monolayers with and without neutrophils. Am J Respir Cell Mol Biol 1991; 4:219–227.

13

Lung Injury Induced by Mechanical Ventilation

JACOB IASHA SZNAJDER and KAREN M. RIDGE

Michael Reese Hospital and
University of Illinois
Chicago, Illinois

GEORGES SAUMON

Institut National de la Santé et de la
Recherche Médicale
Paris, France

DIDIER DREYFUSS

Faculté Xavier Bichat
Hôpital Louis Mourier
Paris, France

I. Introduction

Positive-pressure mechanical ventilation is commonly used to support the oxygenation and ventilatory functions of injured lungs. Even though positive-pressure mechanical ventilation is used as part of the care for respiratory failure, it may under some circumstances cause or worsen lung injury by causing alveolar overdistension. This deleterious effect of positive-pressure mechanical ventilation has been termed "barotrauma." Clinicians define barotrauma as the occurrence of air leaks resulting in the accumulation of extra-alveolar air responsible for a number of manifestations: depression of cardiac output and blood pressure, interstitial emphysema, and pneumothorax. More recently the concept of "volutrauma" has been introduced which comprises the above described deleterious effects and also includes changes in lung permeability and lung injury that may worsen the extent of pulmonary edema.

II. Does Mechanical Ventilation Cause Lung Injury?

In the 1960s it was reported that atelectasis can increase pulmonary surface tension in dogs that were ventilated for 24 hours. There were changes in lung mechanics and peak airway pressures (PAP) (1). In the seventies, Webb and Tierney in a landmark study in rats reported a significant amount of pulmonary edema occurs during intermittent pressure ventilation with high inflation volumes and pressures, whereas in animals ventilated with positive end-expiratory pressure (PEEP) there was less edema (see Fig. 1) (2). Further, recent studies by Dreyfuss et al. demonstrated that ventilation with high inflation pressures (45 cm H_2O for 20) produced lung injury and pulmonary edema in rats (see Fig. 2) (3). These same investigators demonstrated that increased tidal volume excursions, and not PAP, were the important factors determining lung injury (17). In these studies the investigators ventilated rats with small tidal volumes but with a constricted chest wall which increased PAP and compared them to another group of animals where an "extra chest wall or iron lung" was created by ventilating rats to low PAP but high tidal volumes (4). These experiments demonstrated that rats ventilated with high tidal volumes and low PAP

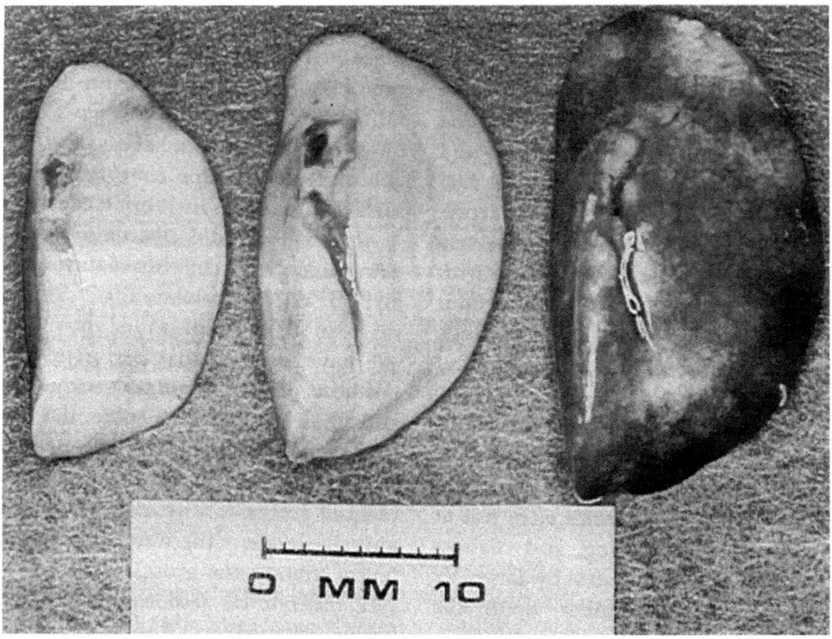

Figure 1 Comparison of left lungs from rats ventilated with intermittant positive pressures/no PEEP (14/0 cm H_2O), high inspiratory pressures/low PEEP (45/10 cm H_2O), and high inspiratory pressures/no PEEP (45/0 cm H_2O) (left to right). Rats ventilated with high inspiratory pressure of 45 cm H_2O and 0 PEEP had hemorhagic edema. (From Ref. 2.)

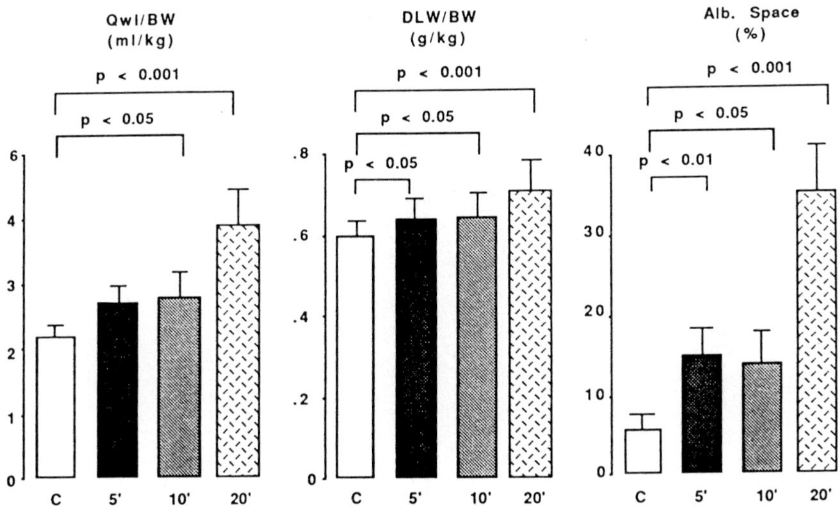

Figure 2 Ventilation of rats with high inflation pressure (45 cm H_2O) for 20 min produced pulmonary edema and injury. Pulmonary edema was assessed by the determination of extravascular lung water content (Qwl/BW). Permeability changes were assessed by the determination of dry lung weight/body weight (DLW/BW) as well as the distribution of ^{125}I-albumin (Alb. Space). (From Ref. 3.)

had lung edema, whereas no lung edema was observed in rats ventilated with low tidal volumes and high PAP (Fig. 3). Although in clinical practice this dissociation between PAP or plateau pressures and tidal volumes occurs infrequently, these and the previous studies demonstrate that ventilating normal lungs with high tidal volumes can cause increased lung permeability, lung injury, and pulmonary edema.

III. Mechanisms and Mediators of Lung Injury During Mechanical Ventilation

Several investigators have reported on the possible mediators of mechanical ventilation-induced lung injury. Recent studies have shown that high tidal volume ventilation may promote lung injury not only by increased volume and overstretching alveoli but by stimulating the release of pro-inflammatory mediators (5–7). Pressure-volume curves and several chemokines were measured in isolated rat lungs ventilated with high tidal volume/high PEEP or high tidal volume/zero PEEP. High tidal volume/high PEEP did not change the P-V curve, in contrast high tidal volume-zero PEEP ventilation resulted in a severalfold

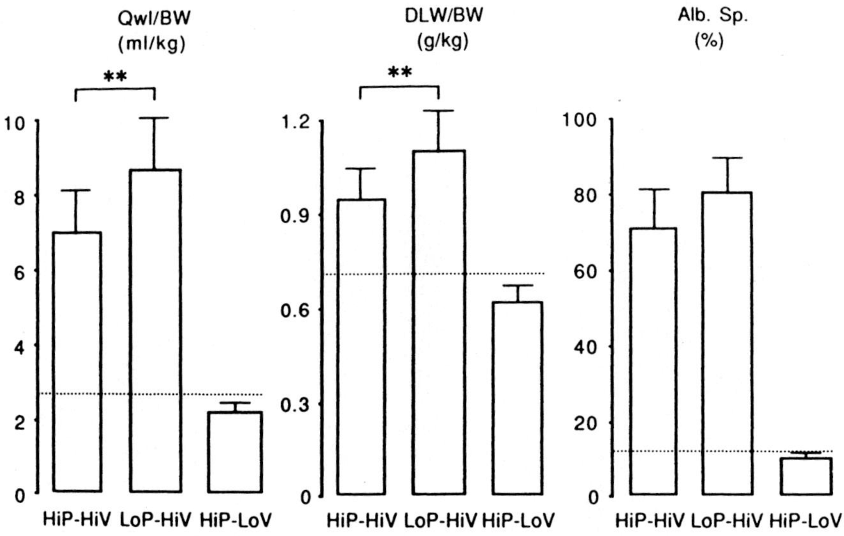

Figure 3 The effects of high peak (45 cm H_2O) positive inspiratory pressure-high tidal volume ventilation (Hip-HiV) was compared to negative inspiratory airway pressure-high tidal volume ventilation (extra chest wall ventilation = LoP-HiV) and high peak (45 cm H_2O) positive inspiratory pressure-low tidal volume ventilation (constricted chest wall = HiP-LoV) in adult rats. Animals ventilated with a high-peak pressure and a normal tidal volume had no edema. High tidal volume ventilation resulted in increased lung permeability and pulmonary edema. Dotted lines represent the upper 95% confidence limit for control values. (From Ref. 4.)

increase of TNFα, IL-1β, IL-6, MIP-2, INFγ, and IL-10 in BALF, with a decrease in compliance and a rightward shift in the P-V curve (6) (Fig. 4). Metalloproteinases have also been implicated in mechanical ventilation-induced lung injury. Rats mechanically ventilated for 20 min had increased metalloproteinases in the bronchoalveolar lavage (BALF) (assessed by gelatinolytic activity and SDS-PAGE zymography), and increased metalloproteinases mRNA expression in the lung interstitium and the alveolar epithelium (5). These animal studies complement the studies in which BALF of mechanically ventilated patients in whom gelatinases were present (8). A role for metalloproteinases in altering permeability has been reported in hyperoxia (9) and interstitial lung diseases (10) as well as in facilitating metastasis in lung cancer (11). Also, in epithelial cells that were stretched in vitro induction of IL1β occurred with 30% of strain by 24 hours (12). Yet other recent studies demonstrated that cyclic strain in endothelial cells induced oxidative stress by increasing thiobarbituric acid (an index of lipid peroxidation) and the reactive oxygen metabolite H_2O_2 production, and in pleural mesothelial caused increased permeability and stimulated the re-

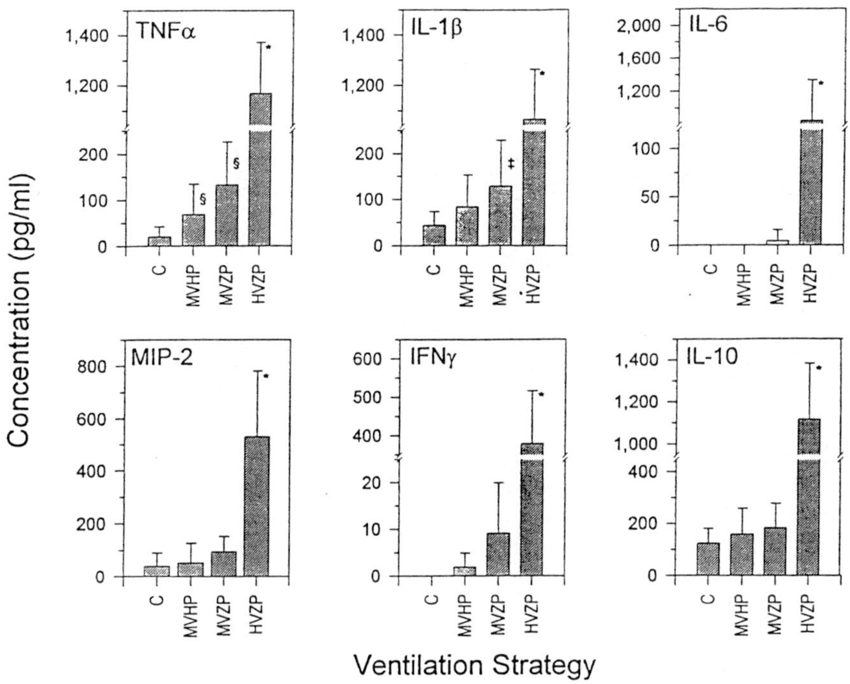

Figure 4 The effect of ventilation strategy on lung inflammatory mediators was assessed BALF from adult rats. The lowest level of cytokines was observed in the control group (C) ventilated with low tidal volume-low PEEP (V_t = 7 cc/kg) and highest levels in high volume-zero PEEP (HVZP) (V_t = 40 cc/kg). (From Ref. 6.)

lease of endothelin-1 (13–15). Although not definite, the sum of these studies suggests that mechanotransduction can stimulate the production of harmful chemokines, oxidants, and metalloproteinases that can induce changes in permeability and start a cascade leading to lung injury and systemic inflammatory response syndrome. The role of the above-described mediators are only recently implicated in the pathogenesis of mechanical ventilation-induced lung injury, introducing new concepts to the understanding of mechanical ventilation-induced lung injury. These concepts are complementary to the previous understanding that mechanical ventilation with high tidal volumes causes direct mechanical "bursting" of the alveolar epithelium, increasing distal airway and alveolar shear forces causing capillary stress failure, pore stretching, and depletion of pulmonary surfactant.

Regardless of which cellular mechanisms cause the ventilation-induced pulmonary edema, several studies have reported changes in the filtration coefficient (K_{fc}) and permeability in both pulmonary capillaries and alveolar

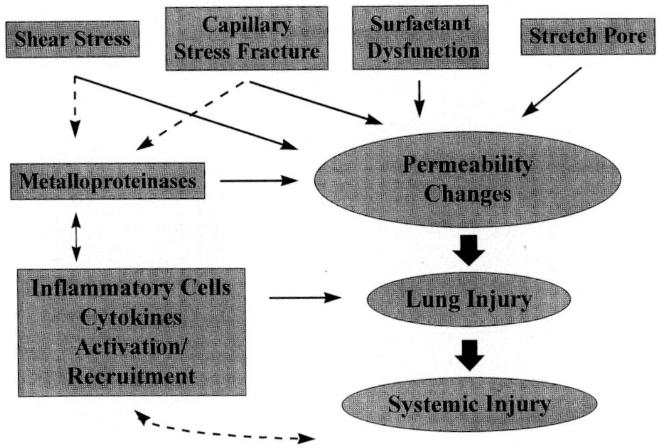

Figure 5 Schematic diagram proposing a sequence of events implicating mechanical ventilation causing shear stress, capillary stress fracture, surfactant dysfunction and stretch pore phenomenon. Some of these events activate metalloproteinases and cytokines by inflammatory cells, thus leading to permeability changes and lung injury which in turn can cause systemic injury.

epithelium with increasing tidal volume ventilation leading to edema accumulation and possibly systemic injury. A recent study reported increased intestinal permeability in rats ventilated with high tidal volumes, suggesting mechanisms for lung activation of inflammatory mediators released to the systemic circulation and causing systemic injury as seen in systemic inflammatory response syndrome (16). This mechanistic approach is proposed in Figure 5 in which a schematic sequence of events is depicted implicating mechanical ventilation in the changes of permeability, lung injury, and systemic injury.

IV. Evidence for Changes of the Filtration Coefficient and Microvascular Permeability

Dreyfuss and colleagues (3,4,17,18) reported that extravascular lung water, dry lung weight, and the distribution space in the lungs of intravenously injected ^{125}I-albumin, an index of the rate of albumin leakage from pulmonary vessels, increased after only 5 min of high-volume-pressure ventilation (see Fig. 2). Lung edema developed very rapidly, accumulating around the perivascular cuffs, and alterations in the microvascular permeability were documented by a significant increase in lung weight and albumin permeability. After 10 min of ventilation, there was increased edema in the interstitial spaces, and after 20 min of ventilation alveolar flooding was apparent in all animals. The severity of the permeability alteration was such that the ratio of ^{125}I-albumin activity in tracheal fluid versus plasma was close to unity.

Parker and colleagues demonstrated that microvascular permeability was not affected by changes in peak airway pressures up to 30 cm H_2O in isolated dog lungs (19). In contrast, capillary filtration coefficient increased in association with increasing inspiratory pressures of 45 to 65 cm H_2O where the estimated protein reflection coefficient decreased only at the highest airway pressures (19) (Fig. 6). Similar observations have been obtained in larger animals (20,21) but only after longer periods of high peak pressure ventilation. For example, the extravascular lung water: dry lung weight ratio was only 19% in lambs ventilated for 6 hours at 58 cm H_2O peak inspiratory pressure (20). Light microscopic examination of the lungs revealed either normal or only mild perivascular edema

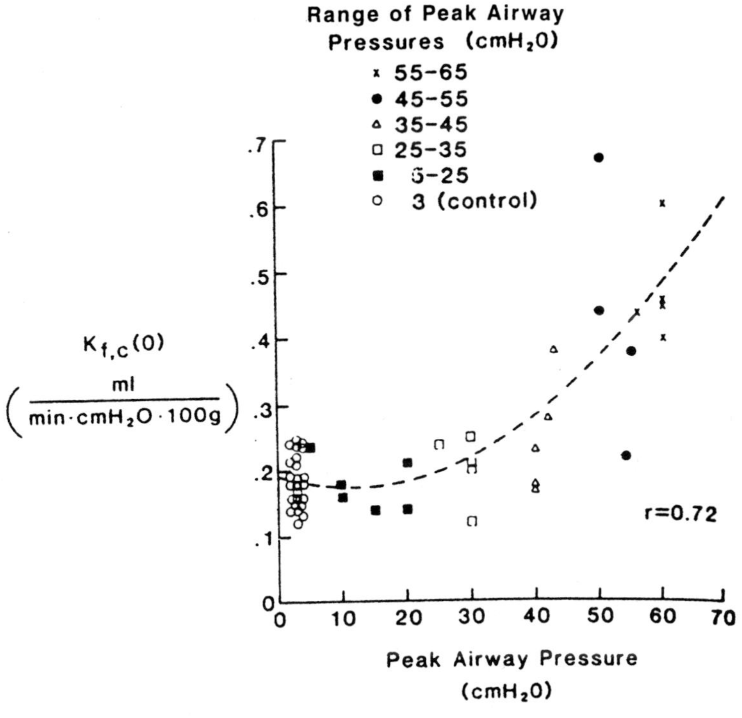

Figure 6 Pulmonary microvascular permeability (K_{FC}) increased in isolated blood-perfused lobes of dog lungs after 20 min ventilation with increasing peak airway pressure. Moderate (up to 30 cm H_2O) increases in peak airway pressure did not affect K_{FC}; conversely, higher levels of peak pressure resulted in a significant increase in K_{FC}. (From Ref. 19.)

with no alveolar edema. In a different study, sheep mechanically ventilated for 18 hours at 50 cm H_2O peak inspiratory pressure developed both interstitial and alveolar edema (22,23). The resulting extravascular lung water: dry lung weight ratio was increased by 136% as compared to controls.

The endothelial cell breaks observed during high tidal volume ventilation have also been described with increases in pulmonary vascular pressures and coined "capillary stress failure" (24–26). These studies demonstrate that different time courses are necessary to produce lung edema, which ranges from ~30 min in rodents to over 24 hours in large animals. The summary of these data suggests that high peak airway pressure pulmonary edema is produced by a combination of increased K_{fc} and altered reflective coefficient for proteins. The hydrostatic component appears to be moderate, at least in closed-chest animals. The rapid onset of pulmonary edema during high tidal volume ventilation may be explained by the synergistic actions of increased hydrostatic forces and alterations in the microvascular barrier.

V. Evidence for Increased Epithelial Permeability

During high tidal volume ventilation there is a concomitant increase in alveolar epithelial permeability to small hydrophilic solutes when lung volume increases. During mechanical (27) or spontaneous (28) ventilation in sheep, increased functional residual capacity was associated with an increase in aerosolized ^{99}mTc-DTPA (di-ethylenetriamine penta-acetic acid) clearance. The increase in clearance was larger than anticipated based on the changes in alveolar exchange surface area. A similar effect has been reported in humans (29), where DTPA clearance increased when the lungs were inflated by either positive-pressure breathing or voluntary hyperinflation (30).

Epithelial permeability in fluid-filled in situ sheep lungs was also significantly increased as a result of overinflation (31). In some instances, there was leakage through epithelial breaks as indicated by increased movement of albumin across the epithelium (31). Subjecting sheep lobes and rabbit lungs to distending pressures of 40 cm H_2O showed that whole-lung static inflation only increased the lung volume three- to fourfold, whereas segmental static inflation caused a 12-fold increase in segmental volume from FRC (32). Further, whole-lung overinflation did not significantly effect albumin permeability. Hence, these studies suggest that changes in epithelial permeability to macromolecules can only be effected by major increases in lung volume. Support for this concept was provided by a study performed in bullfrog lungs showing that epithelial permeability increased only after overinflation and not by inflation within the physiologic range (33).

Alveolar epithelial permeability alterations may be present in varying degrees during mechanical ventilation-induced pulmonary edema. Ultrastructural studies disclosed that rats ventilated with high airway pressures had profound alterations in the epithelial layer. The severity of the alterations varied from alveolar epithelial type I cell swelling to almost complete destruction of alveolar epithelial type I cells, leaving a denuded basement membrane (3,4,34) (see Fig. 7). Previously, it was thought that the alveolar capillary barrier was resistant to moderate increases in pulmonary vascular pressure (35–37). However, recent studies using both transmission and scanning electron microscopy demonstrated that capillary transmural pressures of 40 mm Hg or greater were associated with the disruption of both alveolar epithelial and capillary endothelium (24,25,38). These ultrastructural breaks occur as a result of capillary stress failure. Capillary stress failure is a phenomenon that takes place when capillary wall radial stress is approximately equal to that of the aorta in the presence of a 100 mg Hg transmural pressure (25). The disruption in the alveolar capillary barrier that

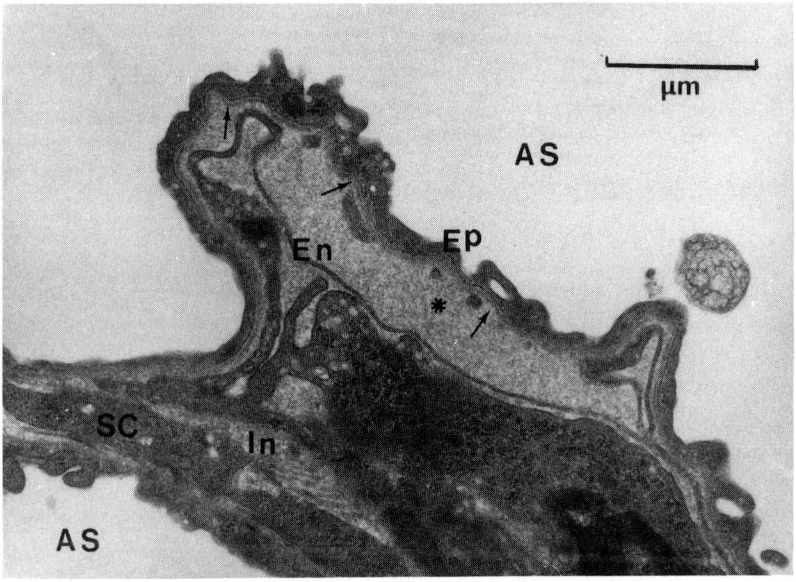

Figure 7 Ultrastructural studies demonstrate that rats ventilated for 5 min to a peak airway pressure of 45 cm H_2O had alterations in the alveolar epithelial and endothelial layer. The arrow indicates the formation of an endothelial bleb due to detachment of the endothelial cell (En) away from the basement membrane. This bleb is filled with electron dense material (*) of the same density as plasma. At this time period, epithelial type I (Ep) cells are still intact. Of note is the interstitial edema (In). SC = septal cell; AS = alveolar space. (From Ref. 3.)

correlates with increased microvascular permeability when microvascular pressures are high (39,40) is referred to as the stretched-pore phenomenon (41,42). Mechanical ventilation-induced injury and capillary stress failure have many of the same "trademarks." The ultrastructural appearance of the endothelial and epithelial cell lesions are nearly identical (25,38). Further, it appears that both insults are reversible to some degree. There are data showing that when high-volume ventilation was halted, albumin leakage from capillaries stopped (18). The number of endothelial and epithelial breaks were reduced when capillary pressure was returned to normal after elevation to a level causing stress failure, resulting in improved microvascular permeability (39,40). Of great importance is the relationship between capillary pressures and lung volume: at a capillary transmural pressure of 32.5 cm H_2O, increasing lung volume by increasing transpulmonary pressure from 5 to 20 cm H_2O resulted in numerous alveolar type I epithelial and capillary endothelial breaks (43). A reported difference between capillary stress failure and high tidal volume-induced lung injury has been the extent of epithelial damage and lysis during mechanical ventilation. These more specific epithelial injury elements may be due to inactivation or displacement of the surfactant and repetitive opening and closing of distal pulmonary units creating higher shear stress. These phenomena are more evident in the dependent areas of injured lungs as reported in dog (44) and rat lungs (unpublished observations, Sznajder and Ridge).

VI. Does PEEP Protect Against Mechanical Ventilation-Induced Lung Injury?

The report of Webb and Tierney and more recent studies have shown that animals ventilated with PEEP to the same peak airway pressures and volumes had less or no edema as compared to animals ventilated without PEEP (2). The beneficial effects of PEEP have been demonstrated by the preservation of gas exchange and the protection of the alveolar epithelium (2,45). Most of these studies attributed the beneficial effects of PEEP to the preservation of surfactant activity; however, a study suggested that hemodynamic changes effected by PEEP could also play a role. Most of the initial studies showing protection by PEEP were in rats, where hemodynamic assessment is difficult; however, a recent study showed that PEEP significantly reduced the blood pressure and possibly the preload and lung perfusion of these rats, therefore decreasing lung edema accumulation. When the decreased blood pressure was restored by the infusion of dopamine, the amounts of edema in the rat lungs with PEEP and without PEEP were similar (4). Also, the prophylactic use of PEEP neither prevented the formation of edema in a oleic acid lung injury model nor prevented ARDS in patients at risk of lung injury (46). Therefore, although the exact mechanisms of the protection with PEEP are not fully defined, they probably include one or a combination of three distinct possibilities: preservation of pulmonary surfactant properties; hemodynamic alterations; and reduction of closing and opening of terminal lung units and thus reduction of lung shear stress.

VII. Positive Effects of Stretch During Mechanical Ventilation

There is considerable evidence regarding the negative effects of overstretching normal lungs; however, there is also evidence to suggest that cyclic lung movement is of benefit. A recent study demonstrated that a single stretch of alveolar epithelial cells in vitro increased surfactant production possibly via a calcium-activated pathway, representing a protective mechanism to decrease alveolar surface tension and keep the alveoli free of edema (47). Also, it has been shown that edema induced by high tidal volume ventilation resolved quite rapidly (18). One possible mechanism for the rapid resolution of pulmonary edema may be stimulation of active Na^+ transport via the upregulation of alveolar epithelial Na,K-ATPase as reported in rats, that were ventilated with high tidal volumes for 20 min (48). Although it is unclear whether the upregulation of the Na,K-ATPase was triggered by the edema or cellular stretch or both. Further studies by Waters et al. (56) suggest that stretching the alveolar epithelial cells upregulates Na,K-ATPase function within 30 min. This increase in Na,K-ATPase function is possibly due to rapid recruitment of Na^+ pumps from inner pools to the cell plasma membrane, and suggests that stretch itself, independent of the edema, elicits this protective effects via yet undescribed mechanisms (49).

VIII. Mechanical Ventilation in Preexisting Lung Injury

In the ICU mechanical ventilation is often used in patients with already injured lungs, so titration of tidal volume in these patients is of paramount importance. For example, a modeling study of pulmonary atelectasis by Mead and colleagues, calculated that the pressure needed to expand an atelectatic region surrounded by a fully expanded lung would be approximately 140 cm H_2O, at transpulmonary pressure of 30 cm H_2O (50). Studies conducted in the oleic acid-injured, isolated rabbit lung demonstrated that ventilation with high tidal volume resulted in significantly greater weight gain than lungs ventilated with small tidal volumes (51). Further, when oleic acid administration was followed by mechanical ventilation, a compounded effect was observed with a significant increase in the capillary filtration coefficient in conjunction with an increase in the wet-dry weight ratio (52). Also, inactivation of surfactant by dioctyl

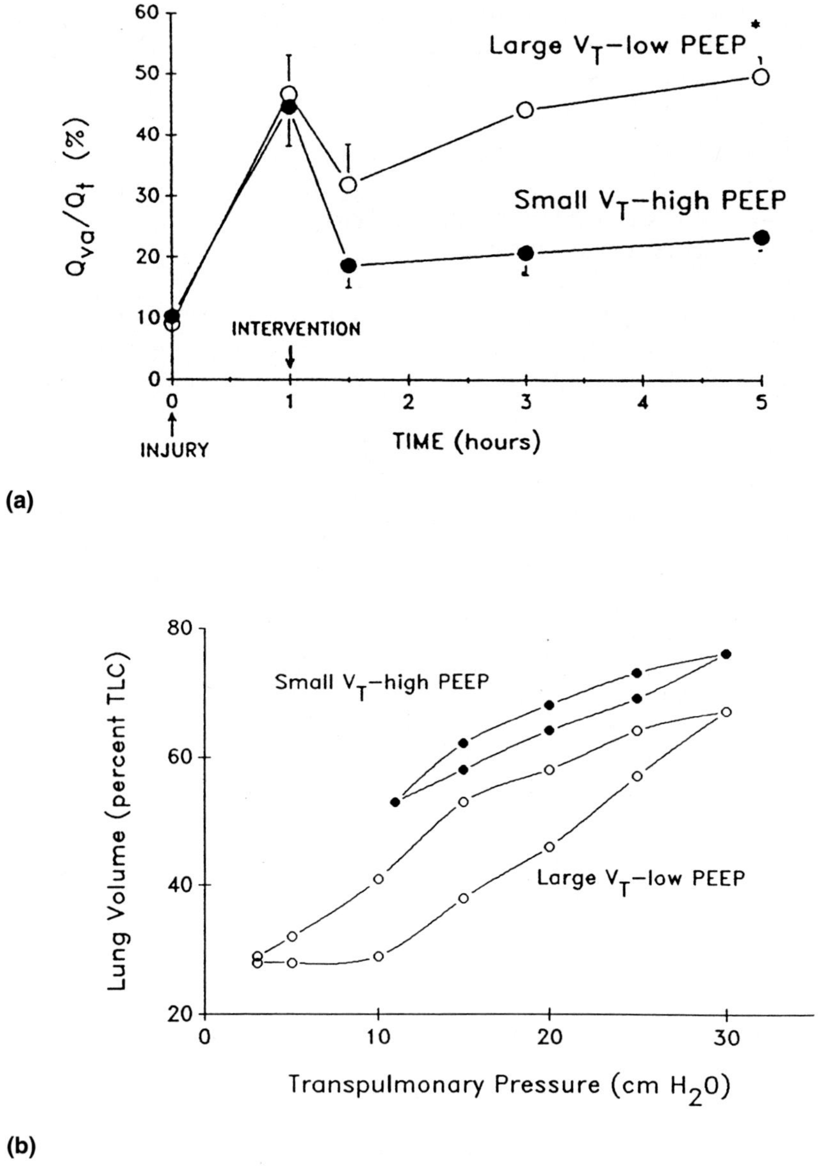

Figure 8 After inducing HCl aspiration, lung edema animals were ventilated with high tidal volume-low PEEP (V_t = 30 mL/kg) and compared to low tidal volume-high PEEP (V_t = 15 mL/kg), both groups were ventilated to the same peak transpulmonary pressure (a). Animals ventilated with high tidal-volume-low PEEP had worse gas exchange (Q_{va}/Q_{vt}) (b). (From Ref. 45.)

succinate prior to high peak pressure ventilation resulted in even greater changes in the filtration coefficient (53). These studies suggest that ventilation-induced lung edema seems to develop at lower airway pressures in lungs with preexisting injury.

In another study, Corbridge et al. demonstrated that in HCl aspiration-induced pulmonary edema in dogs, those animals ventilated with high tidal excursions and low levels of PEEP had worse gas exchange and more edema as than another group of animals ventilated to the same peak transpulmonary pressure but with small tidal excursions and higher levels of PEEP (see Fig. 8a, b) (45). Another study comparing the effects of increasing levels of lung distension during mechanical ventilation in rats injured by α-naphtylthiourea (ANTU) showed that ventilation for 2 min with moderate V_t (25 mL/kg) did not increase significantly lung injury. However, ventilation for 2 min with high tidal volumes (45 mL/kg) caused changes in lung mechanics and severe pulmonary edema to a much greater degree than the predicted additive insults (17) (see Fig. 9). The synergy was dependent upon the degree of lung injury prior to mechanical ventilation. In fact, the amount of edema resulting from high tidal volume ventilation in ANTU-injured rats correlated inversely with the quasistatic respiratory compliance (an index of open nonflooded lung regions) measured during the very first cycles of ventilation before it could add damage. These data suggest that the less distensible the lungs were before ventilation,

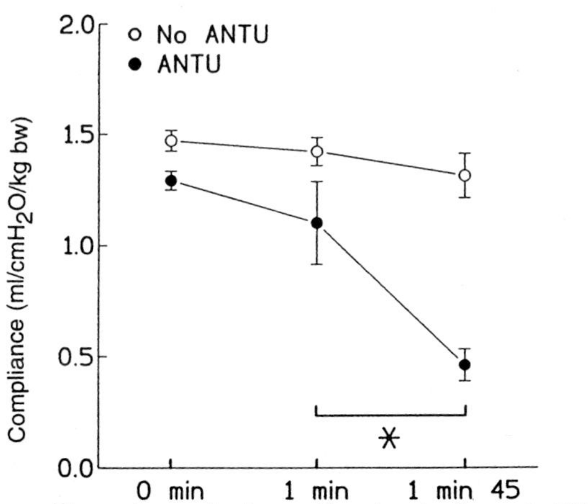

Figure 9 Anesthetized rats injected with ANTU 2 h prior to high tidal volume ventilation (V_t = 45 mL/kg) had significant decrease in quasi-static respiratory system compliance compared to control animals. (From Ref. 17.)

the more severe was the injury induced by high-V_t ventilation and that ventilation during lung injury may have compounding synergistically adverse effects. These studies are clinically relevant because patients with pulmonary edema have parts of their lungs consolidated or filled with fluid and may not be recruitable. Therefore, ventilating even with what may appear to be normal tidal volumes could overstretch the noninjured alveoli, cause volutrauma and compound lung injury.

IX. Rationale for Ventilating ARDS Patients with Low Tidal Volume

The concept of ventilating patients with low Vt, because patients with ARDS had small lungs, was introduced by Gattinoni et al., who showed in serial CT scans that even at high PEEP patients with ARDS have nonrecruitable lung areas (54). This concept is being incorporated in clinical practice in which patients with ARDS are being effectively ventilated with smaller tidal volumes so as not to overstretch their lungs and avoid compounding the lung injury. This issue is discussed in more detail in Chapter 20. Conceivably, this can be accomplished by adjusting the ventilator to smaller tidal volumes and estimating the possible area of the lung that is not injured and available for ventilation. A strategy of ventilation utilizes the "open lung approach" (55,56) where patients are ventilated with higher PEEP and smaller tidal volumes to overcome the lower inflection point and recruit lung volume with PEEP. This approach theoretically could reduce the shear forces associated with repetitive opening and closing of terminal airways. Another approach to avoid volu- and barotrauma is a variation of the former in which patients are ventilated with smaller tidal volumes up to a peak airway pressure of 35 cm H_2O or plateau pressure of 25 cm H_2O, maintaining adequate P_{O_2} and allowing the P_{CO_2} to raise in a controlled way, called "permissive hypercapnia."

In summary, much has been learned since the early studies reported in the 1960s and 1970s that with increased peak airway pressures there may be an increased chance of barotrauma as evidenced by interstitial emphysema, pneumothorax, and perhaps worsening lung injury. Mechanisms that could contribute to the change in lung permeability include cytokines and metalloproteinases which can initiate and propagate a cascade of inflammatory mechanisms that may lead to increased pulmonary permeability, lung injury, and worse lung edema. On the other hand, cyclic stretch of the alveolar cells by mechanotransduction may induce protective mechanisms opposing lung injury and increasing lung edema clearance. A recognition of the possibility of volutrauma or barotrauma while ventilating critically ill patients with apparently normal tidal volumes may be a step forward to adjusting the ventilator management and avoiding compounding lung injury. However, preliminary data from multicenter trials suggest that there is no apparent advantage of ventilating patients with small tidal volumes (5 to 7 mL/kg) as opposed to "normal" tidal volumes (~10 mL/kg) (57–59). On the other hand, studies such as the "open lung approach" which advocate higher PEEP to recruit lung volume and prevent the "shear-stress" of closing and reopening lung units with each breath, as well as ventilation with small tidal volumes of patients with ARDS, may have some benefit, though need further study (21). These approaches need validation and potentially could improve management of patients and attenuate mechanical ventilation induced lung injury. A further discussion of these issues is included in Chapter 20.

References

1. Greenfiled LJ, Ebert PA, Benson DW. Effects of positive pressure ventilation on surface tension properties of lung extracts. Anesthesiology 1964; 25:312–316.
2. Webb HH, Tierney DF. Experimental pulmonary edema due to intermittent positive pressure ventilation with high inflation pressures. Protection by positive end expiratory pressure. Am Rev Respir Dis 1974; 110:556–565.
3. Dreyfuss D, Basset G, Soler P, Saumon G. Intermittent positive-pressure hyperventilation with high inflation pressures produces pulmonary microvascular injury in rats. Am Rev Respir Dis 1985; 132:880–884.
4. Dreyfuss D, Soler P, Basset G, Saumon G. High inflation pressure pulmonary edema. Respective effects of high airway pressure, high tidal volume, and positive end-expiratory pressure. Am Rev Respir Dis 1988; 137:1159–1164.
5. Pardo A, Ridge K, Segura L, Sznajder JI, Selman M. Gelatinase A and interstitial collagenase are upregulated during high tidal volume mechanical ventilation. Am J Respir Crit Care Med 1996; 153:A531.
6. Tremblay L, Valenza F, Ribeiro SP, Li J, Slutsky AS. Injurious ventilatory strategies increase cytokines and c-fos mRNA expression in an isolated rat lung model. J Clin Invest 1997; 99:944–952.
7. Uhlig S, Bethmann AN. Prolonged hyperventilation is required for release of tumor necrosis factor a but not interleukin-6 from isolated perfused mouse lung. AJRCCM 1997; 155:A505.
8. Delclaux C, D'Ortho MP, Delacourt C, Lebargy F, Brun-Buisson C, Brochard L, Lemaire F, Lafuma C, Harf A. Gelatinases in epithelial lining fluid of patients with adult respiratory distress syndrome. Am J Physiol 1997; 272:L442–L451.
9. Pardo A, Selman M, Ridge K, Barrios R, Sznajder JI. Increased expression of gelatinases and collagenase in rat lungs exposed to 100% oxygen. Am J Respir Crit Care Med 1996; 154:1067–1075.
10. Pardo A, Selman M. The Collagenase Gene Family: Relationships Between Collaenolytic Activity and Fibrogenesis. Boca Raton: CRC Press, 1991.
11. Grillo HC. Collagenolytic activity during mammalian wound repair. Dev Biol 1967; 15:300–317.
12. Hubmayr RD, Limper AH, Burton SL, Vlahakis NE, Schroeder MA. Stretch causes IL-8 release from alveolar epithelial cells in vitro. AJRCCM 1997; 155:A500.

13. Howard AB, Alexander W, Nerem R, Griendling K, Taylor R. Cyclic strain induces an oxidative stress in endothelial cells. Am J Physiol 1997; 272:C421–C427.
14. Waters C, Gluksberg M, Depaola N, Chang J, Grotberg J. Shear stress alters pleural mesothelial cell permeability in culture. J Appl Physiol 1996; 81:448–458.
15. Waters C, Chang J, Gluksberg M, Depaola N, Grotberg J. Mechanical forces alter growth factor release by pleural mesothelial cells. Am J Physiol 1997; 272:L522–L557.
16. Guery B, Neviere R, Fialdes P, Chidiac C, Roussel-Delvallez M, Marchandise X, Beaucaire G. Mechanical ventilation regimen induces intestinal permeability changes in a rat model. AJRCCM 1997; 155:A505.
17. Dreyfuss D, Soler P, Saumon G. Mechanical ventilation-induced pulmonary edema. Interaction with previous lung alterations. Am J Respir Crit Care Med 1995; 151: 1568–1575.
18. Dreyfuss D, Soler P, Saumon G. Spontaneous resolution of pulmonary edema caused by short periods of cyclic overinflation. J Appl Physiol 1992; 72:2081–2089.
19. Parker JC, Townsley MI, Rippe B, Taylor AE. Increased microvascular permeability in dog lungs due to high airway pressures. J Appl Physiol 1984; 57:1809–1816.
20. Carlton DP, Cummings JJ, Scheerer RG, Poulain FR, Bland RD. Lung overexpansion increases pulmonary microvascular protein permeability in young lambs. J Appl Physiol 1990; 69(2):577–583.
21. Borelli M, Kolobow T, Spatola R, Prato P, Tsuno K. Severe acute respiratory failure managed with continuous positive airway pressure and partial extracorporeal carbon dioxide removal by an artificial membrane lung. Am Rev Respir Dis 1988; 138: 1480–1487.
22. Eagan EA, Nelson RM, Olver RE. Lung inflation and alveolar permeability to nonelectrolytes in the adult sheep in vivo. J Physiol (Lond) 1976; 260:409–424.
23. Kolobow T, Moretti MP, Fumagalli R, Mascheroni D, Prato P, Chen V, Joris M. Severe impairment in lung function induced by high peak airway pressure during mechanical ventilation. Am Rev Respir Dis 1987; 135:312–315.
24. Costello ML, Mathieu-Costello O, West JB. Stress failure of alveolar epithelial cells studied by scanning electron microscopy. Am Rev Respir Dis 1992; 145:1446–1455.
25. West JB, Tsukimoto K, Mathieu-Costello O, Prediletto R. Stress failure in pulmonary capillaries. J Appl Physiol 1991; 70(4):1731–1742.
26. John E, McDevitt M, Wilborn W, Cassady G. Ultrastructure of the lung after ventilation. Br J Exp Pathol 1982; 63:401–407.
27. Cooper JA, Van der Zee H, Line BR, Malik AB. Relationship of end-expiratory pressure, lung volume, and 99mTc-DTPA clearance. J Appl Physiol 1987; 63:1586–1590.
28. O'Brodovich H, Coates G, Marrin M. Effect of inspiratory resistance and PEEP on 99mTc-DTPA clearance. J Appl Physiol 1986; 60:1461–1465.
29. Nolop KB, Maxwell DL, Royston D, Hughes JMB. Effect of raised thoracic pressure and volume on 99mTc-DTPA clearance in humans. J Appl Physiol 1986; 60: 1493–1497.

30. Marks JD, Luce JM, Lazar NM, Wu JN, Lipavsky A, Murray JF. Effect of increases in lung volume on clearance of aerosolized solute from human lungs. J Appl Physiol 1985; 59:1242–1248.
31. Egan EA. Lung inflation, lung solute permeability, and alveolar edema. J Appl Physiol: Respir Environ Exercise Physiol 1982; 53(1):121–125.
32. Egan EA, Nelson RM, Olver RE. Lung inflation and alveolar permeability to non-electrolytes in the adult sheep in vivo. J Physiol 1976; 260:409–424.
33. Kim KJ, Crandall ED. Effects of lung inflation on alveolar epithelial solute and water transport properties. J Appl Physiol 1982; 52:1498–1505.
34. Dreyfus D, Saumon G. Ventilator-induced injury. In: Tobin M, ed. Principals and Practice of Mechanical Ventilation. New York: McGraw-Hill, 1994:793–811.
35. Cottrell TS, Levine OR, Senior RM, Wiener J, Spiro D, Fishman AP. Electron microscopic alterations at the alveolar level in pulmonary edema. Circ Res 1967; 21:783–797.
36. Defouw DO, Berendsen PB. Morphological change in isolated perfused dog lungs after acute hydrostatic edema. Circ Res 1978; 43:72–82.
37. Montaner JSG, Tsang J, Evans KG, Mullen JBM, Burns AR, Walker DC, Wiggs B, Hogg JC. Alveolar epithelial damage: a critical difference between high pressure and oleic acid-induced low pressure pulmonary edema. J Clin Invest 1986; 77: 1786–1796.
38. Tsukimoto K, Mathieu-Costello O, Prediletto R, Elliott AR, West JB. Ultrastructural appearances of pulmonary capillaries at high transmural pressures. J Appl Physiol 1991; 71:573–582.
39. Nycolaysen G, Waaler BA, Aarseth P. On the existence of stretchable pores in the exchange vessels of the isolated rabbit lung preparation. Lymphology 1979; 12: 201–207.
40. Rippe B, Townsley M, Thigpen J, Parker JC, Korthuis RJ, Taylor AE. Effects of vascular pressure on the pulmonary microvasculature in isolated dog lungs. J Appl Physiol 1984; 57:233–239.
41. Shirley HH, Wolfram CG, Wasserman K, Mayerson HS. Capillary permeability to macromolecules: stretched pore phenomenon. Am J Physiol 1957; 190: 189–193.
42. Fishman AP, Pietra GG. Hemodynamic pulmonary edema. In: Fishman AP, Renkin EM, eds. Pulmonary Edema. Bethesda, MD: American Physiological Society, 1979: 79–96.
43. Fu Z, Costello ML, Tsukimoto K, Prediletto R, Elliott AR, Mathieu-Costello O, West JB. High lung volume increases stress failure in pulmonary capillaries. J Appl Physiol 1992; 73:123–133.
44. Hotchkiss JR, Broccard AF, Kuwayama N, Wangensteen OD, Marini JJ. The influence of gravity on the distribution of lung edema during ventilator induced lung injury in an isolated, perfused rabbit lung preparation. AJRCCM 1996; 153:A378.
45. Corbridge TC, Wood LDH, Crawford GP, Chudoba MJ, Yanos J, Sznajder JI. Adverse effects of large tidal volumes and low PEEP in canine acid aspiration. Am Rev Respir Dis 1990; 142:311–315.
46. Pepe PE, Potkin RT, Reus DH, Hudson LD, Carrico CJ. Clinical predictors of the adult respiratory distress syndrome. Am J Surg 1982; 144(1):124–129.

47. Wirtz HRW, Dobbs LG. Calcium mobilization and exocytosis after one mechanical stretch of lung epithelial cells. Science 1990; 250:1266–1269.
48. Sznajder JI, Ridge KM, Harris ZL, Olivera WG, Curiel C, Rutschman DH. Alveolar type II cell Na,K-ATPase is upregulated during mechanical ventilation-induced pulmonary edema. Chest 1994; 105:116S–117S.
49. Waters CM, Ridge KM, Craig C, Sznajder JI. Mechanical stretching of alveolar epithelial cells increases Na,K-ATPase activity. AJRCCM 1995; 151:A190.
50. Mead J, Takishima T, Leith D. Stress distribution in lungs: a model of pulmonary elasticity. J Appl Physiol 1970; 28:596–608.
51. Bowton DL, Kong DL. High tidal volume ventilation produces increased lung water in oleic acid-injured rabbit lungs. Crit Care Med 1989; 17:908–911.
52. Hernandez LA, Peevy KJ, Moise AA, Parker JC. Chest wall restriction limits high airway pressure-induced lung injury in young rabbits. J Appl Physiol 1989; 66: 2364–2368.
53. Coker PJ, Hernandez LA, Peevy KJ, Adkins K, Parker JC. Increased sensitivity to mechanical ventilation after surfactant inactivation in young rabbit lungs. Crit Care Med 1992; 20:635–640.
54. Gattinoni L, Pesanti A, Macheroni D, Marcolin R, Fumagalli R, Rossi F, Iapicino G, Romagnoli G, Zoff D, Uziel L, Agostini A, Kolobow TH, Damia G. Low frequency positive pressure ventilation with extracorporeal CO_2 removal in severe acute respiratory failure. JAMA 1986; 256:881–886.
55. Amato MB, Barbas CSV, Medeiros DM. Beneficial effects of the "open lung approach" with low distending pressures in acute respiratory distress syndrome. Am J Respir Crit Care Med 1995; 152:1835–1846.
56. Amato M, Barbas C, Medeiros D, Lorenzi FG, Kairalla RA, Deheinzelin D, Magaldi RB, Carvalho CRR. Improved survival in ARDS: beneficial effects of a lung protective strategy. AJRCCM 1996; 153:A531.
57. Brochard L, Roudot-Thoraval F. Tidal volume reduction in acute respiratory distress syndrome: a multicenter randomized study. AJRCCM 1997; 155:A505.
58. Brower R, Shanholtz C, Shade D, Fessler H, White P, Wiener C, Teeter J, Almog Y, Dodd-O J, Piantadosi S. Randomized controlled trial of small tidal volume ventilation in ARDS. AJRCCM 1997; 155:A93.
59. Stewart TE, Meade MO, Granton J, Lapinsky S, Hodder R, McLean R, Mazer D, Rogevin T, Schouten D, Todd T, Cook DJ, Slutsky AS. Pressure and volume limited ventilation strategy in patients at high risk for ARDS—results of a multicenter trial. AJRCCM 1997; 155:A505.

14

Resolution of Alveolar Edema

In Vivo Studies

ETHAN P. CARTER,* YIBING WANG, ANDRE R. CAMPBELL, and MICHAEL A. MATTHAY

University of California at San Francisco
San Francisco, California

CHRYSTELLE GARAT

National Jewish Center for Immunology and Respiratory Medicine
Denver, Colorado

TSUTOMU SAKUMA

Kanazawa Medical University
Ishikawa, Japan

I. Introduction

It is now apparent that active salt transport drives fluid removal from the distal airspaces of the lung. The results of several in vivo studies have demonstrated that changes in hydrostatic or protein osmotic pressures cannot account for the removal of excess fluid from the distal airspaces of the lungs (1,2). The role of active sodium transport in fluid removal from the distal airspaces has been demonstrated in in vivo, ex vivo, and in several in vitro studies (see Chaps. 15, 16, 17). Active sodium transport by the distal airway and alveolar epithelium is present in all species studied, including human lungs (3,4)

This chapter reviews the mechanisms of fluid transport across the distal airway and alveolar epithelium in the adult lung. The first section describes several experimental preparations that have been used to study fluid clearance from the intact lung. The second section describes how the fluid removal process is regulated by catecholamine-dependent and -independent mechanisms. The third section examines several clinically relevant pathologic models of alveolar fluid clearance. The final section considers clinical implications of these new insights into how the alveolar epithelial barrier regulates lung fluid balance.

**Current affiliation:* Colorado Health Sciences Center, Denver, Colorado.

II. Structure and Function of the Alveolar Epithelium

The fundamental structure and function of the alveolar epithelium are well described in Chapters 2 and 5 and will only be briefly discussed in this chapter.

A. Structural Basis for Resolution of Alveolar Edema

The alveolar epithelium is composed of two cell types—thin squamous type I cells, and cuboidal type II cells (5). The tight junctions joining the epithelial cells provide a high resistance barrier to the passage of solutes and water (6,7). Alveolar type I cells are the largest cell in the alveolar septum, but generally do not exceed 0.2 μm thick. Type I cells cover more than 95% of the surface of the alveolar air spaces, but the number of type I cells, due to their large size, is about half that of type II cells in the distal lung of adult mammals. Alveolar type II cells, well characterized in a variety of air breathing mammals, are structurally and functionally polarized. This polarization is essential to their two most important functions, vectorial ion transport and surfactant secretion (8,9). The active transport of sodium by type II cells provides the major driving force for the removal of fluid from the alveolar space. Sodium uptake occurs on the apical surface primarily through amiloride-sensitive sodium channels (10–12) (see Chap. 15). Then, sodium is pumped into the lung interstitium by the Na,K-ATPase located in the basolateral membrane (13) (see Chap. 16). Recent studies also indicate that alveolar type I and II cells contain functional water channels, which may aid in fluid balance across the alveolar epithelial barrier (14–16) (see Chap. 18) (Fig. 1).

B. Functional Evidence of Active Sodium Transport by the Lung

Until relatively recently, the concept that the alveolar epithelium might actively transport ions (with water following passively) into or out of the alveolar air-spaces was not appreciated. In contrast to the kidney or intestinal epithelial barriers, it had been thought that the morphological appearance of the cells in the distal regions of the lung was not well suited for the transport of ions and fluid.

The ability of mammalian lungs to absorb instilled fluid has been recognized for some time (17,18). Kylstra (18) found that 0.9% saline was slowly absorbed from dog lungs, and that distilled water disappeared more rapidly. The issue of fluid removal from the distal airspaces was revisited some years later using improved methods developed in in vivo (1), in situ (2,19), and in ex vivo preparations (20–23). These studies showed conclusively that fluid removal was an active, energy-dependent process. The process responsible for fluid removal

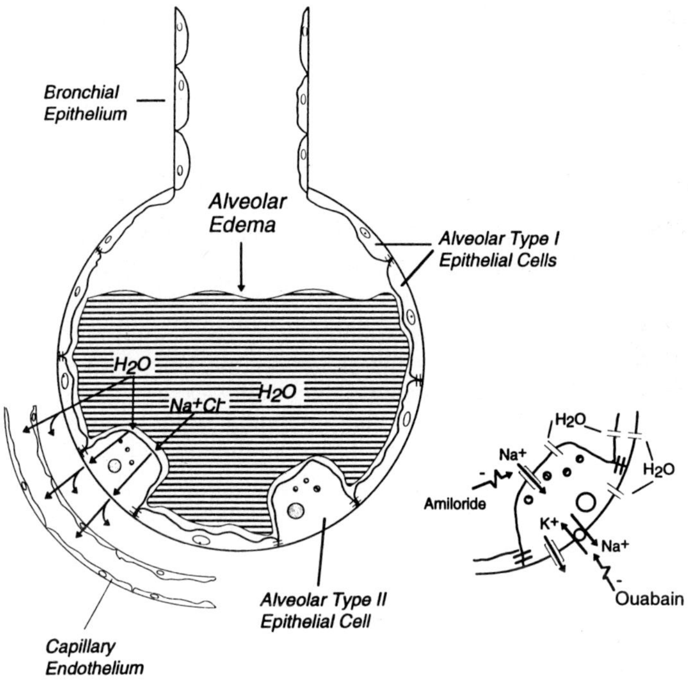

Figure 1 Schematic diagram of the major pathways for ion and water transport across the alveolar epithelium. Other known membrane transports that are not involved directly in vectorial fluid transport, such as Na^+/H^+ antiporter and K^+ conductance, are not shown. See text for further details.

was identified as active sodium transport by the alveolar epithelium. This was confirmed through the use of a variety of in vivo preparations, in situ preparations, isolated perfused lungs, and in vitro models using isolated alveolar type II cells. The major contributions using in vivo and in situ models are summarized below.

In Vivo Lung Studies

In vivo alveolar fluid clearance was first demonstrated using a model developed in sheep (1). The method determining fluid clearance uses the measurement of the protein concentration of a solution instilled into the distal airspaces as an index of alveolar fluid clearance. Because the epithelial barrier is very tight, fluid is removed much more rapidly than protein, and therefore an increase in protein concentration reflects alveolar fluid removal (1,3,4,20). In most preparations the test solution (serum, plasma, or 5% albumin) is instilled into distal airspaces of one lung and the concentration of the instilled labeled (i.e., ^{125}I-albumin) and unlabeled protein (albumin or total protein) is measured over time to estimate alveolar liquid clearance. This technique was used initially to measure clearance from the lungs of anesthetized, ventilated sheep (1). At the end of 4 hours, > 95% of the instilled ^{125}I-albumin was recovered from the airspaces, indicating slow clearance of the protein. In the airspaces, total protein concentration (labeled and unlabeled) increased by 48%. In subsequent studies, protein continued to concentrate in the airspaces up to 24 hours (24) (Fig. 2). The authors proposed that the active metabolic process was dependent on active ion transport with passive water flux.

In several other species, similar properties regarding fluid clearance from the airspaces were observed, although the rates of clearance varied significantly. Berthiaume et al. (25) measured alveolar liquid and protein clearance from

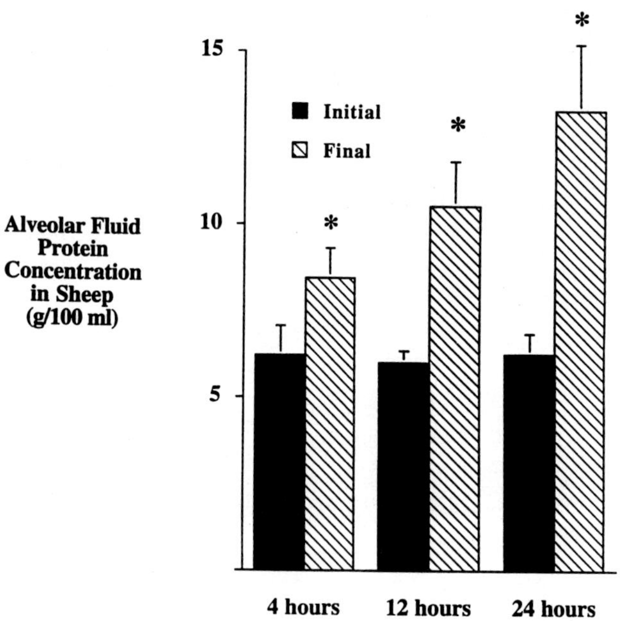

Figure 2 Change in alveolar protein concentration in sheep over 24 hours. One hundred milliliters of autologous serum was instilled into one lower lobe of unanesthetized sheep. At 4, 12, and 24 hours an alveolar sample was obtained for total protein concentration determination. There was a progressive concentration of alveolar protein at each time point, indicating a continuous removal of alveolar fluid. By 24 hours, approximately 80% of the alveolar fluid was removed. Data expressed as mean ± SD, $*P < .05$ compared to the initial protein concentration. (From Ref. 87.)

normal dog lungs using the same methods as described in sheep. Protein clearance was slow, similar to what was observed in sheep. Over 4 hours, the rate of alveolar liquid clearance in dogs was slower than in sheep (12% vs. 33% clearance, respectively). In fact, by 12 hours only 36% of the fluid was cleared. In rabbits, the rates of clearance are quite high, greater than in either sheep or dog (26). Rabbits cleared approximately 50% of the instilled solution over 4 hours. This higher rate of clearance was not due to elevated circulating epinephrine levels, since propranolol treatment did not slow the rate of clearance, as was observed in sheep (27). In rats, alveolar and lung liquid clearance was fast, as in rabbits; 50% of the instilled fluid was cleared over 4 hours (28). As in rabbits and sheep, the basal rate of clearance was not due to endogenous circulating catecholamine levels since propranolol administration had no effect on fluid removal. The mechanism responsible for the different rates of clearance have not been identified. Table 1 compares the rates of basal alveolar fluid clearance in different in vivo preparations.

Alveolar epithelial fluid clearance can be upregulated with β_2-adrenergic agonist stimulation (25,27–28). In anesthetized sheep, both terbutaline (10^{-5} M) and epinephrine (5.5×10^{-6} M) increased lung liquid clearance over 4 hours (27). In dogs, terbutaline (10^{-5} M) doubled the volume of liquid cleared from the lungs over 4 hours (25). However, lung liquid clearance in dogs treated with β-agonists was proportionally (50%) less than in sheep treated with β-agonists. Alveolar fluid clearance can also be stimulated in rats (28). However, clearance cannot be upregulated in rabbits using β-adrenergic agonists (26). Recent evidence demonstrated that β-adrenergic agonists do increase alveolar fluid clearance in the resected human lung (3,4).

To confirm that β-adrenergic agonist administration increased alveolar fluid clearance through a sodium-dependent process, amiloride was used in two in vivo models to inhibit the stimulatory effects of terbutaline. In sheep, amiloride (10^{-4} or 10^{-3} M) inhibits the effect of terbutaline on lung liquid clearance (27). Similarly, in rats, amiloride (10^{-3} M) inhibits the terbutaline stimulated alveolar liquid clearance (28). In rabbits, which do not respond to β-adrenergic stimulation, amiloride inhibits 60% of the basal lung liquid clearance (29). Thus, in in vivo lung preparations, alveolar liquid clearance is the result of sodium entry through apical sodium channels and extrusion through basolateral Na, K-ATPase (30). In addition, β-adrenergic stimulation increases the number and open time of apical sodium channels and possibly the activity of basolateral Na,K-ATPase (12,31).

Other Lung Preparations

Several in situ lung preparations have been developed to measure the contribution of active sodium transport to alveolar fluid clearance. In animals, such as sheep, goats, or rats, perfusion is accomplished by a roller pump and alveolar

Table 1 Comparison of the Rate of Basal Alveolar Fluid Clearance in Several Species

Species	Time of measurement	Initial protein concentration	Final protein concentration	Lung liquid clearance (% of instilled over 4 hrs)	Reference
Sheep	4 h	6.3 ± 0.6	8.4 ± 0.6	33	1
Goats	4 h	6.4 ± 0.6	8.3 ± 1.3	25 ± 6	19
Dogs	4 h	5.5 ± 0.6	6.1 ± 0.4	11 ± 3	25
Rabbits	4 h	4.6 ± 0.8	6.8[a]	48 ± 8	26
Rats	4 h	4.5 ± 0.8	7.1 ± 1.1	42 ± 8	28,60
Humans[b]	4 h	4.9 ± 0.1	5.5 ± 0.1	12 ± 2	3

[a]Estimated from 8-hour experiments.
[b]Based on ex vivo lung studies. *Source*: Refs. 3 and 4.

fluid clearance is measured without removing the lungs from the thorax (2,19). Typically, the animal is rapidly exsanguinated, and the shed blood (often diluted with an isomolar salt solution) is used to perfuse the pulmonary vasculature via the pulmonary artery. The perfusate is collected from the left atrium, heated, and recirculated through the pulmonary circulation. The in situ preparation may be stable for up to 4 hours. This preparation has several unique applications. One is the ability to control the temperature of the preparation, thus making it possible to study the effects of temperature on the active transport mechanisms that regulate alveolar fluid clearance. It is also possible to measure lung lymphatic flow rates in large animals such as sheep and goats using the in situ preparation, as well as manipulate hemodynamics during the clearance period (19,30).

In the in situ goat lung preparation, alveolar clearance was measured under several different perfusion temperatures in order to test the hypothesis that active transport was responsible for fluid removal (19). The rate of alveolar fluid clearance progressively declined as temperature was lowered from 37 to 18°C, with clearance reduced by 50% at 30°C. The temperature dependence of alveolar clearance has also been reported in isolated, perfused rat lungs (23) as well as in the resected human lung (3).

Sodium and fluid resorption in the in situ rat lung was studied by Basset et al. (2). Their preparation was a cross-circulation technique in which the lungs of a recipient rat were perfused with blood from a donor rat. The donor rat was ventilated and the recipient rat was not. The lungs of the recipient rat were instilled with isotonic Ringer's containing [^{125}I]albumin to calculate alveolar volume change and $^{22}Na^{+}$ to trace sodium movement. Active sodium transport out of the airspaces and fluid clearance were correlated. Amiloride (10^{-4} M) inhibited $^{22}Na^{+}$ flux and fluid clearance to the same degree, about a 50% reduction. Basset et al. (2) concluded that fluid transport out the lungs was secondary to active sodium transport by the alveolar epithelium.

A variation of the in situ lung preparation has been developed which demonstrated that alveolar fluid clearance in sheep continues for up to 4 hours in the absence of perfusion and ventilation (30). Alveolar liquid clearance, measured as the percent increase in alveolar protein concentration over 4 hours, was similar between sheep without blood flow (31% ± 8%) compared with sheep with normal blood flow (31% ± 7%). Administration of ouabain inhibited 90% alveolar liquid clearance in this model indicating that this process depends on active transport by Na,K-ATPase located in the alveolar epithelium. Interestingly, this is one of the few intact lung preparations that has been successful in using ouabain to inhibit completely sodium and fluid resorption.

More recently, this nonperfused model was adapted to measure alveolar fluid clearance in mice (32). Mice were exsanguinated followed by instillation of 0.5 ml of a 5% albumin solution into both lungs via a tracheal cannula. Mouse body temperature was kept at 37°C with an infrared heat lamp. After 1 hour, 22% ± 2% of the instillate was cleared from the airspace, while in the presence of 10^{-3} M amiloride, only 13% ± 2% of the instillate was cleared. Isoproterenol, not terbutaline, increased the rate of alveolar fluid clearance in the mice. The development of this novel model will allow for the evaluation of alveolar epithelial transport and barrier properties in transgenic mice (32).

The nonperfused lung preparation laid the groundwork for clearance measurements that were made in nonperfused resected human lungs (3). In the human model, resected lungs were surgically obtained from patients who underwent surgery for lung cancer. The resected lung was placed in a 37°C incubator. Then, a test solution containing 5% albumin was instilled in one segment of a resected lobe within 20 min of resection, and the increase in albumin concentration over 4 hours was used to quantify alveolar liquid clearance. Basal alveolar liquid clearance was 12% over 4 hours. Amiloride and ouabain reduced clearance by 40% and 49%, respectively, while terbutaline doubled the rate of clearance to

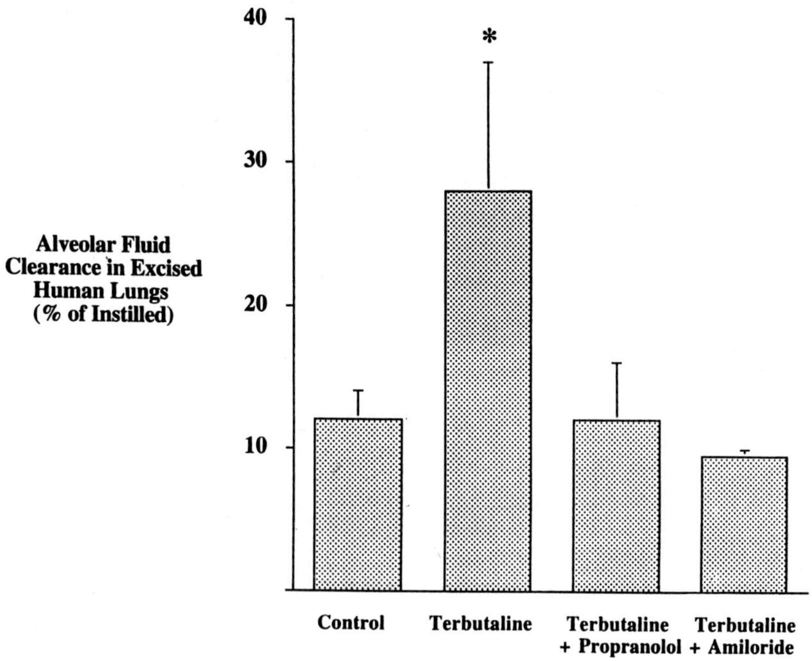

Figure 3 Clearance of alveolar fluid in resected human lung. Alveolar fluid clearance over 4 hours was calculated from the concentration of instilled albumin into the airspaces. Terbutaline (10^{-4} M), a β-adrenergic agonist, more than doubled alveolar fluid clearance, an effect that was inhibited with propranolol (10^{-4} M) or by amiloride (10^{-4} M). Data expressed as mean ± SD, $*P < .05$ compared to other experimental conditions. (From Ref. 87.)

28% over 4 hours (Fig. 3). Therefore, these data provide evidence that the reabsorption of alveolar edema fluid in humans depends on an active sodium transport process (33,34). While the nonperfused model has provided useful information, it does have limitations. First, the preparation is viable for only a few hours. Also, because of the lack of blood flow, pulmonary lymphatic drainage is not normal, which could slow clearance rates.

III. Regulation of Alveolar Fluid Clearance

The following section describes clinically relevant mechanisms that can regulate alveolar fluid clearance and the resolution of pulmonary edema.

A. Catecholamine-Dependent Regulation of Alveolar Fluid Clearance

In all of the models described above, sodium transport and net alveolar fluid clearance can be augmented with β-adrenergic agonists. Terbutaline administration in anesthetized, ventilated sheep, dogs, rats, and mice markedly increases alveolar fluid clearance (25,27,28). Coadministration of propranolol, a β-adrenergic antagonist, prevents all of the β-adrenergic agonist effects (27). Studies in isolated perfused lungs and in in vivo preparations have provided evidence that the β-adrenergic stimulatory pathway is through a cAMP second-messenger pathway but does not involve protein kinase C activation (35,36).

Since β-adrenergic stimulation increases alveolar fluid clearance in the human lung, these data have potential clinical relevance. The magnitude of the stimulatory effect in the human lung is similar to other species; a doubling of β-adrenergic agonist stimulated alveolar fluid clearance. These data are particularly important based on recent evidence indicating that aerosolized β-adrenergic agonist therapy with salmeterol, a long-acting, lipid-soluble β-agonist, can markedly increase the rate of alveolar fluid clearance in sheep (37). Also, recent data indicate that 10^{-6} M salmeterol can accelerate alveolar fluid clearance in the human lung (3). Thus, aerosolized β-adrenergic agonist treatment in some patients with pulmonary edema might be effective in accelerating resolution. In addition, recent work indicates that it is the β_2 receptor in rat and human lungs that mediates the betaadrenergic effects (38). This observation has clinical relevance because dobutamine, a β_2-adrenergic agonist frequently used in clinical medicine, has been shown to increase markedly the rate of alveolar fluid clearance in rats.

B. Catecholamine-Independent Regulation of Alveolar Fluid Clearance

Although endogenous catecholamine stimulation is an important mechanism for upregulating alveolar fluid clearance, recent work indicates that several catecholamine-independent mechanisms can upregulate alveolar fluid clearance. Sodium transport is increased in isolated alveolar type II cells following treatment with epidermal growth factor (39). Transforming growth factor-α (TGF-α) acutely increases alveolar fluid transport in ventilated rats (40). Dexamethasone also upregulates basal alveolar fluid clearance at 24 hours (41), an effect that may be mediated be an upregulation of epithelial sodium channel activity (42). In a rat model of pneumonia, alveolar epithelial fluid transport was markedly upregulated by the pro-inflammatory cytokine, tumor necrosis factor-α (TNF-α) (43). An intriguing possible explanation comes from observations that TNF-α can form ion-permeable channels in planar lipid bilayer membranes and increase the sodium permeability of human U937 histiocytic lymphoma cells (44). Alternatively, TNF-α may release oxidants that could upregulate alveolar fluid clearance (12).

When acute lung injury causes damage to the epithelial barrier with loss of alveolar type I cells, alveolar type II cells proliferate to provide a new epithelial barrier (45,46). Preliminary evidence indicates that restoration of the alveolar epithelial barrier with type II cells following intratracheal administration of bleomycin is associated with a marked increase in the fluid transport capacity of the alveolar epithelium (47). It is not yet known whether the augmented transport capacity is due to an increased number of alveolar type II cells or whether there is also an upregulation of sodium transport per cell. This is an important issue because proliferation of alveolar type II cells following acute lung injury may provide a mechanism for sustained upregulation of the transport capacity of the alveolar epithelium following lung injury. While endogenous release of epinephrine, TGF-α, or TNF-α may upregulate alveolar fluid clearance in the acutely injured lung, their effect is likely to be restricted to the early phase of acute lung injury. However, proliferation of alveolar type II cells may provide a fundamental mechanism of sustained upregulation of alveolar fluid transport that might be critical for the removal of alveolar edema fluid in the injured lung.

C. Downregulation of Alveolar Fluid Clearance

Although the mechanisms that increase alveolar fluid clearance have received considerable attention, there is a growing list of conditions associated with a downregulation of alveolar epithelial fluid clearance.

Since the lung has two extravascular compartments separated by a tight epithelium, a moderate rise in lung vascular pressure is not associated with accumulation of alveolar edema fluid (48). The alveolar space is protected by the tight alveolar epithelium; however, a rapid rise in lung vascular pressure to very high levels can cause a mechanical break in the endothelial and epithelial barriers, as Bachofen (49) and West (50) have proposed. The increased fluid that is filtered across the lung endothelium in the presence of moderately elevated vascular pressures accumulates first in the interstitium, where there are several mechanisms that prevent alveolar flooding (see Chap. 5). There is a pressure gradient in the interstitium from the alveolar to the extra-alveolar interstitium, even in the presence of edema (51). Higher levels of lung inflation produce more negative pressure in the extra-alveolar interstitium (52). Therefore, a significant fraction of the vascular filtrate moves to the extra-alveolar compartment, where lung lymph flow can markedly increase to remove some of the excess interstitial edema fluid (48).

Also, some of the interstitial edema fluid flows across the low-resistance visceral pleural mesothelium into the pleural space (53). Because the extra-alveolar interstitial space is compliant, a large volume of edema fluid, up to 500 ml, can collect in the human lung (48). The pressure in the extra-alveolar interstitium increases from a baseline value of approximately 1 cm H_2O to only 2 to 3 cm H_2O even in moderately severe edema (52). Translocation of interstitial edema to the airspaces may not occur until interstitial pressure sharply increases as the capacity of the interstitial compartment is exceeded. In view of these mechanisms that restrict edema fluid to the lung interstitium, it is possible that net alveolar fluid clearance could continue even in the presence of substantial elevations in lung vascular pressures. If this hypothesis is correct, then alveolar fluid clearance should persist, even with moderate elevations of lung vascular pressure. Preliminary data in sheep with an elevated left atrial pressure of 24 cm H_2O support this hypothesis (54). Under these conditions, alveolar liquid clearance persisted at a normal basal level. Since plasma epinephrine levels were elevated, bilateral adrenalectomy was done which resulted in a 30% decrease in alveolar fluid clearance in the presence of left atrial hypertension to 24 cm H_2O. Therefore, endogenous epinephrine maintained alveolar fluid clearance at basal levels despite elevated left atrial pressure.

There is recent evidence that hypoxia alters the function of the alveolar epithelium by downregulating sodium transport in isolated alveolar type II cells (55). Following exposure to either 3% or 0% oxygen for 18 hours, $^{22}Na^+$ flux through sodium channels was reduced by 32% and 67%, respectively, while 5% oxygen had no effect. The decreased sodium channel function was temporally associated with reductions in mRNAs encoding the α-, β-, and γ-subunits of the rat epithelial NA^+ channel (rENaC). Similar decreases also were observed in the function and expression of the Na,K-ATPase. These hypoxic effects on alveolar epithelial type II cell sodium transport may have clinical implications.

Lung deflation combined with ischemia, as might occur during lung transplantation or pneumothorax, leads to severe alveolar flooding within 1 hour of reinflation and reperfusion in rabbits (56). Although neutrophil depletion did not prevent the injury, continuous inflation with either oxygen or nitrogen during the 4-hour ischemic episode did prevent injury and alveolar flooding upon reperfusion. While the mechanism for this protective effect is not known, it is possible that inflation during ischemia preserves the microvascular architecture between vascular endothelial cells, thus reducing the flooding and edema upon reperfusion. In addition, there is some new evidence that deflation of the isolated rat lung reduces alveolar while inflation restores clearance (57). Thus, there may be mechanosensitive mechanisms that can downregulate alveolar fluid clearance, although effects of deflation on surface area and metabolic substrates needs to be examined.

IV. Alveolar Epithelial Function Under Pathological Conditions

This section considers several experimental studies which provide new insights into the function of the alveolar epithelial barrier under clinically relevant pathological conditions. In each of the studies, the primary focus was to assess the net fluid transport capacity of the alveolar and distal airway epithelium under specific physiologic stresses and well-defined pathological insults. Interestingly, the results indicate that the alveolar and distal airway epithelium is remarkably resistant to injury, particularly compared to the adjacent lung endothelium. Even when mild to moderate alveolar epithelial injury occurs, the capacity of the alveolar epithelium to transport salt and water is often preserved. In addition, several mechanisms may result in an upregulation of the fluid transport capacity of the distal pulmonary epithelium, even after moderate to severe epithelial injury (Table 2).

A. Resistance of the Alveolar Epithelium to Injury

The first evidence to demonstrate the resistance of the alveolar epithelial barrier to injury evolved from studies in which large numbers of neutrophils and monocytes crossed the tight alveolar epithelial barrier without inducing a significant change in either permeability to protein or transport capacity of the alveolar epithelium. In the initial studies, instillation of autologous serum or plasma into the distal airspaces of sheep was associated with an influx of both neutrophils and monocytes. Despite the influx of inflammatory cells, there was no increase in epithelial permeability to plasma protein; in addition, alveolar fluid clearance was normal (24). In a subsequent study in normal human volunteers, large numbers of neutrophils were recruited to the distal airspaces by instillation of the potent neutrophil chemotactic factor, leukotriene B_4; however, there was no influx of plasma protein into the airspaces (58). Finally, to maximize the recruitment of cells to the air spaces of the lung and to stimulate the release of large quantities of proinflammatory cytokines such as tumor necrosis factor, interleukin-1, and interleukin-8, *E. coli* endotoxin (100 to 200 μg/kg) was

Table 2 Effect of Pathological Conditions on Alveolar Epithelial Fluid Clearance in Several Species

Pathological condition	Species	Severity of lung injury		Alveolar epithelial fluid clearance	Reference
		Endothelium	Epithelium		
Saltwater aspiration	Rabbit	Mild	Mild	Normal	62
Hyperoxia	Hamster/rat	Moderate	Moderate	?	66–72
Endotoxin, intravenous	Sheep	Mild	None	Normal	59
Endotoxin, alveolar	Sheep	None	None	Normal	59
	Rat	None	None	Increased	77
Exotoxin, alveolar	Rat	None	None	Increased	76
Bacteria, intravenous[a]	Sheep	Moderate/severe	Mild/severe	Increased/decreased	60
	Rat	Mild	None	Increased	73
	Rabbit	Mild	None	Normal	73
Bacteria, alveolar[a]	Sheep	Mild	Mild	Normal	60
	Rat	Mild	Moderate/severe	Normal/decreased	43
	Rabbit	Mild	Moderate/severe	Normal/decreased	74
Oleic acid, intravenous[b]	Sheep	Moderate	Moderate	Normal	79
Acid aspiration	Rabbit	Severe	Severe	Decreased	78
No pulmonary blood flow	Sheep	None	None	Normal	30
No ventilation	Sheep	None	None	Normal	30
	Human	?	?	Normal	3
Severe cooling followed by rewarming (transplant)	Human	None	None	Normal (after rewarming)	86

[a]The extent of injury to the epithelial and endothelial barriers is dependent on the dose and virulence of bacteria that are administered (43,60,73,74).
[b]Initially the injury after intravenous oleic acid is severe, but the alveolar epithelium recovers after 4 hours sufficiently to remove some of the excess edema fluid (79).

instilled into the distal air spaces in sheep. Although large numbers of neutrophils and monocytes were recruited to the air spaces, there was again no significant increase in epithelial permeability to protein and alveolar fluid clearance was normal as assessed in short-term (4 hours) and longer-term experiments (24 hours) (59). These studies demonstrated conclusively that the alveolar epithelial barrier can remain intact and functional even though large numbers of inflammatory cells migrate through the alveolar epithelial tight junctions.

B. Septic and Hypovolemic Shock

Because exogenous administration of β-adrenergic agonists markedly upregulated alveolar fluid clearance in several animals including the human lung, several studies have been carried out to determine if endogenous release of epinephrine would upregulate sodium and fluid transport in clinically relevant pathological conditions. The first study evaluated alveolar fluid clearance in rats with gram-negative septic shock that were hypotensive without fluid resuscitation (60). Markedly elevated levels of epinephrine were measured in the plasma, and alveolar fluid clearance over 4 hours nearly doubled compared to control rats. The increase in clearance was blocked with intra-alveolar amiloride or propranolol.

To determine if the mechanism of endogenous release of epinephrine was germane to other clinically relevant conditions, the alveolar fluid clearance studies were carried out in rats that had been subjected to 90 min of hemorrhagic shock without resuscitation. The results provided strong evidence for a marked upregulation of alveolar fluid transport that was inhibitable with intra-alveolar amiloride or propranolol (61). In neither the septic-shock nor hypovolemic-shock experiments was there evidence of increased protein flux across the alveolar epithelial barrier, so the upregulation of alveolar fluid clearance occurred in the absence of alveolar epithelial injury. However, these rats were not resuscitated from shock. Additional studies have been done following short-term (15 min) hemorrhagic shock to determine if the upregulation of alveolar fluid clearance would persist for several hours following fluid resuscitation. Although there was evidence of mild to moderate endothelial and epithelial injury, alveolar fluid clearance was increased several hours after shock.

C. Seawater Aspiration

Recent experiments with instillation of a hyperosmolar solution into the airspaces of anesthetized, ventilated rabbits have provided important information on the function of the alveolar epithelial barrier in the presence of an osmotic stress (Table 2). When sea water is used as the hyperosmolar solution (900 mOsm), there is an abrupt translocation of pure water into the airspaces of the lung so that isosmolar conditions are reached within 3 to 5 min and the alveolar volume increases threefold (62). This translocation of water occurs through endothelial and epithelial water channels (14,15,63). Interestingly, this rapid movement of fluid into the airspaces was followed by an influx of neutrophils, but there was only a minimal, transient increase in epithelial permeability to protein. Over the subsequent 6 hours, the rate of alveolar sodium and fluid transport was normal (62), as has been observed in one well-described clinical case (64). Thus, even though a large volume of edema fluid accumulates in the airspaces rapidly, the alveolar epithelial barrier remains intact and functional to remove the edema fluid at a rapid rate.

D. Hyperoxia-Induced Lung Injury

Hyperoxic exposure is widely used for studying acute lung injury because of its clinical relevance to oxygen therapy and the detrimental consequences of prolonged exposure. Exposure of mammals to pure oxygen leads to pulmonary edema, respiratory failure, and eventually death—similar to what is seen clinically in ARDS patients. The morphological changes in the blood-gas barrier with oxygen toxicity are well characterized and will not be discussed (65).

Passive Transport Function of the Alveolar Epithelium During Hyperoxic Lung Injury

Recently two studies measured alveolar epithelial permeability following exposure of hamsters to 100% O_2. Wangensteen and co-workers (66,67) used an isolated perfused lung preparation to measure the permeability $\times$ surface area products of several solutes. The measurements were made during the course of injury (66) and during recovery (67). Bovine serum albumin (BSA) and sucrose PS products began to increase several days into exposure. After 5 days of exposure, the sucrose permeability was 4.7 times control and the BSA permeability was 31 times control (66), which persisted 1 day into recovery (67). By 7 to 14 days following exposure, permeabilities were back to normal. These data indicate that initially there is no change in alveolar permeability in response to breathing pure oxygen, but then permeability progressively increases with time with the greatest change is seen with the largest solutes.

Active Sodium Transport by the Alveolar Epithelium During Hyperoxic Lung Injury

Data regarding sodium transport during hyperoxia-induced acute lung injury have only recently been published. The most complete information is from a subacute exposure model whereby rats are exposed to 85% O_2 for 7 days (68–70). Sznajder and colleagues (69,70) investigated rat lung and isolated type

II cell sodium transport following exposure to 85% O_2 for 7 days. Active sodium resorption was measured in isolated perfused lungs from exposed animals and Na,K-ATPase activity was assessed in type II cells isolated from the lungs of exposed animals. Active sodium transport increased immediately after oxygen exposure and returned to control values by 7 days of recovery in room air. Since both amiloride-inhibitable and ouabain-inhibitable transport were increased, the upregulation was attributed to increased function of both sodium channels and Na,K-ATPase. Increased Na,K-ATPase activity in type II cells isolated from exposed lungs confirmed the perfused lung observations. Haskell et al. (68) also investigated type II cell sodium transport in this model of lung injury. Type II cells were isolated from rat lungs following a similar exposure regimen as Olivera et al. (69). Amiloride-sensitive sodium channel function and expression were assessed using the patch-clamp technique and Western blot analysis, respectively. Mean channel open time as well as channel antigenic protein were increased in the isolated type II cells. Thus, in this model of lung injury, the available evidence indicates that both whole-lung and alveolar type II cell sodium transport is increased as a result of increased function of both sodium channels and Na,K-ATPase.

In a study designed to assess Na,K-ATPase expression during acute lung injury, Nici et al. (71) exposed rats to 60 hours of 100% O_2. Immediately following exposure or after recovery in room air, peripheral lung Na,K-ATPase steady-state mRNA and antigenic protein levels were measured. Increases in the steady-state mRNA signal of both the α_1- and β_1-subunits were observed as early as 36 hours into the 60-hour exposure and diminished toward the unexposed values by 3 days of recovery in room air. Western blot analysis of the peripheral lung membrane α-subunit showed that the antigenic signal did not noticeably change during exposure, but increased by 1 day of recovery and remained elevated for several more days of recovery. It was proposed by Nici et al. (71) that this upregulation of the Na,K-ATPase is an early response to pulmonary edema and/or hyperoxic injury. However, in this acute (100% O_2) model of exposure, the available data indicate that sodium transport and fluid resorption are not significantly increased and may even be decreased. The exact mechanism for this is not known but may involve oxidation of transport proteins or other proteins, combined with tight-junction disruption rendering any remaining sodium transport ineffective.

Interestingly, exposure of rats to 85% oxygen for 7 days immediately followed by exposure to 100% oxygen for 4 days upregulates alveolar type II cell sodium channel expression and function (72). Alveolar type II sodium channel mRNA (αrENaC) expression increased threefold following exposure to 85% oxygen and sixfold after exposure to 85% oxygen followed by exposure to 100% oxygen. Immunoblots revealed a similar response in sodium channel protein. Patch-clamp analysis of type II cells revealed that this hyperoxic exposure sequence increased the sodium channel function as well. Thus, exposure to 85%

oxygen before 100% oxygen elicits a response in sodium transport not seen by exposure to only 100% oxygen.

E. Endotoxin- and Bacterial-Induced Lung Injury

Even when severe lung endothelial injury occurs, the alveolar epithelial barrier may remain normally impermeable to protein and retain its normal fluid transport capacity (Table 2). For example, either intravenous endotoxin or bacteria have been used to produce lung endothelial injury in sheep (59) or rats (60), but permeability to protein across the lung epithelial barrier was not increased. In the rat studies, septic shock occurred, resulting in a marked increase in plasma epinephrine levels. Even though there was endothelial injury and mild interstitial pulmonary edema, alveolar epithelial fluid transport was increased from 45% over 4 hours in control rats to 75% over 4 hours in the septic rats. The effect was inhibited with instillation of either amiloride (10^{-4} M) or propranolol (10^{-4} M) into the distal airspaces, thus proving that the stimulated clearance depended on β-adrenergic agonist stimulation of alveolar epithelial sodium transport. When more severe septic shock was produced in sheep, the alveolar epithelial barrier was resistant to injury in the majority of sheep with confinement of the edema to the pulmonary interstitium (73) (Table 2). In some sheep, however, more severe systemic and pulmonary endothelial injury was associated with alveolar flooding, a marked increase in epithelial permeability to protein, and the inability to transport fluid from the airspaces of the lung. The inability to remove excess fluid from the airspaces in these sheep may have been related to a marked increase in paracellular permeability from injury to the epithelial tight junctions or to a loss salt and water transport capacity of alveolar epithelial cells.

In animal models of pneumonia, the degree injury is dependent, in part, on the size of the bacterial inoculum (see Chap. 7). Severe injury develops when large numbers of virulent bacteria are used, although studies with less virulent bacteria result in less epithelial injury and a preserved capacity to transport fluid from the distal airspaces of the lung (74). It is possible that bacterial products or inflammatory products of neutrophils or macrophages may decrease sodium transport in alveolar epithelial type II cells. One in vitro study did report a downregulation of alveolar epithelial type II cell sodium transport by an L-arginine-dependent product from endotoxin-stimulated alveolar macrophages (75). On the other hand, in vivo studies with alveolar endotoxin and exotoxin A have reported normal or increased rates of alveolar epithelial sodium and fluid transport in two different species (43,76,77).

F. Severe Lung Injury—Acid Aspiration

In some experimental studies, such as severe acid aspiration-induced lung injury (78), the injury to the epithelial barrier is so severe that recovery does not occur

(Table 2). In other types of severe lung injury, as occurs from intravenous oleic acid, the initial injury to the tight junctions results in severe alveolar flooding, although recovery may occur within a few hours, presumably from reestablishment of the normal tight barrier characteristics of the alveolar barrier (79).

V. Clinical Implications of Alveolar Epithelial Fluid Transport

The fluid transport capacity of the alveolar epithelial barrier under pathological conditions, particularly in patients with pulmonary edema and acute lung injury, is of major interest to both basic and clinical investigators. More than 10 years ago, clinical studies indicated that protein-rich pulmonary edema can be collected from patients with acute lung injury, whereas patients with cardiogenic or hydrostatic pulmonary edema have a significantly lower protein concentration in the edema fluid (80,81). However, there was no direct information in these clinical studies regarding the contribution of the epithelial barrier to the resolution of the alveolar edema. Until recently, pathological studies provided the only direct information regarding the status of the alveolar epithelial barrier in patients with acute lung injury. For example, postmortem studies of patients who died with acute lung injury report diffuse alveolar damage to both the endothelial and epithelial barriers of the lung with protein-rich pulmonary edema, inflammatory cells, and intra-alveolar exudate, pathological hallmarks of the pulmonary response to acute lung injury. Ultrastructural studies indicate widespread necrosis and denuding of alveolar type I cells, usually with some evidence of alveolar epithelial type II cell hyperplasia (46). However, these postmortem studies represent a sampling of only the most severe cases of acute lung injury. Recent clinical studies indicate that there is considerable heterogeneity in the fluid transport and barrier properties of the alveolar epithelial barrier of patients with acute lung injury (33,34,82,83).

Two properties of the epithelial barrier can be assessed clinically. First, since the epithelial barrier is normally impermeable to protein, the quantity of protein that accumulates in the distal air spaces is a good index of epithelial permeability. Secondly, since concentration of protein in alveolar fluid reflects net clearance of alveolar fluid (Figs. 2, 3), measurement of protein concentration in sequential alveolar edema fluid samples provides a physiologic index of the ability of the alveolar epithelial barrier to remove edema fluid. In a recent study, patients who died with acute lung injury had threefold more protein lavaged from their distal air spaces than patients who survived (82). In another study, approximately 40% of patients were able to reabsorb some of the alveolar edema fluid within 12 hours of intubation and acute lung injury (33). These patients had a more rapid recovery from respiratory failure and a lower mortality. In contrast, the patients who did not reabsorb any of the alveolar edema fluid in the first 12 hours following acute lung injury had protracted respiratory failure and a higher mortality (Fig. 4). These clinical studies suggest that the function of the alveolar epithelial barrier may be critical in determining the capacity of the lung for recovery from acute lung injury.

Could β-adrenergic agonist therapy be practical and useful in treatment of acute lung injury? Recent data demonstrate that alveolar fluid clearance is increased in anesthetized, ventilated sheep using clinically relevant doses of an aerosolized, long-acting β_2-adrenergic agonist, salmeterol (37). In addition, the

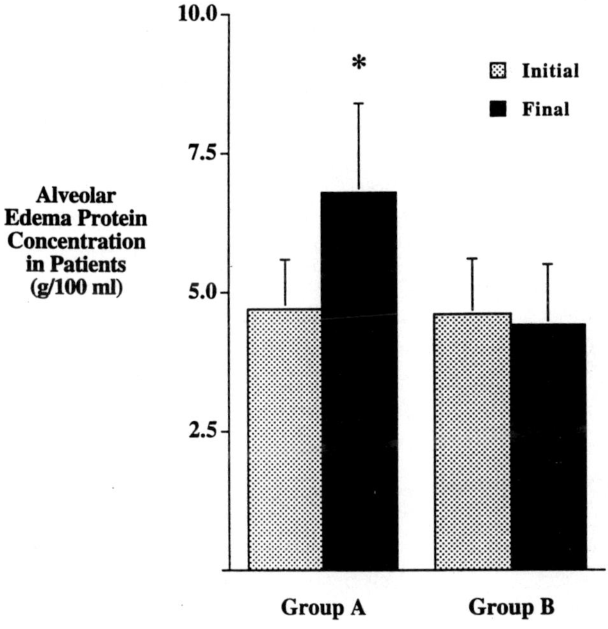

Figure 4 Concentration of protein in alveolar edema fluid obtained from patients with acute lung injury. The initial sample was obtained within 0.5 hours of endotracheal intubation. The subsequent sample was obtained within 12 hours of intubation. (Group A) Patients whose alveolar edema fluid protein concentration increased by 10% or more above their initial value, indicating net alveolar fluid clearance. (Group B) Patients whose alveolar edema fluid protein concentration increased by less than 10% above their initial value, indicating little or no net alveolar fluid clearance. Patients in group A had more repid recovery from respiratory failiure and a lower mortality than patients in group B, suggesting that intact alveolar fluid transport mechanisms in the early phase of acute lung injury provide favorable prognostic indicator. Data expressed as mean ± SD, $*P < .05$ compared to initial value. (From Ref. 87.)

aerosolized β_2-adrenergic treatment did not alter hemodynamics. Thus, aerosolized β-adrenergic therapy may be safe and effective in the treatment of both cardiogenic pulmonary edema resulting from left atrial hypertension and permeability edema from alveolar epithelial injury (see Chap. 20). In fact, hyperoxia-injured lungs are responsive to β-adrenergic stimulation (84,85). Lasnier et al. (84) demonstrated that 10^{-3} M terbutaline stimulated alveolar fluid clearance by 50% in rats exposed to 60 hours of 100% oxygen. Similarly, in rats exposed to 40 hours of 100% oxygen, 10^{-4} M terbutaline increased alveolar liquid clearance by 45%, similar to unexposed rats (85). These reports indicate that even in the face of significant alveolar epithelial and capillary endothelial injury caused by hyperoxia, the alveolar epithelium is capable of vectorial sodium and fluid resorption. Since endogenous catecholamines may already be increased during shock and other clinical conditions, clinical studies that evaluate the effectiveness of exogenous catecholamine therapy, in relation to endogenous plasma catecholamine levels, need to be done. In addition, it is also apparent that catecholamine-independent mechanisms, such as growth factors, cytokines, and alveolar epithelial type II cell hyperplasia, may influence alveolar epithelial fluid transport in the injured lung.

In summary, much has been learned about the resistance of the alveolar epithelial barrier to injury and its ability to maintain vectorial fluid transport after injury. More experimental studies are needed to measure the function of sodium and water transport pathways under pathological conditions. Also, clinical studies should be considered to test the feasibility and clinical value of stimulating alveolar fluid clearance in patients with pulmonary edema (see Chap. 20).

Acknowledgments

This work was supported by National Institutes of Health grants HL51854, HL51856, and DK35124. Dr. Carter was also supported by a fellowship from the American Lung Association and California Lung Association.

References

1. Matthay MA, Landolt CC, Staub NC. Differential liquid and protein clearance from the alveoli of anesthetized sheep. J Appl Physiol 1982; 53:96–104.
2. Basset G, Crone C, Saumon G. Fluid absorption by rat lung in situ: pathways for sodium entry in the luminal membrane of alveolar epithelium. J Physiol 1987; 384: 325–345.
3. Sakuma T, Okaniwa G, Nakada T, Nishimura T, Fujimura S, Matthay MA. Alveolar fluid clearance in the resected human lung. Am J Respir Crit Care Med 1994; 150: 305–310.

4. Sakuma T, Folkesson HG, Suzuki S, Okaniwa G, Fujimara S, Matthay MA. Beta-adrenergic agonist stimulated alveolar fluid clearance in ex vivo human and rat lungs. Am J Respir Crit Care Med 1997; 155:506–512.
5. Staub NC, Albertine KH. The structure of the lungs relative to their principal function. In: Murray JF, Nadel JA, eds. Textbook of Respiratory Medicine. Philadelphia, PA: W.B. Saunders; 1986.
6. Gumbiner BM. Breaking through the tight junction barrier. J Cell Biol 1993; 123:1931–1633.
7. Schneeberger EE, Lynch RD. Structure, function, and regulation of cellular tight junctions. Am J Physiol 1992; 262:L647–L661.
8. Goodman BE, Fleischer RS, Crandall ED. Evidence for active Na^+ transport by cultured monolayers of pulmonary alveolar epithelial cells. Am J Physiol 1983; 245:C78–C83.
9. Wright JR, Clements JA. Metabolism and turnover of lung surfactant. Am Rev Respir Dis 1987; 135:426–444.
10. Matalon S, Bridges RJ, Benos DJ. Amiloride-inhibitable Na^+ conductive pathways in alveolar type II pneumocytes. Am J Physiol 1991; 260:L90–L96.
11. Matalon S. Mechanisms and regulation of ion transport in adult mammalian alveolar type II pneumocytes. Am J Physiol 1991; 261:C727–C738.
12. Matalon S, Benos DJ, Jackson RM. Biophysical and molecular properties of amiloride-inhibitable sodium channels in alveolar epithelial cells. Am J Physiol 1996; 271:L1–L22.
13. Schneeberger EE, McCarthy KM. Cytochemical localization of Na^+-K^+-ATPase in rat type II pneumocytes. J Appl Physiol 1986; 60:1584–1589.
14. Folkesson HG, Matthay MA, Hasegawa H, Kheradmand F, Verkman AS. Transcellular water transport in lung alveolar epithelium through mercury-sensitive water channels. Proc Natl Acad Sci USA 1994; 91:4970–4974.
15. Carter EP, Matthay MA, Farinas J, Verkman AS. Transalveolar osmotic and diffusional water permeability in intact mouse lung measured by a novel surface fluorescence method. J Gen Physiol 1996; 108:133–142.
16. Dobbs L, Gonzalez R, Matthay MA, Carter EP, Allen L, Verkman AS. Highly water-permeable type I alveolar epithelial cells confer high transalveolar water permeability in rat lung. Proc Natl Acad Sci USA. In press.
17. Courtice FC, Phipps PJ. The absorption of fluids from the lungs. J Physiol 1946; 105:186–190.
18. Kylstra JA. Lavage of the lung. Acta Physiol Pharmacol Neerl 1958; 7:163–221.
19. Serikov VB, Grady M, Matthay MA. Effect of temperature on alveolar liquid and protein clearance in an in situ perfused goat lung. J Appl Physiol 1993; 75: 940–947.
20. Basset G, Crone C, Saumon G. Significance of active ion transport in transalveolar water absorption: a study on isolated rat lung. J Physiol 1987; 384: 311–324.
21. Goodman BE, Kim KJ, Crandall ED. Evidence for active sodium transport across alveolar epithelium of isolated rat lung. J Appl Physiol 1987; 62:2460–2466.
22. Effros RM, Mason GR, Hukkanen J, Silverman P. New evidence for active sodium transport from fluid-filled rat lungs. J Appl Physiol 1989; 66:906–919.

23. Rutschman DH, Olivera W, Sznajder JI. Active transport and passive liquid movement in isolated perfused rat lungs. J Appl Physiol 1993; 75:1574–1580.
24. Matthay MA, Berthiaume Y, Staub NC. Long-term clearance of liquid and protein from the lungs of unanesthetized sheep. J Appl Physiol 1985; 59:928–934.
25. Berthiaume Y, Broaddus VC, Gropper MA, Tanita T, Matthay MA. Alveolar liquid and protein clearance from normal dog lungs. J Appl Physiol 1988; 65:585–593.
26. Smedira N, Gates L, Hastings R, Jayr C, Sakuma T, Pittet JF, Matthay MA. Alveolar and lung liquid clearance in anesthetized rabbits. J Appl Physiol 1991; 70:1827–1835.
27. Berthiaume Y, Staub NC, Matthay MA. Beta-adrenergic agonists increase lung liquid clearance in anestherized sheep. J Clin Invest 1987; 79:335–343.
28. Jayr C, Garat C, Meignan M, Pittet JF, Zelter M, Matthay MA. Alveolar liquid and protein clearance in anesthetized ventilated rats. J Appl Physiol 1994; 76:2636–2642.
29. Vejlstrup NG, Boyd CAR, Dorrington KL. Effect of lung inflation on active and passive liquid clearance from in vivo rabbit lung. Am J Physiol 1994; 267:L482–L487.
30. Sakuma T, Pittet JF, Jayr C, Matthay MA. Alveolar liquid and protein clearance in the absence of blood flow or ventilation in sheep. J Appl Physiol 1993; 74: 176–185.
31. Suzuki S, Zuege D, Berthiaume Y. Sodium-independent modulation of NA^+-K^+-ATPase activity by β-adrenergic agonist in alveolar type II cells. Am J Physiol 1995; 268:L983–L990.
32. Garat CV, Carter EP, Matthay MA. New in situ mouse model to quantify alveolar epithelial fluid clearance. J Appl Physiol. In press.
33. Matthay MA, Wiener-Kronish JP. Intact epithelial barrier function is critical for the resolution of alveolar edema in humans. Am Rev Respir Dis 1990; 142:1250–1257.
34. Hastings RH, Grady M, Sakuma T, Matthay MA. Clearance of different-sized proteins from the alveolar space in humans and rabbits. J Appl Physiol 1992; 73:1310–1316.
35. Goodman BE, Anderson JL, Clemens JW. Evidence for regulation of sodium transport from airspace to vascular space by cAMP. Am J Physiol 1989; 257:L86–L93.
36. Berthiaume Y, Sapijaszko M, Mackenzie J, Walsh MP. Protein kinase C activation does not stimulate lung liquid clearance in anesthetized sheep. Am Rev Respir Dis 1991; 144:1085–1090.
37. Campbell AR, Folkesson HG, Osorio O, Cohen-Solal JM, Matthay MA. Alveolar fluid clearance can be accelerated in ventilated sheep with an aerosolized beta-adrenergic agonist (Salmeterol). Am J Respir Crit Care Med 1995; 151:A620.
38. Tibayan FA, Chesnutt AN, Folkesson HG, Eandi J, Matthay MA. Dobutamine increases alveolar fluid clearance in ventilated rats by beta-2 receptor stimulation. Am J Respir Crit Care Med 1997; 156:438–444. Submitted.
39. Borok Z, Hami A, Danto SI, Lubman RL, Kim K-J, Crandall ED. Effects of EGF on alveolar epithelial junctional permeability and active sodium transport. Am J Physiol 1996; 270:L559–L565.
40. Folkesson HG, Pittet J-F, Nitenberg G, Matthay MA. Transforming growth factor-α increases alveolar liquid clearance in anesthetized, ventilated rats. Am J Physiol 1996; 271:L236–L244.

41. Folkesson HG, Matthay MA. Dexamethasone upregulates alveolar epithelial liquid clearance in anesthetized ventilated rats. FASEB J 1997; 11:A561.
42. Lingueglia E, Voilley N, Lazdunski M, Barbry P. Molecular biology of the amiloride-sensitive epithelial sodium channel. Exp Physiol 1996; 81:483–492.
43. Rezaiguia S, Garat C, Delclaux C, Meignan M, Fleury J, Legrand P, Matthay MA, Jayr C. Acute bacterial pneumonia in rats increases alveolar epithelial fluid clearance by a tumor necrosis factor-alpha-dependent mechanism. J Clin Invest 1997; 99:325–335.
44. Baldwin RL, Stocowitz ML, Hood L, Wisnieski BJ. Structural changes of tumor necrosis factor-α associated with membrane insertion and channel formation. Proc Natl Acad Sci USA 1996; 93:1021–1026.
45. Adamson IYR, Bowden DH. The type 2 cell as progenitor of alveolar epithelial regeneration. Lab Invest 1974; 30:35–42.
46. Bachofen M, Weibel ER. Alterations of the gas exchange apparatus in adult respiratory insufficiency associated with septicemia. Am Rev Respir Dis 1977; 116: 589–615.
47. Nitenberg G, Folkesson HG, Osorio O, Cohen-Solal JM, Matthay MA. Alveolar epithelial liquid clearance is markedly increased 10 days following acute lung injury from bleomycin. Am J Respir Crit Care Med 1995; 151:A620.
48. Staub NC. The pathogenesis of pulmonary edema. Prog Cardio Dis 1980; 23:53–80.
49. Bachofen H, Schurch S, Michel RP, Weibel ER. Experimental hydrostatic pulmonary edema in rabbit lungs: barrier lesions. Am Rev Resp Dis 1993; 147:997–1004.
50. West JB, Tsukimoto K, Mathieu-Costello O, Prediletto R. Stress failure in pulmonary capillaries. J Appl Physiol 1991; 70:1731–1742.
51. Bhattacharya J, Gropper MA, Staub NC. Interstitial fluid pressure gradient measured by micropuncture in excised dog lung. J Appl Physiol 1984; 56:271–277.
52. Bhattacharya J, Gropper MA, Shepard JM. Lung expansion and the perialveolar interstitial pressure gradient. J Appl Physiol 1989; 66:2600–2605.
53. Broaddus VC, Wiener-Kronish JP, Staub NC. Clearance of lung edema into the pleural space of volume-loaded anesthetized sheep. J Appl Physiol 1990; 68: 2623–2630.
54. Campbell AR, Folkesson HG, Osorio O, Matthay MA. Alveolar liquid clearance persists even in the presence of moderate left atrial hypertension in anesthetized ventilated sheep. Am J Resp Crit Care Med 1996; 153:A195.
55. Planès C, Escoubet B, Amiel C, Clerici C. Hypoxia decreases expression and activity of amiloride-sensitive sodium channels in adult alveolar epithelial cells. Am J Respir Crit Care Med 1997; 153:A505.
56. Sakuma T, Osorio O, Lam M, Matthay MA. Inflation of ischemic lungs in anesthetized rabbits prevents reperfusion lung injury. Am J Resp Crit Care Med 1996; 153:A387.
57. Sakuma T, Osorio O, Matthay MA. Deflation of the lung downregulates alveolar epithelial fluid transport in isolated rat lungs. Am J Respir Crit Care Med 1997; 155:A858.
58. Martin TR, Pistorese BP, Chi EY, Goodman RB, Matthay MA. Effects of leukotriene B_4 in the human lung. Recruitment of neutrophils into the alveolar spaces without a change in protein permeability. J Clin Invest 1989; 84:1609–1619.

59. Wiener-Kronish J, Albertine KH, Matthay MA. Differential responses of the endothelial and epithelial barriers of the lung in sheep to *Escherichia coli* endotoxin. J Clin Invest 1991; 88:864–875.
60. Pittet J-F, Wiener-Kronish JP, McElroy MC, Folkesson HG, Matthay MA. Stimulation of lung epithelial liquid clearance by endogenous release of catecholamines in septic shock in anesthetized rats. J Clin Invest 1994; 94:663–671.
61. Pittet J-F, Brenner TJ, Modelska K, Matthay MA. Alveolar liquid clearance is increased by endogenous catecholamines in hemorrhagic shock in rats. J Appl Physiol 1996; 81:830–837.
62. Folkesson HG, Kheradmand F, Matthay MA. The effect of salt water on alveolar epithelial barrier function. Am J Respir Crit Care Med 1994; 150: 1555–1563.
63. Schnitzer JE, Oh P. Aquaporin-1 in plasma membrane and caveolae provides mercury-sensitive water channels across lung endothelium. Am J Physiol 1996; 270:H416–H422.
64. Cohen DS, Matthay MA, Cogan MG, Murray JF. Pulmonary edema associated with salt water near-drowning: new insights. Am Rev Respir Dis 1992; 146:794–796.
65. Crapo JD. Morphologic changes in pulmonary oxygen toxicity. Annu Rev Physiol 1986; 48:721–731.
66. Wangensteen D, Piper R, Johnson JA, Sinha AA, Niewoehner D. Solute conductance of blood-gas barrier in hamsters exposed to hyperoxia. J Appl Physiol 1986; 60:1908–1916.
67. Palazzo RM, Wangensteen OD, Niewoehner DE. Time course of functional repair of the alveolar epithelium after hyperoxic injury. J Appl Physiol 1992; 73:1881–1887.
68. Haskell JF, Yue G, Benos D, Matalon S. Upregulation of sodium conductive pathways in alveolar type II cells in sublethal hyperoxia. Am J Physiol 1994; 266: L30–L37.
69. Olivera WG, Ridge KM, Sznajder JI. Lung liquid clearance and Na,K-ATPase during acute hyperoxia and recovery in rats. Am J Respir Crit Care Med 1995; 152: 1229–1234.
70. Sznajder JI, Olivera WG, Ridge KM, Rutschman DH. Mechanisms of lung liquid clearance during hyperoxia in isolated rat lungs. Am J Respir Crit Care Med 1995; 151:1519–1525.
71. Nici L, Dowin R, Gilmore-Hebert M, Jamieson JD, Ingbar DH. Upregulation of rat lung Na-K-ATPase during hyperoxic injury. Am J Physiol 1991; 261:L307–L314.
72. Yue G, Russell WJ, Benos DJ, Jackson RM, Olman MA, Matalon S. Increased expression and activity of sodium channels in alveolar type II cells of hyperoxic rats. Proc Natl Acad Sci USA 1995; 92:8418–8422.
73. Pittet J-F, Wiener-Kronish JP, Serikov V, Matthay MA. Resistance of the alveolar epithelium to injury from septic shock in sheep. Am J Respir Crit Care Med 1995; 151:1093–1100.
74. Wiener-Kronish JP, Sakuma T, Kudoh I, Pittet JF, Frank D, Debbs L, Valil M, Matthay MA. Alveolar epithelial injury and pleural empyema in acute *P. aeruginosa* pneumonia in anesthetized rabbits. J Appl Physiol 1993; 75:1661–1669.

75. Compeau CG, Rotstein OD, Tohda H, Marunaka Y, Rafii B, Slutsky AS, O'Brodovich H. Endotoxin-stimulated alveolar macrophages impair lung epithelial Na^+ transport by an L-Arg-dependent mechanism. Am J Physiol 1994; 266:C1330–C1341.
76. Pittet J-F, Hashimoto S, Pian M, McElroy M, Nitenberg G, Wiener-Kronish JP. Exotoxin A stimulates fluid reabsorption from distal airspaces in anesthetized rats. Am J Physiol 1996; 270:L232–L241.
77. Garat C, Rezaiguia S, Meignan M, D'Ortho M-P, Harf A, Matthay MA, Jayr C. Alveolar endotoxin increases alveolar liquid clearance in rats. J Appl Physiol 1995; 79:2021–2028.
78. Folkesson HG, Matthay MA, Hébert CA, Broaddus VC. Acid aspiration induced lung injury in rabbits is mediated by interleukin-8 dependent mechanisms. J Clin Invest 1995; 96:107–116.
79. Wiener-Kronish JP, Broaddus VC, Albertine KH, Gropper MA, Matthay MA, Staub NC. The relationship of pleural effusions to increased permeability pulmonary edema in anesthetized sheep. J Clin Invest 1988; 88:1422–1429.
80. Fein A, Grossman RF, Jones JG, Overland E, Murray JF, Staub NC. The value of edema fluid protein measurements in patients with pulmonary edema. Am J Med 1979; 67:32–39.
81. Matthay MA, Eschenbacher WL, Goetzl EJ. Elevated concentrations of leukotriene D_4 in pulmonary edema fluid of patients with the adult respiratory distress syndrome. J Clin Immunol 1984; 4:479–483.
82. Clark JG, Milberg JA, Steinberg KP, Hudson LD. Type III procollagen peptide in adult respiratory distress syndrome. Association of increased peptide levels in bronchoalveolar lavage with increased risk for death. Ann Intern Med 1995; 122: 17–23.
83. Matthay MA, Nitenberg G, Jayr C. The critical role of the alveolar epithelial barrier in acute lung injury. In: Vincent JL, ed. Yearbook of Intensive Care and Emergency Medicine. New York: Springer-Verlag, 1993.
84. Garat C, Meignan M, Harf A, Matthay MA, Jayr C. Effect of exposure to 100% oxygen for 40 hours on alveolar and lung liquid clearance in rats. Am Rev Resp Dis 1993; 147:A43.
85. Lasnier J, Wangensteen OD, Schmitz LS, Gross CR, Ingbar DH. Terbutaline stimulates alveolar fluid resorption in hyperoxic lung injury. J Appl Physiol 1996; 81: 1723–1729.
86. Sakuma T, Suzuki S, Usuda K, Handa M, Okaniwa G, Nakada T, Fugimura S, Matthay MA. Preservation of alveolar epithelial fluid transport mechanisms in rewarmed human lung after severe hypothermia. J Appl Physiol 1996; 80:1681–1686.
87. Matthay MA, Folkesson HG, Verkman AS. Salt and water transport across alveolar and distal airway epithelium in the adult lung. Am J Physiol 1996; 270:L487–L503.

15

Biophysical Properties of Na^+ Channels in Alveolar Epithelial Cells

YI GUO, MICHAEL D. DuVALL, and SADIS MATALON

University of Alabama at Birmingham
Birmingham, Alabama

I. Introduction

The major function of the lung is gas exchange. The movement of both oxygen and carbon dioxide across the blood-gas barrier is by simple diffusion. This process is optimized by the large alveolar surface area (between 50 and 100 m^2 in the adult human lung), the proximity of the alveolar and pulmonary capillary membranes, and the lack of any significant amount of fluid in the alveolar space, except for a very thin layer which forms a subphase between the surfactant monolayer and the alveolar epithelium (1).

There have been many attempts to identify the cellular mechanisms responsible for the paucity of alveolar fluid in the healthy lung. The results of various in vivo and ex vivo studies indicate that fluid reabsorption across the alveolar space is at least partly due to the active transport of Na^+ ions across alveolar type II cells (2–5). The importance of active transport in fluid clearance across the injured alveolar epithelium was demonstrated by the studies of Matthay and Wiener-Kronish (6), who found a positive correlation between the ability of the human alveolar epithelium to transport Na^+ actively and the rate of resolution of noncardiogenic pulmonary edema.

More precise information as to the nature and regulation of the specific transport pathways involved has been provided from studies of Na^+ transport across freshly isolated or cultured ATII cells, the most abundant mammalian alveolar epithelial cell (1,7). ATII intracellular Na^+ is less than the equilibrium value predicted from the Nernst equation (8,9). Thus, Na^+ ions diffuse passively across the ATII apical membrane, mainly through cation channels and are then actively transported across the basolateral membrane by the ouabain-sensitive Na^+-K^+-ATPase (10,11).

The recent immunopurification and cloning of various lung Na^+ channel proteins (12–15) have created considerable excitement by providing the tools to study Na^+ transport at a fundamental level. The objectives of this article are: (1) to discuss briefly the properties of epithelial Na^+ channels; (2) to review the evidence for the existence of Na^+ channels in alveolar epithelial cells and describe their biophysical properties; and (3) to summarize the results of molecular biology and biochemical studies reporting the purification of lung Na^+ channel cDNAs and proteins. We will also briefly discuss the physiological relevance of active sodium transport across the alveolar epithelium on lung fluid balance.

II. Epithelial Na^+ Channels

Two different types of Na^+-selective ion channels have been identified: voltage-gated, and epithelial channels. The former, which are inhibited by saxitoxin, or tetrodotoxin, are present in most excitable cells, are voltage-dependent, and are essential for the generation of action potentials. The latter are found in the apical membranes of most reabsorptive epithelial tissues (16–20).

A defining characteristic of epithelial Na^+ channels is their inhibition by the potassium-sparing diuretic amiloride with high affinity (apparent equilibrium dissociation constant $[K_i] \leq 1$ μM). Amiloride is a pyrazine ring compound containing an amino group at ring positions 3 and 5, a chloride at ring position 6, and an acylguanidinium moiety attached to ring position 2 (Fig. 1). Because of this latter group, amiloride is a weak base with pK_a of 8.7 in aqueous solution. Amiloride inhibits Na^+ transport across epithelial tissues rapidly and reversibly. Derivatization of the terminal nitrogen atom of the guanidinium moiety with a benzene ring containing aryl or aralkyl groups results in compounds (such as benzamil and phenamil). On the other hand, alkyl substitution at ring position 5 results in compounds (such as [N-ethyl-N-isopropyl]-2′-amiloride; EIPA).

Sodium channels can be grouped according to their affinity for amiloride and its structural analogs. H-type channels have a high affinity for amiloride ($[K_i] < 0.5$ μM at high external Na^+ concentrations) and display the following structure/inhibitory pattern relationship: phenamil, benzamil > amiloride >>> EIPA (21). They include the so-called classic Na^+ channels present in the apical

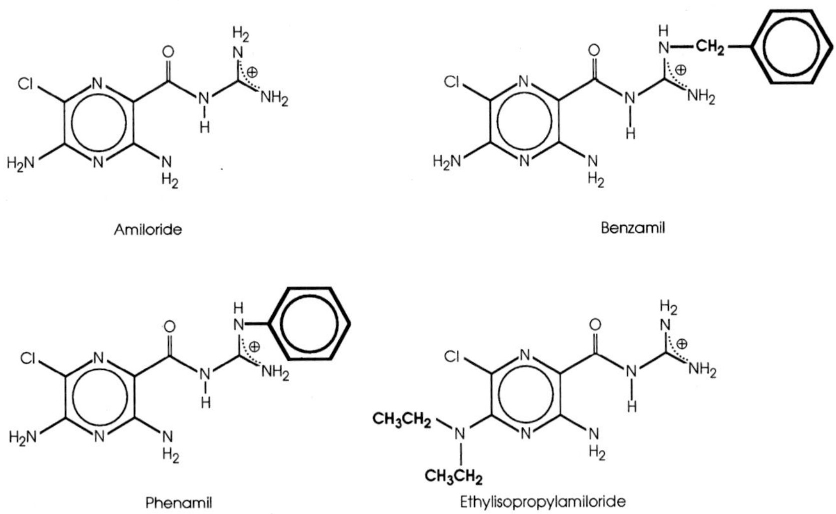

Figure 1 Chemical structures of amiloride and several of its analogs.

membranes of epithelia with high transepithelial electrical resistance, such as frog skin, toad urinary bladder, mammalian colon, bovine renal papilla, and amphibian renal A6 cells. In contrast, L-type channels have somewhat lower affinity for amiloride, with a $K_i \geq 0.5$ μM. Moreover, these channels exhibit a structure/inhibitory pattern distinct from that of H-type Na^+ channels, particularly in that EIPA can inhibit Na^+ transport across them equally, or even more effectively, than amiloride. L-type channels been found in a variety of cells and tissues including LLC-PK_1 and MDCK cells (22), the brush border membranes of rat kidney cortex (23), rabbit blastocyst trophectodermal cells (24), the basolateral membranes of the toad urinary bladder (25), and brain endothelial cells (26).

Additionally, amiloride-sensitive Na^+ channels were classified into three groups on the basis of their ion selectivity and unitary conductance (20): type $Na_{(5)}$, type $Na_{(9)}$, and type $Na_{(28)}$. The $Na_{(5)}$-type channels have low single channel conductance (4 to 5 pS), high permeability selectivity for Na^+ over K^+ ($P_{Na}/P_K > 10$) and long mean open and closed times (0.5 to 5 sec). Moreover, $Na_{(5)}$ channels are voltage-sensitive, as they are activated by hyperpolarization of the cell membrane. The $Na_{(9)}$-type channels have higher conductance values (7 to 15 pS), shorter mean open and closed times (10 to 100 msec), and moderate selectivity for Na^+ over K^+ ($P_{Na}/P_K = 3–4$). In contrast to $Na_{(5)}$, $Na_{(9)}$ channels are activated by membrane depolarization. The third category, type $Na_{(28)}$, consists of poorly selective or nonselective cation channels ($P_{Na}/P_K < 1.5$) with high conductance (> 20 pS) and are voltage-insensitive.

III. Evidence for the Existence of Na^+ Channels in Alveolar Epithelial Cells

The mammalian alveolar epithelium consists of two cell types: (1) large squamous alveolar type I cells (ATI) cover more than 97% of the alveolar surface area, but make up only 30% of the alveolar epithelial cells and 8–10% of all lung cells, and (2) cuboidal type II (ATII) cells, which in the rat make up 14% of all parenchymal cells, 67% of the alveolar epithelial cells but only 3% of the alveolar epithelial surface (1). An important function of ATII cells is the production and storage of pulmonary surfactant, a complex mixture of phospholipid and specific apoproteins (27). In addition, they serve as progenitors to the squamous ATI cells during normal lung development as well as in the reparative response of the alveolar epithelium to injury (28,29). Immunocytochemical and Western blotting studies, utilizing polyclonal antibodies to Na^+ channels and Na^+-K^+-ATPase are consistent with the presence of proteins antigenically related to Na^+ channels and Na^+-K^+-ATPase in the apical and basolateral membranes of ATII cells, respectively (30,31). In addition, Northern blotting studies showed that both adult and late gestational fetal ATII cells contain the mRNA for these transporters (15,32,33). Presently, viable ATI cells cannot be isolated in sufficient numbers to ascertain whether or not these cells are capable of vectorial Na^+ transport.

The fetal lung contains fluid at all stages of intrauterine development. This fluid is formed in the lung and flows out of the trachea. In the last few days before birth, lung fluid secretion rates decrease significantly by about 50% (34). At the same time alveolar epithelial and airway cells are converted from Cl^- secreting to Na^+ absorbing (11). The results of various studies indicate that primary cultures of alveolar epithelial cells isolated from fetal rats at late gestation (20 days; term 22 days) are Na^+-absorbing and not Cl^--secreting cells (11). Late-stage fetal epithelial cells (referred to as FDLE) show specific immunostaining when incubated with a polyclonal antibody to the Na^+ channel protein (35) and demonstrate amiloride-sensitive Na^+ transport. Patch-clamp and lipid bilayer reconstitution studies indicating the presence of various functional types of Na^+ channels in both FDLE and ATII cells are reviewed below.

A. Patch-Clamp Studies

Single-Channel Recordings

Neher and Sakmann first recorded unitary currents through single biological ion channels in cell membranes using the patch-clamp recording technique (36).

This technique relies on the formation of an electrically tight seal between a glass micropipette and a biological membrane, with a resistance around 5 to 50 GΩ (1 gigaohm = 10^9 Ω). Various configurations can be achieved (Fig. 2). In the cell-attached configuration, single-channel recordings can be obtained with the cytoplasmic machinery remaining intact; thus cytoplasmic second messengers (such as cAMP) may be generated in response to the addition of

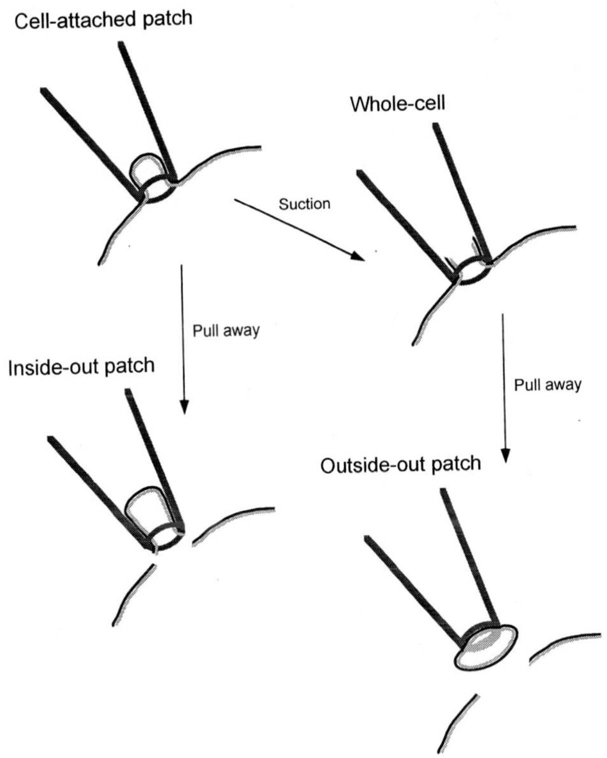

Figure 2 Standard patch-clamp configuration. A specially fabricated glass micropipette is pressed against the cell membrane until a high-resistance seal (> 10^9 GΩ) is formed (cell-attached patch). The patch is then withdrawn, carrying with it a small piece of the membrane (inside-out patch). In this instance the cytoplasmic side of the cell membrane faces the bath solution. Alternatively, while in the cell-attached mode, suction or a high-voltage pulse may be applied, rupturing the cell membrane and allowing for a direct communication between the contents of the pipette and the cell interior (whole-cell patch). Pulling the pipette away from the cell, once a whole-cell patch has been achieved, results in the outside-out patch configuration. In this instance the cell membrane reforms across the pipette tip and the outside of the membrane faces the bath while the inside is in contact with the contents of the pipette.

effectors (i.e., β-agonists) into the bath. In the excised-patch configuration (inside-out or outside-out; see Fig. 2), obtained by withdrawing the pipette tip after the formation of a giga seal, one side of a small patch of the cell membrane is in contact with the bath solution, an ideal configuration for the study of pharmacological agents on ion channel kinetics.

The first evidence for the existence of ion channels in alveolar epithelial cells was provided by Orser et al. (37) (Table 1). These authors harvested distal epithelial cells (FDLE) from the lungs of rats delivered by cesarean section at 20 days' gestation and cultured them on collagen-coated coverslips for 24 to 96 hours. In the presence of symmetrical solutions (140 mM NaCl), inside-out excised patches in the presence of high (Ca^{+2}) (>100 μM) revealed the presence of single channels with conductance of 23 pS, which were equally permeable to Na^+ and K^+ (P_{Na}/P_K = 0.9), but essentially impermeable to Cl^-. When amiloride was present in the pipette solution, the open probability (P_o) of these channels decreased, while their unitary conductance remains unchanged.

A peculiar characteristic of these cation channels was the dependence of their activity on intracellular Ca^{+2}. An increase in intracellular Ca^{+2} from 0.1 μM to 1 mM increased the P_o from almost zero to about 0.4. In contrast, increased Ca^{+2} in A6 cell has been shown to downregulate Na^+ channel activity (38). That these channels were open only at very high intracellular Ca^{+2} concentrations, unlikely to be achieved in vivo, raised questions about their physiological significance. However, Marunaka et al. (39) and Tohda et al. (40) showed that exposure of FDLE cells to terbutaline increased intracellular Ca^{+2} from 35 nM to 3.5 μM, reduced intracellular Cl^- from 45 to 25 mM, and activated these cation channels by increasing their sensitivity to cytosolic Ca^{+2} by 100 to 1000-fold. These observations suggest that these nonselective cation channels may play a role in the increased reabsorption of fluid by alveolar epithelial cells in response to β-agonist stimulation. Ca^{+2}-activated, amiloride-inhibitable cation channels have been identified in adult ATII cells, cultured on collagen-coated coverslips for 24 and 72 hours (41).

Tohda and Marunaka (42) also identified a Na^+-selective, Ca^{+2}-activated channel in the apical membranes of the FLDE cells. This channel had a conductance of 12 pS, was highly selective for Na^+ over K^+ ([P_{Na}/P_K] > 10), and practically nonpermeable to anions ([P_{Na}/P_{Cl}] ≥ 40). Additionally, this channel was blocked by amiloride with an with K_i of 1 to 2 μM, and has a mean P_o which was 10 times higher than the nonselective, Ca^{+2}-activated cation channel at resting membrane potentials. These findings are in agreement with benzamil equilibrium binding studies in membrane vesicles of FLDE cells, indicating the presence of both high- and low-affinity binding sites (35). Single channels exhibiting linear current-voltage relationships and unitary conductances of 4.4 pS and (P_{Na}/P_K > 10) were recorded in outside-out patches of FDLE cells cultured for periods of 24 hours to 8 days (15). Benzamil, phenamil, amiloride, and EIPA

Table 1 Single-Channel Characteristics of Alveolar Epithelial Cation Channels; Mean Values Only

Cell type	Species (# d in cult.)	Type of patch	g (pS)	P_{Na}/P_K	P_{Na}/P_{Cl}	IC_{50} (μM) for P_o		Ca^{2+}	Ref.
						Amil.	EIPA		
FDLE	rat (1–4)	I/O	23 (linear)	0.9–1.1	> 20	< 1	N.D.	> 100 μM	37
FDLE	rat (2–3)	I/O; C.A.	27 (linear)	1.1	> 50	< 1	N.D.	1 mM	42
FDLE	rat (2–3)	I/O; C.A.	12 (inw. rect.)	> 10	40	1–2	N.D.	1 mM	42
FDLE	rat (1–8)	O/O	4 (linear)	> 10	> 20	0.09	100	10 nM	15
FDLE	g. pig (0–0.5)	I/O	11 (linear)	1.8	N.D.	0.4–4	N.D.	100 nM	43
ATII	rat (1–3)	I/O	20 (linear)	1.1	2.0	1	N.D.	> 10 μM	41
ATII	rat (0–1)	I/O; C.A.	27 (linear)	7	8	< 1	< 1	< 10 nM	45

FDLE = fetal distal lung epithelial cells; ATII = adult alveolar type II cells; g = conductance (determined under symmetrical Na^+ (> 100 μM) solutions; Ca^{+2} = minimum intracellular calcium concentration, needed to activate the channels; I/O = inside-out; C.A. = cell attached; O/O = outside out; P_o = open probability; IC_{50} = concentration needed to inhibit variable to 50% of control value; N.D. = not determined.

inhibited the currents with K_i values of 14 nM, 19 nM, 90 nM, and 400 nM, respectively, suggesting that they are H-type Na^+ channels.

A nonselective cation channel was reported in alveolar epithelial cells by MacGregor et al. (43), who isolated FDLE cells from the lungs of fetal guinea pigs 5 days before the end of gestation and measured Na^+ conductance in excised inside-out patches. About 20% of all patches showed single-channel activity with a linear current-voltage relationship, a unitary conductance of 11 pS in symmetrical Na^+ solutions, and a P_{Na}/P_K of 1.8. This channel was blocked completely by the inclusion of 10 μM amiloride in the pipette solution. At lower concentrations (0.4 to 4 μM), amiloride reduced channel density and caused the channels to flicker. Additionally, 0.1 mM guanosine 5′-O-(3-thiotriphosphate) added to the cytoplasmic site of inside-out patches caused activation of single-channel activity in previously quiescent patches and increased channel density in active patches, indicating that this channel is regulated by G proteins. A subunit of the H-type Na^+ channel protein, isolated from A6 cells, also was identified as the α-subunit of the GTP-binding protein $G_{\alpha i3}$ (44); treatment of A6 monolayers, which are known to contain H-type Na^+ channels, with pertussis toxin (PTX), an inhibitor of the G protein, decreased transepithelial Na^+ transport (44).

There is also evidence for the existence of Na^+-selective, Ca^{2+}-independent channels in apical membranes of adult ATII cells (15,45). Yue et al. (45) patched ATII cells, isolated from the lungs of adult rats and kept in primary culture for periods of 12 to 24 hours, in either the cell-attached or inside-out modes. When patched in the cell-attached mode using symmetrical Na^+ solutions (150 mM Na^+), single-channel currents were observed at holding potentials between −80 and 30 mV with a unitary conductance of 27 pS, and a P_o of 0.36. Single-channel currents with a conductance of 25 pS and a P_{Na}/P_K = 7 also were recorded across inside-out excised patches of ATII cells. Inclusion of amiloride or EIPA (1 μM each) in the pipette solution blocked single channel activity almost completely. Taken together, these findings indicate that the apical membranes of adult ATII cells contain Na^+-selective, L-type, and Ca^{+2}-activated cation channels. FDLE cells, on the other hand, contain L-type, Ca^{+2}-activated cation channels and H-type Na^+ channels with different cationic selectivity.

Whole-Cell Currents

Only about 10% of the cell-attached or inside-out patches in ATII cells showed single-channel activity. Furthermore, the contributions of various types of channels with different conductances and densities to overall Na^+ transport are difficult to ascertain. Additional information can be obtained from measurements of current-voltage relationships from ATII cells patch-clamped in the whole-cell configuration. After the formation of a high-resistance, cell-attached seal, application of suction or a voltage pulse ruptures the membrane within the pipette, creating a direct communication between the pipette solution and the cytoplasmic contents of the cell. Under these conditions, the potential across the entire plasma membrane can be set to a given value and all channels in the membrane studied simultaneously.

Several laboratories have reported successful whole-cell recordings in ATII cells. When patched using symmetrical Na^+ solutions, both freshly isolated and cultured rabbit or rat ATII cells exhibited outwardly rectified Na^+ currents (31,46). Addition of 10 mM tetraethyl ammonium (TEA) in the bath solutions did not alter the values of these currents, indicating that the movement of Na^+ ions did not occur through TEA-sensitive K^+ channels, known to exist in cultured ATII cells (47,48). At 0 and 24 hours in culture, $> 60\%$ of the outward currents were reversibly inhibited by amiloride, benzamil, or EIPA with a $K_i \leq 1$ μM (Fig. 3). When patched using bionic solutions (150 mM K^+ in the pipette; 150 mM Na^+ in the bath), amiloride or EIPA (1 μM) reversibly inhibited the inward Na^+, but not the outward K^+ currents; conversely, in this experiment TEA (10 mM) decreased the K^+ but not the Na^+ currents.

A potential limitation of the whole-cell technique is that dilution of the cytoplasmic contents by the pipette solution may cause the concentration of critical cellular factors to fall below a given threshold, thereby modifying the characteristics of ion channels. This limitation is circumvented by the addition

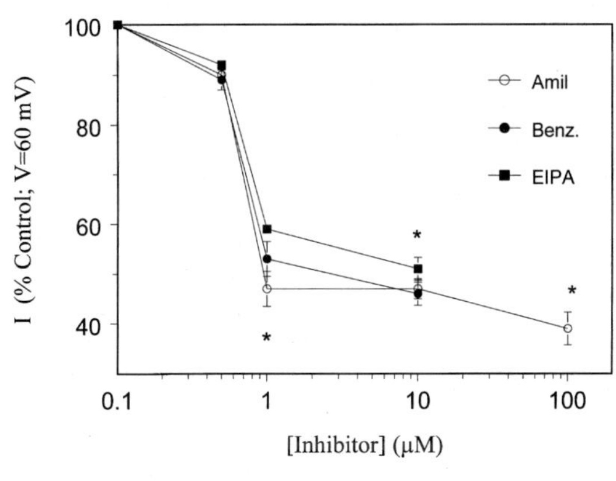

Figure 3 Effects of amiloride, benzamil, and EIPA, added to the bath solution, on whole-cell outward currents of ATII cells cultured for 24 hours and patched using symmetrical solutions (150 mM Na^+-glutamate). Currents were obtained at a membrane potential of 60 mV and expressed as percent from their corresponding control values. All inhibitors were equally effective in reducing the outward currents. Values are means ± SEM for five different cells; $*P < .05$. (Modified from Ref. 46.)

of pore-forming antibiotics, such as nystatin or amphotericin B, in the pipette solution. These ionophores allow the movement of small monovalent ions through the membrane patch, while restricting the movement of larger solutes (perforated patch). Using this technique, Wang et al. (49) showed that Na^+ currents through the Ca^{+2}-activated, nonselective cation channels in FDLE cells were decreased by addition of amiloride, benzamil, and EIPA (20 μM) in the bath solution. Half-maximum whole-cell current inhibition occurred 3 to 4 min following addition of these substances into the bath solution, similar to values obtained in whole-cell currents across adult ATII (31,46) and trophectodermal cells (a nonepithelial cell line containing L-type Na^+ channels [24]). In contrast, Bubien et al. (50) reported considerably faster inhibition of inward Na^+ currents in B-lymphocytes, which are known to contain H-type channels. The reason for this discrepancy is not clear at the present time.

Taken together, the results of these studies indicate that the apical membranes of adult ATII cells contain both Na^+-selective, low-amiloride affinity Na^+

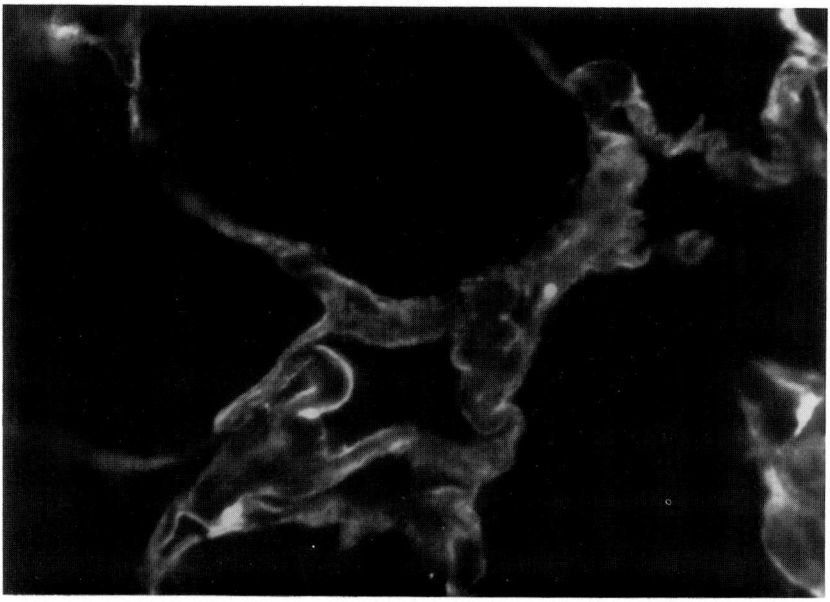

Figure 4 Thin frozen section (5 μM) of normal rat lungs incubated with 1 : 100 dilution of a polyclonal antibody to Na^+ channel protein (NaAb) and the secondary antibody, goat-antirabbit-IgG-conjugated to rhodamine. Intense fluorescence staining is observed on the apical membranes of cells located in the alveolar corners, presumably ATII pneumocytes. When rabbit IgG was substituted for NaAb, only background levels of fluorescence were seen (data not shown). (Modified from Ref. 52.)

channels (L-type) and Ca^{+2}-activated cation channels. FDLE cells, on the other hand, contain L-type, Ca^{+2}-activated cation channels and H-type Na^+ channels with different cationic selectivities.

B. Immunocytochemical Localization of Proteins Antigenically Related to Na^+ Channels

Using antibodies raised against a Na^+ channel protein from A6 cells and bovine kidney papilla (51) and indirect immunofluorescent techniques, several studies demonstrated the presence of proteins antigenically related to Na^+ channels in FDLE and ATII cells both in vivo and in vitro (31,35,46,52). In frozen lung sections, staining was most intense in the apical sides of cuboidal epithelial cells located in the alveolar corners (Fig. 4). Colocalization studies in which freshly isolated ATII cells were colabeled with this antibody and the apical surface marker *Maclura Pomifera Agglutinin* as well as confocal microscopy studies (Fig. 5), showed that antigenic sites were present at the apical surface regions

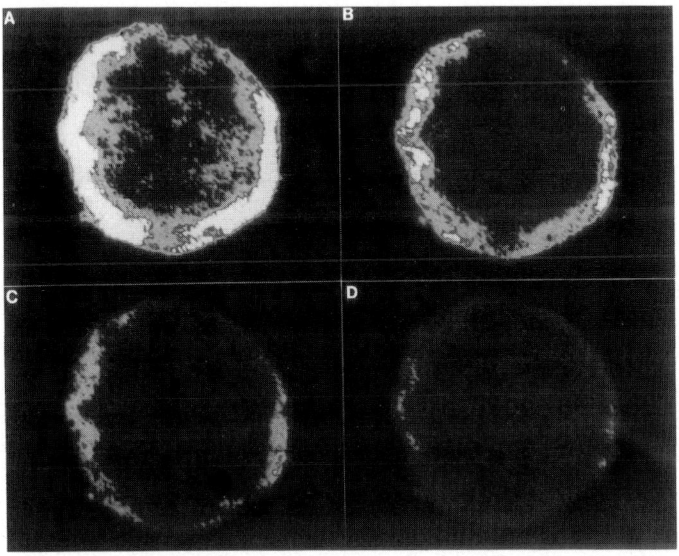

Figure 5 Typical confocal microscopy image of a freshly isolated rat ATII cell incubated with the NaAb followed by goat-antirabbit IgG conjugated to FITC as described in the text. Optical section, 0.4 μm apart, starting with the very top of the cell (A). Fluorescent intensity has been false colored to the following scale: white > red > yellow > blue > black. The apical membrane is viewed *en face*. Notice the lack of fluorescence in the cell interior. (Modified from Ref. 31.)

of ATII cells. In Western blots, the antibodies specifically recognized a 135- to 150-kDa protein of ATII and FDLE membrane vesicles, under both reducing and nonreducing conditions; no specific binding was observed in membrane vesicles of alveolar macrophages, in agreement with patch-clamp data demonstrating the absence of amiloride-sensitive Na^+ currents across alveolar macrophages (31). Antigenic activity for Na^+-K^+-ATPase has been identified in the basolateral membranes of ATII cells (30,53). These findings are consistent with in the results of in vivo and in vitro studies indicating the ability of ATII cells to transport Na^+ in a vectorial fashion.

IV. Purification, Characterization, and Reconstitution of Na^+ Channel Proteins in Lipid Bilayers

Additional proof for the existence of Na^+ channels in ATII cells was obtained by purifying to homogeneity a putative Na^+ channel protein from freshly isolated rabbit ATII cells, using ion-exchange chromatography, followed by immunoaffinity purification over a column to which rabbit polyclonal antibodies raised against purified bovine renal Na^+ channel protein were bound (12). The purified protein consists of two peptides with molecular masses of ~ 130 and 70 kDa under denatured/reduced or nonreduced conditions. In contrast, an H-type Na^+ channel protein purified from A6 cells and bovine kidney papilla has a molecular mass of about 730 kDa under nonreduced conditions and is composed of at least six major polypeptides with average molecular mass values of 315, 150, 95, 71, 55, and 40 kDa, which are covalently attached through disulfide bridges (51). Studies utilizing a photoreactive amiloride analog (2′-methoxy-5′-nitrobenzamil; NMBA) and antiamiloride antibodies, as well as monoclonal anti-idiotypic antibodies (RA 6.3) directed against antiamiloride antibodies, identified the 130-kDa polypeptide as an amiloride-binding protein in both H- and L-type channels (54).

When the ATII cell Na^+ channel protein was reconstituted in lipid bilayers, single-channel Na^+ currents with a linear conductance of 25 pS, and a P_{Na}/P_K of 7:1 were observed (12). The addition of amiloride or EIPA to the extracellular (*trans*) side of the bilayer resulted in a flickering type of block and reduced both the P_o the mean current through the channels, without altering the single-channel conductance; the K_i values for amiloride and EIPA were 8 and 1 μM, respectively (Fig. 6). In contrast, reconstitution of the H-type Na^+ channel protein isolated from kidney papilla or A6 cells into the same type of lipid bilayers resulted in channels with unitary conductances of 56 and 8.5 pS, fully blocked by 0.1 μM amiloride but insensitive to EIPA (55). Addition of the catalytic subunit of protein kinase A (PKA) plus ATP to the presumed cytoplasmic (*cis*) side of the bilayer resulted in a significant increase in the single

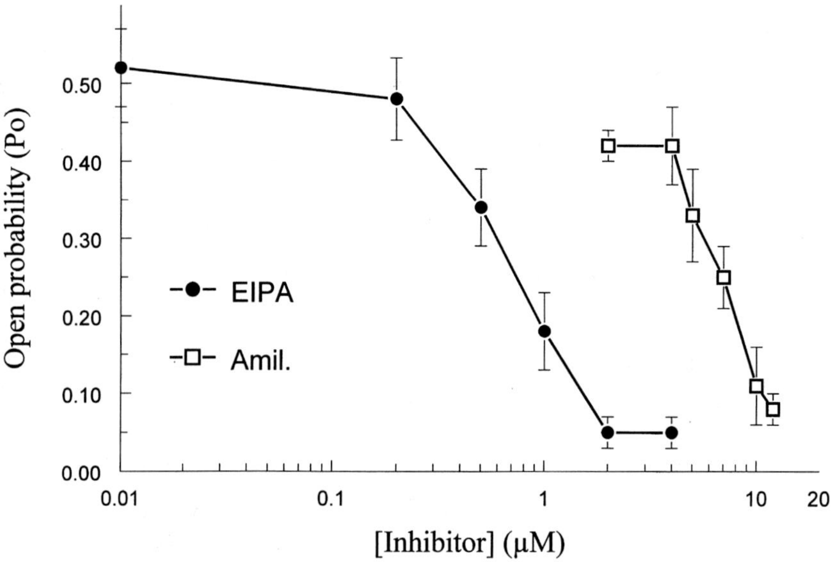

Figure 6 Amiloride or EIPA inhibition of mean current of immunopurified rabbit ATII cell Na^+ channels in planar bilayers. Each point represents means ± SEM for five experiments. (Modified from Ref. 12.)

channel P_O, from 0.4 to 0.8 in a voltage-independent fashion, without altering the single-channel conductance. Recent data indicate that PKA-induced phosphorylation caused a shift to the right in the concentration-response curves for amiloride and EIPA. The apparent K_i for amiloride increased from 8 μM under control conditions to 15 μM after PKA-induced phosphorylation, whereas that for EIPA increased from 1 μM to 2 μM (56). These findings are in excellent agreement with patch-clamp studies in freshly isolated cells, indicating that most likely this protein is an L-type channel (31,45,46). Furthermore, they indicate that the biophysical properties of the ATII cell Na^+ channels are regulated by their phosphorylation state.

An amiloride-binding protein, which presumably represents an amiloride-sensitive Na^+ channel, has been identified from the pig kidney cortex by Barby et al. (23). SDS/PAGE of the purified phenamil-binding protein under nonreducing conditions revealed a single polypeptide of molecular mass 180 kDa, whereas reducing conditions suggests that it is a dimer composed of two identical subunits, each with a molecular mass of 90 to 105 kDa. $^{22}Na^+$ uptake into membrane vesicles derived from pig kidney cortex demonstrate that both amiloride and EIPA inhibited $^{23}Na^+$ uptake with a K_i of 6 to 10 μM (57). Finally, a recent study showed that the absorption of isotonic fluid across the rat alveolar epithelium in vivo is inhibited to the same extent by amiloride and EIPA, suggesting the presence of L-type channels in the alveolar epithelium in vivo (58). Thus, there is considerable biochemical, biophysical, and physiological evidence for the existence of multiple types of Na^+ channel proteins in alveolar epithelial cells.

V. Molecular Cloning of Putative Na^+ Channel Components

A complementary DNA (cDNA) encoding an amiloride-sensitive Na^+ channel was cloned from the colon of salt-deprived rats using functional RNA expression (13,14). This clone, termed αrENaC (for the α subunit of the rat epithelial Na^+ channel) contains a 2094-nt open reading frame corresponding to 698 amino acids with a predicted molecular mass of 79 kDa and shares significant homology with *mec-4* and *deg-1*, members of a family of *Caenorhabditis elegans* genes involved in sensory touch expression. When expressed in *Xenopus* oocytes, αrENaC displayed the characteristics of the H-type, $Na_{(5)}$ Na^+ channels—i.e., much higher affinity to amiloride (K_i = 0.1 μM) than EIPA (K_i = 10 μM), no significant K^+ conductance, and high permeability to Li^+ ions (P_{Li}/P_{Na} = 1.6).

Subsequently Canessa et al. (14) identified and cloned two additional subunits of this channel, named βrENaC and γrENaC, with molecular masses of 72 kDa and 75 kDa, respectively. Coexpression of all three subunits in oocytes generated 100-fold higher amiloride-sensitive currents than αrENaC alone (14). Each subunit has two putative transmembrane domains, yielding a protein with a large (~ 50 kDa) hydrophilic loop and short hydrophilic NH_2 and COOH termini. A recent study suggests that αrENaC spans the membrane twice with the short terminal ends on the cytoplasmic side and a large hydrophilic loop in the extracellular space (59). Sequence analysis revealed that the extracellular loop contains several consensus sequences for N-linked glycosylation, consistent with the functional location of the channel at the plasma membrane.

It was proposed that αrENaC encodes one of the subunits of the H-type epithelial Na^+ channel protein identified by Benos et al. (51), perhaps the 150-kDa amiloride binding subunit, which is present in both H- and L-type channels. The αrENaC message was identified only in organs known to contain Na^+ channels, such as kidney medulla and cortex, and distal colon. O'Brodovich et al. (32) demonstrated that αrENaC mRNA was present in fetal lung tissue, FDLE cells in late-gestation, and adult ATII cells. Furthermore, αrENaC mRNA levels in FDLE cells increased markedly just before birth, in agreement with previous findings that the fetal epithelium becomes Na^+ absorbing shortly before birth. Administration of agents known to accelerate fetal lung development (such as thyroid-releasing hormone and dexamethasone) to pregnant rats early in gestation also increased αrENaC mRNA expression in fetal lungs (32). In a recent report, Hummler et al. (60) showed that neonatal mice, in which αrENaC gene was inactivated, were unable to clear the fetal lung fluid and died within 40 hours of birth with severe respiratory distress. These observations suggest that αrENaC is a vital component of the epithelial Na^+ channels in the fetal lung. Expression of αrENaC mRNA in adult rat ATII cells was also demonstrated by Yue et al. (33), who further showed that its expression increases following exposure of rats to hyperoxia, which is known to damage the alveolar epithelium and increase its permeability to solute (58).

Other subunits of the epithelial Na^+ channel, analogous to αrENaC, have been cloned from both human and bovine cDNA libraries. Voilley et al. (15) used a fragment of the rat colon Na^+ channel cDNA to screen a human lung cDNA library. One of the hybridizing clones contained a 2007-bp open reading frame, encoding a 699-amino acid protein with a mass of 76 kDa. When injected into oocytes, the cloned channel also exhibited the characteristics of a H-type channel, in close agreement to those observed in FDLE cells patched in the inside-out mode. Northern blot analysis with the mRNA of this channel, identified the presence of a 3.8-kb transcript, similar in size to the αrENaC transcript, in both human and rat lung tissue. Furthermore, as in the studies of O'Brodovich et al. (32), expression of the mRNA increased significantly shortly before birth. The sequence shares 81% identity with αrENaC if methionine-27 of the rat colon sequence is aligned with the first methionine of the human sequence. However, because this Na^+ channel subunit was cloned from a whole-lung cDNA library, its relationship to the native alveolar epithelial amiloride-sensitive Na^+ channel has yet to be determined.

Careful analysis of the physiological, biochemical, biophysical, and molecular biological studies reviewed so far point out an apparent important discrepancy: adult ATII cells seem to contain mRNA similar to that for the H-type channels; however, both whole-cell and single-channel currents across these cells are EIPA-inhibitable, indicating the functional expression of L-type and not H-type channels. There are several possible explanations for these findings. First, Western blotting and photoaffinity studies indicate that both the H- and L-type channels contain a 135 kDa peptide that acts as the amiloride-binding site. Thus, since αrENaC may be coding for the amiloride binding site of the Na^+ channel, it may recognize mRNA from either channel protein.

VI. Summary and Conclusions

Information presented herein indicates that ATII cells contain Na^+ channels. Biochemical and patch clamp studies indicate that these channels are equally sensitive to amiloride and EIPA, in sharp contrast to the traditional Na^+ channels, which are EIPA-insensitive. Immunopurification of a putative protein and its reconstitution in lipid bilayers reconfirmed these findings.

The physiological importance of active Na^+ transport is clearly elucidated by work of different laboratories (see Chaps. 14, 16, 17, and 20). For example, exposure of animals to sublethal hyperoxia results in upregulation of both Na^+ channel and Na^+-K^+-ATPase mRNA and activities in ATII cells (10,30,33,61–63). These observations suggest that active Na^+ transport may play an important role in minimizing alveolar edema under conditions in which alveolar epithelial permeability to solute has been increased.

Acknowledgments

This project was supported by NIH grants HL31197 and HL51173, and a grant from the Office of Naval Research (N00014-97-1-0309). Dr. Guo was partially supported by T32 HL07553; Dr. DuVall is a Parker B. Francis Fellow.

References

1. Haies DM, Gil M, Weibel ER. Morphometric study of rat lung cells. Am Rev Respir Dis 1981; 123:533–541.
2. Basset G, Crone C, Saumon G. Fluid absorption by rat lung in situ: pathways for sodium entry in the luminal membrane of alveolar epithelium. J Physiol (Lond) 1987; 384:325–345.
3. Basset G, Crone C, Saumon G. Significance of active ion transport in transalveolar water absorption: a study on isolated rat lung. J Physiol (Lond) 1987; 384: 311–324.
4. Matthay MA, Landolt CC, Staub NC. Differential liquid and protein clearance from the alveoli of anesthetized sheep. J Appl Physiol 1982; 53:96–104.
5. Matthay MA, Folkesson HG, Verkman AS. Salt and water transport across alveolar and distal airway epithelial in the adult lung. Am J Physiol Lung Cell Mol Physiol 1996; 270:L487–L503.
6. Matthay MA, Wiener-Kronish JP. Intact epithelial barrier function is critical for the resolution of alveolar edema in humans. Am Rev Respir Dis 1990; 142:1250–1257.
7. Dobbs LG. Isolation and culture of alveolar type II cells. Am J Physiol 1990; 258: L134–L147.
8. Gallo RL, Finkelstein JN, Notter RH. Characterization of the plasma and mitochondrial membrane potentials of alveolar type II cells by the use of ionic probes. Biochim Biophys Acta 1984; 771:217–227.
9. Jones GS, Miles PR, Lantz RC, Hinton DE, Castranova V. Ionic content and regulation of cellular volume in rat alveolar type II cells. J Appl Physiol 1982; 53: 258–266.

10. Matalon S, Benos DJ, Jackson RM. Biophysical and molecular properties of amiloride-inhibitable Na^+ channels in alveolar epithelial cells. Am J Physiol 1996; 271:L1–L22.
11. O'Brodovich H. Epithelial ion transport in the fetal and perinatal lung. Am J Physiol 1991; 261:C555–C564.
12. Senyk O, Ismailov I, Bradford AL, Baker RR, Matalon S, Benos DJ. Reconstitution of immunopurified alveolar type II cell Na^+ channel protein into planar lipid bilayers. Am J Physiol 1995; 268:C1148–C1156.
13. Canessa CM, Horisberger JD, Rossier BC. Epithelial sodium channel related to proteins involved in neurodegeneration. Nature 1993; 361:467–470.
14. Canessa CM, Schild L, Buell G, Thorens B, Gautschi I, Horisberger JD, Rossier BC. Amiloride-sensitive epithelial Na^+ channel is made of three homologous subunits. Nature 1994; 367:463–467.
15. Voilley N, Lingueglia E, Champigny G, Mattel MG, Waldmann R, Lazdunski M, Barbry P. The lung amiloride-sensitive Na^+ channel: biophysical properties, pharmacology, ontogenesis, and molecular cloning. Proc Natl Acad Sci USA 1994; 91: 247–251.
16. Benos DJ, Saccomani G, Brenner BM, Sariban-Sohraby S. Purification and characterization of the amiloride-sensitive sodium channel from A6 cultured cells and bovine renal papilla. Proc Natl Acad Sci USA 1986; 83:8525–8529.
17. Benos DJ, Hyde BA, Latorre R. Sodium flux ratio through the amiloride-sensitive entry pathway in frog skin. J Gen Physiol 1983; 81:667–685.
18. Bridges RJ, Garty H, Benos DJ, Rummel W. Na^+ uptake into colonic enterocyte membrane vesicles. Am J Physiol 1988; 254:C484–C490.
19. Kleyman TR, Smith PR, Benos DJ. Characterization and localization of epithelial Na^+ channels in toad urinary bladder. Am J Physiol 1994; 266:C1105–C1111.
20. Palmer LG. Epithelial Na channels: function and diversity. Annu Rev Physiol 1992; 54:51–66.
21. Smith PR, Benos DJ. Epithelial Na^+ channels. Annu Rev Physiol 1991; 53: 509–530.
22. Moran A, Asher C, Cragoe EJ Jr, Garty H. Conductive sodium pathway with low affinity to amiloride in LLC-PK1 cells and other epithelia. J Biol Chem 1988; 263: 19586–19591.
23. Barbry P, Chassande O, Vigne P, Frelin C, Ellory C, Cragoe EJ Jr, Lazdunski M. Purification and subunit structure of the [^{3}H]phenamil receptor associated with the renal apical Na^+ channel. Proc Natl Acad Sci USA 1987; 84:4836–4840.
24. Robinson DH, Bubien JK, Smith PR, Benos DJ. Epithelial sodium conductance in rabbit preimplantation trophectodermal cells. Dev Biol 1991; 147:313–321.
25. Garty H, Warncke J, Lindemann B. An amiloride-sensitive Na^+ conductance in the basolateral membrane of toad urinary bladder. J Membr Biol 1987; 95:91–103.
26. Vigne P, Champigny G, Marsault R, Barbry P, Frelin C, Lazdunski M. A new type of amiloride-sensitive cationic channel in endothelial cells of brain microvessels. J Biol Chem 1989; 264:7663–7668.
27. Wright JR, Dobbs LG. Regulation of pulmonary surfactant secretion and clearance. Annu Rev Physiol 1991; 53:395–414.

28. Hackney JD, Spier CE, Anzar UT, Clark KW, Evans MJ. Effect of high concentrations of oxygen on reparative regeneration of damaged alveolar epithelium in mice. Exp Mol Pathol 1981; 34:338–344.
29. Evans MJ, Cabral LJ, Stephens RJ, Freeman G. Transformation of alveolar type 2 cells to type 1 cells following exposure to NO_2. Exp Mol Pathol 1975; 22: 142–150.
30. Nici L, Dowin R, Gilmore-Hebert M, Jamieson JD, Ingbar DH. Upregulation of rat lung Na-K-ATPase during hyperoxic injury. Am J Physiol 1991; 261:L307–L314.
31. Matalon S, Kirk KL, Bubien JK, Oh Y, Hu P, Yue G, Shoemaker R, Crogoe EJ Jr, Benos DJ. Immunocytochemical and functional characterization of Na^+ conductance in adult alveolar pneumocytes. Am J Physiol 1992; 262:C1228–C1238.
32. O'Brodovich H, Canessa C, Ueda J, Rafii B, Rossier BC, Edelson J. Expression of the epithelial Na^+ channel in the developing rat lung. Am J Physiol 1993; 265: C491–C496.
33. Yue G, Russell WJ, Benos DJ, Jackson RM, Olman MA, Matalon S. Increased expression and activity of sodium channels in alveolar type II cells of hyperoxic rats. Proc Natl Acad Sci USA 1995; 92:8418–8422.
34. Barker PM, Markiewicz M, Parker KA, Walters DV, Strang LB. Synergistic action of triiodothyronine and hydrocortisone on epinephrine-induced reabsorption of fetal lung liquid. Pediatr Res 1990; 27:588–591.
35. Matalon S, Bauer ML, Benos DJ, Kleyman TR, Lin C, Cragoe EJ Jr, O'Brodovich H. Fetal lung epithelial cells contain two populations of amiloride-sensitive Na^+ channels. Am J Physiol 1993; 264:L357–L364.
36. Neher E, Sakmann B. Single-channel currents recorded from membrane of denervated frog muscle fibres. Nature 1976; 260:799–802.
37. Orser BA, Bertlik M, Fedorko L, O'Brodovich H. Cation selective channel in fetal alveolar type II epithelium. Biochim Biophys Acta 1991; 1094:19–26.
38. Silver RB, Frindt G, Windhager EE, Palmer LG. Feedback regulation of Na channels in rat CCT. I. Effects of inhibition of Na pump. Am J Physiol 1993; 264: F557–F564.
39. Marunaka Y, Tohda H, Hagiwara N, O'Brodovich H. Cytosolic $Ca(^{2+})$-induced modulation of ion selectivity and amiloride sensitivity of a cation channel and beta agonist action in fetal lung epithelium. Biochem Biophys Res Commun 1992; 187: 648–656.
40. Tohda H, Foskett JK, O'Brodovich H, Marunaka Y. Cl^- regulation of a $Ca(^{2+})$-activated nonselective cation channel in beta-agonist-treated fetal distal lung epithelium. Am J Physiol 1994; 266:C104–C109.
41. Feng ZP, Clark RB, Berthiaume Y. Identification of nonselective cation channels in cultured adult rat alveolar type II cells. Am J Respir Cell Mol Biol 1993; 9:248–254.
42. Tohda H, Marunaka Y. Insulin-activated amiloride-blockable nonselective cation and Na^+ channels in the fetal distal lung epithelium. Gen Pharmacol 1995; 26: 755–763.
43. MacGregor GG, Olver RE, Kemp PJ. Amiloride-sensitive Na^+ channels in fetal type II pneumocytes are regulated by G proteins. Am J Physiol 1994; 267:L1–L8.

44. Ausiello DA, Stow JL, Cantiello HF, de Almeida JB, Benos DJ. Purified epithelial Na^+ channel complex contains the pertussis toxin-sensitive G alpha i-3 protein. J Biol Chem 1992; 267:4759–4765.
45. Yue G, Shoemaker RL, Matalon S. Regulation of low-amiloride-affinity sodium channels in alveolar type II cells. Am J Physiol 1994; 267:L94–L100.
46. Yue G, Hu P, Oh Y, Jilling T, Shoemaker RL, Benos DJ, Cragoe EJ Jr, Matalon S. Culture-induced alterations in alveolar type II cell Na^+ conductance. Am J Physiol 1993; 265:C630–C640.
47. DeCoursey TE. State-dependent inactivation of K^+ currents in rat type II alveolar epithelial cells. J Gen Physiol 1990; 95:617–646.
48. DeCoursey TE, Jacobs ER, Silver MR. Potassium currents in rat type II alveolar epithelial cells. J Physiol (Lond) 1988; 395:487–505.
49. Wang X, Kleyman TR, Tohda H, Marunaka Y, O'Brodovich H. 5-(N-Ethyl-N-isopropyl)amiloride sensitive Na^+ currents in intact fetal distal lung epithelial cells. Can J Physiol Pharmacol 1993; 71:58–62.
50. Bubien JK, Warnock DG. Amiloride-sensitive sodium conductance in human B lymphoid cells. Am J Physiol 1993; 265:C1175–C1183.
51. Benos DJ, Saccomani G, Sariban-Sohraby S. The epithelial sodium channel. Subunit number and location of the amiloride binding site. J Biol Chem 1987; 262: 10613–10618.
52. Matalon S, Yue G, Hu P, Oh Y, Benos DJ. Mechanisms of active Na^+ transport across freshly isolated and cultured adult alveolar type II pneumocytes. In: Effros RM, Chang HK, eds. Fluid and Solute Transport in the Airspaces of the Lungs. New York: Marcel Dekker, 1994:179–217.
53. Schneeberger EE, McCarthy KM. Cytochemical localization of Na^+-K^+-ATPase in rat type II pneumocytes. J Appl Physiol 1986; 60:1584–1589.
54. Oh Y, Matalon S, Kleyman TR, Benos DJ. Biochemical evidence for the presence of an amiloride binding protein in adult alveolar type II pneumocytes. (Published erratum appears in J Biol Chem 1992; 25;267(36):26200.) J Biol Chem 1992; 267: 18498–18504.
55. Oh Y, Benos DJ. Single-channel characteristics of a purified bovine renal amiloride-sensitive Na^+ channel in planar lipid bilayers. Am J Physiol 1993; 264:C1489–C1499.
56. Berdiev BK, Shlyonsky VG, Senyk O, Keeton D, Guo Y, Matalon S, Cantiello HF, Prat AG, Ausiello DA, Ismailov II, Benos DI. Protein kinase A phosphorylation and g-protein regulation of type II pneumocyte Na^+ channels in lipid bilayers. Am J Physiol Cell Physiol 1997; 272:1262–1270.
57. Barbry P, Frelin C, Vigne P, Cragoe EJ Jr, Lazdunski M. [^{3}H]phenamil, a radiolabelled diuretic for the analysis of the amiloride-sensitive Na^+ channels in kidney membranes. Biochem Biophys Res Commun 1986; 135:25–32.
58. Yue G, Matalon S. Mechanisms and sequelae of increased alveolar fluid clearance in hyperoxic rats. Am J Physiol Lung Cell Mol Physiol 1997; 272: L407–L412.
59. Canessa CM, Merillat AM, Rossier BC. Membrane topology of the epithelial sodium channel in intact cells. Am J Physiol 1994; 267:C1682–C1690.

60. Hummler E, Barker P, Gatzy J, Beermann F, Verdumo C, Schmidt A, Boucher R, Rossier BC. Early death due to defective neonatal lung liquid clearance in α*ENaC*-deficient mice. Nat Genet 1996; 12:325–328.
61. Payen DM, Gatecel C, Plaisance P. Almitrine effect on nitric oxide inhalation in adult respiratory distress syndrome. Lancet 1993; 341:1664. Letter.
62. Haskell JF, Yue G, Benos DJ, Matalon S. Upregulation of sodium conductive pathways in alveolar type II cells in sublethal hyperoxia. Am J Physiol 1994; 266: L30–L37.
63. Carter EP, Duvick SE, Wendt CH, Dunitz J, Nici L, Wangensteen OD, Ingbar DH. Hyperoxia increases active alveolar Na^+ resorption in vivo and type II cell Na, K-ATPase in vitro. Chest 1994; 105:75S–77S.

16

Na,K-ATPase and the Clearance of Pulmonary Edema Fluid

DAVID H. INGBAR and CHRISTINE H. WENDT

University of Minnesota School of Medicine
Minneapolis, Minnesota

EDWARD D. CRANDALL

Will Rogers Institute Pulmonary Research Center
University of Southern California
Los Angeles, California

I. Introduction

Clearance of sodium and water from the alveolar space is primarily mediated by active sodium transport by the alveolar epithelium using a combination of an apical amiloride-sensitive sodium channel (1) and the basolateral sodium pump, Na,K-ATPase (2). The importance of this pathway is supported by inhibitor and ion substitution studies in living animals, isolated perfused lungs, cultured type II alveolar epithelial cell monolayers, and patch clamp studies of cell membranes (3,4). The rate of alveolar fluid clearance by this pathway likely is regulated and increases in many conditions with alveolar flooding, as discussed in Chapter 14. This chapter will review the structure and regulation of the sodium pump and then summarize our knowledge of it in the normal lung, in the developing lung, and in injury and lung disease.

The sodium pump, Na,K-ATPase, is a ubiquitous plasma membrane enzyme that plays a critical role in the survival of essentially all cells. It uses ATP to translocate three sodium molecules out of cells against the sodium concentration gradient, while bringing two potassium ions into the cell (5). It plays a central role in many physiological processes, including regulation of cell volume, ion transport, sodium-coupled uptake of many other substrates (glucose, amino acids), and propagation of the action potential of muscle and nerve. In many cells the action of the sodium pump consumes 20% to 30% of cellular ATP. This use of ATP is justified by the critical need to maintain the ion gradients that drive so many other vital cellular processes. While this enzyme is important for all cells, in most transporting epithelial cells it is present in greater quantities and is required for transcellular vectorial transport of sodium and often other ions. For example, renal distal tubular epithelial cells are rich in sodium pump.

Abnormal function of the sodium pump has been described in a variety of disease states. Decreased activity has been reported in diabetes and may contribute to neuropathy, ocular problems, and abnormal lung maturation. Salt loading increases renal sodium pump activity. Chronic renal failure decreases renal sodium pump activity, and this is overcome by hemodialysis. In polycystic kidney disease, the sodium pump is abnormally redistributed to the apical plasma membrane, which may diminish sodium resorption. In addition, augmented sodium pump activity may contribute to hypertension. For example, in rats with spontaneous hypertension, the sodium pump activity of skeletal muscle and red blood cells is increased. Pump activity is diminished in congestive heart failure, but this may be adaptive since it reduces ATP consumption. There also are shifts in the expression of specific isoforms of the subunits. Finally it has been suggested that diminished airway Na,K-ATPase in asthmatics may contribute to bronchoconstriction.

II. Structure of Na,K-ATPase

Since the sodium pump was discovered, approximately 40 years ago (6), it has been intensively studied. The enzyme is a heterodimer of the P1 ATPase class that is composed of alpha and beta subunits in a 1:1 ratio (7) (Fig. 1). Other enzymes in this class include the H^+-K^+ ATPase of the stomach, sarcoplasmic reticulum Ca-ATPase, plasma membrane Ca-ATPase, bacterial copper and cadmium ATPases and magnesium import ATPase, and plant, yeast, and fungal Ca-ATPase and H-ATPase (7). This superfamily of enzymes is transiently phosphorylated during their reaction cycle. They are located in the plasma membrane or membranes of specialized organelles and maintain ionic concentrations in specific cellular compartments. They consist of one or several subunits, with considerable similarity of the phosphorylated catalytic subunit. Most of these enzymes, in contrast to F- or V-type ATPases, are inhibited by vanadate, a chemical analog of phosphate. The structure of Na,K-ATPase is very similar to the dimeric H,K-ATPase, with 60% to 65% homology between the alpha-1 subunits and 30% to 40% homology between the beta-1 subunits.

The sodium pump alpha subunit is a polypeptide of approximately 96,000 to 112,000 daltons with seven to 10 membrane spanning domains (5). Its cat-

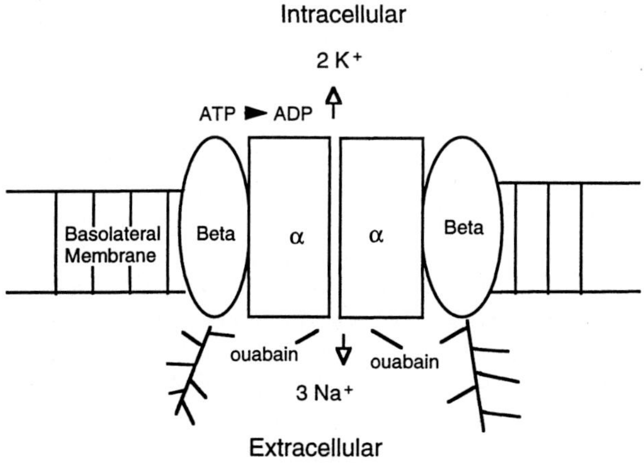

Figure 1 This cartoon depicts the arrangement of the Na,K-ATPase heterotetramer in the plasma membrane. The catalytic alpha subunit has a cytoplasmic ATP binding and phosphorylation site while there is an extracellular ouabain binding site. Only the beta subunit is glycosylated.

alytic mechanism is complicated and remains somewhat uncertain, but it undergoes phosphorylation-dephosphorylation and has states of occlusion with potassium and sodium. The alpha subunit has three isoforms that are tissue-dependent (8). The alpha-1 is the predominant form in epithelial tissues, including type II alveolar epithelial cells (9,10). Although this finding is still controversial, type I-like alveolar epithelial cells in vitro have been reported by one group to express the alpha-2 subunit (11). The functional differences among these three isoforms are uncertain, except that the alpha-2 isoform has a relatively lower affinity for binding selective sodium pump inhibitors, such as ouabain and other digitalis glycosides. The alpha-1 subunit has eight to 10 transmembrane domains and a C-terminal cytoplasmic domain (7). The extracellular portion has the binding site for ouabain, while the cytoplasmic portion has the binding site for ATP. Hence the alpha subunit is considered the catalytic subunit, and it probably forms most of the transmembrane channel for ion passage. The alpha-2 isoform predominates in the brain whereas alpha-3 is found in skeletal muscle and the developing heart.

The beta subunit is a glycosylated polypeptide with a peptide core of approximately 35 kD, with a single membrane spanning segment. The beta subunit also has three isoforms, but the beta-1 isoform is ubiquitous, whereas beta-2 is found only in brain and pineal gland. The beta-1 isoform is highly conserved across different animal species, with approximately 90% homology. The single transmembrane spanning domain is identical in sheep rat, dog, and pig. This subunit has three pairs of disulfide bonds that also are conserved. Unlike the alpha subunit, the beta subunit is glycosylated at N-asparagine groups. The functional significance of this glycosylation is uncertain since the heterodimer can be assembled, transported to the cell membrane, and function without glycosylation. The beta subunit is glycosylated to variable degrees in different cell types, and this makes recognition difficult with some antibodies (12). The beta-2 subunit was originally termed adhesion molecule of glia and plays a role in glial cell adhesion. It has approximately 40% homology with the beta-1 isoform. A third beta isoform also has been reported. Neither beta-2 or beta-3 isoforms have been reported in the lung, and at present the localization of beta-1 in the lung is uncertain. Study of the beta subunit has been somewhat limited by difficulties in producing antibodies that recognize the subunit protein in different glycosylation and conformational states. The beta subunit likely plays a critical role in assembly of alpha-beta heterodimers and targeting them to the plasma membrane (13,14). Both subunits are required for activity of the enzyme in yeast and *Xenopus* oocytes. However, some authorities believe that alpha subunits in the plasma membrane can be enzymatically active alone.

For many years there have been suggestions that there may be additional subunits of the sodium pump. The best characterized of these is the gamma subunit, but its tissue distribution and functional significance are uncertain.

The distribution of the sodium pump within the plasma membrane is a function of the cell type. In nonpolarized cells, such as fibroblasts and endothelial cells (15), the enzyme is on all cell surfaces. In transporting epithelia, the plasma membrane distribution is polarized. In almost all epithelia, it is on the basolateral membrane. The most notable exception is the ciliary epithelium, which moves salt and fluid in a basal to apical direction and on which the pump is located apically. Considerable work has assessed the mechanism of polarity and whether it occurs through initial targeted delivery of the protein or redistribution of the proteins within the membrane. This likely is cell type-dependent (16). While tight junctions probably are not essential for maintenance of this polarity, interaction with a basal matrix surface may be required. Elegant studies utilizing chimeric hybrids of Na,K-ATPase and H,K-ATPase demonstrated that the amino-terminal end of the beta-1 subunit is sufficient for polarized accumulation of the sodium pump in the basolateral plasma membrane (17).

In the plasma membrane, Na,K-ATPase is linked to the subcortical cytoskeleton through sequential interactions with ankyrin, fodrin, and actin. These interactions likely are important in maintaining polarized distribution of the sodium pump to the basolateral membrane of most epithelia. The role of these connections in regulating sodium pump activity is unknown, but this mechanism influences apical sodium channel function, which has similar cytoskeletal attachments.

III. Regulation of Na,K-ATPase

Regulation of Na,K-ATPase occurs at multiple levels (18,19) including transcription (20–22), mRNA stability (23), translation (24), protein degradation rate (25), delivery to the plasma membrane from intracellular vesicle pools (26), basolateral-apical membrane polarity, recycling from the plasma membrane, and modification of pump molecules in the plasma membrane. Short-term regulation can be achieved rapidly by altering the activity of the enzyme already in the plasma membrane or the number of pump molecules recycled into the membrane. Alternatively, long-term regulation occurs more slowly, through one or more of many steps that increase the amount of pump protein available for insertion in the plasma membrane, including increased gene transcription.

A. Short-Term Regulation

Functional activity rapidly is increased by lower K^+ or higher Na^+ intracellular ion concentrations, and by various hormones such as glucocorticoids and mineralocorticoids, adrenergic agonists, and thyroid hormone (27). Most cells are believed to have excess sodium pump capacity; in other words, the pump is working at less than full capacity and can readily increase activity to meet demand for sodium transport. The electrochemical ionic driving forces and the rate of sodium entry can also alter pump activity. For example, increased intracellular sodium concentration will augment pump activity. However, the mechanisms involved are likely complex. Extracellular stimuli also can alter Na,K-ATPase activity through a network of receptormediated signals.

Protein kinases and G protein-linked membrane receptors alter sodium pump activity in many different systems. Roles have been demonstrated for adenosine 3′,5′-cyclic monophosphate (cAMP), c-AMP-dependent protein kinase (protein kinase A; PKA), and protein kinase C (PKC). Study of these factors is complex for several reasons (19). First, purified membrane preparations or particulate fractions often do not demonstrate effects seen in intact cells. Second, even within a single organ, the same protein kinase may have opposite effects on sodium pump activity in different cell types. Third, the same exogenous stimulant may have very different modes of action in different cell types, even within the same organ. For example, exogenous dopamine inhibits activity in the proximal nephron by increasing PKC activity, whereas dopamine inhibits activity in the distal nephron through increased PKA activity.

The effect of PKA activation on sodium pump activity varies in different tissues (19). When activated by cAMP, forskolin, or dopamine in the cortical collecting duct, PKA inhibits enzyme activity. However, this effect does not occur in the proximal convoluted tubule. PKA may act directly through phosphorylation of the pump molecule or via indirect effects. PKA phosphorylates the serine 943 residue of the sodium pump alpha subunit, very close to the carboxy-terminal end of the molecule. In contrast, PKC phosphorylates the serine 23 residue near the amino-terminal end of the molecule and possibly other sites as well. At present it is not possible a priori to predict the functional consequences of phosphorylation in specific cell types.

Eicosanoids, inositol phosphates, angiotensin II, and intracellular calcium also are signal transduction mechanisms that can modify sodium pump activity. In some cell types, Na,K-ATPase function can be inhibited by phosphorylation, dopamine, parathyroid hormone, endothelin, or PGE2 and stimulated by vasopressin or growth factors (19). Pump activity also may be regulated by cell cycle stage. Other compounds reported to stimulate Na,K-ATPase include cyclosporine, FK506, serum, hypertonicity, and prolactin. Many studies have identified an endogenous Na,K-ATPase inhibitor circulating in plasma or in specific tissues, but the chemical nature of the inhibitor has yet to be defined. An endogenous activator also has been reported, but is even less well characterized at present. Thus there is a plethora of potential extracellular regulators of the sodium pump and many intracellular signaling pathways that influence this enzyme.

Few studies have examined the regulation of Na,K-ATPase in normal alveolar or airway epithelial cells. In cultured alveolar type II cells, beta-adrenergic agonists increase sodium resorption and type II cell Na,K-ATPase activity (28).

B. Transcriptional Regulation

The Na,K-ATPase isoforms belong to a multigene family (30,30a). Both alpha and beta subunits have >70% homology between isoforms within each subunit (31), and there is significant interspecies homology of the Na,K-ATPase coding and promoter sequences. For example, rat and sheep have 97% homology of the alpha-1 isoform (32,33). Since the subunit genes are on different chromosomes, transcription may be independently regulated.

In terms of new sodium pump production, the mRNA isoform levels are controlled by tissue specificity, developmental stage, and hormonal milieu (glucocorticoids [GC], mineralocorticoids [MC], and tri-iodothyronine [T3]). Sodium pump transcription also is upregulated by intracellular Na and K levels (26). Most of these transcriptional effects are on the order of two- or threefold changes. This is likely sufficient to markedly alter the amounts of functional protein, since many tissues have relatively high basal expression of this "housekeeping" gene. Unequal amounts of alpha and beta mRNA and protein concentrations are present in many tissues, even though the final sodium pump has a 1:1 stoichiometry of alpha and beta subunits.

For the rat alpha-1 subunit, the major transcription initiation site is 262 base pairs upstream from the translation initiation site and is preceded by a

TATA box at position −32. The factors regulating alpha-1 gene transcription are partially defined. Included in the 5′ flanking region are two Spl TF binding sites, two putative GC response element (GRE) half-consensus sequences (33), and a consensus cAMP response element (CRE). The human gene has a TATA box and five Spl-like elements (34). The rat alpha-1 subunit promoter has positive regulatory regions at −155 and −49 bp and an "ATP1a1" regulatory element or "ARE" at −94 to −69 bp that binds both common (designated ARE C1 and C2) and cell type-specific transcription factors (ARE C3) (35). This part of the promoter sequence is conserved across rat, horse, and human genes, but is not present in other Na,K-ATPase subunit promoters. At least seven ARE-binding factors have been identified by gel mobility shift assays and Southwestern cloning (36). AREB6 is a zinc finger protein related to the interleukin-2 gene regulator Nil-2. It can regulate ATP1A1 positively or negatively, depending on cell type and conformational state of the protein (37). Across multiple cell lines, activating transcription factor-1 (ATF-1)/CRE binding protein (CREB) heterodimers bind to the −61/−72 region of the alpha-1 promoter and are required for transcription (38). Although these transcription factors (TFs) are ubiquitous and probably are required for basal transcription of many genes, they can be regulated by cAMP, calcium, and transforming growth factor-beta (TGFβ). In vivo footprinting identified rat tissue specific transcriptional control involving cooperation between a canonical GC box at −57/−49 that binds an Spl-like TF and the ATF region (−72/−65) (39). Thus a series of transactivating TFs have been identified for the alpha-1 subunit gene, but little is known of their regulation and physiologic roles.

Much less is known about transcriptional regulation of the beta-1 subunit gene. The rat gene's promoter contains a potential TATA box at position −31, four GC-rich boxes, a CRE-like sequence, and two sites with putative half-consensus thyroid response element sequences—TRE-1 and TRE-2 (40). The human gene consists of six exons and has two major and three minor transcription initiation sites. The human beta-1 gene has three potential TREs, but only one is functional (41).

Other TFs active in alveolar epithelial cells (AECs) might regulate cell-specific sodium pump gene transcription, although this is purely speculative. For example, pump regulation may resemble that for surfactant apoprotein genes, since the latter also (1) have active CREs, GREs, and Spl-like binding elements; (2) are upregulated in complex fashion by GCs (42) or oxygen (43); and (3) increase in the lung at approximately the same time as the sodium pump genes. For example, the C/EBPα transcription factor is expressed only in type II AEC that appear in fetal rat lung between fetal days 18 and 20 and may regulate surfactant apoprotein transcription (44), but no data exist about its effects on sodium pump gene transcription.

C. Posttranscriptional Regulation

Since similar increases in steady-state levels of mRNA result in different activity levels of the pump, posttranscriptional steps also play a role in the regulation of Na,K-ATPase (45). The relative amount of beta mRNA is less than alpha mRNA in many tissues, but their half-lives and translational efficiencies are unknown (30,46). During differentiation of HL60 cells, alteration in mRNA stability alters the amount of functional sodium pump (23). The Na,K-ATPase alpha-1 mRNA is translated less efficiently than the beta-1 mRNA due to the influence of 3′ untranslated regions (UTRs) (24). Once the subunits are translated, they are unable to leave the endoplasmic reticulum without folding and assembly into alpha-beta heterodimers with glycosylation and disulfide bond formation (14,47,48). At some point there is removal of five amino acids at the amino-terminal end of the alpha-1 subunit (49). The subunits are assembled shortly after cotranslational insertion into the endoplasmic reticulum, undergo an ill-defined posttranslational maturation, and then, in renal epithelial cells, are transported into the cytoplasmic membrane over 1 to 4 hours to generate active pump that binds ouabain (25,26). There also is an inactive, endogenous pool of Na,K-ATPase that presumably derives from recycled plasma membrane sodium pump. Phosphorylation may play a role in cycling between the plasma membrane and late endosomal compartments. Although pump molecules can be shifted from this intracellular pool to and from the plasma membrane by different stimuli, such as by insulin in muscle, the factors that regulate these shifts are not well understood.

D. Hormonal Regulation

T3 markedly increases sodium pump activity and gene transcription in most tissues (50,51) and may differentially alter expression of alpha and beta subunits (52). However, local factors such as T3 receptor (TR) type, quantity, and location play major roles in determining the effects of T3 (53). In cardiac myocytes, alpha-2 subunit mRNA level is increased by T3 through posttranscriptional mechanisms, but a negative functional TRE is evident when TR is cotransfected (54). Similarly, in alpha-3, binding to TRE inhibits transcription.

Thyroid hormone is vital to the development of many organs, particularly the brain, and it is important for normal lung maturation (55). In the developing or adult lung, T3 may theoretically stimulate Na,KATPase either directly or through promotion of lung maturation and type II cell development. Mice with genetic primary hypothyroidism have thicker septae, smaller alveoli, and fewer type II cell lamellar bodies (56). T3 predominantly acts through binding to its receptor and stimulation of gene transcription (57). The two T3 receptor genes each have alternative mRNA splice products (TR-alpha-1, alpha-2, beta-1, and beta-2). TR levels are developmentally regulated and vary between organs and specific cell types, partly due to transcription (58). TR-alpha is expressed early in multiple tissues, in many species preceding T3, whereas TR-beta is expressed much later, occurring first in brain. TR-beta may be more important after early development, since thyroid hormone resistance syndromes are associated with TR-beta, but not TR-alpha, mutants. Type II AEC nuclei bind T3, but the ontogeny of TR forms in the lung has not been assessed. The role of thyroid hormones in regulating Na,KATPase in the adult or developing lung is currently unknown, but merits definition.

Both glucocorticoids (GCs) and mineralocorticoids (MCs) also can stimulate Na,K-ATPase activity and transcription. For example, there is very rapid stimulation of Na,K-ATPase transcription in the infant rat kidney by GCs (59,60). In fetal rat type II cells, dexamethasone stimulates vectoral sodium transport through both sodium channels and Na,K-ATPase (61,62). Tracheal transport of salt and water also is stimulated by GCs. Maternal rat steroid treatment can accelerate maturation of fetal AEC and the surfactant system and protect against oxidant injury (63), but also can delay postnatal alveolarization. The effect on lung sodium pump can be stimulatory (64,65), but the effect depends on the dosing and timing—as for surfactant apoproteins.

Like T3, GCs bind to a cytosolic corticosteroid receptor (CR) that translocates to the nucleus, binds to a GRE, and acts as a transcription factor (TF). GCs may also activate MR receptors that affect the same DNA response elements. The CR is in the steroid/thyroid receptor superfamily that includes all the steroid receptors, TR, retinoic acid receptors, and some "orphan" receptors. Most receptors in this family are developmentally regulated and in the absence of ligand may silence basal gene transcription (66). Rat lung CR mRNA levels remain persistly high from late fetal life into adulthood, whereas levels vary in other organs (67). However, in isolated rat fetal AECs, CR mRNA increased fivefold from fetal day 18 to 20, followed by increased protein, whereas fibroblast levels of mRNA and protein peaked at FD19 and then fell (68). The timing of this increase in AEC CR is consistent with the period when Na,K-ATPase transcription is upregulated (69,70).

Both GC and T3 may affect the sodium pump indirectly by promoting lung maturation. Both accelerate the appearance of beta-adrenergic receptors (beta-AR) in the lung (71–73), but the receptor level may fall with repeated GC treatment. In the lung, smooth muscle and airway epithelial express β-AR, but AECs respond to adrenergic stimuli with increased surfactant secretion and activity of the sodium channel and pump. Activated beta-AR work through G proteins to stimulate adenyl cyclase, calcium channels, and diacylglycerol formation. In turn, activated cAMP-dependent protein kinase and protein kinase C stimulate CREs and TPA-responsive elements and alter gene transcription. Physiologic studies on fetal type II cells indicate that terbutaline alone stimulates sodium transport and synergizes with GCs and T3 (74). Since sodium pump promoters have CRE-like sequences and the enzyme is activated by beta-adrenergic agonists, this pathway could play a cooperative role in turning on gene expression in late fetal development.

IV. Na,K-ATPase in Normal Lung Solute and Fluid Transport

The importance of Na,K-ATPase, working jointly with the sodium channel and other apical sodium entry pathways, in active salt and water resorption across the alveolar epithelium is supported by studies of intact animals, intact lungs, and cultured cells (2–4). Beta-adrenergic agonists and cAMP stimulate fluid clearance in situ in human (75) and rat lungs (76–78) and sodium transport in type II cells (28). In both cardiogenic and ARDS edema, there is active sodium and water resorption against an oncotic gradient, and higher rates of resorption are associated with better patient outcomes (80).

The ion transport properties of adult type II cells have been reviewed (2,3) and are discussed elsewhere in this volume. At the apical membrane, sodium may enter by at least three mechanisms: Na channels (81), Na-glucose cotransport, or Na^+-H^+ exchange. Hypothetically, there also may be basal sodium entry via a different form of Na^+-H^+ antiporter and/or a Na,K,C12 cotransporter, but these pathways have not been established in adult type II cells. Na channels are quantitatively the predominant path of sodium entry, at least in adult type II cells (2,3; Chap. 15). Both high and low amiloride affinity forms of the sodium channel have been reported in type II cells, although only high-affinity channels are present in cultured AEC (1). Both the sodium pump and channel are needed for Na transport; not surprisingly, their activities usually change in parallel. In addition to clearing the alveoli of fluid, the low intracellular sodium concentration maintained by Na,K-ATPase allows sodium-coupled cotransport of amino acids and/or glucose into type II cells.

In alveoli of normal rat lung, this ubiquitous enzyme is detected primarily on the basolateral surface of type II cells, based on cytochemistry and immunolocalization of the alpha-1 isoform (9,10). Based on one study of rat type I-like cells in culture, it was suggested that type I cells may express the alpha-2 isoform of Na,K-ATPase (11), but this has not yet been confirmed in vivo. The beta subunits have not been localized in the lungs of any species. The density of sodium pumps on type II cells supports their importance in maintaining a dry alveolus. The lack of detectable density of sodium pump and sodium channel on type I cells in situ leads to uncertainty about their relative function as transporters. However, they almost certainly have low densities of sodium pumps for their survival, but below the current histologically detectable threshold. Since they occupy 20 times the alveolar surface area per cell relative to type II cells, it still is possible that they contribute significantly to net alveolar sodium resorption. For example, if type I cell ion transporter densities were 20-fold less than on type II cells and they functioned with equal efficiency, then the two cell types would contribute equally to net active sodium resorption.

As discussed in Chapter 14, many factors can stimulate sodium resorption in the normal adult lung or type II cells, including arginine vasopressin, growth factors (transforming growth factor alpha [TGF alpha], hepatocyte growth factor [HGF], keratinocyte growth factor [KGF], and epidermal growth factor [EGF] [83]), cytokines (tumor necrosis factor alpha [TNF alpha]), endotoxin, mineralocorticoids, dopamine, dobutamine (84), and beta-adrenergic agonists. These factors may stimulate the function of both sodium channels and sodium pumps in alveolar epithelial cells, but this has not been established at the molecular level, except for catecholamines (28).

V. Na,K-ATPase and Ion Transport in the Developing Lung

Through most of fetal development, the airspace epithelium secretes Cl and fluid, presumably using apical Cl channels and basal Na,K,Cl2 cotransport. Late in gestation, Cl secretion decreases and sodium and fluid resorption predominates, as required for effective gas exchange after the first breath (85–87). The amounts of Na channel and Na pump mRNA, protein, and function increase at approximately fetal day 20 in the rat (69,88,89) and mRNA at neonatal day (ND) 1 in the mouse (90). In contrast, isolated sheep type II cells bind ouabain before birth, but do not have active ouabain-inhibitable pumping of rubidium until after birth (91,92).

Developing lung AECs have a variety of sodium entry pathways, including high and low amiloride affinity-sodium selective cation channels (ENaC) (1), non-cation-selective channels, and Na,K,2Cl cotransporter (93). Oxygen tension and fetal lung matrix also can influence the levels of sodium transporter expression in fetal type II cells (95). Dexamethasone can increase sodium channel expression with differential effects on the isoform expression (94) and, if increased at specific times, also Na,K-ATPase (65). Functional sodium channel is required for survival after birth, since mice with an alpha isoform renal epithelial Na channel (alpha-rENaC) knockout mutation die within minutes of birth and exhibit normal lung morphology except for fluid-filled alveoli (96). Transgenic mice with selective knockout of the GC receptor have a very high perinatal mortality due to respiratory failure with atelectasis and also lower lung Na channel mRNA levels (97). However, these mice also may have impaired development of beta-adrenergic receptors and surfactant function.

Recent reviews proposed that the presence and then activation of the sodium channel are the requisite steps for perinatal fluid resorption (85–87). Activation probably results from a combination of the increased GC levels and beta-adrenergic stimulation that occur late in gestation and with labor. However, other factors are probably also important, since beta-adrenergic receptor blockade does not prevent the decrease in lung water content. The late-gestational switch to alveolar fluid resorption requires active Na,K-ATPase. Thus it is not surprising that the pump seems to be expressed and regulated in parallel with the sodium channel.

Abnormal fluid transport likely contributes to the neonatal lung diseases known as infant respiratory distress syndrome (RDS) and transient tachypnea of the newborn (TTN) (98). Infants with TTN have increased lung water content, but normal surfactant protein and lipid levels. They also have smaller amiloride-inhibitable potential differences across their apical nasal epithelium, consistent with lesser Na channel function. The risk of RDS in prematurely born human infants is decreased by prenatal maternal treatment with GCs or combined GCs and TRH (99,100). In animal models, combined T3 and GC treatment is required to normalize the sodium absorptive response to beta-adrenergic agonists in thyroidectomized lambs (101,102). These hormones also synergistically promote lung maturation (103) and surfactant phospholipid function (104). Infants of diabetic mothers are at increased risk of RDS and in animal models have diminished Na,K-ATPase mRNA and activity (105). T3 or dexamethasone reverses the diabetic rat fetus' delayed surfactant system maturation (106). Which components of the fluid resorptive system are abnormal with immaturity or TTN are not defined but may include the beta-adrenergic receptor, GTP-binding proteins, adenyl cyclase, cAMP-dependent kinase, Na channel, or Na pump. Further exploration of the role of deficient Na,K-ATPase function and aveolar fluid resorption in contributing to infant RDS and TTN is important.

VI. Lung Na,K-ATPase and Fluid Transport During Lung Injury and Recovery

The impact of lung injury on fluid transport has been studied in many models of lung injury and recovery, as discussed in Chapter 14. The injury model studied in greatest detail is acute (>95% oxygen) or chronic (70% to 80% oxygen) hyperoxia. In these models, there are variable effects of acute injury on active sodium resorption, but resorption typically is increased during recovery and in more chronic, subacute injury. Since resorption requires activity of both sodium channel and sodium pump, these data suggest increases in sodium pump activity in these settings. However, in vitro exposure of cells or membranes to oxidants can significantly decrease Na,K-ATPase activity. Thus oxidants are capable of either inhibiting or stimulating the sodium pump, depending upon many specific aspects of the oxidants, the target system (animal, tissues, intact cells, or membranes), and the Na,K-ATPase parameters measured. The complexity of the impact of oxidants and the potential for oxidants to simultaneously affect the pump in multiple ways has been reviewed (106).

The results reported in studies of the acute hyperoxic model of lung injury illustrate this complexity; the results are apparently conflicting, but closer examination of the reports indicates that the data may not be in direct conflict. When older rats, who are more susceptible to injury, are exposed to 100% oxygen for 64 hours, both Na,K-ATPase activity and active sodium resorption decrease (107,108). However, when younger rats with better antioxidant defenses are exposed for 60 hours, a different pattern is seen. There is no change in the mean active sodium resorption (109,110); however, there is significant heterogeneity in the degree of injury (111). The rats with less severe injury have decreased active alveolar sodium resorption, while the more severely injured rats have normal or increased resorption. For either the older or younger rats, the maximal sodium pump activity in lung membranes decreases—but these techniques measure the maximal capacity which probably is not used under steady-state conditions.

Studies of alveolar type II cells isolated from rats with moderate injury reveal decreases in maximal pump activity of the membranes, but maintained pump activity in intact cells (112). This suggests that there is oxidative inhibition of the type II cells' maximal pump capacity when rats are exposed to hyperoxia, but that up to a point the type II cells are able to compensate and at least maintain normal steady-state levels of transport. The observation that sodium pump mRNA levels in the lung and in the alveolar type II cells increase early with hyperoxic exposure (10,112) is consistent with a homeostatic increase in gene expression. Indeed, renal epithelial cells exposed in vitro to hyperoxia have increased beta-1 gene transcription, and the portion of the rat beta-1 gene promoter required for this effect has been localized to a 60-bp region (113). However, the effects of hyperoxia at the protein level are less clear-cut, with decreases in alpha-1 and normal beta-1 subunit levels in the isolated type II cells. These data are most consistent with multiple simultaneous effects of hyperoxia on different aspects of Na,K-ATPase transcription, protein synthesis, and function.

In contrast, the chronic hyperoxic model shows consistent increases in alveolar sodium resorption, sodium channel quantity and function (114,115), and Na,K-ATPase quantity and activity (116). This may result from the less severe nature of the injury or the presence of hyperplastic type II cells as part of the response to injury. The increases in sodium channel are present on a per-cell basis and thus are not solely due to the increased number of type II cells. Interestingly, there is some heterogeneity of the physiologic responses in active sodium resorption in these rats, as occurs in acute hyperoxia (116a). The reason for this heterogeneity remains unexplained.

The impact of hyperbaric hyperoxia also has been studied. Rats exposed for 2.5 hours to 2.8 atm pressure of 100% oxygen increased the amounts of lung Na,K-ATPase mRNA fourfold and activity twofold (117) during recovery. No studies have examined fluid resorption or sodium channel function in these animals.

The function of the sodium pump has been studied in very few other in vivo models of lung injury. Permeability pulmonary edema induced by thiourea increases active sodium resorption and the Na,K-ATPase activity and alpha-1 subunit protein level (118). Interestingly, alveolar flooding with a proteinaceous solution, without injury, induces a similar increase in fluid resorption and Na,K-ATPase; this suggests that alveolar flooding per se plays a role in triggering the homeostatic increase in sodium pump function. Intratracheal dibutyryl cAMP decreases the severity of phosgene-induced lung injury, even when given more than an hour after the injury (119). It significantly decreases the degree of pulmonary edema and the extent of glutathione and lipid oxidation. Much of the protection is due to changes in arachidonic acid metabolites that potentially could alter Na,K-ATPase function.

Recently the impact of mechanical ventilatory patterns on alveolar edema formation and clearance has drawn much interest. When living rabbits were ventilated with one fluid-filled lung at low and high degrees of inflation, greater inflation was accompanied by less active sodium resorption. This suggested that overinflation decreased alveolar fluid clearance. In contrast, alveolar type II cells isolated from rats ventilated with high tidal volumes for 25 min had increases in the amount of Na,K-ATPase that bound ouabain, suggesting that there could be rapid upregulation in sodium pump activity (120).

In many in vitro cell culture systems, oxidants inhibit the function of alveolar epithelial cell sodium channel and/or the sodium pump. For example, hydrogen peroxide inhibits the function of both transporters, but particularly the sodium pump (121). Peroxynitrite causes greater inhibition of sodium channel function (122), especially when on the apical surface, but also can inhibit the sodium pump. Hydrogen peroxide-generating systems can induce biphasic effects on alveolar type II cell Na,K-ATPase, with an initial decrease followed by an increase to either baseline or supranormal levels (123). The degree of the initial decrease was dependent on the hydrogen peroxide concentration. As with the acute hyperoxia model, this suggests that initial pump inhibition by oxidants may induce a compensatory response. Other physiologic stresses also can inhibit sodium pump activity. For example, endotoxin-stimulated macrophages impair type II cell ion transport through a nitric oxide-mediated mechanism (124). Renal tubular epithelial cells can downregulate sodium pump through autocrine production of nitric oxide products (125). Hypoxia can inhibit both Na,K-ATPase and sodium channel function of alveolar epithelial cells, independent of the decrease in ATP concentration (126,127).

Oxidants can also stimulate Na,K-ATPase and sodium transport in certain cell types. For example, airway epithelial cells exposed to nitrogen dioxide doubled their sodium pump activity with increased affinity of ouabain binding (128). The results were most consistent with increased turnover rate for the sodium pump molecules in the membrane. Several studies of intact endothelial cells demonstrated increased Na,K-ATPase activity after oxidant exposure (15,129). The increase could not be directly attributed to changes in PKA or PKC activity (15). In alveolar epithelial cells, lipopolysaccharides simulate sodium-dependent transport and likely Na,K-ATPase, while protecting against oxidant injury (130). Thus there are clearly some systems in which oxidants stimulate Na,K-ATPase activity, particularly in intact cell systems.

The mechanisms by which oxidants impact on Na,K-ATPase are not yet defined, but this subject has been reviewed (106). Chemical modification of the sodium pump itself may occur. For example, the disulfide bonds of either subunit are potential targets for oxidation that could result in inhibition of enzyme function (131). Ventricular myocytes with oxidized sulfhydryl groups have diminished sodium pump current (132). In the presence of neutrophils, activated macrophages and inflammation, nitrotyrosine, nitrosothiol, or chlorotyrosine groups could be formed that alter enzyme function. Neutrophils inhibit the Na,K-ATPase activity of renal tubular epithelial membranes (133). Alternatively, oxidation of specific amino acids could accelerate enzyme degradation via the ubiquitin pathway. Peroxidation of nearby lipids also indirectly inhibits the Na,K-ATPase activity in some experimental systems. It is likely that different mechanisms of pump alteration will be found depending on the particular stresses to which the lung and, based on their antioxidant defense profiles, the specific cell types are involved.

VII. Summary

Our knowledge of the regulation of the lung Na,K-ATPase is in its infancy, and many questions remain open. However, it is clear that this enzyme plays a major role in normal cellular homeostasis and in the stress response and likely could be an important target for therapeutic manipulation in the future. In particular, understanding the regulation of the sodium pump during development, injury, and repair should permit development of strategies to speed recovery. Already strategies such as treatment with EGF (83), KGF, and beta-adrenergic agonists are reasonable to test in animal models of lung injury or in abnormal lung development.

Acknowledgments

The experimental work of the authors in this area has been supported by grants from the National Institutes of Health (HL-50152 SCOR in Acute Lung Injury for D.H.I.; K08 HL03114 for C.H.W., and HL38621 and HL 38578 for E.C.), the American Heart Association (research grants-in-aid to D.H.I. and C.H.W.), and the American Lung Association (Career Investigator Award to D.H.I.).

References

1. Matalon S, Benos DJ, Jackson RM. Biophysical and molecular properties of amiloride-inhibitable Na channels in alveolar epithelial cells. Am J Physiol (Lung) 1996; 271:L1–L22.
2. Matthay MA, Folkesson HG, Verkman AS. Salt and water transport across alveolar and distal airway epithelia in the adult lung. Am J Physiol (Lung) 1996; 270: L487–L503.
3. Matalon S. Mechanisms and regulation of ion transport in adult mammaliam alveolar type II pneumocytes. Am J Physiol 1991; 261:C727–C738.
4. Saumon G, Basset G. Electrolyte and fluid transport across the mature alveolar epithelium. J Appl Physiol 1993; 74:1–15.
5. Skou JC. Overview: the Na,K-Pump. Meth Enzymol 1988; 156:1–25.
6. Robinson JD. Steps to the Na-K pump and Na-K-ATPase (1939–1962). NIPS 1995; 10:184–188.
7. Horisberger J-D. The Na.K-ATPase: Structure-Function Relationship. Austin: R.G. Landes Co., 1994.
8. Sweadner KJ. Isozymes of the Na,K-ATPase. Biochim Biophys Acta 1989; 988: 185–220.
8a. Jewell EA, Shamraj OI, Lingrel JB. Isoforms of the alpha subunit of Na, K-ATPase and their significance. Acta Physiol Scand 1992; 146:161–169.
9. Schneeberger EE, McCarthy KM. Cytochemical localization of NaK-ATPase in rat type II pneumocytes. J Appl Physiol 1986; 60:1584–1589.
10. Nici L, Dowin R, Jamieson JD, Ingbar DH. Upregulation of rat type II pneumocyte Na,K-ATPase during hyperoxic lung injury. Am J Physiol (Lung) 1991; 261: L307–L314.
11. Ridge KM, Rutschman DH, Factor P, Katz AI, Bertorello AM, Sznajder JI. Differential expression of Na-K-ATPase isoforms in rat alveolar cells. Am J Physiol (Lung) 1997; 273:L246–L255.
12. Zhang XL, Danto SI, Borok Z, Eber JT, Martin-Vasallo, Lubman RL. Identification of Na-K-ATPase beta-subunit in alveolar epithelial cells. Am J Physiol (Lung) 1997; 272:L85–L94.
13. Fambrough DM, Lemas MV, Hamrick M, Emerick M, Renaud KJ, Inman EM, Hwang B, Takeyasu K. Analysis of subunit assembly of the Na-KATPase. Am J Physiol (Cell) 1994; 266:C579–C589.
13a. Geering K. Subunit assembly and posttranslational processing of Na^+-pumps. Acta Physiol Scand 1992; 146:177–181.
14. Geering K, Beggah A, Good P, Girardet S, Roy S, Schaer D, Jaunin P. Oligomerization and maturation of Na,K-ATPase: functional interaction of the cytoplasmic NH_2 terminus of the beta subunit with the alpha subunit. J Cell Biol 1996; 133:1193–1204.

15. Charles A, Dawicki DD, Oldmixon E, Kuhn C, Cutaia M, Rounds S. Studies on the mechanism of short-term regulation of pulmonary artery endothelial cell Na/K pump activity. J Lab Clin Med 1997; 130:157–168.
16. Mays RW, Siemers KA, Fritz BA, Lowe AW, van Meer G, Nelson WJ. Hierarchy of mechanisms involved in generating Na/K-ATPase polarity in MDCK epithelial cells. J Cell Biol 1995; 130:1105–1115.
17. Gottardi CJ, Caplan MJ. Molecular requirements for the cell-surface expression of multisubunit ion-transporting ATPases. J Biol Chem 1993; 268:14342–14347.
18. Ewart HS, Klip A. Hormonal regulation of the Na-K-ATPase: mechanisms underlying rapid and sustained changes in pump activity. Am J Physiol 1995; 269: C295–C311.
19. Bertorello AM, Katz AI. Short-term regulation of renal Na,K-ATPase activity: physiological relevance and cellular mechanisms. Am J Physiol 1994; 265:GF743–F755.
20. Herrera VLM, Emanuel JR, Ruiz-Opazo N, Levenson R, Nadal-Ginard B. Three differentially expressed Na, K-ATPase alpha subunit isoforms: structural and functional implications. J Cell Biol 1987; 105:1855–1865.
21. Schneider J, Mercer RW, Gilmore-Hebert M, Benz EJ. Tissue specificity, localization in brain and cell-free translation of mRNA encoding the alpha-3 isoform of NaK-ATPase. Proc Natl Acad Sci USA 1988; 85:284.
22. Shull GE, Greeb J, Lingrel JB. Molecular cloning of three distinct forms of the Na^+,K^+-ATPase alpha-subunit from rat brain. Biochemistry 1986; 25:8125–8132.
23. Chambers SK, Gilmore-Hebert M, Kacinski BM, Benz EJ. Changes in Na,K-ATPase gene expression during granulocytic differentiation of HL60 cells. Blood 1992; 80:1559–1564.
24. Devarajan P, Gilmore-Hebert M, Benz EJ. Differential translation of the Na,K-ATPase subunit mRNAs. J Biol Chem 1992; 267:22435–22439.
25. Mircheff AK, Bowen JW, Yiu SC, McDonough AA. Synthesis and translocation of Na,K-ATPase alpha and beta subunits to plasma membrane in MDCK cells. Am J Physiol 1992; 262:C470–C483.
26. Caplan MJ, Forbush B, Palade GE, Jamieson JD. Biosynthesis of the Na,K-ATPase in MDCK cells: activation and cell surface delivery. J Biol Chem 1990; 265: 3528–2534.
27. McDonough AA, Tang M-J, Lescale-Matys L. Ionic regulation of the biosynthesis of Na,K-ATPase subunits. Semin Nephrol 1990; 10:400–409.
28. Suzuki S, Zuege D, Berthiaume Y. Sodium-independent modulation of Na,K-ATPase activity by beta-adrenergic agonist alveolar type II cells. Am J Physiol 1995; 268:L983–L990.
29. Shull MM, Lingrel JB. Multiple genes encode human Na^+,K^+-ATPase catalytic subunit. Proc Natl Acad Sci USA 1987; 84:4039–4043.
30. Lingrel JB, Orlowski J, Shull MM, Price EM. Molecular genetics of Na,K-ATPase. Progress Nucl Acid Res 1990; 38:37–89.
30a. Modyanov NN, Petrukhin KE, Sverdlov VE, Grishin AV, Orlova MY, Kostina MB, Makarevich OI, Broude NE, Monastyrskaya GS, Sverdlov ED. The family of human Na,K-ATPase genes. FEBS Lett 1991; 278:91–94.

31. Shull GE, Lane LK, Lingrel JB. Amino-acid sequence of the beta-subunit of the (Na^+-K^+)ATPase deduced from a cDNA. Nature 1986; 321:429–431.
32. Kawakami K, Nojima H, Ohta T, Nagano K. Molecular cloning and sequence analysis of human Na,K-ATPase alpha-subunit. Nucleic Acids Res 1986; 14:2833–2844.
33. Yagawa Y, Kawakami K, Nagano K. Cloning and analysis of the 5′-flanking region of rat Na^+/K^+-ATPase alpha-1 subunit gene. Biochim Biophys Acta 1990; 1049:286–292.
34. Shull MM, Pugh DG, Lingrel JB. The human Na,K-ATPase alpha-1 gene: characterization of the 5′-flanking region and identification of a restriction fragment length polymorphism. Genomics 1990; 6:451–460.
35. Yagawa YS, Kawakami K, Nagano K. Housekeeping Na,K-ATPase alpha-1 subunit gene promoter is composed of multiple cis elements to which common and cell type-specific factors bind. Molec Cell Biol 1992; 12:4046–4055.
36. Watanable YU, Kawakami K, Hirayama Y, Nagano K. Transcription factors positively and negatively regulating the Na,K-ATPase alpha-1 subunit gene. J Biochem 1993; 114:849–855.
37. Ikeda K, Kawakami K. DNA binding through distinct domains of zinc-finger-homeodomain protein AREB6 has different effects on gene transcription. Eur J Biochem 1995; 233:73–82.
38. Kobayashi M, Kawakami K. ATF-1CREB heterodimer is involved in constitutive expression of the housekeeping Na,K-ATPase alpha-1 subunit gene. Nucl Acids Res 1995; 23:2848–2855.
39. Nomoto M, Gonzales FJ, Mita T, Inoue N, Kawamura M. Analysis of cis-acting regions upstream of the rat Na/K-ATPase alpha-1 subunit gene by in vivo footprinting. Biochim Biophys Acta 1995; 1264:35–39.
40. Liu B, Gick G. Characterization of the 5′ flanking region of the rat Na,K-ATPase beta-1 subunit gene. Biochim Biophys Acta 1992; 1130:336–338.
41. Feng J, Orlowski J, Lingrel JB. Identification of a functional thyroid hormone response element in the upstream flanking region of the human Na,KATPase alpha-1 gene. Nucl Acids Res 1993; 21:2619–2626.
42. Schellhase DE, Shannon JM. Effects of maternal dexamethasone on expression of SP-A, SP-B and SP-C in the fetal rat lung. Am J Respir Cell Mol Biol 1991; 4: 304–312.
43. Accaregui MJ, JM Snyder, Mendelson CR. Oxygen modulates the differentiation of human fetal lung in vitro and its responsiveness to cAMP. Am J Physiol 1993; 264:L465–L474.
44. Li F, Rosenberg E, Smith CI, Notarfrancesco K, Reisher SR, Shuman H, Feinstein SI. Correlation of expression of transcription factor C/EBPalpha and surfactant protein genes in lung cells. Am J Physiol 1995; 269:L241–L247.
45. Gick GG, Ismail-Beigi F, Edelman IS. Thyroidal regulation of rat renal and hepatic Na,K-ATPase gene expression. J Biol Chem 1988; 263:16610–16618.
47. Geering K, Beggah A, Good P, Girardet S, Roy S, Schaer D, Jaunin P. Oligomerization and maturation of Na,K-ATPase: functional interaction of the cytoplasmic NH_2 terminus of the beta subunit with the alpha subunit. J Cell Biol 1996; 133:1193–1204.

48. Beggah AT, Jaunin P, Geering K. Role of glycosylation and disulfide bond formation in the beta subunit in the folding and functional expression of Na,K-ATPase. J Biol Chem 1997; 272:10318–10326.
49. Pressley TA, Allen JC, Clarke CH, Odebunmi T, Higham SC. Amino terminal processing of the catalytic subunit from Na-K-ATPase. Am J Physiol 1996; 271: C825–C832.
50. Ismail-Beigi F. Thyroid hormone regulation of Na,K-ATPase expression. Trends Endocrinol Metab 1993; 4:152–155.
51. McDonough AA, Brown TA, Horowitz B, Chiu A, Schlotterbeck J, Bowen J, Schmitt CA. Thyroid hormone coordinately regulates Na-K-ATPase alpha and beta subunit mRNA levels in kidney. Am J Physiol 1988; 254:C323–C329.
52. Orlowski J, Lingrel JB. Thyroid and glucocorticoid hormones regulate the expression of multiple Na,K-ATPase genes in cultured neonatal rat cardiac myocytes. J Biol Chem 1990; 265:3462–3470.
53. Nomura T, Borges M, Ingbar SH, Silva JE. Factors determining the differential tissue response of Na.K-ATPase to thyroid hormone in the neonatal rat. Metabolism 1990; 39:1049–1055.
54. Huang F, He H, Gick G. Thyroid hormone regulation of Na,K-ATPase alpha-2 gene expression in cardiac myocytes. Cell Mol Biol Res 1994; 40:41–52.
55. Ingbar DH. The respiratory system in hyperthyroidism. In: Braverman LE, Utiger RD, eds. Werner and Ingbar's The Thyroid. 7th ed. Philadelphia: Lippincott Raven Publishers, 1996.
56. deMello DE, Heyman S, Govindarajan R, Sosenko IRS, Devaskar UP. Delayed ultrastructural lung maturation in the fetal and newborn hypothyroid (hyt/hyt) mouse. Pediatr Res 1994; 36:380–386.
57. Oppenheimer JH, Schwartz HL, Strait KA. The molecular basis of thyroid hormone actions. In: Braverman LE, RD Utiger, eds. Werner & Ingbar's The Thyroid. 7th ed. New York: Lippincott-Raven Publishers, 1996:162–184.
58. Strait KA, Schwartz HL, Seybold VS, Ling NC, Oppenheimer JH. Immunofluorescence localization of thyroid hormone receptor protein beta-1 and variant alpha-2 in selected tissues. Proc Natl Acad Sci USA 1991; 88:3887–3891.
59. Celsi G, Nishi A, Akusjarvi G, Aperia A. Abundance of Na^+-K^+-ATPase mRNA is regulated by glucocorticoid hormones in infant rat kidneys. Am J Physiol 1991; 260:F192–F197.
60. Wang Z-M, Yasui M, Celsi G. Glucocorticoids regulate the transcription of Na-K-ATPase genes in the infant rat kidney. Am J Physiol (Cell) 1994; 267:C450–C455.
61. Cott GR, Rao AK. Hydrocortisone promotes the maturation of Na^+-dependent ion transport across the fetal pulmonary epithelium. Am J Respir Cell Mol Biol 1993; 9:166–171.
62. Rao AK, Cott GR. Ontogeny of ion transport across fetal pulmonary epithelial cells in monolayer culture. Am J Physiol 1991; 261:L1678–L187.
63. Frank L. Prenatal dexamethasone treatment improves survival of newborn rats during prolonged high O_2 exposure. pediatr Res 1992; 32:215–221.
64. Celsi G, Wang Z-M, Akusjarvi G, Aperia A. Sensitive periods for glucocorticoids' regulation of Na^+,K^+-ATPase mRNA in the developing lung and kidney. Pediatr Res 1993; 33:5–9.

65. Ingbar DH, Duvick SE, Savick SK, Schellhase DE, Detterding R, Jamieson JD, Shannon JM. Developmental changes of fetal rat lung Na,K-ATPase following maternal treatment with dexamethasone. Am J Physiol 1997; 272:L665–L672.
66. Perlmann T, Vennstrom B. Nuclear receptors: the sounds of silence. Nature 1995; 377:387–388.
67. Kalinyak JE, Friffin CA, Hamilton RW, Bradshaw JG, Perlman AJ, Hoffman AR. Developmental and hormonal regulation of glucocorticoid receptor mRNA in the rat. J Clin Invest 1989; 84:1843–1848.
68. Sweezey N, Mawdsley C, Ghibu F, Song L, Buch S, Moore A, Antakly T, Post M. Differential regulation of glucocorticoid receptor expression by ligand in fetal rat lung cells. Pediatr Res 1995; 38:506–512.
69. Ingbar DH, Weeks CB, Gilmore-Hebert M, et al. Developmental regulation of Na,K-ATPase in rat lung. Am J Physiol (Lung) 1996; 270:L619–L629.
72. Mak JCW, Nishikawa M, Barnes PJ. Glucocorticoids increase beta-2-adrenergic receptor transcription in human lung. Am J Physiol 1995; 268:L41–L46.
73. Whitsett JA, Darovec-Beckerman C, Adams K, et al. Thyroid dependent maturation of beta-adrenergic receptors in the rat lung. Biochem Biophys Res Commun 1980; 97:913–917.
74. Krochmal EM, Barker PM, Gatzy JT. Effects of hormones on potential difference and liquid balance across explants from proximal and distal fetal rat lung. J Physiol 1993; 463:647–665.
75. Sakuma T, Folkesson HG, Suzuki S, Okaniwa G, Fujimura S, Matthay MA. Beta-adrenergic agonist stimulated alveolar fluid clearance in ex vivo human and rat lungs. Am J Respir Crit Care Med 1997; 155:506–512.
76. Berthiaume Y. Effects of exogenous cAMP and aminophylline on alveolar and lung liquid clearance in anesthetized sheep. J Appl Physiol 1991; 70:2490–2497.
77. Crandall ED, Heming TA, Palombo RL, Goodman BE. Effects of terbutaline on sodium transport in isolated perfused rat lung. J Appl Physiol 1986; 60:289–294.
78. Lasnier J, Wangensteen OD, Schmitz LS, Gross CR, Ingbar DH. Terbutaline stimulates alveolar fluid resorption in hyperoxic lung injury. J Appl Physiol, 1996; 81:1723–1729.
80. Matthay MA, Wiener-Kronish JP. Intact epithelial barrier function is critical for the resolution of alveolar edema in humans. Am Rev Respir Dis 1990; 142:1250–1257.
81. Russo RM, Lubman RL, Crandall ED. Evidence for amiloride-sensitive sodium channels in alveolar epithelial cells. Am J Physiol 1992; 262:L405–L411.
83. Borok Z, Hami A, Danto SI, Lubman RL, Kim KJ, Crandall ED. Effects of EGF on alveolar epithelial junctional permeability and active sodium transport. Am J Physiol (Lung) 1996; 270:L559–L565.
84. Tibayan FA, Chesnutt AN, Folkesson HG, Eandi J, Matthay MA. Dobutamine increases alveolar liquid clearance in ventilated rats by beta O_2 receptor stimulation. Am J Respir Crit Care Med 1997; 156:438–444.
85. Bland RD. Lung epithelial ion transport and fluid movement during the perinatal period. Am J Physiol (Lung) 1990; 259:L30–L37.
86. Bland RD, Nielson DW. Developmental changes in lung epithelial ion transport and liquid movement. Annu Rev Physiol 1992; 54:373–394.
86a. Gross I. Regulation of fetal lung maturation. Am J Physiol (Lung) 1990; 259: L337–L344.

87. O'Brodovich H. Epithelial ion transport in the fetal and perinatal lung. Am J Physiol (Cell) 1991; 261:C555–C564.
88. O'Brodovich H, Staub O, Rossier BC, Geering K, Kraehenbul J-P. Ontogeny of alpha-1 and beta-1 isoforms of Na-K-ATPase in fetal distal rat lung epithelium. Am J Physiol 1993; 264:C1137–C1143.
89. O'Brodovich H, Canessa C, Ueda J, Rafii B, Rossier BC, Edelson J. Expression of the epithelial Na channel in the developing rat lung. Am J Physiol 1993; 265:C491–C496.
89a. Orser BA, Bertlik M, Fedorko L, O'Brodovich HM. Non-selective cation channel in fetal alveolar type II epithelium. Biochim Biophys Acta 1991; 1094:1926.
90. Crump RG, Askew GR, Wert SE, Lingrel JB, Joiner CH. In situ localization of sodium-potassium ATPase mRNA in developing mouse lung epithelium. Am J Physiol (Lung) 1995; 269:L299–L308.
91. Bland RD, Boyd CAR. Cation transport in lung epithelial cells derived from fetal, newborn, and adult rabbits. J Appl Physiol 1986; 61:507–515.
92. Chapman DL, Widdicombe JH, Bland RD. Developmental differences in rabbit lung epithelial cell Na,K-ATPase. Am J Physiol 1990; 259:L481–L487.
93. Tessier GJ, Lester GD, Langham MR, Cassin S. Ion transport properties of fetal sheep alveolar epithelial cells in monolayer culture. Am J Physiol 1996; 270: L1008–L1016.
94. Tchepichev S, Ueda J, Canessa C, Rossier BC, O'Brodovich HM. Lung epithelial Na channel subunits are differentially regulated during development and by steroids. Am J Physiol 1995; 269:C805–C812.
95. Pitkanen O, Tanswell AK, Downey G, O'Brodovich H. Increased PO_2 alters the bioelectric properties of fetal distal lung epithelium. Am J Physiol 1996; 270: L1060–L1066.
96. Hummler E, Barker P, Gatzy J, Beermann F, Verdumo C, Schmidt A, Boucher R, Rossier BC. Early death due to defective neonatal lung liquid clearance in alpha-ENaC-deficient mice. Nature Genet 1996; 12:325–329.
97. Cole TJ, Blendy JA, Monaghan AP, Krieglstein K, Schmid W, Aguzzi A, Fantuzzi G, Hummler E, Unsicker K, Schutz G. Targeted disruption of the glucocorticoid receptor gene blocks adrenergic chromaffin cell development and severely retards lung maturation. Genes Dev 1995; 9:1608–1621.
98. O'Brodovich HM. The role of active Na transport by lung epithelium in the clearance of airspace fluid. New Horizons 1995; 3:240–247.
99. Ballard RA, Ballard PL, Creasy RK, Padbury J, Polk DH, Bracken M, Moya FR, Gross I. Respiratory disease in very low birthweight infants after prenatal TRH and glucocorticoid. Lancet 1992; 330:510–515.
100. Moya FR, Gross I. Combined hormonal therapy for the prevention of respiratory distress syndrome and its consequences. Semin Perinatol 1993; 17:267–274.
101. Barker PM, Markiewicz M, Parker KA, Walters DV, Strang LB. Synergistic action of triiodothyronine and hydrocortisone on epinephrine-induced reabsorption of fetal lung liquid. Pediatr Res 1990; 27:588–591.
102. Barker PM, Strang LB, Walters DV. The role of thyroid hormones in maturation of the adrenaline-sensitive lung liquid reabsorptive mechanism in fetal sheep. J Physiol 1990; 424:473–485.

103. Liggins GC, Schellenberg J, Manzai M, Kitterman JA, Lee CC. Synergism of cortisol and TRH in lung maturation in fetal sheep. J Appl Physiol 1988; 65:1880–1884.
104. Warburton D, Parton L, Buckley S. Combined effects of corticosteroid, thyroid hormones and beta-agonist on surfactant, pulmonary mechanics & beta-receptor binding in fetal lamb lung. Pediatr Res 1988; 24:166–170.
105. Pinter E, Peyman JA, Snow K, Jamieson JD, Warshaw JB. Effects of maternal diabetes on fetal rat lung ion transport. Contribution of alveolar and bronchiolar epithelial cells to Na,K-ATPase. J Clin Invest 1991; 87:821–830.
106. Ingbar DH, Wendt CH. The sodium pump and oxidant stress: if only it were so simple. J Lab Clin Med 1997; 130:119–122.
106a. Rotenberg M, Gewolb IH. Reversal of lung maturational delay in the fetus of the diabetic rat using T3 or dexamethasone. Biol Neonate 1993; 64:318–324.
107. Olivera WG, Ridge KM, Sznajder JI. Lung liquid clearance and Na,K-ATPase during acute hyperoxia and recovery in rats. Am J Respir Crit Care Med 1995; 152:1229–1234.
108. Sznajder JI, Olivera WG, Ridge KM, Ruschman DH. Mechanisms of lung liquid clearance during hyperoxia in isolated rat lungs. Am J Respir Crit Care Med 1995; 151:1519–1525.
109. Zheng LP, Du RS, Goodman BE. Effects of acute hyperoxic exposure on solute fluxes across the blood-gas barrier in rat lungs. J Appl Physiol 1997; 82:240–247.
110. Garat C, Meignan M, Matthay MA, Luo DF, Jayr C. Alveolar epithelial fluid clearance mechanisms are intact after moderate hyperoxic lung injury in rats. Chest 1997; 111:1381–1388.
111. Carter EP, Wangensteen OD, O'Grady SM, Ingbar DH. Effects of hyperoxia on type II cell Na,K-ATPase function and expression. Am J Physiol (Lung) 1997; 272:L542–L551.
112. Carter EP, Wangensteen OD, Dunitz JM, Ingbar DH. Hyperoxic effects on alveolar sodium resorption & lung Na,K-ATPase. Am J Physiol (Lung) 1997; 273: L1191–L1202.
113. Wendt CH, Towle H, Sharma R, Gick G, Kawakami K, Ingbar DH. Regulation of Na, K-ATPase gene expression in hyperoxia. Am J Physiol (Cell) 1998; 273: C356–C364.
114. Haskell JF, Yue G, Benos DJ, Matalon S. Upregulation of sodium conductive pathways in alveolar type II cells in sublethal hyperoxia. Am J Physiol 1994; 266: L30–L37.
115. Yue G, Russell WJ, Benos DJ, Jackson RM, Olman MA, Matalon S. Increased expression of sodium channels in alveolar type II cells of hyperoxic rats. Proc Natl Acad Sci USA 1995; 92:8418–8422.
116. Olivera W, Ridge K, Wood LDH, Sznajder JI. Active sodium transport and alveolar epithelial Na-K-ATPase increase during subacute hyperoxia in rats. Am J Physiol 1994; 266:L577–L584.
116a. Yue G, Matalon S. Mechanisms and sequelae of increased alveolar fluid clearance in hyperoxic rats. Am J Physiol (Lung) 1997; 272:L407–L412.
117. Harris ZL, Ridge KM, Gonzalez-Flecha B, Gottlieb L, Zucker A, Sznajder JI. Hyperbaric oxygenation upregulates rat lung Na,K-ATPase. Eur Respir J 1996; 9: 472–477.

118. Zuege K, Suzuki S, Berthiaume Y. Increase of lung Na-K-ATPase activity during recovery from high permeability pulmonary edema. Am J Physiol 1996; 271: L896–L909.
119. Sciuto AM, Strickland PT, Kennedy TP, Guo YL, Gurtner GH. Intratracheal administrating of DBcAMP attenuates edema formation in phosgene-induced acute lung injury. J Appl Physiol 1996; 80:149–157.
120. Sznajder JI, Ridge KM, Harris AL, Olivera W, Curiel C, Rutschman DH. Alveolar type II cell Na,K-ATPase is upregulated during mechanical ventilation-induced pulmonary edema. Chest 1994; 105:115S–117S.
121. Kim KJ, Suh DJ. Asymmetric effects of H_2O_2 on alveolar epithelial barrier properties. Am J Physiol 1995; 264:L308–L315.
122. Hu P, Ischiropoulos H, Beckman JS, Matalon S. Peroxynitrite inhibition of oxygen consumption and sodium transport in alveolar type II cells. Am J Physiol (Lung) 1994; 266:L628–L634.
123. Gonzalez-Flecha B, Evelson P, Ridge K, Sznajder JI. Hydrogen peroxide increases Na/K-ATPase function in alveolar type II cells. Biochim Biophys Acta 1996; 1290: 46–52.
124. Compeau DG, Rotstein OD, Tohda H, Marunaka Y, Rafii B, Slutsky AS, O'Brodovich H. Endotoxin-stimulated alveolar macrophages impair lung epithelial Na transport by an L-Arg-dependent mechanism. Am J Physiol (Cell) 1994; 266:C1330–C1341.
125. Guzman MJ, Fang MZ, Tan SS, Ingelfinger JR, Garg LC. Autocrine inhibition of Na/K-ATPase by nitric oxide in mouse proximal tubule epithelial cells. J Clin Invest 1995; 95:2083–2088.
126. Planes C, Friedlander G, Loiseau A, Amiel C, Clerici C. Inhibition of Na-K-ATPase activity after prolonged hypoxia in an alveolar epithelial cell line. Am J Physiol 1996; 271:L70–L78.
127. Planes C, Escoubet B, Blot-Chabaud M, Friedlander G, Farman N, Clerici C. Hypoxia downregulates expression and activity of epithelial sodium channels in rat alveolar epithelial cells. Am J Respir Cell Mol Biol 1997; 17:508–518.
128. Robison T, Kim KJ. Enhancement of airway epithelial Na,K-ATPase activity by NO_2 and protective role of nordihydroguaiaretic acid. Am J Physiol (Lung) 1996; 270:L266–L272.
129. Elliott SJ, Schilling WP. Oxidant stress alters Na pump and Na-K-Cl cotransporter activities in vascular endothelial cells. Am J Physiol 1992; 263:L613–L621.
130. Azarian R, Clerici C, Couette S, Griedlander G, Amiel C. Lipopolysaccharides stimulate Na-dependent transport in alevolar cells and protect against oxidant injury. J Cell Physiol 1995; 163:328–338.
131. Lutsenk S, Daoud S, Kaplan JH. Identification of two conformationally sensitive cysteine residues at the extracellular surface of the Na,K-ATPase alpha subunit. J Biol Chem 1997; 272:5249–5255.
132. Haddock PS, Shattock MJ, Hearse DJ. Modulation of cardiac Na-K pump current: role of protein and nonprotein sulfhydryl redox status. Am J Physiol 1995; 269: H297–H307.
133. Julin CM, Zimmerman JJ, Sundaram V, Chobanian MC. Activated neutrophils inhibit Na-K-ATPase in canine renal basolateral membrane. Am J Physiol 1992; 262:C1364–C1370.

17

Use of Isolated Lungs to Clarify the Mechanisms by Which Alveolar Edema Is Resolved

GEORGES SAUMON

Institut National de la Santé et de la Recherche Médicale
Paris, France

I. Introduction

The complex architecture of the distal lung makes it difficult to study transport properties of the alveolar epithelium using the usual methods (e.g., Ussing chambers) employed for other epithelia. Therefore, cultures of alveolar type II cells have been used as a model of the native epithelium in studies designed to understand the fundamental mechanisms of alveolar transepithelial solute transport and the resulting movement of water. However, type II cells cover only 5% of alveolar surface in vivo and undergo a phenotypic shift in culture that may influence their transport properties. The rate of active transport by monolayers of cultured alveolar pneumocytes is low (a few microampere/cm^2) and depends on the culture conditions. The tightness of these monolayers is similarly affected, with resistances ranging from a few hundred to 2000 ohm cm^2 (1,2).

The use of fluid-filled, isolated lungs goes some way to overcome these limitations. The slow rate of transport is offset by the huge exchange surface area of the lungs, which allows easier measurement of solute and water fluxes. The isolated lung is advantageous compared to in vivo studies because it allows the use of toxic compounds and enables the composition and volume of the basolateral medium (perfusate) to be controlled, so that the fluxes across the distal airspace epithelia in both the apical-to-basolateral and the reverse direction can be measured. Limiting the volume of perfusate produces a system suitable for obtaining precise estimates of the fluxes of high-molecular-weight solutes and for studying the relationship between altered permeability and fluid clearance. The main cause of variability in isolated lung studies is nonuniformity. Nonuniform perfusion is not important when measuring fluid absorption, because it is unaffected by complete interruption of perfusion (3). However, nonuniform perfusion may influence solute flux measurements by reducing the effective exchange surface area, resulting in basolateral solute concentrations or tracer activities differing from those of the perfusate. The fluid instilled into airspaces may not evenly fill the lungs, and both perfusion and the epithelial transport rate probably vary from place to place. For example, there appears to be no or minimal fluid absorption in subpleural alveoli (4). Passive fluxes in the apical-to-basolateral direction have sometimes been found slightly larger than those measured in the other direction (5), a difference that has been ascribed to nonuniform filling of alveoli facing a more homogeneous perfusion distribution. However, the acceptable reproducibility within and between laboratories, despite somewhat different methods, together with the stability of the preparation (as indicated by the reproducibility of most measurements over 1 to 2 hours), suggests that nonuniformity has no important consequences. One of its usual significant causes, unstirred layers, is probably absent from fluid-filled lungs because of the small size of the alveoli.

II. Methods for Studying Alveolar Transport Using Isolated Lungs

Most studies have been performed with isolated-perfused rat lungs. The lungs and heart are generally removed en bloc from the thorax of the animal and placed under humidified and thermostated conditions. The alveoli are filled with an artificial solution via the trachea. These lungs are usually perfused via the pulmonary artery, the venous effluent either flowing out freely or being recirculated. There are minor differences between preparations used in different studies. These concern how perfusion and tracheal instillation are performed and how the alveolar instillate is recovered. Lungs have sometimes been perfused with whole blood oxygenated by a donor rat (6,7). This preparation resembles fluid-filled lobes in vivo. Bronchial perfusion and lymphatic drainage are maintained. However, the precise composition of the basolateral medium is not set, and certain inhibitors of ion transport cannot be used because of their cardiac effects.

The more general form of isolated lungs makes it easy to control the composition of the media bathing the two (apical-alveolar and basolateral-vascular) sides of the distal lung epithelium. Airway pressure and the flow rate of perfusate can be controlled and monitored. The perfusion rate is determined by the physiological condition of the donor rat in the cross-circulation preparation. Lungs are usually instilled and perfused with the same physiological solution buffered with bicarbonate, phosphate, or in some instances N-2-hydroxyethylpiperazine-N′-2-ethanesulfonic acid (HEPES). Albumin is always added to the perfusate to preserve capillary permeability, sometimes together with another macromolecule, or a small proportion of whole blood. The lungs are perfused by gravimetric pressure or by using a roller pump at a rate of 8 to 12 ml/min. When perfusate is recirculated there is a risk of interference from the accumulating metabolites. Perfusion volumes ranged from 12 to 300 ml. When bicarbonate was used as the buffer, perfusate was equilibrated with 95% O_2/5% CO_2. Differences between protocols have only limited influence on the results obtained and the conclusions drawn from these experiments.

A. Transepithelial Transport

Fluid Transport

Several methods have been used to estimate fluid movements across the distal airspace barrier. These movements are usually assessed by the dilution method, in which changes in instillate volume are deduced from changes in the concentration of an impermeable tracer (8). The gravimetric method does not allow precise estimation of alveolar fluid transport, but may indicate whether fluid enters or leaves the lungs (9). Airspace fluid absorption has recently been obtained by direct measurement of the amount of fluid contained in a reservoir tightly sealed to a large airway (10,11).

The basic assumption of the dilution method is that the distal lung epithelium is quite impermeable to macromolecules. This assumption is reasonable for exchange times of up to 2 hours. The liquid flow out of airspaces, J_w, is thus given by the equation:

$$J_w = V_{i(o)}\,({}^*C_{i(t)} - {}^*C_{i(o)})/({}^*C_{i(t)}\,\Delta t) \qquad (1)$$

where $V_{i(o)}$ is the instilled volume and ${}^*C_{i(o)}$ and ${}^*C_{i(t)}$ the (impermeable) tracer concentration or activity at the beginning and end of a period Δt.

To compare this liquid flow among species or animals of various sizes, it is expressed as a percentage of the instilled fluid, as a flux by division with the assumed exchange surface area of airspaces (5000 cm^2 for a 300-g rat, for example), or standardized by the dry weight of lungs.

Passive Solute Transport

Several models have been developed to calculate the unidirectional movement of solutes across the alveolar barrier. More often, a two-compartment model is used to describe the transport of species between airspace instillate and perfusate:

$$d^*C_i/dt = PA\ (^*C_p - {^*C_i})/V_i \tag{2}$$

$$d^*C_p/dt = PA\ (^*C_i - {^*C_p})/V_p \tag{3}$$

in which $^*C_i$ and $^*C_p$ are tracer activities in the instillate and perfusate, respectively, PA is the apparent permeability-surface area product of the traced species (unidirectional flux), and V_p is perfusate volume. Because fluid resorption rate is slow, the instillate volume V_i is sometimes assumed to be constant. Small solute unidirectional fluxes are sometimes derived from the rate at which tracers added to alveolar instillate appear in the perfusate (9,12,13):

$$C_p = V_i\ C_i(1 - e^{-kt})/(V_i + V_p) \tag{4}$$

where $k = PA/(1/V_i + 1/V_p)$. A symmetrical equation has been used to describe the appearance of tracers added to the perfusate in alveolar instillate (5).

Unidirectional fluxes have also been calculated from the rate at which tracer disappears from the instillate (8,13–15). A simple equation for PA was derived (8) assuming that perfusate volume was infinite and taking into account alveolar volume changes (symbols as in Eq. 1):

$$PA = -\ Jw\ [1 + \ln\ (*C_{i(t)}/*C_{i(o)})/\ln((V_{i(o)} + Jw\Delta t)/V_{i(o)}] \tag{5}$$

Equations 4 and 5 give "apparent" PA products that sum the active and passive fluxes. If the tracer does not enter cells, these equations describe the passive transport properties of the epithelium.

The passive unidirectional flux of a species transported by the epithelial cells can be obtained when active transport is inhibited (for example for Na^+ by adding, as detailed below, the inhibitors amiloride and phlorizin to the instillate). However, the assumptions that fluid absorption is isosmotic and that the luminal Na^+ or Cl^- concentration does not vary significantly during alveolar fluid clearance (which has been verified consistently), allow calculation of the Na^+ or Cl^- passive permeability in the absence of inhibitors (8):

$$\text{passive PA component} = -Jw\ [\ln(*C_{i(t)}/*C_{i(o)})/\ln((V_{i(o)} + Jw\Delta t)/V_{i(o)})] \tag{6}$$

This approach provides estimates that are reasonably close to those obtained when ion transport is inhibited. Tracer activities in the perfusate may not be negligible when fluxes are high. The differential system (Eqs. 1, 2) must then be numerically integrated to solve for PA (16).

Active Solute Transport

Knowledge of changes in instillate volume can be used to calculate net ion fluxes (the mass equation using the "cold" ion concentrations and the change in instilled volume). Assuming that fluid transport is isosmotic and the consequence of net NaCl transport, net Na^+ or Cl^- fluxes are considered to reflect the rate of active transport (6).

The active Na^+ transport rate can also be deduced from the total, unidirectional Na^+ flux out of the alveoli (apparent PA) and the PA for mannitol. This calculation is based on several assumptions, the most fundamental being that passive Na^+ transport takes place through the same aqueous pathways across the epithelium as that of small hydrophilic solutes like mannitol. The main advantage of this analysis is that it allows comparison of active Na^+ transport rates between experimental conditions in which the passive permeability differs. It is assumed that the departures from linearity of the relationship between Na^+ and mannitol PAs due to size and charge selectivity and to transepithelial Na^+ electrochemical potential difference can be neglected for limited changes in passive permeability. The resulting estimates of the rate of active Na^+ transport under different experimental conditions i are obtained by covariance analysis of Na^+ PA (dependent variable) with mannitol PA as the covariate (16). Covariance analysis provides a common slope, b, of the relationship between unidirectional fluxes of Na^+ and mannitol, which reflects the size selectivity of the aqueous passive pathway (b would be 2 for free diffusion in water) and elevations, a_i, which represent the active Na^+ transport rate under each experimental condition:

$$\text{Active Na}^+\ \text{PA}_i + \text{Passive Na}^+\ \text{PA}_i = a_i + b\ \text{mannitol PA}_i \qquad (7)$$

Attempts to estimate alveolar ion transport by electrophysiological methods have been disappointing. The potential in fluid-filled subpeural alveoli reflects more airway transport than alveolar epithelium transport (17).

III. Application to Studies on Ion Transport

A. Alveolar Sodium Transport

Apical Pathways

Amiloride-Sensitive Transport

Amiloride and its analogs are widely used to interfere with Na^+ transport because they efficiently block epithelial Na^+ channels and inhibit Na^+-H^+

exchange. If amiloride is placed in the alveolar instillate of rat lungs at concentrations of at least 10^{-4} M, the unidirectional (total, sum of the active and passive components) flux of Na^+ out of the alveoli is reduced by 10% (8) to 35% (9) and net Na^+ efflux falls by 30% to 70% in isolated rat lungs (8,14) and by 60% in lungs in situ (6). This effect of amiloride is ascribed to the depression of transcellular, active Na^+ transport because either passive permeability is unaffected (Fig. 1) or after correcting for paracellular permeability changes by the covariance analysis model, amiloride decreases active Na^+ transport by about 60% (16). Na^+ transport is similarly inhibited in hamster lungs (18) by luminal amiloride. The presence in the apical membrane of adult alveolar epithelial cells of Na^+ channels with low sensitivity to the inhibitor (19) accounts for this effect.

Amiloride-Insensitive Transport

However, even high amiloride concentrations do not completely abolish active epithelial Na^+ transport; there is always a residual 40% in rats (6). This incomplete inhibition suggests that there are other pathways for removing Na^+ from airspaces. One striking observation is that the glucose concentration of the instillate of isolated rat lungs always rapidly falls well below that of the perfusate (3,6) or remains low when it is initially absent (20). Several lines of evidence suggest that there is apical Na-glucose cotransport, as in the intestinal or kidney epithelia. Glucose is no longer removed when Na^+ is replaced by choline in the instillate or when phlorizin, a specific inhibitor of this cotransport system, is added to the solution (6). The strongest evidence is that the glucose analog alpha-methylglucose, which is specifically cotransported with Na^+ but does not

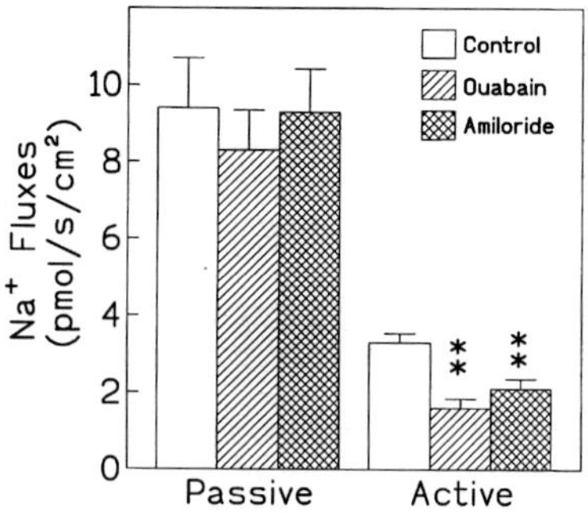

Figure 1 Effect of inhibiting Na^+ transport on alveolar fluid absorption in isolated rat lungs. Active Na^+ flux is significantly inhibited by basolateral ouabain or apical amiloride (** $P < .01$). The inhibitors do not affect passive Na^+ fluxes (or mannitol PA, not shown). (Redrawn from Ref. 8.)

enter cells by facilitated diffusion, is removed faster from airspaces than are other analogs that do not share this pathway (21). Finally, luminal glucose stimulates transepithelial Na^+ transport (18,22). The cotransporter is also present in the rat tracheal epithelium (23).

Basolateral Pathways

Ouabain, which inhibits Na,K-ATPase, significantly reduces the net and unidirectional Na^+ fluxes out of airspaces (8,9) when it is added to the perfusate of isolated lungs. Paracellular permeability remains unaffected, indicating that it is transcellular Na^+ transport that is actually depressed. However, inhibition of Na^+ transport is incomplete, probably because the rat enzyme is resistant to ouabain.

Rate of Na^+ Transport

Most of estimates of unidirectional Na^+ fluxes (expressed as apparent Na^+ permeability) have been obtained in isolated rat lungs (6,8,9,13,14,16,21,24). There is no appreciable difference between the estimates obtained from measuring the rate of appearance of tracer in the perfusate and those based on the disappearance of tracer from the instillate (13,14,16). The unidirectional Na^+ flux is 10 to 15 pmol/sec/cm^2 assuming the alveolar surface 5000 cm^2. Active Na^+ transport is estimated to be 3 mL/h/g dry lung weight, or 6 pmol/sec/cm^2 using the covariance analysis model (16), which compares favorably with the estimated rate of net Na^+ removal slightly over 4 pmol/s/cm^2 (6,8,14). Values for unidirectional Na^+ fluxes have also been obtained in dogs (25), hamsters (18), and mice (26). Comparison with the rat data requires precise estimation of the exchange alveolar surface area which depends on the size of the animal for a given amount of lung tissue (27).

B. Potassium Transport

Potassium movements across the alveolar epithelium are complex, and their connection with the mechanism of alveolar fluid clearance is unclear. The potassium concentration in the epithelial lining fluid has been estimated to be twice that of plasma by direct puncture of alveoli (28) in rabbits and three times the plasma concentration by bronchoalveolar lavage in rats (29). These observations, together with the low transepithelial electrical potential difference across alveolar epithelium (28), suggest that K^+ is secreted into the aerated alveoli. However, a small K^+ absorption, rather than secretion, has been reported for rabbit (30) and rat (7) fluid-filled isolated lungs.

Addition of the K^+ channel blocker Ba^{2+} to the airspace instillate increases K^+ absorption from 0.23 to 0.37 pmol/sec/cm^2 (7), suggesting that there are two opposite K^+ fluxes, and that inhibition of a masked K^+ secretion with Ba^{2+} causes this K^+ absorption enhancement. The K^+ absorption from alveoli turns into a secretion when ouabain is added to the instillate. Luminal ouabain also decreases the unidirectional flux of ^{86}Rb (which traces K^+ movement) out of airspaces by more than 50%, without affecting passive permeability or fluid absorption. These results suggest that alveolar K^+ is continuously pumped out of airspaces by an active mechanism which is sensitive to ouabain (7). This pump may be a Na,K-ATPase. However, a Na,K-ATPase has only been demonstrated in the basolateral membrane of alveolar epithelial cells to date (31,32). It is also possible that the apical K^+ pump is a K,H-ATPase, since a form of this pump has been described in the apical membrane of guinea pig colon epithelial cells, which is inhibited by ouabain (33). The presence of a K,H-ATPase would account for both K^+ absorption from and H^+ secretion into alveoli, and could explain why the pH of the epithelial lining fluid is low (34). This possibility was suggested by Effros et al. (30). However, whereas there is an omeprazole-sensitive ^{86}Rb influx in guinea-pig pneumocytes, suggesting the presence of a K,H-ATPase in this species, no such transport activity has been demonstrated in rat pneumocytes (35).

A model of the of alveolar epithelium (7,36) has been proposed to account for the complexity of K^+ transport across the rat alveolar epithelium. This model includes two epithelial cell populations—one for Na^+ absorption, the other for K^+ absorption. Interestingly, this corresponds well with the finding of two populations of type II cells that differ in the specific properties of their K^+ channels (37).

C. Alveolar Chloride Transport

None of the studies using isolated lungs have demonstrated transcellular Cl^- transport. Indeed, neither bumetanide (which inhibits Na^+ -K^+ -$2Cl^-$ cotransport), DIDS, or SITS (which interfere with anion exchange systems) nor acetazolamide (which inhibits carbonic anhydrase) affects Cl^- unidirectional flux, whether they are placed in the instillate or in the perfusate (unpublished observations). The unidirectional Cl^- flux out of rat alveoli was estimated to be 15 pmol/sec/cm^2 (6).

IV. Alveolar Liquid Absorption

A. Relationship to Active Solute Transport

Isolated lungs have provided compelling evidence that the absorption of alveolar liquid is linked to transepithelial Na^+ transport. Interference with any of the above Na^+ transport pathways affects the rate of absorption (Fig. 2). The relative change in fluid absorption usually corresponds to that of the Na^+ flux. Inhibition

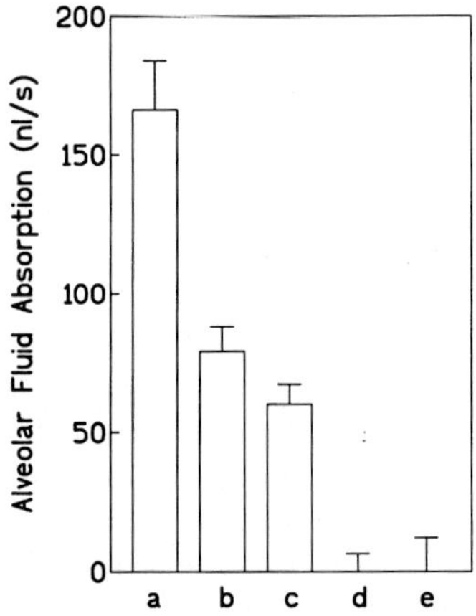

Figure 2 Influence of interference with apical epithelial Na^+ transport pathways on alveolar fluid absorption. (a) Control conditions; (b) replacement of glucose by mannitol in the alveolar instillate; (c) addition of 10^{-4} M amiloride to the instillate; (d) no glucose + amiloride; (e) replacement of Na^+ by choline in the instillate. (Redrawn from Ref. 6.)

of the amiloride-sensitive and amiloride-insensitive (by phlorizin or the omission of glucose) apical Na^+ pathways, or replacing Na^+ in the instillate with choline, completely abolishes alveolar fluid clearance (6). These results suggest that Na^+ transport is the main, if not the only, determinant of the absorption. The finding that active Na^+ (obtained by covariance) and fluid fluxes are significantly correlated (Fig. 3) provides additional evidence. Finally, inhibition of enzymatic

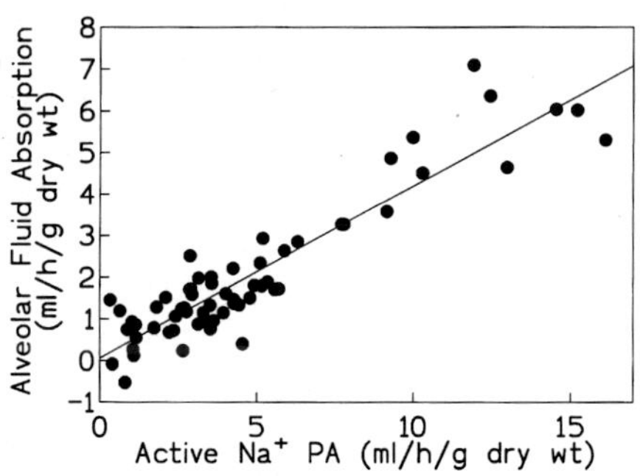

Figure 3 Correlation between alveolar fluid absorption in isolated rat lungs and active epithelial Na^+ transport (expressed as a PA product) determined with the covariance model ($r = .92$, $P < .001$). (Redrawn from Ref. 16.)

activity by cooling rat lungs to 4°C results in the complete arrest of alveolar fluid absorption (15).

Fluid absorption is the consequence of the difference in osmotic pressure developed across the epithelium by the active transport of Na^+. It has been shown in isolated lungs that the reflection coefficient of the epithelium to small hydrophilic solutes like electrolytes is probably close to unity (25,38), suggesting that transport by solvent drag is negligible. Thus, a concentration difference of Na across the epithelium of only 1 mmol/L would result in a pressure difference of nearly 25 cm H_2O. Even if the overall rate of Na^+ transport is low, it may be higher in places (for example, near type II cells) and be a powerful force for driving water. The permeability of the alveolar epithelium to water is several hundred times greater than its permeability to Na^+ or small hydrophilic solutes (13,39), probably because of the presence of aqueous channels in epithelial cell membranes (40). This is why a concentration difference of solutes across the epithelium results in the movement of pure water, and the difference is lost in less than 5 min (38).

All studies report similar rates of fluid absorption for a given instilled volume. Rat lungs resorb bicarbonate solutions at about 30 pl/sec/cm^2 (6,8,13,14). Increasing the volume of instillate increases fluid absorption proportionally (41) probably because of recruitment of empty alveoli. Fluid absorption is lower when HEPES is used as the buffer (3,30) in both rat and rabbit lungs. However, it is not affected by replacing bicarbonate with phosphate (6). The rate of alveolar fluid absorption (and Na^+ transport) is low compared, for example, to that of the proximal tubule, which is 65,000 pl/sec/cm^2 (42). The net K^+ transport rates are too low to significantly affect alveolar fluid movements (7,36). However, the long-term effect of interference with K^+ transport has not been evaluated.

There are probably interspecies differences in both the mechanisms and the rate of alveolar fluid absorption. Isolated rabbit lungs transport fluid slightly more slowly than rat lungs (30), while mouse lungs rapidly clear the fluid instilled into airspaces—about twice as fast as rats for the same amount of lung tissue (26). It may be that the exchange surface area per unit volume of these lungs is greater than that of the rat lungs because the mouse alveolus is smaller (27). Surprisingly, although SGLT1 mRNA is detected in mouse lungs, suggesting the presence of Na-glucose cotransport, luminal glucose has no influence on alveolar fluid resorption (26). In hamsters, only amiloride-sensitive Na^+ absorption was evidenced (18). Species also differ in their response to hormonal stimulation (see Sec. VI).

Using rat lungs, several studies have demonstrated that airspace glucose influences fluid absorption (6,22,43). The rate of fluid absorption is 15.4 pl/sec/cm^2 when the amiloride-sensitive pathway is blocked. It has been calculated that the absorption of glucose alone would have produced absorption at a rate of only 2.5 pl/sec/cm^2 (6). The remaining absorption is the consequence of cotransport of Na^+ with glucose: Na^+ that enters the apical cell membrane with glucose is actively pumped out by the basolateral Na,K-ATPase. The enhancement of transepithelial Na^+ transport accounts for four-fifths of the glucose-induced increase in fluid absorption; the removal of glucose alone is responsible for the remaining one-fifth (43). It is unlikely that Na^+ and fluid fluxes are affected by luminal glucose because of increased glucose consumption and ATP availability because these fluxes are not depressed by inhibiting lung glycolysis (16).

The influence of lung Na^+ and ion transport on the formation of pulmonary edema has been studied in isolated rat lungs using a model of ischemia/reperfusion lung injury (44). Inhibition of lung Na^+ transport by amiloride and of Na^+ pump by ouabain significantly increases ischemia-reperfusion edema, whereas phlorizin is without effect. These inhibitors were added to the perfusate and reached the epithelial surface through alveolar edema fluid. Their effects might thus have not been restricted to epithelial cells. However, these observations suggest that ion transport acts as a further safety factor to attenuate the development of pulmonary edema.

B. Role of the Passive Movement of Solutes

Passive leakage through the paracellular pathway may be a shunt through which a backward Na^+ flux may alter the efficiency of transepithelial transport. It may also be the main, if not the only, way by which some solutes are removed from airspaces. Knowledge of the properties and possible modulation of the passive pathway is thus essential.

It has long been known that the alveolar epithelium is much tighter than the endothelium facing it (45). Some studies using isolated lungs concluded that there is no size selectivity of the alveolar barrier, because small hydrophilic solutes escaped from airspaces at rates proportional to their diffusion coefficients in free water (46), whereas other characterized the passive permeability as formed of one or several populations of aqueous pores (13,25). Berg et al. (13) calculated that the permeability to small hydrophilic solutes of rat alveolar barrier may be accounted for by a large population of very small pores (0.5 nm radius) and a small population of larger pores (3.4 nm radius). The size of these larger pores agrees with the value of the ratio of passive Na^+ to mannitol permeability (16). The passive permeability of the epithelium is remarkably small, comparable to that of other tight epithelia such as the urinary bladder. The electrical resistance deduced from permeability measurements is 18,000 $ohm.cm^2$ in rat lungs (6). However, this high value may be due to the huge surface covered by type I cells and the scarcity of intercellular junctions.

Despite this low permeability, the passive Na^+ flux was estimated to be $> 40\%$ unidirectional Na^+ flux under basal conditions, representing a significant parallel shunt (6,8) (Fig. 1). Passive Cl^- permeability is 1.5 times larger (6,8) than that of Na^+. Comparison of passive Na^+ and Cl^- permeability values suggest that the charge selectivity of this pathway is small.

The tightness of the epithelium explains why fluid movements are not governed by the same forces across the epithelium and the endothelium. As discussed above, a concentration difference of small solutes such as ions (or glucose) develops a large hydrostatic pressure difference across the alveolar epithelium, but not the endothelium. Whereas differences in protein concentrations play an important role in fluid balance across the microvasculature, these have negligible effects across the alveolar epithelial barrier. Macromolecule concentrations are too small (a few mmol/L) to counteract the differences in ion concentration resulting from transepithelial transport. In keeping with this deduction, fluid absorption rate does not differ when the alveolar instillate is Ringer solution or plasma (6). A striking illustration of this phenomenon was obtained by Effros et al. (47), who showed that transepithelial oncotic pressure differences of −65 to 65 mm Hg produced by manipulating airspace or perfusate albumin concentration did not influence alveolar fluid transport. This suggests that the increase in luminal protein concentration resulting from the resorption of alveolar edema has little influence on the clearance rate, at least during the first few hours of the process. Late removal of proteins from alveoli may, however, be a key event for the complete resolving of alveolar edema. Long-term alveolar fluid clearance in vivo is negatively correlated with alveolar oncotic pressure (48), suggesting that large concentrations of protein may have some influence.

Another consequence of the low passive permeability is that the luminal glucose concentration decreases during fluid absorption, the passive entry of glucose into airspaces down its concentration gradient being insufficient to compensate for its active removal by cotransport with Na^+. The steady alveolar glucose concentration in fluid-filled rat lungs is estimated to be 0.1 to 0.5 mmol/L, less than one-twentieth the perfusate concentration, and well below the apparent affinity constant of the cotransport system for glucose (20). A consequence of this low steady-state concentration is that the proportion of alveolar fluid resorption resulting from glucose removal progressively vanishes unless the glucose concentration into airspaces is somehow restored. This will be discussed in Section VIB. The low steady-state glucose concentration in fluid-filled lungs explains why inhibition of Na-glucose cotransport does not affect the fetal fluid absorption rate in newborn guinea-pigs (49).

V. Metabolic Requirements for Alveolar Fluid Absorption

Fluid absorption from alveoli is not markedly affected by the discontinuation of perfusion (3), indicating that pulmonary blood flow is not crucial for transepithelial solute transport. It also suggests that there is still considerable alveolar Na^+ transport under conditions of low O_2 supply and, thus, that the ATP produced by glycolysis may be sufficient to fuel epithelial transport. Lung tissue glycolytic activity and lactate production rate are high, even under aerobic conditions, for reasons not yet elucidated (50). This high glycolytic rate is not an absolute metabolic necessity for deep lung fluid balance because inhibition of glycolysis does not result in pulmonary edema (51). Lungs also tolerate complete anoxia well (52).

The Na^+ pump activity relies preferentially on glycolysis-derived ATP in some cell types with a high rate of aerobic glycolysis (53). In lungs, inhibition of glycolysis does not markedly affect alveolar Na^+ and fluid transport under baseline (i.e., in the absence of hormonal stimulation; see Sec. VI.A) conditions. Lipids are probably the alternative energy source for epithelial transport when glycolysis is inhibited. As pointed out by Tierney (54), the intense lipid metabolism of type II cells may be sufficient to supply mitochondria for hours. Inhibiting respiration (chemical anoxia) slows but does not abolish alveolar fluid absorption. Chemical anoxia results in a massive stimulation of lactate production (Pasteur effect). The ATP produced by the glycolytic pathway allows epithelial Na^+ transport to continue for at least 1 hour following metabolic inhibition (16). There is some increase in permeability to mannitol, but this is not sufficient to severely alter the barrier properties of the epithelium and, particularly, its reflection coefficient. Indeed, large increases in permeability do not seem to affect the capacity of Na^+ transport to drive alveolar fluid absorption (55,56) (Fig. 4b). Alveolar fluid absorption decreases after 1 hour of chemical anoxia, probably because of the lack of integrity of the endothelial layer and the development of pulmonary edema, as there is still a high level of active Na^+ transport by the alveolar epithelium.

Thus, alveolar epithelium transport properties, which are essential to life, are retained under severe metabolic conditions. A strong Pasteur effect allows the alveolar epithelium to maintain active Na^+ transport and fluid clearance for at least 1 hour under anoxic conditions.

VI. Modulation of Alveolar Ion and Fluid Transport in Isolated Lungs

A. Hormonal Modulation and Second Messengers

Few agents have been shown to affect alveolar ion and fluid transport in isolated lungs. The most extensively studied hormonal mediators are the β-adrenergic agonists (such as terbutaline or isoproterenol) and cell-permeable analogs of its intracellular second messenger cAMP, such as dibutyryl-cAMP (DBcAMP). The response to β-adrenergic agonists includes an increase in unidirectional Na^+

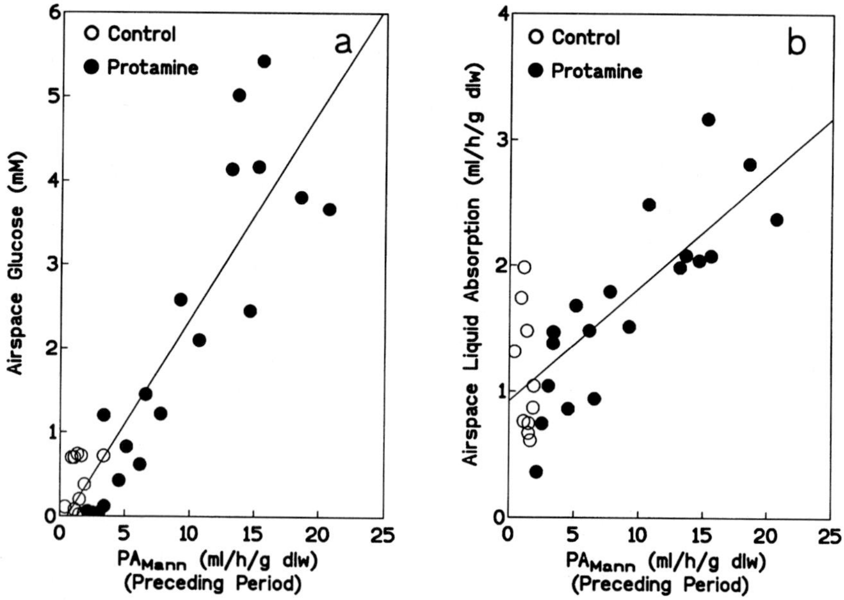

Figure 4 Effect of the apical application of 20 μM protamine in isolated rat lungs instilled with fluid that does not contain glucose. Glucose concentration in airspaces remains low in the absence of protamine (open circles). Protamine increases permeability to mannitol (PA_{Mann}) and disturbs glucose balance, allowing glucose to enter airspaces from the perfusate and raising the alveolar glucose concentration (a). As a consequence, alveolar fluid absorption is stimulated (b) by the start up of Na-glucose cotransport. (From Ref. 43.)

flux out of alveoli (9,12), alterations in alveolar K^+ transport (36), and stimulation of alveolar fluid resorption (3,13,14,24) in rat lungs. The rates of Na^+ and fluid transport are usually increased three- to fourfold over the basal level (Fig. 5). The response to terbutaline is inhibited by the β-adrenergic antagonist propanolol (3). β-adrenergic agonists increase glucose consumption and lactate production by the lung (16). However, the stimulation of fluid absorption is due to an increase in Na^+ transport through the amiloride-sensitive pathway, whereas Na^+ cotransport with glucose is unaffected or even slightly depressed (24). Thus, the increase in glucose uptake associated with this increased glycolysis probably does not occur by cotransport but by facilitated diffusion. Na^+ and fluid transports decrease significantly when glycolysis is inhibited with iodoacetate in the presence of isoproterenol, in contrast to the lack of effect of iodoacetate on these transports in the absence of hormonal stimulation. Further, inhibition of epithelial Na^+ transport with amiloride or ouabain also decreases lung lactate produc-

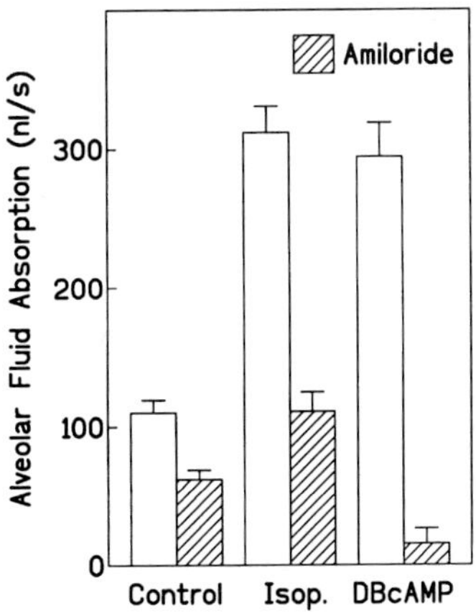

Figure 5 Stimulation of alveolar fluid absorption in isolated rat lungs by isoprotrerenol (Isop.) or 10^{-3} M DBcAMP ($P < .001$). Stimulation is abolished by inhibiting apical Na^+ transport with amiloride. (Redrawn from Ref. 24.)

tion under stimulated conditions (16). These observations suggest that alveolar fluid clearance during β-adrenergic stimulation depends more on extracellular glucose than in the unstimulated state.

The analog DBcAMP closely reproduces the effects of β-adrenergic agonists, with a large increase in fluid absorption (24,36) (Fig. 5) due to stimulation of Na^+ transport (57). The effect of DBcAMP depends on its concentration: 10^{-3} M always stimulates Na^+ transport, whereas 10^{-4} M does not elicit a complete response (24). This response is completely abolished by amiloride. The response to these mediators is species-specific: β-adrenergic agonists do not cause increase in alveolar Na^+ and fluid transport in isolated rabbit lungs (30) or hamster lungs (18).

The only humoral mediator that seems to depress alveolar Na^+ and liquid absorption is atrial natriuretic factor (ANF) (58). ANF induces the release of cGMP from the tissue and decreases the clearance rate by about 30% when added to the perfusate of isolated rat lungs. The unidirectional Na^+ flux is unaffected, probably because of an increase in the passive, paracellular component, since ANF increases mannitol permeability (by 50%) and the entry of fluorescein-labeled albumin into airspaces. It is unlikely that the small increase in the shunt, paracellular permeability, is responsible for this depressing effect. Greater changes do not alter alveolar fluid clearance (55,56). Adding ANF to the alveolar instillate slightly increases passive fluxes but does not affect fluid absorption.

Dystrophic hamsters have multiple abnormalities, including skeletal and cardiac muscle degeneration and alveolar hypoventilation. These hamsters also have low rates of alveolar sodium transport, greater passive alveolar permeability, and greater lung wet/dry weight ratios than normal animals (59). Cardiomyopathic hamsters have been shown to produce high amounts of ANF in response to hypoxia (60). It may be that the deep lung fluid balance abnormalities observed in dystrophic hamsters are due to increased ANF production.

The modulation of K^+ transport by β-adrenergic agonists is less well understood than that of Na^+ because of the complex movements of K^+ across alveolar epithelium. The response of isolated lungs to isoproterenol is time-dependent (36). K^+ is secreted into airspaces during the first 30 min after addition of the agonist to the perfusate, whereas secretion later turns into absorption. The effect of isoproterenol is reproduced by 10^{-3} M DBcAMP, whereas only K^+ secretion occurs with 10^{-4} M DBcAMP. As previously mentioned, 10^{-3} M DBcAMP increases Na^+ and fluid transport, whereas 10^{-4} M does not. The transitory K^+ secretion that occurs in response to isoproterenol or 10^{-3} M DBcAMP, as well as that produced by 10^{-4} M DBcAMP, is abolished when apical K^+ channels are blocked with Ba^{2+}, whereas the stimulation of K^+ absorption that occurs later is abolished by adding ouabain to the instillate. Thus, there seems to be a dose-dependent response to cAMP, with low concentrations resulting in the opening of apical K^+ channels and K^+ secretion, while higher concentrations stimulate both Na^+ and K^+ absorption (36). Because of this coordinated effect, alveolar K^+ concentration does not notably increase during the stimulation of alveolar fluid absorption. These results suggest that the alveolar epithelium may secrete K^+ when intracellular cAMP is moderately increased. Whether such a secretory mechanism is responsible for the elevated K^+ concentration in epithelial lining fluid (28) remains to be elucidated. The significance of these K^+ movements is not understood; they appear to be too small to significantly affect the resorption of alveolar edema.

Stimulation of the alveolar epithelium with β-adrenergic agonists or large doses of cAMP analogs sometimes increases paracellular permeability (24,36), but some researchers have not found such an effect (12,57). This increase in permeability occurred in isolated lungs perfused with blood or 4% blood cells. It may have been due to an indirect rather than a direct effect on alveolar epithelium. It has been reported that the polyamine spermine, which interferes with different signaling pathways (e.g., 61), increases both alveolar fluid absorption and paracellular permeability (56) in isolated rat lungs (see Sec. VI.B).

B. Physical and Chemical Agents

Hyperoxia is a widely used model of lung injury. Submitting rats to hyperoxia results in the proliferation of alveolar epithelial cells and upregulation of the expression of several genes in type II cells, including Na,K-ATPase (62) and Na^+ channels (63). Alveolar Na^+ transport and fluid absorption have been evaluated in isolated lungs (41,64) from rats subjected to 7 days of subacute (85%) hyperoxia. Unidirectional Na^+ flux is increased by 40% immediately after the hyperoxic period and remains above the control value for 7 more days. This increased flux is due both to the stimulation of active transport that parallels the upregulation of Na,K-ATPase expression in type II cells and to moderate changes in the passive permeability. The increased Na^+ flux occurs through the amiloride-sensitive pathway (64). Even more severe hyperoxia (95% for 60 hours) (11), sufficient to produce pulmonary edema and neutrophil infiltration, does not impair the resorption of fluid from airspaces. Alveolar resorption is higher that in control, normoxic animals and can be even more efficiently stimulated by terbutaline. This stimulation may be one mechanism by which lungs are protected against alveolar edema and maintain gas exchange during injury.

Several physical and chemicals agents increase the permeability of the alveolar epithelium. Lung inflation, even within the physiological range, results in an increase in alveolar permeability that exceeds the recruitment of alveolar surface area in aerated lungs (65). Static overinflation sometimes produced large leaks (66) (see Chap. 13). The rate of active alveolar fluid absorption, measured with the reservoir method, is slowed by lung inflation in vivo (10). Active fluid absorption stops when the inflating pressure is 9 cm H_2O, which corresponds to a total lung volume of 16 to 17 mL/kg body weight in these fluid-filled lungs—thus far from total lung capacity. These observations suggest that moderate stretching may influence lung liquid clearance. Repeated overinflation in vivo during mechanical ventilation results in permeability edema, with reversible increases in both endothelial and epithelial permeability, provided lesions are not too severe (29). Overinflation during mechanical ventilation also induces upregulation of Na,K-ATPase in type II cells (67). The effect of this type of lung injury on alveolar fluid clearance has not been evaluated.

Some leukocyte bactericidal secretory peptides (such as defensins) and histones (that may be released by damaged tissue) are strongly cationic. In addition to the erratic effect of β-adrenergic agonists, or DBcAMP on paracellular permeability mentioned above, polycationic compounds, whatever their properties (organic or inorganic, hydrophylic or amphiphilic), produce more consistent changes. Instillation of protamine or polylysine into airspaces causes a rapid (within 10 min), transient increase in the passive permeability of the alveolar-airway barrier (55). This response is dose-dependent and correlated with the charge density conveyed by the compound. It is not due to cytotoxicity, because the ultrastructural appearance of the alveolar epithelium is normal, as well as its ability to respond to β-adrenergic stimulation by an increase in active Na^+ transport and liquid clearance. For a given level of active transepithelial

Na^+ transport, fluid absorption is preserved, despite the increase in permeability. The same response is observed with the wasp venom peptide mastoparan, a G-protein activator. The effect of polycations on alveolar epithelium differs from their action on the endothelium because adding protamine to the perfusate of isolated lungs produces microvascular injury and permeability edema.

Recent results obtained with the polyamine spermine reinforce the idea that there are pathways to modulate paracellular permeability. Spermine is a strong base with four positive charges and a molecular weight of only 202. Spermine has been shown to have several extracellular and intracellular targets (NMDA receptors, K^+ channels, intracellular Ca^{2+} pools, phospholipase C . . .). It is also readily transported into alveolar epithelial cells, as these cells have efficient membrane polyamine transport systems (68). Luminal spermine causes dose-dependent, saturable increase in both alveolar fluid clearance and paracellular permeability to albumin 1 hour after instillation. There is often a 40-fold increase in mannitol permeability and a 10-fold increase in albumin permeability without impairment of alveolar fluid clearance and, thus, without profound alteration of the coupling between Na^+ and fluid transport (56). Clearance and passive permeability seem to be positively correlated. Spermine on the vascular side did not produce microvascular injury and edema, as do other polycations (55), suggesting that its effect, while apparently similar, is not produced in the same way.

Increasing paracellular permeability without impairing fluid clearance may allow easier resolution of alveolar edema by accelerating the outward movement of high-molecular-weight solutes that are not actively transported. Another possible interaction between paracellular permeability and the clearance of alveolar edema may take place through glucose movement (22,43). The glucose concentration in airspace fluid falls rapidly to a low level in rats, which considerably reduces clearance efficiency by lowering Na^+ transepithelial transport. A similar decrease may also occur a few hours after the resorption of alveolar edema begins. One way by which alveolar fluid may be cleared more rapidly would be to increase its glucose concentration when this becomes too low. This may happen if the entry of glucose into airspaces is facilitated by an increase in the passive permeability. Experiments have been carried out in isolated lungs filled with glucose-free instillate in which the permeability of the airspace epithelium was made to vary with protamine (43). Protamine by itself does not influence alveolar fluid clearance. The increase in permeability results in an increase in luminal glucose concentration and in airspace liquid clearance (Fig. 4), in agreement with a mathematical model describing glucose and liquid transport in distal airspaces. These experiments suggest that, in addition to hormonal stimulation of active Na^+ transport, modulation of the passive pathway properties may positively influence alveolar edema clearance.

VII. Perspectives

Isolated lungs will remain a useful tool because they make it easy to study some of the transport properties of the native alveolar epithelium, and, in particular, fluid absorption. They are a valuable model for assessing the acute effects of toxic or therapeutic agents. It would be worthwhile developing isolated mouse lung preparations that provide reproducible estimates of alveolar epithelial barrier properties and deep lung fluid balance, as these could be used to study transgenic mice or the effects of gene therapy. The main disadvantage of isolated lungs is that they are rather short-lived with a good physiological condition for less than 3 hours.

Many aspects on the way alveolar edema is removed remain unclear. For example, plasma proteins concentrate within airspaces during resorption, and some of them interfere with surfactant function. Most plasma proteins are probably not cleaved in the airspaces and are eliminated passively and slowly (69) (see Chap. 19). Increasing protein clearance may be one way to accelerate edema resolution, because plasma in the airspaces alters surfactant surface properties (70). Isolated lungs may be useful for investigating whether albumin clearance can be accelerated, and if there are other pathways for modulating the transport properties of the distal lung epithelia. They may also be used to determine whether there is coordination between alveolar fluid absorption and surfactant secretion to optimize distal airway reopening.

Lastly, airspace fluid-filled preparations are a tool for investigating the mechanism by which alveolar edema is cleared rather than epithelial lining fluid homeostasis. It is worth mentioning that only the fundamental mechanisms of fluid absorption from distal airspaces have been delineated so far. How this absorption rate may be slowed down or reversed to control epithelial lining fluid depth or volume is still unknown. Clearly, the fluid thickness should be kept at some minimum to optimize gas exchange, and its composition should be maintained such that free luminal cells can satisfy their needs. The arbitrary composition of the fluid instilled into airspaces to study deep lung fluid balance may have altered the normal function of the alveolar epithelium (20). Elucidation of the physiological mechanisms that govern the transition between fluid-filled and air-filled lungs is a great challenge for future studies.

References

1. Mason RJ, Williams MC, Widdicombe JH, Sanders MJ, Misfeldt DS, Berry LC Jr. Transepithelial transport by pulmonary alveolar type II cells in primary culture. Proc Natl Acad Sci USA 1982; 79:6033–6037.

2. Cheek JM, Kim KJ, Crandall ED. Tight monolayers of rat alveolar epithelial cells: bioelectric properties and active sodium transport. Am J Physiol 1989; 256: C688–C693.
3. Effros RM, Mason GR, Sietsema K, Silverman P, Hukkanen J. Fluid reabsorption and glucose consumption from edematous rat lungs. Circ Res 1987; 60: 708–719.
4. Ballard ST, Gatzy JT. Volume flow across alveolar epithelium of the adult rat lung. J Appl Physiol 1991; 70:1665–1676.
5. McLaughlin GE, Kim KJ, Berg MM, Agoris P, Lubman RL, Crandall ED. Measurement of solute fluxes in isolated rat lungs. Respir Physiol 1993; 91:321–334.
6. Basset G, Crone C, Saumon G. Fluid absorption by rat lung in situ: pathways for sodium entry in the luminal membrane of alveolar epithelium. J Physiol (Lond) 1987; 384:325–345.
7. Basset G, Bouchonnet F, Crone C, Saumon G. Potassium transport across rat alveolar epithelium: evidence for an apical Na^+ K^+ pump. J Physiol (Lond) 1988; 400:529–543.
8. Basset G, Crone C, Saumon G. Significance of active ion transport in transalveolar water absorption: a study on isolated rat lung. J Physiol (Lond) 1987; 384: 311–324.
9. Goodman BE, Kim KJ, Crandall ED. Evidence for active sodium transport across alveolar epithelium of isolated rat lung. J Appl Physiol 1987; 62:2460–2466.
10. Vejlstrup NG, Boyd CAR, Dorrington KL. Effect of lung inflation on active and passive liquid clearance from in vivo rabbit lung. Am J Physiol 1994; 267:L482–L487.
11. Lasnier JM, Wangensteen OD, Schmitz LS, Gross CR, Ingbar DH. Terbutaline stimulates alveolar fluid resorption in hyperoxic lung injury. J Appl Physiol 1996; 81:1723–1729.
12. Crandall ED, Heming TA, Palombo RL, Goodman BE. Effects of terbutaline on sodium transport in isolated perfused rat lung. J Appl Physiol 1986; 60:289–294.
13. Berg MM, Kim KJ, Lubman RL, Crandall ED. Hydrophilic solute transport across rat alveolar epithelium. J Appl Physiol 1989; 66:2320–2327.
14. Effros RM, Mason GR, Hukkanen J, Silverman P. New evidence for active sodium transport from fluid-filled rat lungs. J Appl Physiol 1989; 66:909–919.
15. Rutschman DH, Olivera W, Sznajder JI. Active transport and passive liquid movement in solated perfused rat lungs. J Appl Physiol 1993; 75:1574–1580.
16. Saumon G, Martet G. Effect of metabolic inhibitors on Na^+ transport in isolated perfused rat lungs. Am J Respir Cell Mol Biol 1993; 9:157–165.
17. Ballard ST, Gatzy JT. Alveolar transepithelial potential diffrence and ion transport in adult rat lung. J Appl Physiol 1991; 70:63–69.
18. Goodman BE, Anderson JL, Clemens JW, Kircher KJ, Stormo ML, Waltz JS, Waltz WF, White JW. Differences in sodium and D-glucose transport between hamster and rat lungs. J Appl Physiol 1994; 76:2578–2585.
19. Matalon S, Benos DJ, Jackson RM. Biophysical and molecular properties of amiloride-inhibitable Na^+ channels in alveolar epithelial cells. Am J Physiol 1996; 271:L1–L22.

20. Saumon G, Martet G, Loiseau P. Glucose transport and equilibrium across the alveolar-airway barrier of rat. Am J Physiol 1996; 270:L183–L190.
21. Basset G, Saumon G, Bouchonnet F, Crone C. Apical sodium-sugar transport in pulmonary epithelium in situ. Biochim Biophys Acta 1988; 942:11–18.
22. Saumon G, Dreyfuss D. Luminal glucose enhances transepithelial Na^+ and fluid transports in rat lungs. Pflügers Arch 1991; 417:571–576.
23. Saumon G, Seigné E, Clérici C. Evidence for a sodium-dependent sugar transport in rat tracheal epithelium. Biochim Biophys Acta 1990; 1023:313–318.
24. Saumon G, Basset G, Bouchonnet F, Crone C. cAMP and β-adrenergic stimulation of rat alveolar epithelium. Effects on fluid absorption and paracellular permeability. Pflügers Arch 1987; 410:464–470.
25. Taylor AE, Gaar KA Jr. Estimation of equivalent pore radii of pulmonary capillary and alveolar membranes. Am J Physiol 1970; 218:1133–1140.
26. Icard P, Bergeron A, Loiseau P, Saumon G. Alveolar fluid clearance mechanisms in mice. Am J Respir Crit Care Med 1997; 155:A832.
27. Mercer RR, Russell ML, Crapo JD. Alveolar septal structure in different species. J Appl Physiol 1994; 77:1060–1066.
28. Nielson DW. Electrolyte composition of pulmonary alveolar subphase in anesthetized rabbits. J Appl Physiol 1986; 60:972–978.
29. Dreyfuss D, Soler P, Saumon G. Spontaneous resolution of pulmonary edema caused by short periods of cyclic overinflation. J Appl Physiol 1992; 72:2081–2089.
30. Effros RM, Mason GR, Hukkanen J, Silverman P. Reabsorption of solutes and water from fluid-filled rabbit lungs. Am Rev Respir Dis 1987; 136:669–676.
31. Schneeberger EE, McCarthy KM. Cytochemical localization of Na^+K^+ATPase in rat type II pneumocytes. J Appl Physiol 1986; 60:1584–1589.
32. Ingbar DH, Weeks CB, Gilmore-Hebert M, Jacobsen E, Duvick S, Dowin R, Savik SK, Jamieson JD. Developmental regulation of Na,K-ATPase in rat lung. Am J Physiol 1996; 270:L619–L629.
33. Suzuki Y, Kaneko K. Ouabain sensitive H^+ -K^+ exchange mechanism in the apical membrane of guinea pig colon. Am J Physiol 1989; 256:G979–G988.
34. Nielson DW, Goerke J, Clements JA. Alveolar subphase pH in the lungs of anesthetized rabbits. Proc Natl Acad Sci USA 1981; 78:7119–7123.
35. Kemp PJ, Roberts GC, Boyd CAR. Identification and properties of pathways for K^+ transport in guinea-pig and rat alveolar epithelial type II cells. J Physiol (Lond) 1994; 476:79–88.
36. Saumon G, Basset G, Bouchonnet F, Crone C. Cellular effects of β-adrenergic and of cAMP stimulation on potassium transport in rat alveolar epithelium. Pflügers Arch 1989; 414:340–445.
37. Peers C, Kemp PJ, Boyd CAR, Nye PCG. Whole-cell K^+ currents in type II pneumocytes freshly isolated from rat lung: pharmacological evidence for two subpopulations of cells. Biochim Biophys Acta 1990; 1052:113–118.
38. Effros RM, Mason GR, Sietsema K, Hukkanen J, Silverman P. Pulmonary epithelial sieving of small solutes in rat lungs. J Appl Physiol 1988; 65:640–648.
39. Taylor AE, Guyton AC, Bishop VS. Permeability of the alveolar membrane to solutes. Circ Res 1965; 16:353–362.

40. Matthay MA, Folkesson HG, Verkman AS. Salt and water transport across alveolar and distal airway epithelia. Am J Physiol 1996; 270:L487–L503.
41. Sznajder JI, Olivera WG, Ridge KM, Rutschman DH. Mechanisms of lung liquid clearance during hyperoxia in isolated rat lungs Am J Respir Crit Care Med 1995; 151:1519–1525.
42. Windhager EE. Sodium chloride transport. In: Giebish G, Tosteson DC, Ussing HH, eds. Membrane Transport in Biology. IV.A. Transport Organs. Berlin: Springer-Verlag, 1979:145–213.
43. Saumon G, Martet G. Effect of changes in paracellular permeability on air-space liquid clearance: role of glucose transport. Am J Physiol 1996; 270:L191–L198.
44. Khimenko PL, Barnard JW, Moore TM, Wilson PS, Ballard ST, Taylor AE. Vascular permeability and epithelial transport effects on lung edema formation in ischemia and reperfusion. J Appl Physiol 1994; 77:1116–1121.
45. Chinard FP. The permeability characteristics of the pulmonary blood-gas barrier. In: Caro CG, ed. Advances in Respiratory Physiology. London:Arnold, 1966: 106–147.
46. Wangensteen D, Wittmers LE, Johnson JA. Permeability of the mammalian blood-gas barrier and its components. Am J Physiol 1969; 216:719–727.
47. Effros RM, Hacker A, Silverman P, Hukkanen J. Protein concentrations have little effect on reabsorption of fluid from isolated rat lungs. J Appl Physiol 1991; 70: 416–422.
48. Matthay MA, Berthiaume Y, Staub NC. Long-term clearance of liquid and protein from the lungs of unanesthetized sheep. J Appl Physiol 1985; 59:928–934.
49. O'Brodovich H, Hannam V, Rafii B. Sodium channel but neither Na^+-H^+ nor Na-glucose symport inhibitors slow neonatal water clearance. Am J Respir Cell Mol Biol 1991; 5:377–384.
50. Fischer AB, Dodia C. Lactate and the regulation of lung glycolytic rate. Am J Physiol 1984; 246:E426–E429.
51. Bolin R, Guest RJ, Albert RK. Glycolysis is not required for fluid homeostasis in isolated rabbit lung. J Appl Physiol 1988; 64:2517–2521.
52. Bassett DJP, Fischer AB. Metabolic response to carbon monoxide by isolated rat lungs. Am J Physiol 1976; 230:658–663.
53. Paul RJ. Smooth muscle energetics. Ann Rev Physiol 1989; 51:331–349.
54. Tierney DF. Lung metabolism and biochemistry. Ann Rev Physiol 1974; 36: 209–231.
55. Saumon G, Soler P, Martet G. Effect of polycations on barrier and transport properties of alveolar epithelium in situ. Am J Physiol 1995; 269:L185–L194.
56. Saumon G. Martet G. Spermine increases alveolar fluid clearance and paracellular permeability in isolated rat lungs. Am J Respir Crit Care Med 1997; 155:A647.
57. Goodman BE, Anderson JL, Clemens JW. Evidence for regulation of sodium transport from airspace to vascular space by cAMP. Am J Physiol 1989; 257:L86–L93.
58. Olivera W, Ridge K, Wood LDH, Sznajder JI. ANF decreases active sodium transport and increases alveolar epithelial permeability in rats. J Appl Physiol 1993; 75: 1581–1586.

59. Waltz WF, Burbach JA, Schenker EH, Goodman BE. Sodium transport and fluid balance in lungs from normal and dystrophic hamsters. J Appl Physiol 1994; 74: 1750–1754.
60. Dinardo P, Minieri M, Sampaolesi M, Carbone A, Loreni F, Samuel JL, Lauro R. Atrial natriuretic factor (ANF) and ANF receptor C gene expression and localization in the respiratory system: effects induced by hypoxia and hemodynamic overload. Endocrinology 1996; 137:4339–4350.
61. Periyasamy S, Kothapalli MR, Hoss W. Regulation of the phosphoinositide cascade by polyamines in brain. J Neurochem 1994; 63:1319–1327.
62. Nici L, Dowin R, Gilmore-Hebert M, Jamieson JD, Ingbar DH. Upregulation of Na-K-ATPase during hyperoxic lung injury. Am J Physiol 1991; 261:L307–L314.
63. Haskell JF, Yue G, Benos DJ, Matalon S. Upregulation of sodium conductive pathways in alveolar type II cells in sublethal hyperoxia. Am J Physiol 1994; 266: L30–L37.
64. Olivera W, Ridge KM, Wood LDH, Sznajder JI. Active sodium transport and alveolar epithelial Na,K-ATPase increase during hyperoxic injury. Am J Physiol 1994; 266:L577–L584.
65. Marks JD, Luce JM, Lazar NM, Ngao-Sun WJ, Lipavsky A, Murray JF. Effect of increases in lung volume on clearance of aerosolized solute from human lung. J Appl Physiol 1985; 59:1242–1248.
66. Egan EA. Response of alveolar epithelial solute permeability to changes in lung inflation. J Appl Physol 1980; 49:1032–1036.
67. Sznajder JI, Ridge KM, Harris ZL, Olivera W, Curiel C, Rutschman DH. Alveolar type II cell Na,K-ATPase is upregulated during mechanical ventilation-induced pulmonary edema. Chest 1994; 105:116S–117S.
68. Rannels DE, Kameji R, Pegg AE, Rannels SR. Spermidine uptake by type II pneumocytes: interactions of amine uptake pathways. Am J Physiol 1989; 257:L346–L353.
69. Folkesson HG, Matthay MA, Weström BR, Kim KJ, Karlsson BW, Hastings RH. Alveolar epithelial clearance of protein. J Appl Physiol 1996; 80:1431–1445.
70. Tierney DF, Johnson RP. Altered surface tension of lung extracts and lung mechanics. J Appl Physiol 1965; 20:1253–1260.

18

Water Transport and Molecular Water Channels in Lung

ALAN S. VERKMAN

Cardiovascular Research Institute
University of California at San Francisco
San Francisco, California

I. Introduction

The movement of fluid between the airspace and vascular compartments in lung plays an important physiological role in a number of processes, including the maintenance of proper airway hydration, the reabsorption of alveolar fluid in the neonatal period in preparation for alveolar respiration, and the resolution of pulmonary edema (1,2). The general paradigm for the transport of fluid across various epithelia in lung is that active salt transport drives osmotic water movement. Although considerable effort has focused on the mechanisms of salt movement across epithelia in lung, including the recent identification of sodium and chloride transporters involved in transepithelial ion transport (3–5), less attention has been given to the mechanisms of water transport.

It was recognized for many years that various cell plasma membranes, including those in red blood cells and kidney epithelia, have a high water permeability that is inhibited by mercurial compounds (6,7). Although the existence of molecular water-transporting proteins was suggested by these observations, as well as the finding that expression of mRNA from reticulocytes and kidney increased water permeability in *Xenopus* oocytes (8), the first protein that functioned as a water-selective transporter was not cloned until 1991 (9).

Subsequently, a family of molecular water channels (aquaporins) has been identified which are present in many fluid-transporting tissues in mammals as well as in lower animals, plants, and bacteria (10–13). At least four members of the family are expressed in trachea and/or lung. This chapter reviews recent data on water permeability in lung tissues and the evidence for a role of molecular water channels in lung.

II. Anatomy of Water Transport in Lung

Figure 1 depicts the principle barriers to transport of water between airspace, interstitial, and vascular compartments in lung. The trachea and large airways contain an epithelial cell layer but represent only a small fraction of the total surface area available for movement of fluid into and out of the airspaces. The more numerous smaller airways also contain an epithelial cell layer but still represent a relatively small surface area. In human lung, the total airway surface area is ~ 1.4 m^2, which represents only about 1% of the alveolar surface area of 143 m^2 (14). The alveolar epithelium thus provides the major surface for the movement of salt and water. The alveolar epithelium contains two cell types: type I cells, which make up the majority of the alveolar epithelial surface but whose function is relatively poorly understood; and type II cells, which appear to transport salt actively. Movement of water between the airspace and capil-

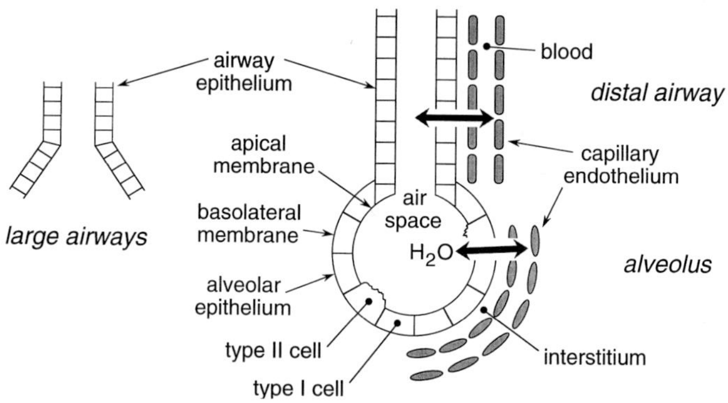

Figure 1 Barriers to water movement in lung. Transport of water between the airspace and capillary compartments involves movement across the alveolar epithelium, interstitium, and endothelium, or across airway epithelium and capillary endothelium. The epithelium is polarized so that transcellular transport involves serial passage across apical and basolateral plasma membranes.

lary compartments through the alveolar epithelium also encounters potential permeability barriers in the interstitium and capillary endothelium. The starting point in evaluation of the role of water transporters in lung is the determination of water transport rates across various epithelial and endothelial barriers. As described in the next section, recent experiments have begun to provide information about these rates; however, questions remain concerning the relative water permeabilities of epithelial vs. endothelial barriers of apical vs. basolateral cell plasma membranes and of type I versus type II alveolar epithelial cells.

III. Functional Measurements of Water Transport in Lung

A. Airspace-to-Capillary Water Transport in Intact Lung

The movement of fluid into and out of the airspace compartment has been a topic of considerable interest because of its importance in mechanisms of formation and resolution of pulmonary edema. More that 20 years ago, Effros (15) suggested that the hypertonic extraction of water from lung tissue occurs by a transcellular route, although the existence of molecular water channels was not recognized at that time. In 1994, Folkesson et al. (16) estimated the osmotic water permeability (P_f) between the airspace and capillary compartments using an airspace "instillation and sample" approach. The in situ perfused sheep lung was used as a model in which cannulation of the large airways permitted instillation of hypertonic saline and serial sampling of airspace fluid. The vascular compartment was perfused continuously with isosmolar saline (300 mOsm), and the airspace was filled rapidly with hypertonic saline (900 mOsm). Serial samples of airspace fluid showed that osmolality equilibrated rapidly to 300 mOsm with a half-time of ~45 sec (Fig. 2). This equilibration time was slowed approximately threefold upon addition to the perfusate of $HgCl_2$, a known inhibitor of water transport in erythrocytes and kidney tubules. The $HgCl_2$ inhibition was reversed by the reducing agent 2-mercaptoethanol, indicating that the inhibition was not a nonspecific toxic effect of the mercurial compound. P_f was estimated to be 0.02 cm/sec, a very high value that was similar to that of erythrocytes and kidney tubule epithelial cell membranes. It was concluded that water movement between the airspace and capillary compartments in the intact lung was transcellular and facilitated by mercurial-sensitive water channels. However, these studies did not define the location or the contribution of various barriers to water permeability, nor were they able to provide precise P_f values because of limitations in the rate of hypertonic fluid instillation and the accurate sampling of alveolar fluid by cannulation of large airways.

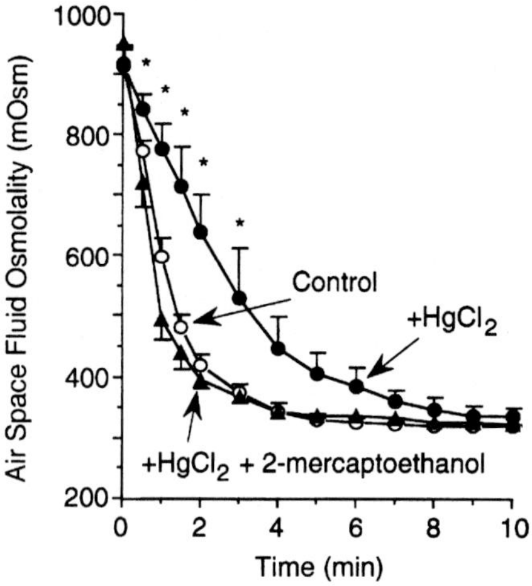

Figure 2 Osmotic water permeability of the airspace-to-capillary barrier in sheep lung. The pulmonary artery in sheep lung was perfused in situ with isosmolar saline. At zero time, hypertonic saline was infused into the lung to induce osmotic water transport into the airspace. Serial airspace fluid samples were obtained by cannulation and assayed for osmolality. Where indicated, $HgCl_2$ (0.5 mM) without or with β-mercaptoethanol (5 mM) was present in the perfusate.

For studies in small animals, where rapid airspace fluid instillation and sampling is not practical, a pleural surface fluorescence method was recently developed in which airspace osmolality was deduced from the fluorescence of an indicator dissolved in the airspace fluid (17). The principle of the method is shown in Figure 3A. The airspace is filled with fluid containing a membrane-impermeant fluorophore at low concentrations in which there is no self-quenching or absorption of excitation light or emitted fluorescence. Because of the finite penetration depth of the excitation light, only lung tissue within 100 to 200 μm of the pleural surface is illuminated. Under these conditions, the surface fluorescence signal is directly proportional to the airspace fluorophore concentration. In response to an osmotic gradient, water flows between the airspace and perfusate compartments, resulting in a change in fluorophore concentration which is "sampled" by measurement of pleural surface fluorescence. This approach has the advantage of excellent time resolution without the need for invasive sampling. Figure 3B shows the instrumentation for measurement of pleural surface fluorescence. The trachea and pulmonary artery are cannulated, the heart and lungs are placed en bloc onto an open perfusion chamber, and pleural surface fluorescence is recorded in an epifluorescence configuration.

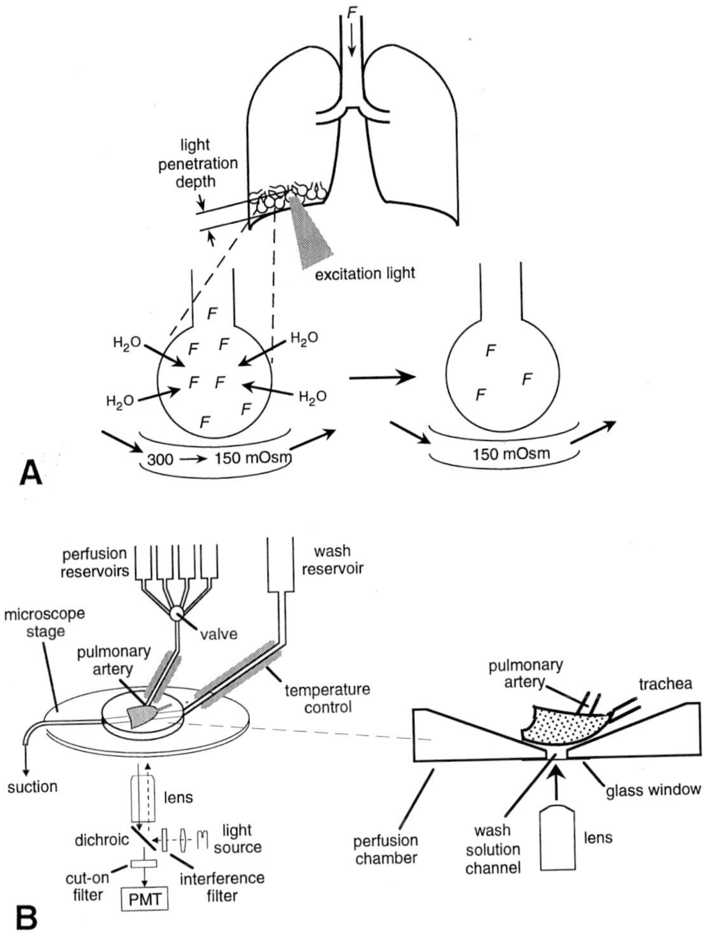

Figure 3 Measurement of osmotic water permeability in intact lung by a pleural surface fluorescence method. (A) The airspace is filled with saline containing a membrane-impermeant fluorescent probe (F) and pleural surface fluorescence is monitored by epifluorescence microscopy ("excitation light"). In response to a decrease in osmolality in fluid perfused into the pulmonary artery, water moves into the airspace and dilutes the fluorophore. Surface fluorescence provide a quantitative measure of intra-alveolar fluorophore concentration. (B) Instrumentation for measurement of pleural surface fluorescence. Cannulae are inserted for intratracheal fluid instillation and pulmonary artery perfusion. The lung is positioned on a perfusion chamber in which pleural surface fluorescence is recorded.

As shown in Figure 4A, the pleural surface fluorescence signal is very stable and the data contain remarkably little experimental noise. In response to doubling of perfusate osmolality from 300 to 600 mOsm, pleural surface fluorescence signal approximately doubles as predicted theoretically. When perfusate osmolality was decreased from 300 to 150 mOsm, pleural surface fluorescence was decreased by approximately twofold. Analysis of the fluorescence time course provides quantitative information about water permeability. P_f in mouse lung was 0.017 $\pm$ 0.008 cm/sec at 23°C, independent of the solute used to induce osmosis, independent of osmotic gradient size and direction, weakly temperature-dependent (activation energy 5.3 kcal/mol) (Fig. 4B), and inhibited by $HgCl_2$.

Measurement of pleural surface fluorescence also provides an approach for measurement of diffusional water permeability (P_d) as well as the transport of various solutes like Na^+ and Cl^- for which suitable fluid phase indicators exist (18). Figure 4C shows the measurement of diffusional water movement between the airspace and capillary compartments in mouse lung. The airspace was filled with isosmolar saline containing the D_2O-sensitive fluorophore ami-

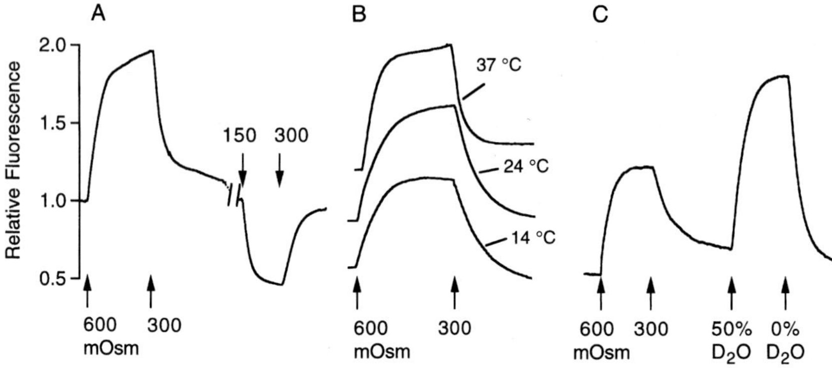

Figure 4 Time course of pleural surface fluorescence in mouse lung. (A) Osmotic water permeability. The airspace was filled with isosmolar saline containing FITC-dextran and the pulmonary artery was perfused with solutions of indicated osmolalities. Pleural surface fluorescence was monitored continuously by epifluorescence microscopy. (B) Dependence of osmotic water permeability on temperature. (C) Diffusional water permeability. The airspace was filled with isosmolar saline (in H_2O buffer) containing the fluorophore ANTS (see text). First, osmotic water permeability was measured from the time course of ANTS fluorescence in response to a change in perfusate osmolality. Then, diffusional water permeability was measured by switching the perfusate to isosmolar saline in 50% D_2O. ANTS fluorescence increases as the concentration of D_2O in the airspace fluid increases.

nonapthalene trisulfonic acid (ANTS) (17). The perfusate was switched from an isosmolar H_2O-containing buffer to an isosmolar buffer containing 50% D_2O. As H_2O exchanges for D_2O across the alveolar epithelium, alveolar fluid D_2O concentration rises and ANTS fluorescence increases. Analysis of the time course of ANTS pleural surface fluorescence in response to addition and removal of D_2O from the perfusate gave a P_d of 1.3×10^{-5} cm/sec. This P_d value is very low, as anticipated, because unstirred layers pose a significant restriction to water diffusion in intact epithelial tissues. The pleural surface fluorescence method was also used to quantify the rates of proton movement across the alveolar epithelium by introduction of a pH-sensitive fluorescent indicator into the alveolar compartment (17).

B. Alveolar Epithelial Versus Endothelial Barriers to Water Transport

The studies described above establish the empirical characteristics of water permeability between the airspace and capillary compartments in intact lung but provide no information about the contributions of epithelial vs. endothelial barriers. From previous studies on salt movement, it was predicted that the alveolar epithelial water permeability should be rate-limiting because the endothelium is relatively leaky. Our laboratory has begun to develop methods to measure the individual epithelial and endothelial permeabilities in intact lung. The strategy to measure endothelial water permeability is to fill the airspace with an inert, water-insoluble perfluorocarbon to restrict lung water to two compartments—the interstitium and the capillaries—and thus establish a single rate-limiting permeability barrier—the capillary endothelium (19). The pulmonary artery is perfused with solutions of specified osmolalities containing equal concentrations of high molecular weight fluorescein-dextran (Fig. 5A). In response to a change of perfusate osmolality, water is osmotically driven into or out of the capillaries, resulting in fluorophore dilution or concentration, respectively. The change in fluorophore concentration is recorded as a prompt change (decrease for fluorophore dilution) in pleural surface fluorescence. The magnitude of the prompt deflection in fluorescence signal increases with increased water permeability or decreased pulmonary artery flow. The prompt deflection is followed by a slower return of fluorescence signal to the original level as interstitial and capillary osmolalities equilibrate; the area under the curve is related to the interstitial volume, and the rate of equilibration is related to a combination of endothelial water permeability, pulmonary artery flow, and interstitial volume.

As shown in Figure 5B, an increase in pulmonary artery perfusate osmolality from 300 to 600 mOsm gave a prompt decrease in pleural surface fluorescence followed by the predicted decrease back to baseline. Return of osmolality to 300 mOsm gave a prompt increased in signal followed by relaxation.

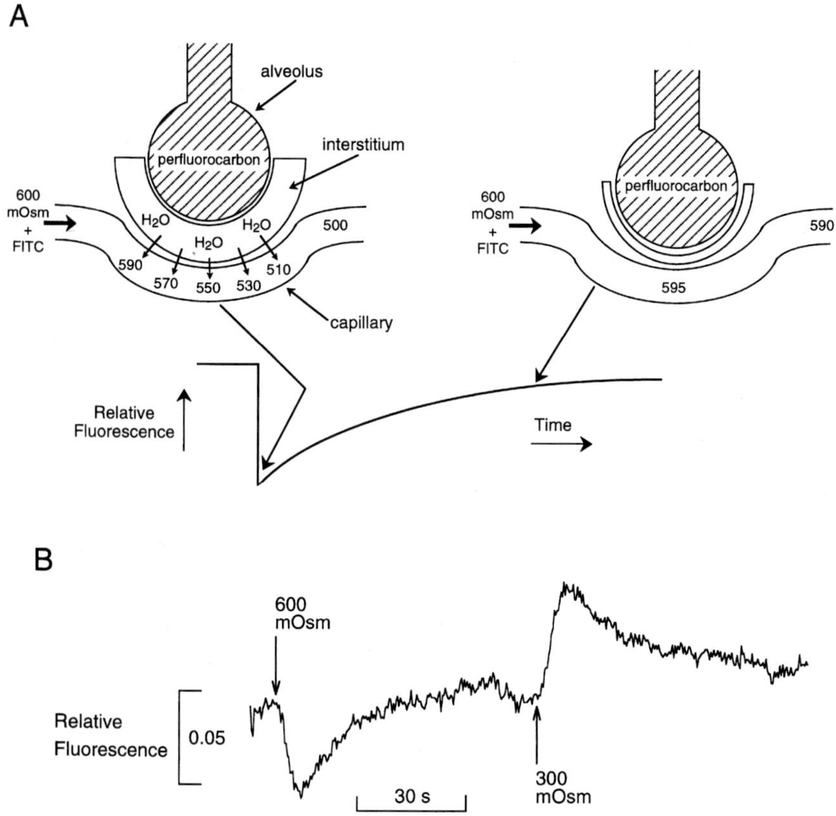

Figure 5 Measurement of transcapillary endothelial water permeability. (A) Principle of method. The airspace is filled with an inert perfluorocarbon and the pulmonary artery is perfused with solutions of specified osmolalities containing equal concentration of a fluorescent probe. In response to an increase in perfusate osmolality, water moves into the capillaries, resulting in decreased osmolality (as depicted) and fluorophore concentration. This causes a prompt fall in pleural surface fluorescence signal, followed by return to the initial level as osmotic equilibrium is established between capillary fluid and the interstitium. (B) Surface fluorescence data obtained from mouse lung. See text.

A mathematical model was developed to determine capillary P_f from the fluorescence data. Temperature dependence experiments showed that the magnitude of the deflection in response to a change in perfusate osmolality increased with increasing temperature, as expected; an increase in perfusate flow gave the expected decrease in signal amplitude. It may also be possible to measure the water permeability of the alveolar epithelial barrier selectively. The capillary compartment (rather than the airspace) is filled with an inert perfluorocarbon to establish a single rate-limiting permeability barrier—the alveolar epithelium. The rate of water transport is determined by pleural surface fluorescence after rapid instillation of hypertonic fluid into the alveolar space. The movement of water from the interstitium into the alveolar space results in fluorophore dilution and decreased pleural surface fluorescence. Preliminary measurements suggest that the alveolar epithelium is the principal barrier for osmotic water movement between airspace and capillary compartments.

C. Water Transport Across Distal Airways

Small airways provide the other major epithelial layer in lung for the movement of water into and out of the airspaces. It is not possible to measure airway water permeability in the intact lung because the alveolar epithelium comprises the majority of surface area. To measure the water transport properties of small airways directly, a microperfusion technique was established based on methods established previously for perfusion of isolated kidney tubules. Distal airways were microdissected and perfused in vitro (20). Small airways from rat, rabbit, mouse, and guinea pig were evaluated; the guinea pig was chosen for the initial studies because relatively long segments of viable distal airway (up to 2 mm length, 0.1 to 0.2 mm diameter) without bifurcations could be microdissected. The approach for measurement of P_f is shown in Figure 6A and is based on a method developed originally for kidney tubules (21,22). The airway lumen is perfused at constant nanoliter/min flow rates with a membrane-impermeant fluorophore. The osmolality of the bath solution surrounding the airway is changed from isosmolar saline to a solution of different osmolality. For example, when bath osmolality is set to 50 mOsm, there is movement of solute-free water from the bath to the airway lumen, resulting in a steady-state profile of increasing fluorophore concentration along the axis of the airway. The fluorescence signal at any point along the airway, proportional to lumen osmolality, is related to transepithelial P_f airway size, and lumen flow rate. Representative experimental data are shown in Figure 6B. Perfusion with hypo-osomolar solution produced a prompt fluorescence decrease which returned to the original level upon reperfusion with isosmolar buffer. The magnitude of the fluorescence decrease was dependent on the size and direction of the osmotic gradient—an increase of bath osmolality to 600 mOsm produced a large increase in fluorescence. Quantitative analysis of the data gave a P_f of 4.5×10^{-3} cm/sec at 23°C which was independent of lumen flow rate (10 to 100 nl/min) and the magnitude and direction of the osmotic gradient. Temperature-dependence measurements between 15 and 37°C gave a low activation energy of 4.4 kcal/mol. Unlike the alveolar water permeability, airway P_f was not inhibited by $HgCl_2$, consistent with a role for the mercury-sensitive water channel AQP4 (discussed later). Transepithelial airway

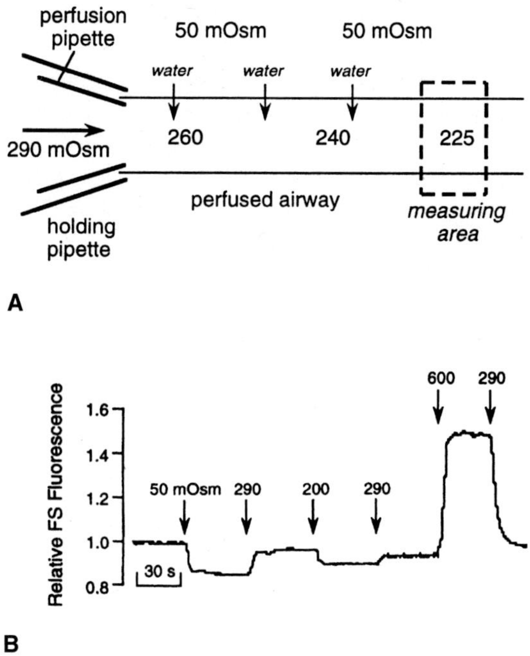

Figure 6 Measurement of water permeability in isolated perfused small airways. (A) Principle of method. A microdissected airway is perfused slowly by cannulation with a glass micropipette and bathed initially in an isosmolar solution. When the bathing solution is replaced by a hypo-osmolar solution (50 mOsm shown here), a steady state is rapidly established in which the osmolality of lumen perfusate decreases along the axis of the airway. Perfusate osmolality at a fixed position is measured from the fluorescence of a probe dissolved in the lumen perfusate. (B) Measurement of osmotic water permeability in a perfused small airway from guinea pig lung. The airway was perfused at 10 nl/min with isosmolar solution containing fluorescein sulfonate. Where indicated, bath osmolality was changed. Osmotic water permeability is deduced from signal amplitude, lumen flow, and airway geometry.

P_f could be increased strongly by the pore-forming agent amphotericin B, indicating that osmosis was not limited by unstirred layers under the conditions of the microperfusion experiment.

The in vitro microperfusion method with fluorescence detection is also applicable to the study of diffusional water transport, as well as transport of ions such as Cl^-, provided that suitable membrane-impermeable fluorescent indicators are available (18). Diffusional water permeability in small airways was measured by perfusion of the airway lumen with isosmolar H_2O-containing saline containing ANTS, and the bath was changed from an isosmolar H_2O buffer to an isosmolar solution containing in which 50% of the H_2O was replaced by D_2O. The diffusional exchange of H_2O for D_2O across the airway epithelium produces an increase in D_2O concentration and ANTS fluorescence along the axis of the airway. Measurement of ANTS fluorescence at a fixed point near the distal end of the airway gave a P_d of 5×10^{-6} cm/sec, indicating significant unstirred layers for diffusional movement of water. It is noted that osmotic movement of water is the process of physiological importance because net volume transport occurs; diffusional water permeability does not produce net volume movement, and describes only the rate at which labeled water (such as ^3H_2O) exchanges with unlabeled water across a membraneous barrier.

D. Water Permeability of Lung Cell Plasma Membranes

The measurement of water permeability in isolated cells or plasma membrane vesicles can provide information about the contributions of specific cell types and individual plasma membranes in the overall water permeability measured in intact lung or airways. Only a few experiments of this type have been done to date. The stop-flow light-scattering technique has become the principal method to measure water permeability in vesicles or cells in suspension. Cell or vesicle suspensions are subjected to an osmotic gradient by rapid (generally less than 1 msec) mixture with a solution of different osmolality in a stop-flow apparatus. Osmotic water movement across the cell plasma membrane produces a change in cell volume and an instantaneous change in the scattered light intensity. Osmotic water permeability is computed from the time course of the light-scattering signal and cell geometry. This approach was used recently to measure P_f in isolated type II alveolar epithelial cells from rat lung. In response to an increase in osmolality from 300 to 500 mOsm, light scattering increased with an apparent half-time of ~1 sec. The deduced high P_f of 0.015 cm/sec suggested the involvement of molecular water channels. Further evidence for water channels was the weak temperature dependence of type II cell P_f and the reversible inhibition of P_f by $HgCl_2$. Recently, a method was developed to isolate purified type I alveolar epithelial cells freshly from rat lung. Osmotic water permeability measurements indicate a remarkably high P_f in the type I cells with a half-time for osmotic equilibration of <100 msec (23).

Water permeability measurements in intact epithelial cells in suspension provide information about the composite water permeabilities of apical and basolateral membranes. However, measurements using suspended cells cannot resolve the individual permeabilities of the two membranes which form serial barriers in the intact epithelium. To measure P_f in individual cell membranes, either purified membrane vesicles must be generated and studied or water permeability must be measured in polarized epithelial layers. Cell membrane water permeability in epithelial cell layers is determined from the time course of cell volume in response to osmotic gradients across the apical or basolateral surfaces. There are no data yet on this issue in lung epithelia. Our laboratory recently developed several methods suitable for the measurement of cell membrane water permeability in epithelial cell layers that are cultured on rigid supports or mounted in an Ussing-type chamber. A total internal reflection (TIR) fluorescence method was developed for quantitative determination of the relative cell volume for cells on a transparent rigid support (24). Cell cytoplasm was stained a polar fluorescent indicator such as calcein, and relative cell volume (inversely proportional to indicator concentration) was deduced from the TIR fluorescence from a thin (<200 nm) layer of cytoplasm near the transparent support. A novel strategy to measure the volume of nonadherent epithelial cell layers was developed utilizing laser interferometry (25). A laser interferometer was used to quantify the small changes in optical path length of a laser beam passing through a cell layer. The method is based on the change in intracellular refractive index as cell volume changes. Recently, the interference principle was applied to develop a relatively simple method to estimate relative cell volume in epithelial layers by quantitative phase-contrast microscopy (26). These methods should permit the assessment of the role of apical versus basolateral membrane water permeabilities in epithelial cells from alveoli and airways as well as the direct measurement plasma membrane water permeability across capillary endothelial cells from lung.

IV. Molecular Water Channels and Lung Water Transport

There are at present at least six water-transporting proteins identified in mammalian tissues. The properties and expression patterns of these proteins are summarized in Table 1. The original names of the first six of these proteins as reported in the initial cloning papers are given, as well as the official gene database names (containing the prefix AQP for aquaporin). Each of the proteins is small (28 to 31 kDa) and related to MIP, the major intrinsic protein of lens fiber; the proteins contain several conserved amino acid sequences, including two NPA motifs, with overall amino acid identities of 28% to 52% after sequence alignment. Hydropathy plots of the proteins are similar and suggest six transmembrane helical segments. In addition, homology in amino acid sequence between the first and second halves of each protein suggests genesis from tandem, intragenic duplication of a three-transmembrane segment (27).

Table 1 Properties of Mammalian MIP Homologs

Original names Official gene symbol	MIP	CHIP28 AQP1	WCH-CD AQP2	WCH-3/hKID AQP6	MIWC AQP4	GLIP AQP3	AQP5 AQP5
Protein size (amino acids)	263	268	265	271	301	285	282
mRNA size (kb)	1.4	2.8	1.9	2.2	5.5	5.5	1.6
N-linked glycosylation	−	+	+	−	−	+	+
Mercurial inhibition	−	+	+	+	−	+/−	+
Tissue expression	lens	wide	kidney	kidney	wide	wide	wide
Transport function	?	water	water	water	water	glycerol urea/water	water
Gene locus	12q13	7p14	12q13	12q13	18q22	9p13	12q13

MIP family members expressed in mammalian tissues are listed (left to right) in the order in which they were identified and cloned. Data on mRNA and protein are given for rat and genetic information for human.
Source: Data taken from Refs. 12, 40, 46, 49, 51,54

A. Structure and Function of the Aquaporins

With the exception of AQP3, the proteins listed in Table 1 appear to be selective for the passage of water. Most of the information about water channel structure comes from studies on AQP1 because it is readily purified in large quantities from human erythrocytes. When purified and reconstituted in proteoliposomes, AQP1 increases water permeability approximately 100-fold, without increased permeability to protons, urea, and other small solutes (28). In addition, various transfected cell culture models have been developed to study water channel function (29–31). Residue cysteine 189 in AQP1 is the site at which mercurials inhibit water permeability (32,33). Freeze-fracture electron microscopy indicated that AQP1 forms tetramers in reconstituted proteoliposomes and biological membranes (34). Two out of four of the monomeric units in the AQP1 tetramer are glycosylated by a complex polylactosaminyl sugar at residue asparagine 42; however, AQP1 glycosylation is required neither for its tetrameric structure nor its water transporting function (35). Although AQP1 forms tetramers in membranes, each of the monomers functions independently as a water channel (36). AQP1 monomers are synthesized at the endoplasmic reticulum in an immature form containing four principal membrane-spanning domains (37); each matured AQP1 monomer at the plasma membrane probably contains six transmembrane helical domains (38). Water movement through individual AQP1 monomers has been proposed to involve an aqueous channel formed by polar residues of helical domains (37) and/or by beta-sheet protein structure involving the NPA residues (39).

The initial biophysical model of the AQP1 water pathway was that of a single-file pore with a diameter of 0.25 nm (40), which was based on single-channel water permeability measured in reconstituted proteoliposomes and hydrodynamic equations describing single-file water pores (41). Recent structural studies of two-dimensional crystals of AQP1 by electron cryocrystallography suggest that each monomer (in the tetramer) contains six helical domains which span the bilayer in an approximately perpendicular orientation and that the helices appear to surround a central cavity, which may represent the entrance to the aqueous pore (42) (Fig. 7). Similar conclusions have been reached by electron crystallography of glucose-preserved crystals of human (43) and bovine (44) AQP1. High-resolution structure information by x-ray diffraction of three-dimensional AQP1 crystals are needed to visualize the precise route of water movement through the protein.

Recent membrane topology studies of AQPs 2 and 4 suggest that each of the aquaporin family homologs contain six helical domains (45,46). When expressed heterologously in *Xenopus* oocytes, AQPs 1, 2, 4, 5, and 6 form water-selective channels that are inhibited reversibly by mercurials (47–52). Water movement through AQP4 is not mercury-sensitive (49) because of the absence

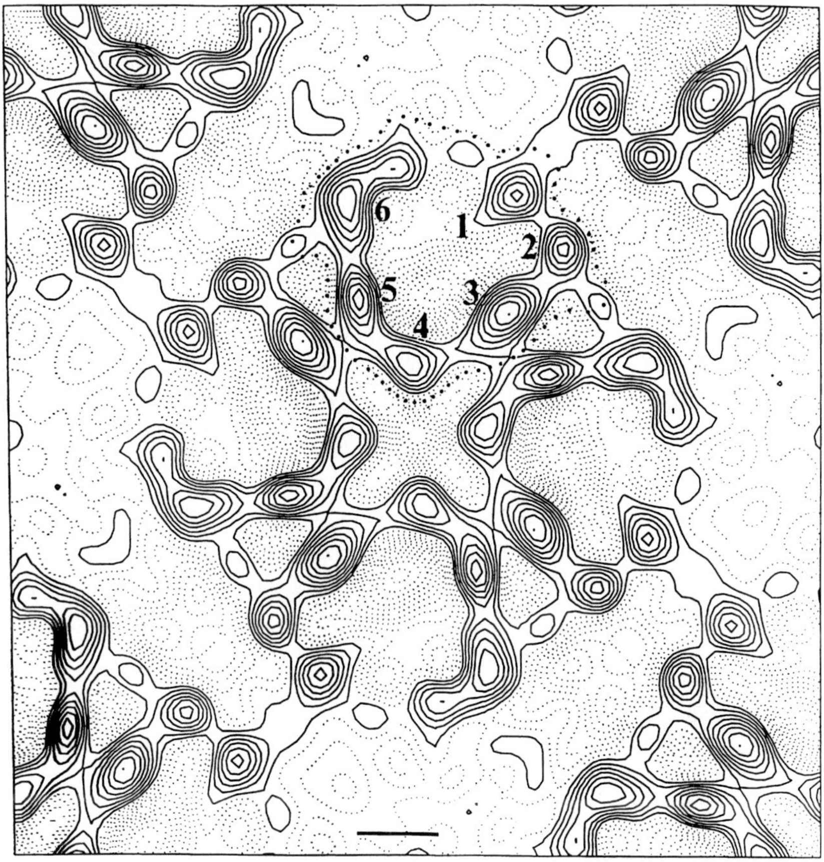

Figure 7 Structure of AQP1 water channel in projection. Purified AQP1 was reconstituted at high density in liposomes for determination of structure by electron cryocrystallography (42). An AQP1 tetramer is shown at the center, in which six putative helical domains are numbered in one monomer of the tetramer. The central opening in each monomer may represent the entrance to the transmembrane water pore. Scale bar: 1 nm.

of a cysteine residue at a position equivalent to cysteine 189 in AQP1; interestingly, mercury sensitivity can be conferred to AQP4 by mutating to cystein-specific residues just proximal to each of the NPA motifs (53). The three laboratories reporting the cloning of AQP3 found strongly increased glycerol permeability in the *Xenopus* oocyte expression system, but lower transport of water (54–56). There are no data on whether the proteins other than AQP1 form tetramers in membranes. Interestingly, freeze-fracture studies indicate that AQP4 forms regular orthogonal arrays of particles when expressed in CHO cells (31). It was proposed that AQP4 is the protein constituent of OAPs found in many mammalian tissues, including basolateral membrane of kidney collecting duct, gastric parietal cells, astrocytes, and others. Recent studies with AQP4 knockout mice confirm that AQP4 is the OAP protein (80).

B. Tissue Distribution of the Aquaporins

Four of the aquaporin family proteins are present in trachea and lung as shown by the RNA protection assay (57). The first localization of an aquaporin in lung was reported by in situ hybridization studies of AQP1 in alveolar cells (58). Subsequent immunolocalization experiments showed that AQP1 is strongly expressed at the plasma membrane of capillary endothelial cells (16,59–61) and to lesser extent on some pneumocytes including type II alveolar epithelial cells. AQP4 is expressed at the basolateral plasma membrane surface in epithelial cells throughout the trachea and the small and large airways (62). AQP5 is expressed at the apical membrane of type I alveolar epithelial cells (63). AQP3 is coexpressed with AQP4 at the basolateral membrane of tracheal epithelial cells but is not present in smaller airways or elsewhere in the lung (62). Of note, water channels have not yet been identified at the basolateral surface of alveolar epithelial cells or at the apical surface of airway epithelial cells. Additional lung water channels are likely to be identified, and it is quite possible that unrelated transporting proteins that are not selective for transport of water may contribute to water permeability in these membranes. For example, the glucose-transporting protein GLUT-1 and the cystic fibrosis chloride channel CFTR have been shown to permit transport of water when expressed at high densities in *Xenopus* oocytes (64–66). A new water channel (AQP8) was cloned recently (78); AQP8 is expressed at low levels in lung but localization has not yet been done.

As summarized in Table 2, several of the aquaporins are expressed widely in mammalian tissues. Most of the tissues containing water channels are clearly involved in fluid movement; however, several are not, such as erythrocytes, which express AQP1, and neuromuscular cells, which express AQP4. The localization of aquaporins to cells involved in vectorial fluid transport suggests but does not prove a role for aquaporins in fluid movement. To date, a definitive role for an aquaporin in mammalian physiology has been demonstrated only for AQP2, the vasopressin-sensitive water channel expressed at the apical membrane of principal cells in kidney collecting duct epithelium (46). Intracellular vesicles containing AQP2 fuse with the apical plasma membrane upon binding of vasopressin to V2 receptors at the basolateral cell membrane surface. Mutations of the AQP2 gene in humans result in a rare disease, hereditary non-X-linked nephrogenic diabetes insipidus, producing a defect in the urinary concentrating

Table 2 Tissue Distribution of Mammalian MIP Homologs

Respiratory system	
alveolus	endothelium: AQP1; type I cells: AQP5; type II cells: AQP1
airways	small airways: AQP4; trachea/large airways: AQP3, AQP4
Neuromuscular system	
brain	choroid plexus: AQP1; ependymal cells: AQP4; pia mater: AQP3, AQP4 supraoptic and paraventricular nuclei: AQP4; astrocytes: AQP4
spinal	astrocytes: AQP4
eye	iris epithelium: AQP1, AQP4; ciliary body: AQP1, AQP4 retina: nuclear layer AQP4; cornea: endothelium AQP1; epithelium AQP5 conjunctiva: AQP3; lens epithelium: AQP1; lens fiber: MIP
muscle	myocytes: AQP4
Cardiovascular system	
	myocardium: AQP1; capillary endothelium: AQP1
Digestive system	
	salivary gland: excretory duct AQP4; secretory lobule AQP5 stomach: gastric parietal cells AQP4 colon: crypt epithelium AQP1; villus epithelium AQP3, AQP4 pancreas: AQP1; gallbladder: AQP1
Genitourinary system	
kidney	proximal tubule and thin descending limb of Henle: AQP1 collecting duct apical membrane: AQP2 collecting duct basolateral membrane: AQP3, AQP4
urinary bladder	transitional epithelium AQP3
Reproductive system	
	testis efferent ductules, seminal vesicles, prostate: AQP1 uterus: AQP1; placenta: AQP1
Other	liver: interlobular bile duct AQP1 hematopoietic: spleen red pulp AQP1; erythrocytes AQP1 skin: epidermis AQP3; sweat gland AQP1

Source: Data are summarized from Refs. 58–60, 62, 76, 77.

mechanism (67). For AQP1, naturally occurring mutations have been identified because AQP1 is the Colton blood group antigen in human erythrocytes. Subjects lacking functional AQP1 protein were reported to be phenotypically normal, suggesting that AQP1 does not have an important physiological role (68). However, recent phenotype analysis of an AQP1 knockout mouse showed a severe defect in urinary concentrating ability (79). Lung phenotype analysis is in progress.

C. Water Transport in Lung Development and Expression of Aquaporins

One approach to study the physiological role of aquaporins is the measurement of aquaporin expression around the time of birth and correlation of expression with water transport function. In preparation for alveolar respiration, the lung at birth undergoes a transition from a fluid secreting to a fluid reabsorbing organ (69,70). It was postulated that this transition is accompanied by an increase in expression of aquaporins and a corresponding increase in water permeability between the airspace and alveolar compartments. An initial study of aquaporin transcript expression was carried out in rat lungs obtained at fetal day 19 to adult (71). By the RNAse protection assay, it was found that AQP1 transcript expression was very low and increased slowly through fetal life, and then strongly increased just after birth. Steroid treatment was associated with increased AQP1 transcript expression (72). AQP4 expression had a similar temporal pattern (71). In contrast, AQP5 transcript expression increased slowly and monotonically between fetal day 20 and day 7 after birth. Quantitative immunoblot analysis showed a progressive increase in AQP1 protein over the first week of life. To address the functional consequences of these observations, the pleural surface fluorescence method was used to measure transalveolar osmotic water permeability in the developing lung (73). There was a significant increase in osmotic water permeability in the first 24 hours after birth, suggesting role for aquaporins in the maintenance of a dry airspace during the first few days of postnatal life.

V. Summary and Perspective

From the recent data summarized in this chapter, it is now known that water permeabilities across epithelia and endothelia in lung are quite high and that several water-transporting proteins are expressed in lung cell membranes. New water channels are likely to be identified that are expressed in lung, and existing proteins may be assigned a water-transporting role, particularly in those lung cell membranes in which water permeability is high and water channels have not yet been identified. An unresolved question in lung physiology is the role of molecular water channels and of high water permeability in normal physiology and clinical disease. One approach to study this question is the use of specific pharmacological blockers of water-transporting proteins; however, specific nontoxic inhibitors of water channels are not at present available for any of the aquaporins. Definitive analysis of the role of aquaporins in lung physiology will probably come from studies on transgenic mice lacking specific aquaporin proteins. Our laboratory recently completed the genomic cloning of mouse AQP4 for generation of AQP4 knockout mice (74). Homozygous knockout

AQP4(−/−) mice were found to be grossly normal and to have a mild defect in urinary concentrating ability (75). In addition to studies on transgenic animals, experiments are needed to quantify the regulation of water channel expression under physiological stress and in various clinically relevant states, including pulmonary edema. Although it is speculative at this time, the pharmacological and genetic manipulation of water channels may provide a novel approach to treat states of defective fluid accumulation in lung and extrapulmonary tissues.

Acknowledgments

I thank Drs. Ethan Carter, Hans Folkesson, Michael Matthay, Tonghui Ma, Fuminori Umenishi, and Baoxue Yang for their continued collaboration on studies of water channels in lung and for their critical reading of this manuscript. This study was supported by National Institutes of Health grants HL51854, DK35124, HL42368, and DK43840, and grant R613 from the National Cystic Fibrosis Foundation.

References

1. Matthay MA, Folkesson H, Verkman AS. Salt and water transport across alveolar and distal airway epithelia in the adult lung. Am J Physiol 1996; 270:L487–L503.
2. Basset G, Crone C, Saumon G. Significance of active ion transport in transalveolar water absorption: a study on isolated rat lung. J Physiol 1987; 384:311–324.
3. Murray CB, Morales MM, Flotte TR, McGrath-Morrow SA, Guggino WB, Zeitlin PL. ClC-2—a developmentally dependent chloride channel expressed in the fetal lung and downregulated after birth. Am J Respir Cell Mol Biol 1995; 12:597–604.
4. Boucher RC. Human airway ion transport. Part one. Am J Respir Crit Care Med 1994; 150:271–281.
5. Hummler E, Barker P, Gatzy J, et al. Early death due to defective neonatal lung liquid clearance in alpha-ENaC-deficient mice. Nature Genet 1996; 12:325–328.
6. Macey RI. Transport of water and urea in red blood cells. Am J Physiol 1984; 246: C195–C203.
7. Verkman AS. Mechanisms and regulation of water permeability in renal epithelia. Am J Physiol 1989; 257:C837–C850.
8. Zhang R, Logee K, Verkman AS. Expression of mRNA coding for kidney and red cell water channels in *Xenopus* oocytes. J Biol Chem 1990; 265:15375–15378.
9. Preston GM, Agre P. Isolation of the cDNA for erythrocyte integral membrane protein of 28 kilodaltons: member of an ancient channel family. Proc Natl Acad Sci USA 1991; 88:11110–11114.
10. Agre P, Preston GM, Smith BL, et al. Aquaporin CHIP—the archetypal molecular water channel. Am J Physiol 1993; 265:F463–F476.
11. Van Os CH, Deen PMT, Dempster JA. Aquaporins—water selective channels in biological membranes—molecular structure and tissue distribution. Biochim Biophys Acta Rev Biomembr 1994; 1197:291–309.

12. Verkman AS, Van Hoek AN, Ma T, et al. Water transport across mammalian cell membranes. Am J Physiol 1996; 270:C12–C30.
13. Knepper MA. The aquaporin family of molecular water channels. Proc Natl Acad Sci USA 1994; 91:6255–6258.
14. Weibel ER. Lung morphometry and models in respiratory physiology. In: Chang HK, Paiva M, eds. Respiratory physiology. New York: Marcel Dekker, 1989:1–56.
15. Effros RM. Osmotic extraction of hypotonic fluid from the lungs. J Clin Invest 1974; 5:935–947.
16. Folkesson HG, Matthay MA, Hasegawa H, Kheradmand F, Verkman AS. Transcellular water transport in lung alveolar epithelium through mercury-sensitive water channels. Proc Natl Acad Sci USA 1994; 91:4970–4974.
17. Carter EP, Matthay MA, Farinas J, Verkman AS. Transalveolar osmotic and diffusional water permeability in intact mouse lung measured by a novel surface fluorescence method. J Gen Physiol 1996; 108:133–142.
18. Verkman AS. Optical methods to measure membrane transport processes. J Membrane Biol 1995; 148:99–110.
19. Carter EP, Ölveczky BP, Matthay MA, Verkman AS. High alveolar capillary water permeability in mouse lung measured by pleural surface fluorescence. Biophys J. In press.
20. Folkesson H, Matthay M, Frigeri A, Verkman AS. High transepithelial water permeability in microperfused distal airways: evidence for channel-mediated water transport. J Clin Invest 1996; 97:664–671.
21. Kuwahara M, Berry CA, Verkman AS. Rapid development of vasopressin-induced hydroosmosis in kidney collecting tubules measured by a new fluorescence technique. Biophys J 1988; 54:595–602.
22. Kuwahara M, Verkman AS. Direct fluorescence measurement of diffusional water permeability in the vasopressin-sensitive kidney collecting tubule. Biophys J 1988; 54:587–593.
23. Dobbs L, Gonzalez R, Matthay MA, Carter EP, Verkman AS. Highly water-permeable type I alveolar epithelial cells confer high transalveolar water permeability in rat lung. Proc Natl Acad Sci USA 1998. In press.
24. Farinas J, Simenak V, Verkman AS. Cell volume measured in adherent cells by total internal reflection microfluorimetry: application to permeability in cells transfected with water channel homologs. Biophys J 1995; 68:1613–1620.
25. Farinas J, Verkman AS. Measurement of cell volume and water permeability in epithelial cell layers by interferometry. Biophys J 1996; 71:3511–3522.
26. Farinas J, Moore M, Verkman AS. Water permeability in intact cell layers measured by quantitative phase-contrast microscopy. J Gen Physiol 1997; 110:283–296.
27. Reizer J, Reizer A, Saier MH. The MIP family of integral membrane channel proteins: sequence comparisons, evolutional relationships, reconstructed pathway of evolution, and proposed functional differentiation of two repeated halves of the protein. Crit Rev Biochem Mol Biol 1993; 28:235–257.
28. Van Hoek AN, Verkman AS. Functional reconstitution of the isolated erythrocyte water channel CHIP28. J Biol Chem 1992; 267:18267–18269.
29. Ma T, Frigeri A, Tsai ST, Verbavatz JM, Verkman AS. Localization and functional analysis of CHIP28k water channels in stably transfected CHO cells. J Biol Chem 1993; 268:22756–22764.

30. Katsura T, Verbavatz J-M, Farinas J, et al. Constitutive and regulated membrane expression of aquaporin-CHIP and aquaporin-2 water channels in stably transfected LLC-PK1 cells. Proc Natl Acad Sci USA 1995; 92:7212–7216.
31. Yang B, Brown D, Verkman AS. The mercurial-insensitive water channel (AQP-4) forms orthogonal arrays in stably transfected CHO cells. J Biol Chem 1996; 271: 4577–4580.
32. Zhang R, Van Hoek AN, Biwersi J, Verkman AS. A point mutation at cysteine 189 blocks the water permeability of rat kidney water channel CHIP28k. Biochem 1993; 32:2938–2941.
33. Preston GM, Jung JS, Guggino WB, Agre P. The mercury-sensitive residue at cysteine 189 in the CHIP28 water channel. J Biol Chem 1993; 268:17–20.
34. Verbavatz JM, Brown D, Sabolic I, et al. Tetrameric assembly of CHIP28 water channels in liposomes and cell membranes. A freeze-fracture study. J Cell Biol 1993; 123:605–618.
35. Van Hoek AN, Wiener MC, Verbavatz JM, et al. Purification and structure-function analysis of PNGase F- and endo-b-galactosidase-treated CHIP28 water channels. Biochem 1995; 34:2212–2219.
36. Shi LB, Skach WR, Verkman AS. Functional independence of monomeric CHIP28 water channels revealed by expression of wild type-mutant heterodimers. J Biol Chem 1994; 269:10417–10422.
37. Skach WR, Shi LB, Calayag MC, Frigeri A, Lingappa VR, Verkman AS. Topology and biogenesis of the CHIP28 water channel at the endoplasmic reticulum. J Cell Biol 1994; 125:803–816.
38. Preston GM, Jung JS, Guggino WB, Agre P. Membrane topology of aquaporin CHIP—analysis of function epitope-scanning mutants by vectorial proteolysis. J Biol Chem 1994; 269:1668–1673.
39. Jung JS, Preston GM, Smith BL, Guggino WB, Agre P. Molecular structure of the water channel through aquaporin CHIP. The hourglass model. J Biol Chem 1994; 269:14648–14654.
40. Zhang R, Skach W, Hasegawa H, Van Hoek AN, Verkman AS. Cloning, functional analysis and cell localization of a kidney proximal tubule water transporter homologous to CHIP28. J Cell Biol 1993; 120:359–369.
41. Finkelstein A. Water movement through lipid bilayers, pores, and plasma membranes: theory and reality. New York: Wiley & Sons, 1987.
42. Mitra AK, Van Hoek AN, Wiener MC, Verkman AS, Yaeger M. The CHIP28 water channel visualized in ice by electron crystallography. Nature Struct Biol 1995; 2: 726–729.
43. Walz T, Typke D, Smith BL, Agre P, Engel A. Projection map of aquaporin-1 determined by electron crystallography. Nature Struct Biol 1995; 2:730–732.
44. Jap BK, Li H. Structure of the osmo-regulated H_2O channel, AQP-CHIP at 3.5 A resolution. J Mol Biol 1995; 251:413–420.
45. Shi LB, Skach WR, Ma T, Verkman AS. Distinct biogenesis mechanisms for water channels MIWC and CHIP28 at the endoplasmic reticulum. Biochem 1995; 34: 8250–8256.
46. Bai LQ, Fushimi K, Sasaki S, Marumo F. Structure of aquaporin-2 vasopressin water channel. J Biol Chem 1996; 271:5171–5176.

47. Preston GM, Carroll TP, Guggino WB, Agre P. Appearance of water channels in *Xenopus* oocytes expressing red cell CHIP28 protein. Science 1992; 256:385–387.
48. Fushimi F, Uchida S, Hara Y, Hirata Y, Marumo F, Sasaki S. Cloning and expression of apical membrane water channel of rat kidney collecting tubule. Nature 1993; 361:549–552.
49. Hasegawa H, Ma T, Skach W, Matthay MA, Verkman AS. Molecular cloning of a mercurial-insensitive water channel expressed in selected water-transporting tissues. J Biol Chem 1994; 269:5497–5500.
50. Yang B, Ma T, Verkman AS. cDNA cloning, gene organization and chromosomal localization of a human mercurial-insensitive water channel: evidence for distinct transcriptional units. J Biol Chem 1995; 270:22907–22913.
51. Raina S, Preston GM, Guggino WB, Agre P. Molecular cloning and characterization of an aquaporin cDNA from salivary, lacrimal, and respiratory tissues. J Biol Chem 1995; 270:1908–1912.
52. Ma T, Yang B, Kuo WL, Verkman AS. cDNA cloning and gene structure of a new water channel expressed exclusively in human kidney: evidence for a gene cluster of aquaporins at chromosome locus 12q13. Genomics 1996; 35:543–550.
53. Shi LB, Verkman AS. Selected cysteine point mutations confer mercurial sensitivity to the mercurial-insensitive water channel MIWC. Biochem 1996; 35:538–544.
54. Ma T, Frigeri A, Hasegawa H, Verkman AS. Cloning of a water channel homolog expressed in brain meningeal cells and kidney collecting duct that functions as a stilbene-sensitive glycerol transporter. J Biol Chem 1994; 269:21845–21849.
55. Ishibashi K, Sasaki S, Fushimi K, et al. Molecular cloning and expression of a member of the aquaporin family with permeability to glycerol and urea in addition to water expressed at the basolateral membrane of kidney collecting duct cells. Proc Natl Acad Sci USA 1994; 91:6269–6273.
56. Echevarria M, Verkman AS. Optical measurement of osmotic water transport in cultured cells: evaluation of the role of glucose transporters. J Gen Physiol 1992; 99:573–589.
57. Umenishi F, Carter EP, Yang B, Olivier B, Matthay MA, Verkman AS. Sharp increase in rat lung water channel expression in the perinatal period. Am J Resp Cell Mol Biol 1996; 15:673–679.
58. Hasegawa H, Zhang R, Dohrman A, Verkman AS. Tissue-specific expression of mRNA encoding the rat kidney water channel CHIP28k by in situ hybridization. Am J Physiol 1993; 264:C237–C245.
59. Nielsen S, Smith BL, Christensen EI, Agre P. Distribution of the aquaporin CHIP in secretory and resorptive epithelia and capillary endothelia. Proc Natl Acad Sci USA 1993; 90:7275–7279.
60. Hasegawa H, Lian SC, Finkbeiner WE, Verkman AS. Extrarenal tissue distribution of CHIP28 water channels by in situ hybridization and antibody staining. Am J Physiol 1994; 266:C893–C903.
61. King LS, Nielsen S, Schnitzer JE, Oh P. Aquaporin-1 in plasma membrane and caveolae provides mercury-sensitive water channels across lung endothelium. Am J Physiol 1996; 39:H416–H422.
62. Frigeri A, Gropper M, Turck CW, Verkman AS. Immunolocalization of the mercurial-insensitive water channel and glycerol intrinsic protein in epithelial cell plasma membranes. Proc Natl Acad Sci USA 1995; 92:4328–4331.

63. Ling, LS, Nielsen S, Agre P. Aquaporin-5 is expressed in rat type I pneumocytes. Am J Respir Crit Care Med 1996; 153:A508. Abstract.
64. Hasegawa H, Skach W, Baker O, Calayag MC, Lingappa V, Verkman AS. A multifunctional aqueous channel formed by CFTR. Science 1992; 258:1477–1479.
65. Zhang R, Alper S, Thorens B, Verkman AS. Evidence from oocyte expression that the erythrocyte water channel is distinct from band 3 and the glucose transporter. J Clin Invest 1991; 88:1553–1558.
66. Fischbarg J, Kunyan K, Vera JC, et al. Glucose transporters serve as water channels. Proc Natl Acad Sci USA 1990; 87:3244–3247.
67. Deen PM, Verkijk MA, Knoers NV, et al. Requirement of human renal water channel aquaporin-2 for vasopressin-dependent concentration of urine. Science 1994; 264:92–95.
68. Preston GM, Smith BL, Zeidel ML, Moulds JJ, Agre P. Mutations in aquaporin-1 in phenotypically normal humans without functional CHIP water channels. Science 1994; 265:1585–1587.
69. Bland RD. Lung epithelial ion transport and fluid movement during the perinatal period. Am J Physiol 1990; 259:L30–L37.
70. Olver RE. Fluid secretion and absorption in the fetus. In: Effros RM, Chang HK, eds. Fluid and Solute Transport in the Airspaces of the Lung. New York: Marcel Dekker, 1994:281–302.
71. Umenishi F, Verkman AS, Gropper M. Quantitative analysis of aquaporin mRNA expression in rat tissues. DNA Cell Biol 1996; 15:475–480.
72. King LS, Nielsen S, Agre P. Aquaporin-1 water channel protein in lung-ontogeny, steroid-induced expression, and distribution in rat. J Clin Invest 1996; 97:2183–2191.
73. Carter EP, Umenishi F, Farinas J, Matthay MA, Verkman AS. Transcapillary endothelial water permeability in intact mouse lung measured by pleural surface fluorescence. 1997. Submitted.
74. Ma T, Yang B, Verkman AS. Gene structure, cDNA cloning and expression of a mouse mercurial-insensitive water channel. Genomics 1996; 33:382–388.
75. Ma T, Yang B, Gillespie A, Carlson EJ, Epstein CJ, Verkman AS. Generation and phenotype of a transgenic knock-out mouse lacking the mercurial-insensitive water channel aquaporin-4. J Clin Invest 1997; 100:957–962.
76. Bondy C, Chin E, Smith BL, Preston GM, Agre P. Developmental gene expression and tissue distribution of the CHIP28 water-channel protein. Proc Natl Acad Sci USA 1993; 90:4500–4504
77. Frigeri A, Gropper M, Umenishi F, Kawashima M, Brown D, Verkman AS. Localization of MIWC and GLIP water channel homologs in neuromuscular, epithelial and glandular tissues. J Cell Sci 1995; 108:2993–3002.
78. Ma T, Yang B, Verkman AS. Cloning of a novel water and urea-permeable aquaporin from mouse expressed strongly in colon, placenta, liver and heart. Biochim Biophys Res Comm 1997; 240:324–328.
79. Ma T, Yang B, Gillespie A, et al. Severely impaired urinary concentrating ability in transgenic mice lacking aquaporin-1 water channels. J Biol Chem. In press.
80. Verbavatz JM, Ma T, Gobin R, Verkman AS. Absence of orthogonal arrays in kidney, brain and muscle from transgenic knockout mice lacking water channel aquaporin-4. J Cell Sci. In press.

19

Alveolar Protein Clearance

RANDOLPH H. HASTINGS

San Diego VA Medical Center
San Diego, California

KWANG-JIN KIM

University of Southern California
Los Angeles, California

I. Introduction

Alveolar protein clearance over short periods of time has been studied extensively, but the rate, route, and mechanisms of protein clearance over long periods after alveolar flooding have not been defined. Passive mechanisms appear to be responsible for the bulk of short-term clearance, while recent data suggest that cellular mechanisms may be important for long-term clearance. Alveolar protein clearance is fundamental to resolution of the transudate and exudate following hydrostatic or permeability pulmonary edema. Inability to clear alveolar protein may be associated with a poor prognosis in patients with pulmonary edema. For example, patients dying with adult respiratory distress syndrome (ARDS) have large quantities of precipitated protein in their airspaces (1) (see Chap. 2). Nonsurvivors of lung injury with ARDS have three times more protein in their airspaces than survivors (2). Protein in the airspaces may be a factor in the progression from alveolar edema to end stage fibrosis in ARDS because hyaline membranes form the framework for growth of fibrous tissue (3,4). Thus, alveolar protein clearance is a physiologically interesting and a clinically relevant topic.

In this chapter we will review protein clearance under normal and pathologic conditions and evaluate the role of alveolar cells in protein uptake and clearance. We will discuss characteristics of protein clearance, such as rate, size dependence, temperature dependence, effects of pharmacologic agents, amount of protein degradation, and apparent changes in mechanism with time. Sections will be devoted to cellular mechanisms, albumin-binding proteins, and scavenger receptors in the alveolar epithelium and alveolar macrophages. We will cover pathologic conditions, including inflammatory reactions, immune reactions, and alveolar proteinosis, and therapeutic use of the lung for drug delivery. Protein transport in the upper airways has been reviewed elsewhere (5).

II. Protein Clearance from the Airspaces Under Normal Conditions

Pulmonary edema fluid contains a high concentration of protein. In hydrostatic edema, the protein concentration may approach 65% of the concentration in serum. The concentration is even higher in permeability edema (6–10). Thus, resolution of alveolar edema requires clearance of both liquid and protein from the alveolar space. Alveolar protein clearance is slow in the normal lung, no more than 1% to 2%/hour for serum proteins. Clearance rate does not vary appreciably between species and is similar for sheep, rabbits, and rats (10–13). Indirect evidence suggests that a similar rate holds for humans, as well (10). The rate of elimination for exogenously instilled protein is remarkably persistent over time. For example, Berthiaume et al. found that ^{125}I-albumin was eliminated from the airspaces of lungs of awake sheep at a monoexponential rate over the course of 6 days (11). In contrast, alveolar liquid is cleared more rapidly than protein, at a rate of 10% to 25%/h, depending on the species (12,14,15). The protein concentration in the edema fluid rises with time because liquid is cleared more rapidly than protein. Liquid clearance then slows as the protein becomes concentrated, due to the increase in protein oncotic pressure (15–18). For example, Matthay et al. instilled 3 mL/kg autologous serum into the lungs of unanesthetized sheep (17). The rate of liquid clearance declined from 8.3%/h in the first four hours to 3.3%/h from 4 to 12 hours. Over the same period, the calculated protein oncotic pressure increased from 40 to 53 cm H_2O. Accordingly, protein clearance is an essential step in the resolution of pulmonary edema.

Morphologic and physiologic techniques have been used to examine the relative resistance of the alveolar epithelium and the capillary endothelium to passage of protein. Horseradish peroxidase and ferritin instilled into the air spaces do not appear to penetrate the epithelium into the interstitium, even over periods as long as 6 hours (19–22). In contrast, the same tracers rapidly enter the pulmonary interstitium from the bloodstream but then do not cross into the airspaces (19–23). Taylor and Gaar calculated reflection coefficients for small solutes and estimated that the pore radii were 0.5 to 0.9 nm in the alveolar epithelium, compared to 6.5 to 7.5 nm in the capillary endothelium (24). Gorin and Stewart estimated the relative barrier properties of the capillary endothelium and alveolar epithelium to passage of ^{125}I-albumin in adult sheep with chronic lung lymph fistulas. The epithelium was responsible for 92% of the resistance to albumin flux across the alveolar-capillary barrier (25). Berthiaume et al. studied protein clearance from the lungs of sheep over 144 hours and found that 75% or more the ^{125}I-albumin remaining in the lung was located in the airspaces (11). Thus, the distal pulmonary epithelium is the principal barrier to protein clearance from the normal lung.

The rate of protein absorption from the distal airspaces appears to be size-dependent. Effros and Mason (26) compared measurements of alveolar epithelial protein permeability published in many sources. The combined data demonstrated an inverse relationship between molecular weight and the rate of lung clearance of different-size molecules. Theodore and colleagues reported that the alveolar epithelial permeabilities of urea, sucrose, inulin, and dextran (60 to 90 kDa) in saline-filled dog lungs varied inversely with molecular size and commensurately with the free diffusion coefficient of the solutes in water (27). Wangensteen and Yankovich found a larger permeability surface area product for sucrose than for albumin in rabbit lungs (28). Folkesson and co-workers found that the bioavailability of intratracheally instilled protein was inversely related to the solute molecular weight (29). For the nonapeptide 1-desamino-8-D-arginine vasopressin (dDAVP) (1.1 kDa), the period of peak passage into blood was 1 to 3 hours, while about 24 hours was required for albumin to pass across the alveolar epithelium (66 kDa) (29,30).

Hastings and colleagues showed that large proteins were cleared from the lungs of rabbits more slowly than small proteins, suggesting an inverse correlation between the Stokes radius and protein clearance (Fig. 1) (10). The same

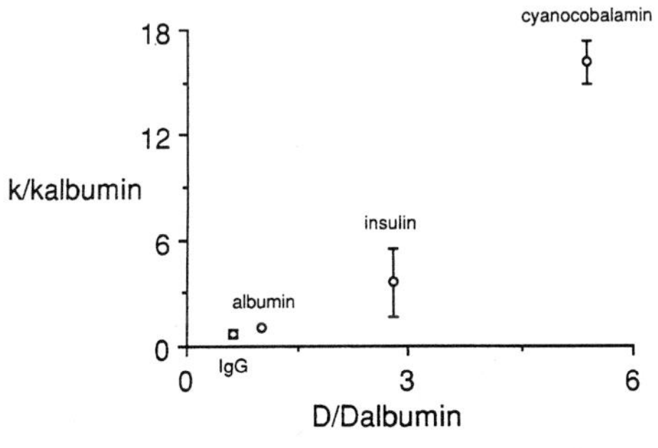

Figure 1 Rate constant for lung tracer clearance (k) plotted versus free diffusion coefficient (*D*), referenced to albumin. *D/D*albumin was calculated assuming *D* was inversely proportional to the Stokes radius of the molecule. Line of identity is shown. (From Ref. 10.)

study investigated size selectivity of protein clearance in humans during the resolution phase of pulmonary edema. Initially, the ratio of albumin concentration to total protein concentration was greater in edema fluid than plasma (10). Over 10 hours, the edema fluid albumin fraction decreased from 0.62 ± 0.12 to 0.58 ± 0.10 ($P < .05$ by paired t-test) in 10 patients with resolving pulmonary edema, presumably because albumin was cleared from the airspaces more rapidly than the larger immunoglobulins (Fig. 2). Thus, rat, rabbit, dog, and human studies provide evidence that protein clearance from the airspaces of the lung is size-dependent (10,27,29).

The concept that proteins are degraded in the airways and then absorbed as smaller protein fragments was first proposed by Drinker and Hardenbergh (31). This process may occur to some extent, but it plays a minimal part in protein clearance under normal conditions. Generally, > 95% of the protein instilled into the distal air spaces of the normal lung reaches the blood circulation intact (10,11,14–17,28–20,32). Berthiaume and colleagues followed clearance of intact radioiodinated albumin for 6 days after intratracheal instillation in sheep (11). Trichloroacetic acid-soluble radioiodine in lung lavage, urine, thyroid, and

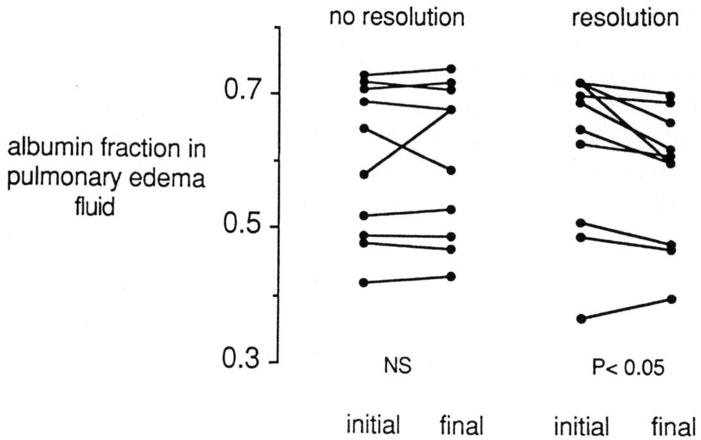

Figure 2 Albumin fraction, the ratio of albumin to total protein, in pulmonary edema fluid consistently decreased during the resolution phase of alveolar edema (n = 10). Albumin fraction did not change consistently if there was no resolution of alveolar edema (n = 10), even though a longer period of time was generally available for protein clearance to occur in the no-resolution group than in the resolution group. Initial and final samples were separated by 22 ± 18 hours (range 6 to 47 hours) in the no-resolution group and 10 ± 5 hours (range 6 to 22 hours) in the resolution group, respectively. Patients were placed in the resolution group if total protein concentration increased > 5%/h between the initial and final samples. (From Ref. 10.)

feces increased after 2 days, suggesting some breakdown, but over 80% of the extrapulmonary radioiodine was still associated with the parent molecule. Schultz et al. (33) and Braley et al. (34) found high levels of protein degradation using perfused dog and rabbit lungs. This may have occurred from protein degradation on the bronchial epithelium (35). However, another group using the same technique found that 95% of the tracer protein was cleared into the perfusate as an intact molecule (36). However, degradation may be the mechanism for clearing some specific proteins from the airspaces. For example, vasoactive intestinal peptide (VIP) is cleared from the air spaces more rapidly than expected for its size and is found to be completely degraded during the clearance process (37). Gastrin (2.2 kDa) is almost entirely degraded during clearance from the air spaces as well (Hastings, unpublished observations). On the other hand, insulin and dDAVP are cleared intact at rates consistent with size (10,29), and aerosolized calcitonin reaches the bloodstream of patients immunologically and biologically intact (38). It is not known whether degradation of small proteins occurs through the action of proteases in the alveolar cell plasma membrane or because of endocytosis, followed by lysosomal proteolysis in the epithelium.

III. Protein Transport by Alveolar Cells

Cellular transport processes, such as endocytosis or phagocytosis, could contribute to alveolar protein clearance. Bignon's immunocytochemical studies provided the first evidence that alveolar epithelial cells could take up protein. He showed that alveolar type I epithelial cells in rat lung contained albumin in vesicles (39). Other investigators have shown that type I and type II cells take up ferritin and horseradish peroxidase in vesicles (19–22). Type II cells take up surfactant protein A (SP-A) from the alveolar space by receptor-mediated endocytosis (40). Both type I and type II cells are capable of phagocytosis (41–44).

Information on the cellular pathways and mechanisms for protein transport specific to the alveolar epithelium is scarce. The numerous vesicles on the alveolar epithelial and capillary barriers could be involved in transport of proteins by pinocytosis (45). Gee and Staub (46) suggested that perivascular cuffs in the bronchoalveolar region may be the leakage site for plasma protein. Similarly, West and colleagues reported that expansion of vascular space volume probably leads to increased leak of protein into alveolar and interstitial spaces (47), although the effect of expansion of vascular beds on overall alveolar epithelial transport is unknown. The exact loci of protein transport or leak across the distal respiratory epithelial tract from the interstitium and vascular spaces are not clearly defined. Furthermore, quantitatively significant protein transport by alveolar epithelial endocytosis has not been established.

Receptor-mediated or adsorptive endocytosis could be involved in translocation of serum proteins and related substances such as surfactant proteins across the epithelial barrier. Maclura pomifera agglutinin and cationic ferritin bind the surface of alveolar type II pneumocytes (22,48), decorating coated and uncoated pits as well as the insides of vesicles. When natural surfactant was instilled intratracheally, Wright et al. (49) reported that subfractions containing proteins of molecular weights ranging from 26 to 36 kDa were preferentially taken up by intact rat lungs to a greater extent than were subfractions that did not contain these apoproteins. The specific mechanisms for enhanced uptake of surfactant fractions containing low-molecular-weight proteins are not known. The alveolar surfaces also contain IgG in alveolar epithelial cell coats, tubular myelin, and free granular deposits, and autologous albumin is present on the surfaces of type II pneumocytes and in vesicles located in type I cells (39,50).

IV. Lung Albumin-Binding Proteins

Lung capillary endothelium expresses a cell plasma membrane protein with albumin-binding specificity. This protein, known as albondin (gp60), is a 60-kDa glycoprotein with a K_d for albumin of about 150 nM (51–53). Endothelial albondin contains only O-linked glycans, but its peptide backbone shares epitopes with the transmembrane spanning region of glycophorin (gp3) (54). Endothelial albondins appear to be localized largely in caveolae—large, uncoated plasmalemmal vesicles that have received much attention recently in terms of potocytosis, endocytosis, and transcytosis (55). Albondins mediate transcytosis of intact (>90%) albumin across the endothelium (56,57). This may account for >40% of total endothelial albumin translocation (56–58). Greater than 90% of endothelial transcytosis of albumin is blocked in the presence of an antibody to albondin (58).

Photoaffinity-labeling of endothelial cells freshly isolated from rat epididymal fat yields two major plasma membrane albumin-binding proteins with apparent molecular weights at 30 and 18 kDa (accounting for >70% of the albumin-binding proteins) and two minor protein bands at 73 and 56 kDa (59, 60). It is not known whether the 56-kDa albumin receptor is the same as albondin. The 30- and 18-kDa albumin-binding proteins (gp30/18) preferentially bind conformationally modified (e.g., maleylated or formaldehyde-treated) albumin, with K_d 6 nM–1 μM, but not native albumin (59–63). The gp30/18 albumin-binding proteins exhibit the characteristics of scavenger-type receptors, which play a role in receptor-mediated endocytosis of heavily modified protein ligands. Uptake by scavenger receptors results in eventual ligand protein degradation in lysosomes with no transcytosis of intact ligand across the endothelium (55,58–63). Separate from these cell membrane-associated albumin receptors, serum contains a secreted albumin-binding protein called SPARC

(~43 kDa) (64,65), as well as specific binding-proteins for senescent albumins that are heavily glycosylated or glycated (66). These albumin-binding proteins are not thought to participate in endothelial transcytosis of native albumin (56,61).

An endothelial albondin antibody reacts with cellular proteins of freshly isolated and primary cultured alveolar epithelial cells from rat lungs (67,68). Moreover, photoaffinity labeling of freshly isolated and cultured alveolar epithelial cells identified a membrane albumin-binding protein of ~60 kDa. Thus, alveolar epithelial cells express albondin-like binding sites for native albumin. The same photoaffinity study did not detect albumin-binding activity in 18- or 30-kDa proteins. Accordingly, alveolar epithelial cells may not express the gp30/18 scavenger receptors found in endothelial cells. Alternatively, the affinity of gp30/18 in alveolar epithelial cells for the photoprobe of native albumin may be extremely low, as is the case in endothelial cells (69). Kim and colleagues have discovered saturable, asymmetric, and rapid fluxes of intact (>85%) albumin across cultured rat alveolar epithelial cell monolayers (67). Thus, albondin or a protein related to albondin may mediate net intact albumin absorption across the alveolar epithelial barrier. Translocation of intact albumin across the alveolar epithelial barrier via nonspecific adsorptive endocytosis is highly unlikely, since the net negative charge on cell plasma membranes would be expected to hinder adsorption of albumin, a negatively charged molecule at physiological pH. Nonspecific fluid-phase endocytosis, which does not require adsorption of ligands, may account for <1% of total albumin flux, based on a recent report on alveolar epithelial pinocytosis rates estimated with horseradish peroxidase (70). Caveolae-like uncoated pits and vesicles are abundant in the type I cells of the distal airspaces of the lung.

Proteins in alveolar fluid may play major roles in numerous homeostatic functions, including immune defense, protection against oxidant stress, and maintaining oncotic pressure (8,42,71–75). Specific information on how these serumborne macromolecules traverse the alveolar epithelium is sparse. Other biologically important molecules, such as surfactant proteins or lipids, DNA-conjugated macromolecules, cytokines, and protein drugs, may adsorb to albumin and enter the pneumocytes or be translocated across the epithelium via the same route(s) as albumin. For example, albumin-binding sites on pneumocytes could serve as a portal of entry for processed or degraded surfactant apoproteins, lipids, or fatty acids (49,76). Thus, mechanistic information on protein transport may improve understanding of processes such as transport of other macromolecules, systemic delivery of inhaled drugs, and trafficking of cytokines, and may support airway approaches to gene therapy (69,77–79).

In summary, the alveolar epithelium contains protein transport organelles and binding proteins similar to the endothelium (56). Endocytosed albumin and other proteins can be demonstrated immunohistochemically and measured in cell culture. This evidence suggests that endocytosis should have a physiological role in alveolar homeostasis. However, it is difficult to envision that albondin, with its high affinity for albumin, would contribute to all aspects of alveolar protein transport. For example, the rate of alveolar clearance of instilled albumin is proportional to albumin concentration over a range of 10 to 300 mg/mL (17,29), orders of magnitude greater than saturating concentrations for binding to albondin (51–53). Proof of the importance of endocytosis requires physiologic investigations, most likely in animals or intact lung preparations, directed specifically toward normal or pathologic conditions and toward specific proteins. Some physiologic investigations have been completed, proceeding in parallel with the in vitro studies.

V. Temperature Dependence of Alveolar Protein Clearance

One strategy has been to examine temperature dependence, attempting to distinguish between active and passive transport mechanisms. Cooling is the classic physiologic approach for blocking metabolic processes. As biologic tissues cool, energy-dependent processes slow and eventually cease. Endocytic vesicles do not form at temperatures below about 13°C. In contrast to endocytosis, diffusion would not exhibit a break point at about 18°C. Passive transport by diffusion through water-filled channels decreases monotonically with temperature because of a decrease in the diffusion coefficient and an increase in the viscosity of the medium (80). Several investigators have examined the temperature dependence of alveolar protein clearance in isolated lung preparations. Hostetter and colleagues (81) showed that clearance of aerosolized albumin from isolated rabbit lungs decreased 89% when the temperature was decreased from 37°C to 12°C. This observation suggests that transport occurs by endocytosis. Diffusive transport should only decrease by about 50% over this fall in temperature. However, Serikov and co-workers found contradictory temperature effects on clearance of albumin from isolated goat lungs (82). In that study, albumin clearance decreased by 80% when temperature was reduced from 37°C to 30°C. If the predominant clearance mechanism were endocytosis, the decrease in clearance should have been much less for a 7°C fall in temperature in that range. More information (such as the activation energy for epithelial transcytosis) is needed to explain the striking temperature dependence of alveolar epithelial protein clearance.

VI. Effect of Endocytosis Inhibitors on Alveolar Protein Clearance

The importance of endocytosis for alveolar protein clearance has also been investigated using pharmacologic inhibitors of endocytosis. Hastings et al. administered monensin or nocodazole into the airspaces of rabbits in an attempt to inhibit endocytosis by the alveolar epithelium (83). Both drugs are active against endocytosis in cell culture systems. Monensin inhibits receptor-mediated endocytosis in human hepatoma cells, hepatocytes, fibroblasts, and pancreatic acini (84–87). The mechanism works through inhibition of acidification of endocytic vesicles and endosomes, a necessary step for receptor-ligand dissociation, transport of ligands to lysosomes, and recycling of endosomal membrane and uncoupled receptors to the plasma membrane. Nocodazole, a microtubule-disrupting drug, inhibits transcytosis in MDCK cell and Caco-2 intestinal epithelial cell monolayers (88,89). Several observations suggested that monensin and nocodazole inhibited endocytosis in the alveolar epithelium. First, nocodazole increased the number of intracellular vesicles in the alveolar epithelium and capillary endothelium, suggesting that it disrupted microtubules. Monensin increased vesicle density in the endothelium, possibly by interrupting cellular membrane traffic. Second, immunohistochemical studies showed that both inhibitors decreased lung parenchymal uptake of instilled human albumin (Fig. 3). Third, monensin and nocodazole inhibited albumin uptake in cultured alveolar type II cells. Fourth, both inhibitors increased the amount of ^{125}I-surfactant protein A (SP-A) associated with the lungs relative to the quantity remaining in the air space 2 hours after instillation, suggesting that they reduced return of endocytosed SP-A to the alveolar space. Although the endocytosis inhibitors decreased alveolar epithelial protein uptake, they did not reduce alveolar clearance of ^{125}I-IgG or ^{131}I-albumin in anesthetized rabbits. Thus, monensin- and nocodazole-sensitive protein uptake pathways do not appear to be crucial for clearance of bulk quantities of serum protein from the rabbit alveolar space in vivo. It is unknown if these inhibitors activate other mechanisms or pathways for alveolar protein clearance.

VII. Protein Transport by Alveolar Macrophages and Neutrophils

Alveolar protein clearance could also be mediated by bloodborne cells. Instillation of a protein solution causes a substantial influx of these cells into the airspaces. Neutrophils predominate initially, but the number of alveolar macrophages increases over several days (11,17). Alveolar macrophage numbers remain elevated for at least 30 days after challenge with inert particles (90). Alveolar macrophages are well-recognized for their endocytic and phagocytic ability. They scavenge and degrade surfactant and other proteinaceous material (91,92). In contrast, neutrophils do not appear to be important in the clearance of protein. Recruitment of neutrophils into the airspaces by endotoxin or LTB4 has no effect on the movement of protein into or out of the alveolar space (93,94). Thus, alveolar macrophages and epithelial cells are the most likely

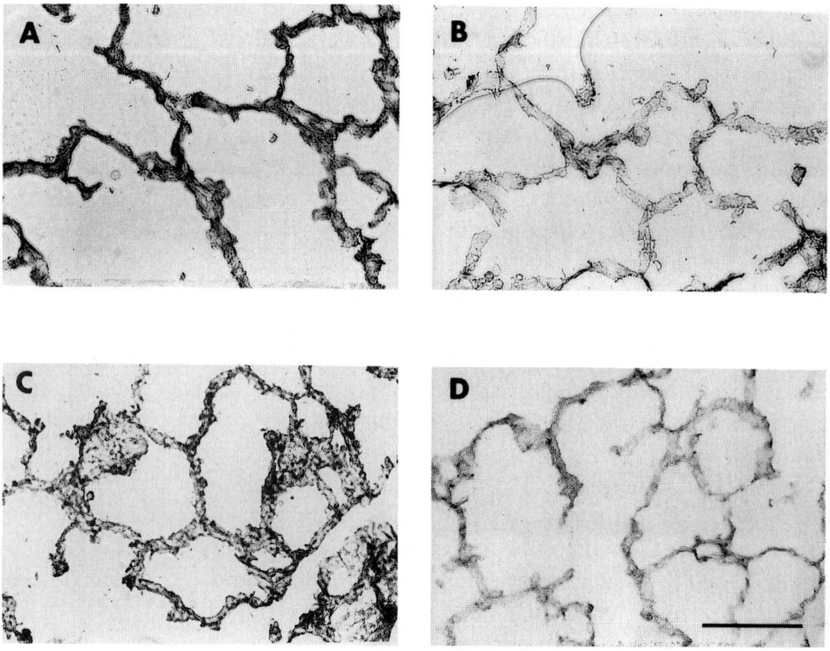

Figure 3 Light micrographs of rabbit lungs instilled with human albumin. Lungs were fixed 2 hours after instillation and stained for human albumin with an immunoperoxidase technique and 3,3′-diaminobenzidine HCl. (A) Ethanol added to instillate as a control for monensin. (B) 3×10^{-5} M monensin. (C) Dimethylsulfoxide control. (D) 3×10^{-5} M nocodazole. Presence of human albumin is marked by dark reaction product. Monensin and nocodazole prevented alveolar epithelial uptake of albumin. However, they did not block alveolar clearance of albumin (not shown). The conclusion is that transcytosis is not the major mechanism for clearing bulk quantities of albumin from the alveolar space. Bar = 0.2 mm.

candidates for ingestion and/or clearance of proteins from the distal airspaces of the lung.

Alveolar macrophages have a phenomenal capacity for endocytosis and phagocytosis. Macrophages take up a fluid volume equal to their own by fluid-phase endocytosis every 30 min (95). Hastings and colleagues compared uptake of albumin by alveolar macrophages and epithelial cells in anesthetized rabbits over periods of 1 to 8 hours using electron microscopic immunohistochemical techniques (Fig. 4) (96). Albumin immunoreactivity appeared in vesicles and endosomes in all three cell types, but alveolar macrophages took up albumin earlier and more avidly than the epithelial cells. Similarly, cultured

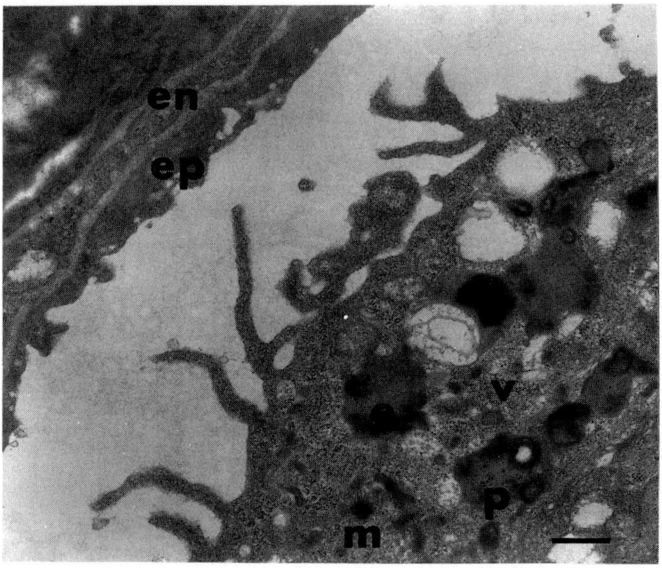

Figure 4 Uptake of colloidal gold-conjugated albumin by rabbit alveolar macrophages in vivo. This macrophage is from a lung instilled with colloidal-gold albumin and fixed by instillation after 2 hours. A labeled macrophage (m) is adjacent to unlabeled alveolar epithelium (ep). Gold-conjugated albumin particles were never found in epithelial or endothelial (en) cells, even 8 hours after instillation (not shown). In contrast, macrophages contained gold particles in vesicles (v), phagosomes (p), and endosomes (e) as early as 2 hours after instillation. Bar = 400 nm. (From Ref. 96.)

alveolar macrophages took up albumin more rapidly than cultured type II cells. Macrophages also demonstrated more rapid phagocytosis than the epithelial cells in vivo. Alveolar macrophages phagocytosed insoluble albumin in the form of colloidal gold-albumin conjugates within two hours of intratracheal instillation, while alveolar epithelial cells did not, even over eight hours. These results are consistent with Williams' observations that alveolar macrophages took up a variety of instilled soluble and insoluble tracers, including neutral and charged dextrans, anionically and cationically derivatized ferritin, and carbon particles more avidly and rapidly than alveolar epithelial cells (22). Other investigators have also found phagocytosis by alveolar epithelial cells to be slower and less pronounced than alveolar macrophage phagocytosis (41,43,97,98). Thus, protein clearance by macrophages appears to be a more rapid and larger-capacity pathway than epithelial cell uptake.

Data on the quantitative contribution of macrophages to alveolar protein clearance is lacking, but qualitative information can be derived from

Berthiaume's study of lung protein clearance over 6 days in sheep (11), using indices of alveolar protein degradation and cellular uptake. The influx of macrophages into the airspaces increased substantially between days 2 and 6. Increased quantities of tracer were associated with macrophages by day 4, and phagolysosomes with staining characteristics similar to those of the instilled serum were present in the macrophage cytoplasm. The quantities of protein-free ^{125}I in lung lavage, urine, and feces increased four- to fivefold from day 2 to day 6. Thus, as time progressed, resident cells in the airspaces appeared to catabolize more protein.

Cell-mediated mechanisms might gain importance with time if protein were modified during its residence in the airspaces. For example, protein might precipitate over the course of days because of the increased protein concentration that occurs as alveolar liquid is cleared. Protein will precipitate if the concentration exceeds its solubility limits. With permeability edema, insoluble protein may form from deposition of fibrin in the alveolar space (1). Insoluble proteins (e.g., precipitated or clotted proteins) cannot be cleared by passive mechanisms and are probably eliminated by phagocytosis. In a recent study, the effects of protein precipitation on alveolar clearance and the role of macrophages in clearing precipitated protein were investigated by instilling rats with tracer ^{125}I-albumin in either 5% or 15% albumin or 15% albumin plus dichloromethylene diphosphonate (Cl_2MDP) liposomes (99). The rationale for this experiment was that albumin will precipitate sooner as liquid is cleared if the starting concentration is higher. Liposome-encapsulated Cl_2MDP causes alveolar macrophage numbers to decline by 70% to 85% within 1 day and to remain depressed for 1 week (100). Table 1 presents the results for 3-day recoveries. Lung recoveries for the three rats in the 15% albumin groups were greater than recoveries in the 5% group. This observation supports the hypothesis that the more concentrated albumin should precipitate earlier than the 5% albumin and then be cleared more slowly. Cl_2MDP liposomes decreased the number of macrophages recovered by lavage by about 30%. This partial depletion of macrophages was enough to increase lung albumin recovery and decrease urine tracer recovery in the Cl_2MDP group ($P < .05$). Cl_2MDP also decreased the quantity of TCA-soluble ^{125}I appearing in plasma and lung lavage (data not shown). Finally, 7.5% ± 0.9% of the airspace tracer was cell-associated in the Cl_2MDP group, compared to 65.1% ± 8.7% in the other groups ($P < .05$). The data indicate that alveolar macrophages degrade protein and have a measurable effect on the clearance of protein from the alveolar space.

Endocytosis of soluble protein by alveolar macrophages may increase if the protein is chemically or physically modified after it enters the alveolar space. Modified protein molecules are ligands for macrophage scavenger receptors, as discussed earlier. Scavenger receptors are known for uptake of oxidized LDL (101). Macrophages express several different receptors that bind aggregated

Table 1 Tracer Recoveries (% of Instilled, Mean ± SEM) 3 Days After Instillation

Albumin	N	Lungs	Plasma	Other organs	Urine	Feces	Total
5%	3	2.3 ± 0.6	1.8 ± 0.6	5.1 ± 1.0	52.8 ± 4.5	1.9 ± 0.9	63.9 ± 6.1
15%	3	4.2 ± 1.6	1.6 ± 0.4	4.0 ± 1.4	47.4 ± 4.4	1.7 ± 0.5	58.9 ± 2.1
15%, $C1_2MDP$	3	10.7 ± 2.9[a]	2.8 ± 0.6	6.9 ± 2.4	32.4 ± 3.9[a]	4.1 ± 1.4	56.7 ± 8.9

[a]Significantly different from 5% albumin group; $P < .05$.
Source: From Ref. 99.

LDL, maleylated albumin, aldehyde-conjugated albumins, or various acylated or oxidized proteins (102–105). Scavenger receptors recognize heavily modified proteins because of alterations in secondary and tertiary structure due to oxidation-induced changes in charge, aggregation, or crosslinking. Airspace proteins could be transformed into ligands for scavenger receptors by Schiff base formation with lipid peroxidation products (such as malondialdehyde), oxidation with superoxide or hydroxyl free radicals, alkylation by arachidonic acid metabolites (such as leukotriene A4 [101,106]), or precipitation or coagulation, since the macrophage scavenger receptor also plays a role in phagocytosis (107). $Alpha_1$ proteinase inhibitor is a well-known example of a protein that may be modified in the airspaces (108). A methionine residue at the active site is oxidized by reactive species contained in cigarette smoke or released by activated neutrophils and macrophages. Inactivation of α_1 proteinase inhibitor may result in unrestrained proteolytic activity in the lung extracellular matrix, leading to emphysema (109). Modification of serum proteins in the airspaces under basal conditions and in pulmonary edema liquid has not been studied. Further work is necessary to explore the mechanisms of alveolar protein clearance over long time periods and the mechanisms under pathologic conditions.

VIII. Protein Clearance Under Pathologic Conditions

Clearance of solutes, liquid, and protein from the airspaces has been studied under a variety of pathologic conditions that can be categorized as injury and inflammation, immune response, or alveolar proteinosis. In disease states involving lung injury, changes in the barrier function of the alveolar epithelium have a major impact on protein clearance. In immune responses, alterations in cellular transport by the epithelium may be important. Finally, in experimental models of alveolar proteinosis, the scavenging function of alveolar macrophages may play a predominant role.

The most striking discovery from studies of lung injury has been the high relative resistance of the alveolar epithelium to molecular traffic. The ability of the epithelium to act as a barrier to liquid and solute flux remains normal in the absence of pulmonary blood flow or ventilation (110,111). The pulmonary epithelium is also resistant against injury by infectious agents. Intravenous *E. coli* endotoxin in rats and sheep, intravenous *Pseudomonas aeruginosa* bacteria in goats and sheep, and alveolar endotoxin in goats and sheep do not alter epithelial albumin permeability or in liquid transport capability, even with concomitant large increases in endothelial permeability (112,113). Pittet and co-workers found that it was necessary to instill 10^{10} live *P. aeruginosa* bacteria into the alveolar space of sheep to injure both the epithelium and the endothelium (13). At these high titers, the rate of movement of tracer albumin across the epithelium into and out of the alveoli doubled. Interestingly, intratracheal instillation of IgG antibody to *P. aeruginosa* prevented the increase in respiratory epithelial permeability, while systemic perfusion of antibody protected the endothelial barrier. Thus, the integrity of the epithelial and endothelial barriers can be altered independently.

Injury to the epithelium under inflammatory conditions appears to be graded. Folkesson and colleagues investigated the effects of pulmonary inflammation induced by intratracheal *E. coli* endotoxin or ferritin in rats (114). The inflammatory agents caused dose-dependent increases in the lung passage of bovine IgG, bovine serum albumin (BSA), and dDAVP. The changes in lung passage were greater for IgG and BSA than for dDAVP. With intermediate degrees of inflammation, caused by endotoxin, lung clearance of BSA approached that of dDAVP. With the greater inflammation induced by ferritin, IgG clearance approached the clearance of the two smaller tracers. Since dDAVP normally crosses the alveolar epithelium by passive diffusion, the results suggest that the increased clearance was due to increases in paracellular transport, with bigger effects on large molecules that are normally restricted over this route. The study could not exclude effects on transcellular passage, however.

Damage to the epithelial barrier effectively prevents net clearance of excess liquid and protein from the airspaces. Clearance fails in injured lungs because airspace liquid and protein move readily into the vascular space, while liquid and protein from the vascular space readily enters the alveoli. Resolution of pulmonary edema requires a functional alveolar epithelial barrier. Strikingly, the epithelium appears to have the capacity to recover rapidly from injury. For example, net clearance of alveolar liquid begins as early as 4 hours after oleic acid-induced permeability edema in sheep (93). Similarly, patients with increased-permeability pulmonary edema can begin to clear the edema fluid within 12 hours of onset, marked by increasing concentration in edema fluid protein, a parallel decrease in edema on the chest radiograph, and an improvement in oxygenation (9). The resolution phase of pulmonary edema is marked by size selectivity (see Fig. 2) (10). This observation is consistent with the size selectivity seen for protein clearance in normal lungs.

The respiratory tract is an important route by which environmental antigens may enter the body. The transport of proteins across the alveolar epithelium in the face of immunization is a fascinating, but not completely understood, subject. If a protein tracer is insufflated into the lungs of an animal specifically immunized against that protein, passage of the protein into the circulation is blocked completely and transport of protein degradation products is increased severalfold (34,115). The phenomenon occurs even with passive immunization due to intravenous administration of antibody (116). Blockade of immunogen transport across the air–blood barrier is not due to rapid reuptake of immune complexes formed in the pulmonary circulation, since immune complexes infused into an isolated lung preparation are not taken up by the lung (116). Therefore, the transport blockade occurs within the lung parenchyma or alveolar space. The effect is quite robust; if protein permeability is increased by inducing inflammation in the immunized lung, the specific antigen still does not leave the alveolar space intact, even though permeability should be greatly increased by the inflammation (117). Interestingly, degradation of nonspecific proteins instilled with the antigen into immunized lungs is also increased, although passage of intact nonspecific protein is not affected (34,116,117). Teleologically, preventing systemic absorption of immunogenic proteins is important in avoiding untoward effects of the immune system. However, the mechanism(s) preventing absorption of intact antigen and stimulating its degradation are unknown.

Recent studies with granulocyte/macrophage–colony-stimulating factor (GM-CSF) knockout mice have suggested that defective macrophage function is important in the pathology of alveolar proteinosis. Alveolar proteinosis is a rare disease of characterized by accumulation of large amounts of pulmonary surfactant, apoproteins, and protein in the alveoli (118). Dranoff and colleagues used homologous recombination techniques in embryonic stem cells to design mice lacking GM-CSF (119). GM-CSF stimulates proliferation and chemotaxis of alveolar macrophages. Mutant mice developed pulmonary disease with progressive accumulation of surfactant apoproteins and lipids in the alveolar space. These are characteristic features of alveolar proteinosis. Surfactant apoprotein mRNA levels and synthesis were normal, but SP-A clearance was reduced.

Surfactant apoprotein recycling pathways also may have been affected. The alveolar space contained enlarged, foamy macrophages laden with lipids, suggesting that the condition may have resulted from a defect in macrophage surfactant clearance or catabolism. To further discern the role of GM-CSF in surfactant homeostasis, these investigators restored GM-CSF selectively into the type II cells of knockout mice. Genetically engineered mice were produced that overexpressed GM-CSF in their type II cells, driven by the SP-C promoter (120). These mice were crossed with the GM-CSF knockout mice, resulting in offspring that only expressed GM-CSF in the alveolar type II cells. GM-CSF corrected the abnormalities of surfactant homeostasis in the bitransgenic mice. Alveolar macrophage numbers increased and SP-A, SP-B, and phospholipid levels were normalized without associated changes in SP-A, SP-B, or SP-C lung mRNA levels. These data indicate that the GM-CSF regulates clearance or catabolism of surfactant apoproteins and that endocytosis or phagocytosis by alveolar macrophages is essential for this process.

IX. Therapeutic Delivery of Proteins via the Distal Airspaces

The lung is a potentially important route for systemic delivery of therapeutic peptides and proteins. The need for parenteral administration restrains the clinical use of a variety of peptides. Nasal and other transmucosal routes have been successful, but the small surface area limits the bioavailability of peptides delivered in this manner. The distal pulmonary epithelium represents an enormous surface compared to the nasal epithelium, with areas roughly equal to the size of a doubles tennis court and a postage stamp, respectively. Considerable research has been focused on pulmonary clearance of proteins and peptides administered for systemic effects, such as thyrotropin-releasing hormone, human growth hormone, enkephalins, insulin, and calcitonin (38,121–126). Peptide and protein drugs targeted locally to the lung, such as immunoglobulins (13) and α_1-antitrypsin (127), have also been administered intratracheally.

Alveolar clearance of exogenous protein drugs is generally similar to other proteins with respect to size dependence and lack of degradation, but determination of mechanisms for translocation of specific drugs across the epithelium will require individual study. For example, thyrotropin-releasing hormone crosses cultured alveolar epithelial cell monolayers predominantly intact (121), but arginine vasopressin and insulin undergo partial degradation that is blocked by alveolar aminopeptidase inhibitors (128–130). Effective drug delivery will be aided by the absence of proteolysis, rapid clearance for systemically targeted drugs, and slow clearance for pulmonary targets. Furthermore, the drug must exert the desired effect after alveolar delivery. Several drugs are known to produce successful effects when administered via the distal airspaces. In rats, intratracheal growth hormone and insulin cause increased growth and hypoglycemia, respectively (122,126). Aerosolized calcitonin causes hypocalcemia in humans (38). Finally, intratracheal instillation of IgG antibody to *Pseudomonas aeruginosa* in sheep protected the alveolar epithelium against injury from live *P. aeruginosa* bacteria and prevented dissemination of the bacteria to the pleural space (13). Thus, prophylactic or therapeutic administration of intra-alveolar immunoglobulin may speed the recovery or improve the prognosis for patients with *Pseudomonas* pneumonia. Successful utilization of the lung for drug delivery awaits further studies of the alveolar clearance mechanisms for specific drugs, studies of biologic effect, and modifications in drug design (such as alterations in size, lipid solubility, and susceptibility to degradation) to improve bioavailability.

X. Summary

Cellular and paracellular mechanisms have been proposed for alveolar protein clearance (Fig. 5). Most proteins and peptides are cleared as intact molecules across the alveolar epithelium of the uninjured lung, in contrast to protein transport across other epithelia (tracheal, gastrointestinal, and proximal renal tubules) that degrade protein. Protein clearance from the airspaces is slow, about 1% to

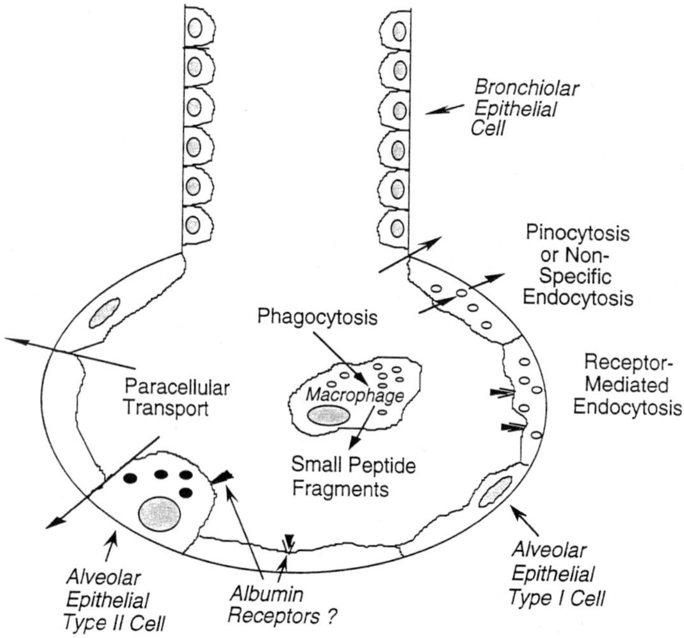

Figure 5 Putative mechanisms for alveolar protein clearance. In the uninjured lung, bulk quantities of serum protein are cleared predominantly by passive mechanisms across the tight junctions of the epithelium in the alveoli or at the bronchial-alveolar junction. Fluid-phase pinocytosis and receptor-mediated endocytosis (possibly involving scavenger-type receptors) may become important over long time periods or in the injured lung. Pulmonary resident cell-mediated transport processes may also be involved in homeostatic mechanisms in the alveolar space. (From Ref. 5.)

2%/h for proteins the size of albumin. Furthermore, transport rates are inversely related to molecular weight and shape of the instilled protein. These characteristics suggest that short-term clearance of bulk serum proteins after alveolar flooding occurs predominantly by passive diffusion through paracellular routes. Interest in pulmonary delivery of therapeutic peptides depends on size-dependent clearance and lack of degradation as well. Some proteins, such as human growth hormone, VIP, and gastrin, are cleared from the lungs much faster than expected for their size, indicating the presence of either specific receptor-mediated transport pathways or degradative pathways. Interestingly, alveolar type II cells and alveolar macrophages also express albumin-binding proteins and scavenger-like receptors. Thus, cellular protein transport mechanisms could be important in long-term alveolar protein clearance, in clearance under pathologic conditions (such as lung injury and inflammation, pulmonary immune response, and alveolar proteinosis), and in some homeostatic processes. Further mechanistic investigations are needed to clarify the processes responsible for alveolar epithelial clearance of protein.

Acknowledgments

The authors thank John Berg, Ph.D., and Edward M. Crandall, Ph.D., M.D., for critical review of the manuscript. Dr. Hastings was supported by a Department of Veterans Affairs Merit Review grant. Dr. Kim was supported by National Institutes of Health grant R01 HL38658 and the Hastings Foundation.

References

1. Bachofen M, Weibel ER. Alterations of the gas exchange apparatus in adult respiratory insufficiency associated with septicemia. Am Rev Respir Dis 1977; 116:589–615.
2. Clark J, Milberg J, Steinberg K, Hudson LD. Type III procollagen peptide in adult respiratory distress syndrome. Association of increased peptide levels in bronchoalveolar lavage fluid with increased risk for death. Ann Intern Med 1995; 122: 17–23.
3. Kobashi Y, Manabe T. The fibrosing process in so-called organized diffuse alveolar damage. Virchows Archiv A 1993; 422:47–52.
4. Tomasehefski JF. Pulmonary pathology of the adult respiratory distress syndrome. Clin Chest Med 1990; 11:593–619.
5. Folkesson HG, Matthay MA, Westrom BR, Kim KJ, Karlsson BW, Hastings RH. Alveolar epithelial clearance of protein. J Appl Physiol 1996; 80:1431–1445.
6. Carlson RW, Schaeffer RC, Michaels SG, Weil MH. Pulmonary edema fluid. Spectrum of features in 37 patients. Circulation 1979; 60:1161–1169.
7. Fein A, Grossman RF, Jones JG, et al. The value of edema fluid protein measurement in patients with pulmonary edema. Am J Med 1979; 67:32–38.
8. Sprung CL, Long WM, Marcial EM, et al. Distribution of proteins in pulmonary edema. The value of fractional concentrations. Am Rev Respir Dis 1987; 136: 957–963.
9. Matthay MA, Wiener-Kronish JP. Intact epithelial barrier function is critical for the resolution of alveolar edema in humans. Am Rev Respir Dis 1990; 142:1250–1257.
10. Hastings RH, Grady M, Sakuma T, Matthay MA. Clearance of different-sized proteins from the alveolar space in humans and rabbits. J Appl Physiol 1992; 73: 1310–1317.
11. Berthiaume Y, Albertine KH, Grady M, Fick G, Matthay MA. Protein clearance from the airspaces and lungs of unanesthetized sheep over 144 h. J Appl Physiol 1989; 67:1887–1897.
12. Berthiaume Y, Broaddus VC, Gropper MA, Tanita T, Matthay MA. Alveolar liquid and protein clearance from normal dog lungs. J Appl Physiol 1988; 65:585–593.

13. Pittet JF, Matthay MA, Pier G, Grady M, Wiener-Kronish JP. *Pseudomonas aeruginosa*-induced lung and pleural injury in sheep: differential protective effect of circulating versus alveolar immunoglobulin G antibody. J Clin Invest 1993; 92: 1221–1228.
14. Berthiaume Y, Staub NC, Matthay MA. Beta-adrenergic agonists increase lung liquid clearance in anesthetized sheep. J Clin Invest 1987; 79:335–343.
15. Smedira N, Gates L, Hastings R, et al. Alveolar and lung liquid clearance in anesthetized rabbits. J Appl Physiol 1991; 70:1827–1835.
16. Matthay MA, Landolt CC, Staub NC. Differential liquid and protein clearance from the alveoli of anesthetized sheep. J Appl Physiol 1982; 53:96–104.
17. Matthay MA, Berthiaume Y, Staub NC. Long-term clearance of liquid and protein from the lungs of unanesthetized sheep. J Appl Physiol 1985; 59:928–934.
18. Mackersie RC, Durelle J. Differential clearance of colloid and crystalloid solutions from the lung. J Trauma 1993; 35:448–453.
19. Schneeberger-Keeley EE, Karnovsky MJ. The ultrastructural basis of alveolar-capillary membrane permeability to peroxidase used as a tracer. J Cell Biol 1968; 37:781–793.
20. Schneeberger EE, Karnovsky MJ. The influence of intravascular fluid volume on the permeability of newborn and adult mouse lungs to ultrastructural protein tracers. J Cell Biol 1971; 49:310–334.
21. Gonzalez-Crussi F, Boston RW. The absorptive function of the neonatal lung: ultrastructural study of horseradish peroxidase uptake at the onset of ventilation. Lab Invest 1972; 26:114–121.
22. Williams MC. Endocytosis in alveolar type II cells: effect of charge and size of tracer. Proc Natl Acad Sci USA 1984; 81:6054–6058.
23. Pietra GG, Sampson P, Lanken PN, Hansen-Flaschen J, Fishman AP. Transcapillary movement of cationized ferritin in the isolated perfused rat lung. Lab Invest 1983; 49:54–61.
24. Taylor AE, Guyton AC, Bishop VS. Permeability of the alveolar membrane to solutes. Circ Res 1965; 16:353–362.
25. Gorin AB, Stewart PA. Differential permeability of endothelial and epithelial barriers to albumin. J Appl Physiol 1979; 47:1315–1324.
26. Effros RM, Mason GR. Measurements of pulmonary epithelial permeability in vivo. Am Rev Respir Dis 1983; 129(suppl):S59–S65.
27. Theodore J, Robin ED, Gaudio R, Acevedo J. Transalveolar transport of large polar solutes (sucrose, inulin, and dextran). Am J Physiol 1975; 229:989–996.
28. Wangensteen D, Yankovich R. Alveolar epithelium transport of albumin and sucrose: concentration difference effect. J Appl Physiol 1979; 47:846–850.
29. Folkesson HG, Westrom BR, Karlsson BW. Permeability of the respiratory tract to different-sized macromolecules after intratracheal instillation in young and adult rats. Acta Physiol Scand 1990; 139:347–354.
30. Folkesson HG, Westrom BR, Pierzynowski SG, Svendsen J, Karlsson BW. Respiratory tract passage of different-sized macromolecules in developing pigs. Acta Physiol Scand 1993; 147:173–178.
31. Drinker CK, Hardenbergh E. Absorption from the pulmonary alveoli. J Exp Med 1947; 86:7–18.

32. Bensch KG, Dominguez EAM, Liebow AA. Absorption of intact protein molecules across the pulmonary air-tissue barrier. Science 1967; 157:1204–1206.
33. Schultz AL, Grisme JT, Wada S, Grande F. Absorption of albumin from alveoli of perfused dog lung. Am J Physiol 1964; 207:1300–1304.
34. Braley J, Dawson C, Moore V, Cozzini B. Adsorption of inhaled antigen into the circulation of isolated lungs from normal and immunized rabbits. J Clin Invest 1978; 61:1240–1246.
35. Johnson LG, Cheng PW, Boucher RC. Albumin absorption by canine bronchial epithelium. J Appl Physiol 1989; 66:2772–2777.
36. Goodale RL, Goetzman B, Visscher MB. Hypoxia and iodoacetic acid and alveolocapillary barrier permeability to albumin. Am J Physiol 1970; 219:1226–1230.
37. Barrowcliffe MP, Morice A, Jones JG, Sever PS. Pulmonary clearance of vasoactive intestinal peptide. Thorax 1986; 41:88–93.
38. Deftos LJ, Nolan JJ, Selly BL, et al. Intrapulmonary drug delivery of bone-active peptides: bioactivity of inhaled calcitonin approximates injected calcitonin. J Bone Min Res 1996; 11(suppl 1):S95.
39. Bignon J, Jaurand MC, Pinchon MC, Sapin C, Warner JM. Immunoelectron microscopic and immunochemical demonstrations of serum proteins in the alveolar lining of the rat lung. Am Rev Respir Dis 1976; 113:104–120.
40. Ryan RM, Morris RE, Rice WR, Ciraolo G, Whitsett JA. Binding and uptake of pulmonary surfactant protein (SP-A) by pulmonary type II epithelial cells. J Histochem Cytochem 1989; 37:429–440.
41. Karrer HE. Electron microscopic study of the phagocytosis process in lung. J Biophys Biochem Cytol 1960; 7:357–365.
42. Corrin B. Phagocytic potential of pulmonary alveolar epithelium with particular reference to surfactant metabolism. Thorax 1970; 25:110–115.
43. Heppleston AG, Young AE. Uptake of inert particulate matter by alveolar cells: an ultrastructural study. J Pathol 1973; 111:159–164.
44. Lauweryns JM, Baert JH. Alveolar clearance and the role of the pulmonary lymphatics. Am Rev Respir Dis 1977; 115:625–683.
45. Gil J, Silage DA. Morphometry of pinocytotic vesicles in the capillary endothelium of rabbit lungs using automated equipment. Circ Res 1980; 47:384–391.
46. Gee MH, Staub NC. Role of bulk fluid flow in protein permeability of the dog lung alveolar membrane. J Appl Physiol 1977; 50:144–149.
47. Tsukimoto K, Mathieu-Costello O, Prediletto R, Elliot AR, West JB. Ultrastructural appearances of pulmonary capillaries at high transmural pressures. J Appl Physiol 1991; 71:573–582.
48. Williams MC. Uptake of lectins by pulmonary alveolar type II cells: subsequent deposition into lamellar bodies. Proc Natl Acad Sci USA 1984; 81:6383–6387.
49. Wright JR, Wager RE, Hamilton RL, Huang M, Clements JA. Uptake of lung surfactant subfractions into lamellar bodies of adult rabbit lungs. J Appl Physiol 1986; 60:817–825.
50. Bignon J, Chahinian P, Feldmann G, Sapin C. Ultrastructural immunoperoxidase demonstration of autologous albumin in the alveolar capillary membrane and in the alveolar lining material in normal rats. J Cell Biol 1975; 64:503–509.

51. Schnitzer JE, Carley WW, Palade GE. Albumin interacts specifically with a 60-kDa microvascular endothelial glycoprotein. Proc Natl Acad Sci USA 1988; 85: 6773–6777.
52. Schnitzer JE, Carley WW, Palade GE. Specific albumin binding to microvascular endothelium in culture. Am J Physiol 1988; 254:H425–H438.
53. Schnitzer JE. gp60 is an albumin-binding glycoprotein expressed by continuous endothelium involved in albumin transcytosis. Am J Physiol 1992; 262:H246–H254.
54. Schnitzer JE, Ulmer JB, Palade GE. Common peptide epitopes in glycophorin and the endothelial sialoglycoprotein gp60. Biochem Biophys Res Commun 1992; 187:1158–1165.
55. Schnitzer JE, Oh P, Pinney E, Allard J. Filipin-sensitive caveolae-mediated transport in endothelium: reduce transcytosis, scavenger endocytosis, and capillary permeability of select macromolecules. J Cell Biol 1994; 127:1217–1232.
56. Schnitzer JE. Update on the cellular and molecular basis of capillary permeability. Trends Cardiovasc Med 1993; 3:124–130.
57. Siflinger-Birnboim A, Schnitzer JE, Lum H, et al. Lectin binding to gp60 decreases specific albumin binding and transport in pulmonary artery endothelial monolayers. J Cell Physiol 1991; 149:575–584.
58. Schnitzer JE, Oh P. Albondin-mediated capillary permeability to albumin. Differential roles of receptors in endothelial endocytosis of native and modified albumins. J Biol Chem 1994; 269:6072–6082.
59. Ghinea N, Eskenasy M, Simionescu M, Simionescu N. Endothelial albumin binding proteins are membrane-associated components exposed on the cell surface. J Biol Chem 1989; 264:4755–4758.
60. Ghinea N, Fixman A, Alexandru D, et al. Identification of albumin-binding proteins in capillary endothelial cells. J Cell Biol 1988; 107:231–239.
61. Schnitzer JE, Bravo J. High affinity binding, endocytosis, and degradation of conformationally modified albumins. Potential role of gp30 and gp18 as novel scavenger receptors. J Biol Chem 1993; 268:7562–7570.
62. Schnitzer JE, Sung A, Horvat R, Bravo J. Preferential interaction of albumin-binding proteins, gp30 and gp18, with conformationally modified albumins. Presence in many cells and tissues with a possible role in catabolism. J Biol Chem 1992; 267:24544–24553.
63. Popov D, Hasu M, Ghinea N, Simionescu N, Simionescu M. Cardiomyocytes express albumin binding proteins. J Cell Mol Cardiol 1992; 24:989–1002.
64. Sage H, Johnson C, Bornstein P. Characterization of a novel serum albumin-binding glycoprotein secreted by endothelial cells in culture. J Biol Chem 1984; 259:3993–4007.
65. Schnitzer JE, Oh P. Antibodies to SPARC inhibit albumin binding to SPARC, gp60, and microvascular endothelium. Am J Physiol 1992; 263:H1872–H1879.
66. Neeper M, Schmidt AM, Brett J, Yan SD, Wang F, Pan YC, Elliston K, Stern D, Shaw A. Cloning and expression of a cell surface receptor for advanced glycosylation end products of proteins. J Biol Chem 1992; 267:14998–14504.
67. Kim KJ, Matsukawa Y, Lee VHL, Crandall ED. Characteristics of albumin absdorption across rat alveolar epithelial cell monolayers. FASEB J 1995; 9:A569. Abstract.

68. Kim KJ, Rattan V, Oh P, Schnitzer J, Kalra VK, Crandall ED. Specific albumin-binding protein in alveolar epithelial cell monolayers (abstr). Am J Respir Crit Care Med 1995; 151:A190.
69. Curiel DT, Agarwal S, Romer MU, Wagner E, Birnstiel ML, Boucher RC. Gene transfer to respiratory epithelial cells via the receptor-mediated endocytosis pathway. Am J Respir Cell Mol Biol 1992; 6:247–252.
70. Matsukawa Y, Yamahara H, Lee VHL, Crandall ED. Transport of horseradish peroxidase across alveolar epithelial cell monolayers. Pharm Res 1996; 1330–1334.
71. Bell DY, Haseman JA, Spock A, McLennan G, Hook GER. Plasma proteins of the bronchoalveolar surface of the lungs of smokers and nonsmokers. Am Rev Respir Dis 1981; 124:72–79.
72. Merrill WW, Naegel GP, Olchowske JJ, Reynolds HY. Immunoglobulin G subclass proteins in serum and lavage fluid of normal subjects. Am Rev Respir Dis 1985; 131:584–589.
73. Holter JF, Weiland JE, Pacht ER, Gadek JE, Davis WB. Protein permeability in the adult respiratory distress syndrome. Loss of size selectivity of the alveolar epithelium. J Clin Invest 1986; 78:1513–1518.
74. Lykens MG, Davis WB, Pacht ER. Antioxidant activity of bronchoalveolar lavage fluid in the adult respiratory distress syndrome. Am J Physiol 1992; 262:L169–L175.
75. Gelb AF, Klein E. Hemodynamic and alveolar protein studies in noncardiogenic pulmonary edema. Am Rev Respir Dis 1976; 114:831–838.
76. Galis Z, Ghitescu L, Simionescu M. Fatty acid binding to albumin increases its uptake and transcytosis by the lung capillary endothelium. Eur J Cell Biol 1988; 47:358–365.
77. Wearly LL. Recent progresses in protein and peptide delivery by noninvasive routes. Crit Rev Ther Drug Carrier Sys 1991; 8:331–394.
78. Allam H, Martinet N. Gallati H, Vaillant P, Hosang M, Martinet Y. Platelet-derived growth factor AA and BB dimers are present in normal human epithelial lining fluid. Eur Resp J 1993; 6:1162–1168.
79. Ferko T, Perales JC, Eckman E, Kaetzel CS, Hanson RW, Davis PB. Gene transfer into the airway epithelium of animals by targeting the polymeric immunoglobulin receptor. J Clin Invest 1995; 95(2):493–502.
80. Chinard FP, DeFouw DO. Ultrastructural changes in the air-blood barrier after spontaneous development of edema in isolated dog lungs perfused at 15°C. Microvasc Res 1981; 21:48–56.
81. Hostetter MW, Dawson CA, Moore VL. Influence of temperature on the absorption of inhaled bovine serum albumin through isolated rabbit lungs. Proc Soc Exp Biol Med 1981; 167:412–418.
82. Serikov VB, Grady M, Matthay MA. Effect of temperature on alveolar liquid and protein clearance in an in situ perfused goat lung. J Appl Physiol 1993; 75: 940–947.
83. Hastings RH, Wright JR, Albertine KH, Ciriales R, Matthay MA. Effect of endocytosis inhibitors on alveolar clearance of albumin, immunoglobulin G, and SP-A in rabbits. Am J Physiol 1994; 266:L544–L552.
84. Potau N, Bailey AC, Roach E, Williams JA, Goldfine IA. Methylamine and monensin do not block insulin internalization but do influence the intracellular

distribution and action of insulin in pancreatic acini from diabetic mice. Endocrinol 1984; 115:205–213.

85. Whittaker J, Hammond VA, Taylor R, Alberti KG. Effects of monensin on insulin interactions with isolated hepatocytes. Evidence for inhibition of receptor recycling and insulin degradation. Biochem J 1986; 234:463–468.
86. Merion M, Sly WS. The role of intermediate vesicles in the adsorptive endocytosis and transport of ligand to lysosomes by human fibroblasts. J Cell Biol 1983; 96: 644–650.
87. Tycko B, Keith CH, Maxfield FR. Rapid acidification of endocytic vesicles containing asialoglycoprotein in cells of a human hepatoma line. J Cell Biol 1983; 97:1762–1768.
88. Breitfeld PP, McKinnon WC, Mostov KE. Effect of nocodazole on vesicular traffic to the apical and basolateral surfaces of polarized MDCK cells. J Cell Biol 1990; 111:2365–2373.
89. Matter K, Bucher K, Hauri HP. Microtubule perturbation retards both the direct and indirect apical pathway but does not affect sorting of plasma membrane proteins in intestinal epithelial cells (Caco-2). EMBO J 1990; 9:3163–3170.
90. Lehnert BE, Valdez YE. Lung and pleural "free-cell responses" to the intrapulmonary deposition of particles in the rat. J Toxicol Environ Health 1985; 16:823–829.
91. Young SL, Wright JR, Clements JA. Cellular uptake and processing of surfactant lipids and apoprotein SP-A in rat lung. J Appl Physiol 1989; 66:1336–1342.
92. Ward DM, Kaplan J. The rate of internalization of different receptor-ligand complexes in alveolar macrophages is receptor-specific. Biochem J 1990; 270: 369–374.
93. Wiener-Kronish JP, Broaddus VC, Albertine KH, Gropper MA, Matthay MA. The relationship of pleural effusions to increased permeability pulmonary edema in anesthetized sheep. J Clin Invest 1988; 82:1422–1429.
94. Martin TR, Pistorese BP, Chi EY, Goodman RB, Matthay MA. Effects of leukotriene B4 in the human lung. Recruitment of neutrophils into the alveolar spaces without a change in protein permeability. J Clin Invest 1989; 84:1609–1619.
95. Steinman RM, Brodie SE, Cohn ZA. Membrane flow during pinocytosis. A stereologic analysis. J Cell Biol 1976; 68:665–687.
96. Hastings RH, Folkesson HG, Petersen V, Ciriales R, Matthay MA. Cellular uptake of albumin from the lungs of anesthetized rabbits. Am J Physiol 1995; 266:L544–L552.
97. Sorokin SP, Brain JD. Pathways of clearance in mouse lungs exposed to iron oxide aerosols. Anat Rec 1974; 181:581–626.
98. Adamson IYR, Bowden DH. Dose response of the pulmonary macrophagic system to various particulates and its relation to transepithelial passage of free particles. Exp Lung Res 1981; 2:165–175.
99. Hastings RH, Summers-Torres D. Precipitation and clearance of concentrated alveolar protein. FASEB J 1995; 9:A569.
100. Berg JT, Lee ST, Thepen T, Lee CY, Tsan M-F. Depletion of alveolar macrophages by liposome-encapsulated dichloromethylene diphosphonate. J Appl Physiol 1993; 74:2812–2819.

101. Brown MJ, Goldstein MS. Lipoprotein metabolism in the macrophage: implications for cholesterol deposition in atherosclerosis. Annu Rev Biochem 1983; 52: 223–261.
102. Horiuchi S, Murakami M, Takata K, Morino Y. Scavenger receptor for aldehyde-modified proteins. J Biol Chem 1986; 261:4962–4966.
103. McCusker K, Hoidal J. Characterization of scavenger receptor activity in resident human lung macrophages. Exp Lung Res 1989; 15:651–661.
104. Khoo JC, Miller E, McLoughlin P, Steinberg D. Enhanced macrophage uptake of low density lipoprotein after self-aggregation. Arteriosclerosis 1988; 8:348–358.
105. Sparrow CP, Parthasarathy S, Steinberg D. A macrophage receptor that recognizes oxidized low density lipoprotein but not acetylated low density lipoprotein. J Biol Chem 1989; 264:2599–2604.
106. Steinberg D, Parthasarathy S, Carew TE, Khoo JC, Wiztum JL. Beyond cholesterol: modifications of low-density lipoprotein that increase its atherogenicity. N Engl J Med 1989; 320:915–924.
107. Sambrano GR, Parthasarathy S, Steinberg D. Recognition of oxidatively damaged erythrocytes by a macrophage receptor with specificity for oxidized low density lipoprotein. Proc Natl Acad Sci USA 1994; 91:3265–3269.
108. Carp H, Miller F, Hoidal JR, Janoff A. Potential mechanisms of emphysema: α_1 proteinase inhibitor recovered from the lungs of smokers contains oxidized methionine and has decreased elastase inhibitor. Proc Natl Acad Sci 1982; 79: 2041–2045.
109. Janoff A. Elastases and emphysema: current assessment of the protease-antiprotease hypothesis. Am Rev Respir Dis 1985; 132:417–433.
110. Jayr C, Matthay MA. Alveolar and lung liquid clearance in the absence of pulmonary blood flow in sheep. J Appl Physiol 1991; 71:1679–1687.
111. Sakuma T, Pittet JF, Jayr C, Matthay Ma. Alveolar liquid and protein clearance in the absence of blood flow in sheep. J Appl Physiol 1993; 74:176–185.
112. Pittet JF, Wiener-Kronish JP, McElroy MC, Folkesson HG, Matthay MA. Stimulation of lung epithelial liquid clearance by endogenous release of catecholamines in septic shock in anesthetized rats. J Clin Invest 1994; 94:663–671.
113. Pittet JF, Wiener-Kronish JP, Serikov V, Matthay MA. Resistance of the alveolar epithelium to injury from septic shock in sheep. Am J Respir Crit Care Med 1995; 151:1093–1100.
114. Folkesson HG, Westrom BR, Pierzynowski SG, Karllson BW. Lung to blood passage of different-sized molecules during lung inflammation in the rat. J Appl Physiol 1991; 71:1106–1111.
115. Thrall RS, Peterson LB, Linehan JH, Abramoff P, Moore VL. The effect of immunization on the uptake of intratracheally-administered antigen. Clin Immunol Immunopathol 1978; 10:136–147.
116. Hostetter MW, Dawson CA, Moore VL, Ju-Ger CK. Effect of passive immunization on absorption of antigen through the respiratory tract. Int Arc Allergy Appl Immunol 1982; 69:179–187.
117. Braley JF, Peterson LB, Dawson CA, Moore VL. Effect of hypersensitivity on protein uptake across the air-blood barrier of isolated rabbit lungs. J Clin Invest 1979; 63:1103–1109.

118. Honda Y, Takahashi H, Shijubo N, Kuroki Y, Akino T. Surfactant protein-A concentration in bronchoalveolar lavage fluids of patients with pulmonary alveolar proteinosis. Chest 1993; 103:496–499.
119. Dranoff G, Crawford AD, Sadelain M, et al. Involvement of granulocyte-macrophage colony-stimulating factor in pulmonary homeostasis. Science 1994; 264:713–716.
120. Huffman JA, Hull WM, Dranoff G, Mulligan RC, Whitsett JA. Pulmonary epithelial cell expression of GM-CSF corrects the alveolar proteinosis in GM-CSF-deficient mice. J Clin Invest 1996; 97:649–655.
121. Morimoto K, Yamahara H, Lee VH, Kim KJ. Transport of thyrotropin-releasing hormone across rat alveolar epithelial cell monolayers. Life Sci 1994; 54:2083–2092.
122. Folkesson HG, Hedin L, Westrom BR. Lung to blood passage of human growth hormone (hGH) after intratracheal instillation: stimulation of growth in hypophysectomized rats. J Endocrinol 1992; 134:197–203.
123. Patton JS, McCabe JG, Hansen SE, Daugherty AL. Absorption of human growth hormone from the rat lung. Biotechnol Ther 1990; 1:213–228.
124. Wang L, Toledo-Velasquez D, Schwegler-Berry D, Ma JKH, Rojanasakul Y. Transport and hydrolysis of enkephalins in cultured alveolar epithelial monolayers. Pharmaceut Res 1993; 10:1662–1667.
125. Kim KJ, Yamahara H, Lehr CM, Lee VHL, Crandall ED. Fate of insulin during alveolar epithelial transit. FASEB J 1993; 7:A436. Abstract.
126. Liu FY, Shao Z, Kildsig DO, Mitra AK. Pulmonary delivery of free and liposomal insulin. Pharmaceut Res 1993; 10:228–232.
127. Hubbard RC, Casolaro MA, Mitchell M, et al. Fate of aerosolized recombinant DNA-produced α_1-antitrypsin: use of the epithelial surface of the lower respiratory tract to administer proteins of therapeutic importance. Proc Natl Acad Sci USA 1989; 86:680–684.

20

Treatment of Acute Pulmonary Edema and the Acute Respiratory Distress Syndrome

YVES BERTHIAUME

University of Montreal
Montreal, Quebec, Canada

LORRAINE B. WARE and MICHAEL A. MATTHAY

Cardiovascular Research Institute
University of California at San Francisco
San Francisco, California

I. Introduction

Nearly 80 years ago Sir William Osler provided detailed recommendations for the rational management of acute pulmonary edema (1). As is often the case, most of his recommendations have stood the test of time. For example, he recognized the importance of decreasing venous return (rotating tourniquets) and inhibiting sympathetic tone (morphia sulfate) in acute cardiogenic pulmonary edema. He also recognized the value of supplemental oxygen therapy. After Osler's clinical observations, the next major advance in treating acute pulmonary edema was the availability of positive pressure ventilation in specialized critical care units. The rational basis for treatment of acute pulmonary edema evolved further from experimental studies by Guyton, Staub, Taylor, and others (see Chap. 1). All of these investigators recognized the important distinction between pulmonary edema that was caused either by high pressure in the pulmonary circulation or by injury to the lung endothelial barrier resulting in increased permeability pulmonary edema.

Hydrostatic pulmonary edema can often be managed pharmacologically, without positive pressure ventilation, although patients with severe or fulminant hydrostatic pulmonary edema usually do require emergent endotracheal intubation and positive pressure ventilation. Increased-permeability pulmonary edema leads to the clinical syndrome known as clinical acute lung injury or the acute respiratory distress syndrome (ARDS). Mortality remains high in patients with ARDS, although in the past 15 years much has been learned about the mechanisms that lead to acute lung injury and the complex pathophysiology of the acute, subacute, and chronic phases of ARDS. It is clear that patients with ARDS often die because of associated nonpulmonary organ dysfunction, but the core of the clinical problem is usually the patient's severe respiratory failure. The clinical syndrome begins with protein-rich pulmonary edema that may evolve to a fibrosing alveolitis. Many of the issues related to the pathogenesis and pathophysiology of ARDS have been extensively discussed in prior chapters in this book, with a focus on specific clinical disorders that lead to clinical acute lung injury. This chapter will refer frequently to these earlier chapters, especially when the data are germane to current or future treatment strategies.

The first section of this chapter reviews the principles for treatment of acute respiratory failure from hydrostatic pulmonary edema that is severe enough to require positive pressure ventilation. The second section considers standard supportive therapy for increased-permeability pulmonary edema, or ARDS. The third section critically evaluates new therapeutic strategies for the treatment of ARDS.

II. Treatment for Hydrostatic Pulmonary Edema

As explained in Chapters 1 and 5, the physiological basis for the development of hydrostatic pulmonary edema depends primarily on an elevation in pulmonary microvascular pressure. Clinically, hydrostatic pulmonary edema occurs most commonly in patients with left ventricular dysfunction or valvular heart disease. Hydrostatic pulmonary edema may also occur in the setting of intravascular volume overload, frequently following major surgical procedures that require intravenous administration of large volumes of blood products and crystalloid fluid. Hydrostatic pulmonary edema may also occur in the setting of septic shock in patients who are volume-overloaded during resuscitation in an effort to improve systemic blood pressure and cardiac output. Hydrostatic pulmonary edema may also be an important mechanism for the development of pulmonary edema in the setting of high-altitude pulmonary edema (see Chap. 11) as well as in the setting of neurogenic pulmonary edema (see Chap. 10).

A. Physiological Basis for Treatment of Cardiogenic Pulmonary Edema

The treatment for hydrostatic pulmonary edema that develops in the setting of left ventricular failure depends primarily on reducing preload to the heart. This objective can be accomplished by several different approaches. In Osler's textbooks, the value of placing the patient in the sitting position as well as using rotating tourniquets to reduce venous return was emphasized. The more modern approach is to use pharmacological agents to reduce preload. First, sublingual or intravenous nitrates (nitroglycerin) are effective in reducing venous return or ventricular preload in patients with cardiogenic edema. If the patient's cardiac insufficiency is complicated by systemic hypertension, then intravenous nitroprusside can be used to reduce both preload and afterload. Diuretic administration with intravenous loop diuretics provides some immediate venodilating effect as well as induction of negative fluid balance through diuresis. The administration of morphine sulfate intravenously also has a beneficial effect, reducing venous return and sympathetic tone, as well as reducing systemic arterial pressure and afterload on the left ventricle. All of these pharmacological approaches can be used to reduce pulmonary microvascular pressure, and thus reverse the primary cause of hydrostatic pulmonary edema (2).

B. Positive Pressure Ventilation for Cardiogenic Pulmonary Edema

In some patients, positive pressure ventilation is required to manage the acute respiratory failure that accompanies the development of cardiogenic pulmonary edema. Usually, positive pressure ventilation is provided following endotracheal intubation although some patients can be managed without intubation with noninvasive positive pressure ventilation delivered by a tight-fitting face mask (3). In these patients, positive pressure ventilation helps to reverse the physiological derangements that contribute to the development of pulmonary edema. First, positive pressure ventilation reduces preload, thus lowering pulmonary microvascular pressure. Second, positive pressure ventilation decreases afterload on the left heart because positive pleural pressure replaces the wide negative swings in pleural pressure that occur in the presence of spontaneous ventilation, which result in an increase in left ventricular afterload. Third, positive pressure ventilation guarantees adequate oxygenation, thus potentially improving myocardial oxygen supply. Finally, positive pressure ventilation decreases the work of breathing so that the oxygen demand on the failing heart is reduced. These mechanisms are summarized in Table 1.

There is no evidence that positive pressure ventilation itself hastens the reabsorption of alveolar edema beyond the indirect hemodynamic and physiological effects described above. Several experimental studies have demonstrated that positive airway pressure does not accelerate the resolution of alveolar edema (4,5). It is possible that a more expanded lung could increase the capacitance of the extra-alveolar interstitial space to store edema fluid (6), but the clinical significance of this effect is uncertain.

Table 1 Mechanisms That Account for the Beneficial Effect of Positive Pressure Ventilation in Cardiogenic (Hydrostatic) Pulmonary Edema

1. Reduced preload on the right and left ventricle
2. Reduced afterload on the left ventricle
3. Decreased work of breathing (decrease in myocardial oxygen consumption)
4. Guarantee adequate oxygenation
5. Reduced endogenous catecholamine production

C. Resolution and Treatment of Hydrostatic Pulmonary Edema

The resolution of hydrostatic pulmonary edema has recently been studied in patients at the University of California, San Francisco, by serial sampling of undiluted pulmonary edema fluid. Interestingly, patients with cardiogenic pulmonary edema that was sufficiently severe to require positive pressure ventilation fell into three groups in terms of their ability to reabsorb alveolar edema fluid. Maximal alveolar fluid clearance (defined as $> 14\%$ per hour) occurred in approximately 35% of the patients. In another 45% of the patients, alveolar fluid clearance proceeded at an intermediate rate (3% to 14%). Finally, there was a group of patients, approximately 20%, in whom alveolar fluid clearance occurred very slowly, at a rate $< 3\%$ per hour. The slow rate of alveolar fluid clearance could not be explained by elevated pulmonary microvascular pressure or elevated systemic arterial pressure. Also, measurement of epinephrine levels did not identify which patients were more likely to have rapid alveolar fluid clearance. Thus, endogenous catecholamine-dependent mechanisms alone may not be the most important mechanism driving alveolar fluid clearance in patients with hydrostatic pulmonary edema. Indeed, as described in several chapters in this book (Chaps. 14, 15, 16, 17), catecholamine-independent mechanisms are also important in upregulating alveolar fluid clearance.

In this clinical study, there was some circumstantial evidence that the resolution of hydrostatic pulmonary edema might be accelerated with the administration of inhaled beta-2 adrenergic therapy. Patients who had been treated with aerosolized beta-2 adrenergic agonists seemed to have evidence of a higher rate of alveolar fluid clearance. This possibility is supported by experimental studies which have demonstrated that beta-2 adrenergic agonists can increase the rate of alveolar fluid clearance in the ex vivo isolated human lung (see Chap. 14), as well as new preliminary work indicating that alveolar fluid clearance can be accelerated by aerosolized beta-2 adrenergic therapy in sheep. In any case, prospective studies will be needed to evaluate aerosolized beta-2 adrenergic agonists as a treatment for hydrostatic pulmonary edema. Also, in the Future Therapies section at the end of this chapter, the potential for using vasoactive therapy with dobutamine (7) or dopamine (8) to increase the rate of alveolar edema fluid clearance will be discussed.

In patients who develop hydrostatic pulmonary edema primarily from intravascular volume overload, treatment should be focused on inducing negative fluid balance with potent diuretics. The combination of a loop diuretic with a thiazide diuretic can promote brisk diuresis. If renal failure is contributing to volume overload, then either ultrafiltration, hemodialysis, or continuous venovenous hemofiltration can be used to reduce pulmonary microvascular pressure.

In the setting of neurogenic pulmonary edema, recent evidence indicates that at least 50% of patients have a hydrostatic mechanism for pulmonary edema (9). Pulmonary venoconstriction may be the primary mechanism for the hydrostatic stress in neurogenic pulmonary edema (see Chap. 10). Most of the patients with a hydrostatic pattern have a rapid resolution of pulmonary edema spontaneously, so specific treatment is not normally needed. The rapid resolution may be related to elevated endogenous catecholamine levels, as Maron's laboratory has reported in experimental studies (see Chap. 10). Neurogenic pulmonary edema is normally treated with positive pressure ventilation, gentle diuresis, and an attempt to control systemic blood pressure in a normal range. In some patients with subarachnoid hemorrhage, systemic blood pressure needs to be maintained at higher-than-normal levels to overcome cerebral vasospasm. In that circumstance, modest diuresis and maintenance of adequate oxygenation with positive pressure ventilation are the principal therapeutic interventions. Experimentally, alpha adrenergic blockade has been used to prevent or treat neurogenic pulmonary edema, but clinically this therapy cannot be used because of the potential problems with systemic hypotension.

The pathogenesis of high-altitude pulmonary edema (HAPE) is probably multifactorial, possibly including an increase in vascular permeability as well as elevation in pulmonary vascular pressure (see Chap. 11). The treatment of choice for patients with high-altitude pulmonary edema is descent from high altitude and supplemental oxygen. These measures are usually sufficient for the resolution of HAPE. Diuretics are sometimes used, but oxygen therapy and removal of the patient from the hypobaric atmosphere are the mainstays of treatment. The current recommendations for prevention of HAPE are reviewed in Chapter 11.

III. Standard Supportive Therapy for Increased-Permeability Pulmonary Edema or ARDS

Overall mortality for patients with increased-permeability pulmonary edema from acute lung injury ranges from approximately 40% to 60% (10–12). The lowest mortality rates tend to be reported in patients who have suffered acute lung injury from trauma, usually a younger and healthier group of patients; also, lower mortality rates are found in studies in which patients with hepatic failure or renal failure have been excluded. Mortality in patients with acute lung injury clearly occurs from both pulmonary and nonpulmonary organ failure (Table 2) (11,13,14).

Table 2 Multivariate Model of Variables Associated with Mortality in Patients with Acute Lung Injury

Variable	Odds ratio	95% CI[a]	*P* value
Nonpulmonary organ system dysfunction between hospital admission and admission to intensive care unit	8.1	(2.1–30.8)	<.0001
Chronic liver disease	5.2	(1.5–18.1)	<.01
Sepsis	2.8	(1.0–7.7)	<.05

[a]CI = confidence interval.
Source: Ref 11.

A. Treatment of the Inciting Clinical Disorder in ARDS

It is important to identify, if possible, the underlying cause of clinical acute lung injury. Several chapters in this book are devoted in detail to the most common causes of acute lung injury, including sepsis (Chap. 6), pneumonia (Chap. 7), aspiration of gastric contents (Chap. 8), hemorrhagic shock and trauma (Chap. 9), and ischemia reperfusion (Chap. 12). In some circumstances, the underlying cause of acute lung injury can be directly treated. For example, patients with pneumonia from bacterial or opportunistic infections will often respond to specific antimicrobial therapy. A careful search for a treatable cause of acute lung injury, such as bacterial pneumonia, atypical pneumonias from *Mycoplasma* or *Legionella,* or an opportunistic infection from fungi, tuberculosis, or *Pneumocystis carinii* is warranted. In other patients, an infectious cause of acute lung injury may be related to an extrapulmonary site of infection, such as biliary infection, peritonitis, or a urologic source of infection. Although the prognosis for recovery from sepsis-induced lung injury is worse than from any other cause (11,13), specific medical and surgical treatment of the pulmonary or extrapulmonary source of sepsis is obviously needed to increase the chance of survival. In most of the other clinical causes of acute lung injury, such as aspiration or multiple transfusions following shock and trauma, the specific cause of lung injury has already occurred and cannot be further treated beyond providing the patient with normal supportive care.

B. Mechanical Ventilation—Optimization of Gas Exchange in ARDS

The mainstay of standard supportive treatment of acute lung injury is positive pressure ventilation (15). Judicious use of positive pressure ventilation and supplemental oxygen is a crucial element of standard supportive treatment for patients with increased-permeability edema, allowing for appropriate respiratory support while the lung recovers from lung injury (16). However, prolonged exposure to high concentrations of oxygen can produce lung injury that is similar to the pathological changes that are observed with ARDS itself (16,17).

In normal human lungs, some lung impairment from oxygen toxicity develops after 40 hours of breathing 100% oxygen (18); no detectable toxicity develops when the FiO_2 is $< 50\%$ (19). However, lungs that are already damaged may be more susceptible to hyperoxic injury (20), making a safe level of oxygen exposure more difficult to determine. Some experimental work with a dog model of lung injury (oleic acid) has shown that exposure to an FiO_2 of 0.5 continuously for 8 days after the injury did not produce any significant superimposed injury due to hyperoxia (21). Although no clinical studies have clearly established which level of FiO_2 is safe in humans with ARDS, an FiO_2 < 0.6 is generally considered safe and probably may not cause additional lung injury (22).

Shortly after the original description of ARDS by Petty and colleagues (23), it was realized that intermittent positive pressure ventilation alone was often insufficient to correct the severe hypoxemia. The addition of positive end–expiratory pressure (PEEP) was observed to significantly improve oxygenation in patients with ARDS (15,23), thereby permitting the same oxygen delivery at a lower FiO_2. By lowering the FiO_2, PEEP may reduce further lung injury from oxygen toxicity. Although multiple mechanisms have been proposed to explain the improved pulmonary function and gas exchange following PEEP therapy, the best-documented effect of PEEP on the lung is an increase in the functional residual capacity (FRC) (15). The increase in FRC could be secondary to an increase in alveolar volume or to alveolar recruitment. Some animal experiments have shown that PEEP can increase alveolar diameter, thus improving gas exchange in previously nonaerated alveolar units.

Recent clinical studies have further defined the effect of PEEP in ARDS. computerized axial tomography (CT) scanning of the lungs of patients with ARDS has shown an inhomogeneous distribution of lung lesions (24–26). The lesions are concentrated in the dependent regions of affected lungs (24–26) (see Chap. 3). Further evaluation of this observation has revealed different zones in the lung. One zone in a nondependent region of the lung has a normal compliance and is normally aerated. A second zone in the most dependent region of the lung is not aerated and the application of PEEP cannot recruit significant lung volume. Finally, the third zone is poorly aerated, but a significant air volume recruitment can be achieved in this zone with the application of PEEP. Thus, the application of PEEP in ARDS patients leads to more alveolar recruitment in this third zone and alveolar distention in the zone corresponding to the normal lung (25). However, the predominant changes in gas exchange correlate with alveolar recruitment and not with the alveolar overdistension in the normal lung zone (25). Thus, PEEP appears to improve gas exchange by increasing FRC by alveolar recruitment (26,27).

Although initially it had been suggested that PEEP may have other beneficial effects besides improving oxygenation, these other benefits have not be confirmed. For example, PEEP does not decrease lung water (28), reduce vascular permeability (5), or hasten the resolution of pulmonary edema (28). Furthermore, prophylactic PEEP does not protect against the development of ARDS (29). PEEP may shift some edema fluid from the alveolar to the extra-alveolar interstitial space, but PEEP does not reduce the overall degree of pulmonary edema (28).

The clear-cut benefits of PEEP on oxygenation are tempered by its major disadvantage: a reduction in cardiac output (30). Several mechanisms have been proposed to account for this phenomenon (31,32). However, the most accepted mechanism of decreased cardiac output associated with PEEP therapy is a decrease in venous return secondary to an increase in intrathoracic pressure (33,34). This decrease in cardiac output is often treated by volume infusion in patients who are volume-depleted or by inotropic agents in patients in whom a tighter control of pulmonary arterial wedge pressure is needed (30).

Since pulmonary benefits of PEEP therapy must be balanced against the potential for a physiologically significant decrease in cardiac output and resultant changes in organ perfusion, many investigators have tried to define clinical criteria that would predict the best PEEP level. Some have suggested using the maximal PEEP possible to minimize FiO_2 (35) or intrapulmonary shunt (36). However, given the risk of barotrauma and the depression of cardiac output associated with high levels of PEEP, some investigators recommend using the lowest level of PEEP to maintain the $FiO_2 < 0.6$ (22,37). More recently, Gattinoni suggested that the maximal PEEP to be applied in a supine patient to recruit alveolar volume that underwent compression atelectasis should not exceed the ventral–dorsal height of the lung in centimeters (37). However, objective data confirming the best strategy for selecting the level of optimal PEEP do not exist.

Although the application of PEEP will be able to improve the oxygenation in most patients with ARDS, it may not be sufficient in some ARDS patients. Over the years, a significant number of other therapeutic strategies have been tried. These strategies have focused on methods that modify the ventilatory strategy (change in body position, inverse-ratio pressure-control ventilation) or on methods that try to limit edema formation (negative fluid balance) or strategies to improve lung compliance (administration of surfactant), or pharmacological methods to improve oxygenation (inhaled nitric oxide). These newer strategies will be discussed later in this chapter in the section, Future Treatments.

C. Fluid Management in ARDS

The question of fluid balance in ARDS has been a contentious issue for many years. The controversy mainly originates from the fact that most of the data suggesting that fluid restriction may be appropriate in ARDS derive from acute animal experiments; no clinical trials have unequivocally demonstrated the advantages of this therapeutic strategy.

The justification for restricting fluid administration or decreasing pulmonary arterial pressure in patients with ARDS relies on the observation that fluid accumulation in lungs with increased vascular permeability occurs at lower pulmonary capillary pressures than in normal lungs (30,38–41). If lung microvascular pressure is elevated in the presence of an increase in lung vascular permeability, then the quantity of pulmonary edema increases substantially (Fig. 1) (41). The short-term effects of volume manipulation were addressed in a study by Prewitt et al. (39) in a canine oleic acid lung injury model. The animals were managed for 4 hours with either (1) PEEP 10 cm H_2O; (2) intravenous albumin; (3) phlebotomy to reduce the pulmonary arterial wedge pressure (PAWP); or (4) nitroprusside to reduce blood pressure by 25% (39). Neither the addition of PEEP nor the administration of albumin decreased extravascular lung water

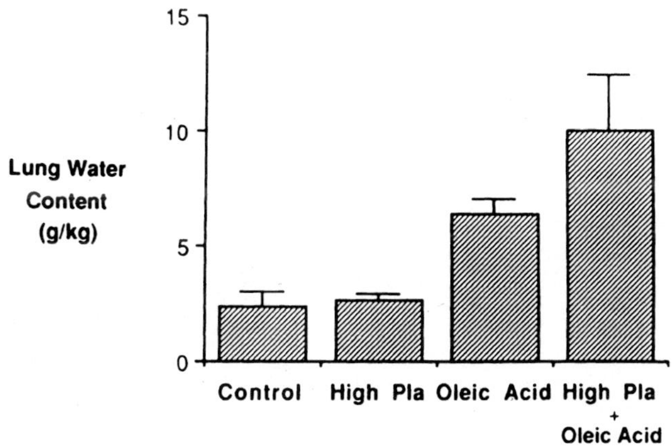

Figure 1 The interaction between increased lung vascular permeability and an elevated lung microvascular pressure on lung water content was studied in in situ perfused canine lungs. Lung water content was not different between control experiments and those in which left atrial pressure (Pla) was elevated to 25 cm H_2O for 60 min. With lung injury caused by oleic acid (0.05 mL/kg body weight), lung water content more than doubled even at normal microvascular pressure. When the same doses of oleic acid were given but left atrial pressure was elevated to 25 cm H_2O, there was a further marked increase in lung water content. (From Ref. 41.)

content; however, phlebotomy and nitroprusside reduced the PAWP by 4 mm Hg and resulted in a 50% reduction in edema (Fig. 2). Reducing hydrostatic pressure with a diuretic such as furosemide is also associated with a reduction in extravascular lung water (38,40). However, it has been suggested that improvement in oxygenation following the utilization of furosemide is not necessarily linked to a change in extravascular lung water but to a redistribution of blood flow to nonflooded lung units (38). Finally, other approaches that reduce hydrostatic pressure, like plasmapharesis and hemofiltration, can also decrease extravascular lung water (42).

The above experimental data are also supported by a few observational and retrospective clinical studies. Treatment of ARDS patients with diuretics or dialysis has been shown to improve oxygenation and respiratory system lung compliance (43). One study reported that survival in ARDS patients was related to negative fluid balance (44); another study reported that survival was greater in patients in whom there was a 25% reduction in pulmonary arterial wedge pressure (45). Finally, one group of investigators observed that patients who gained < 1 L of fluid after 36 hours of being recruited into a study of acute

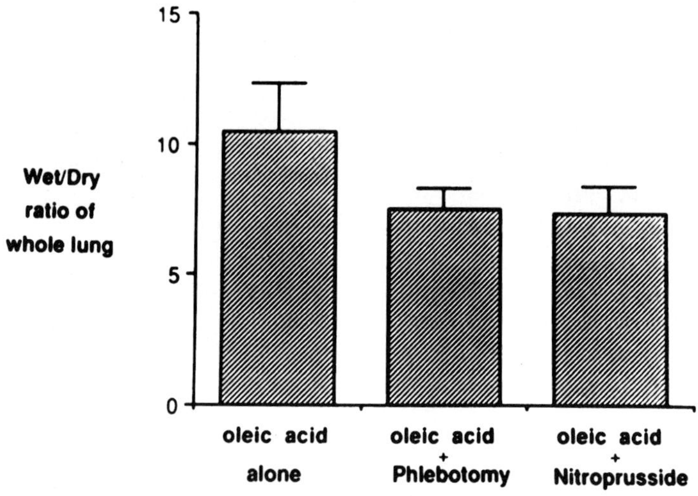

Figure 2 Data from an experimental canine study illustrating the effect of lowering pulmonary microvascular pressures on lung edema after acute lung injury. The extravascular water content is represented as the wet/dry ratio of the whole lung. With oleic acid alone, the wet/dry ratio was more than double the normal wet/dry ratio of 4.6. With either phlebotomy or nitroprusside therapy, both of which lowered pulmonary capillary wedge pressure from 10 mm Hg to 6 mm Hg, there was 50% less lung edema. (From Ref. 39.)

lung injury had a better survival (74%) than the others (50%) (46). However, these observational studies, although supportive of the concept that fluid restriction might be beneficial, do not prove that this therapeutic approach is efficacious. It is possible that the group of patients with less fluid accumulation simply reflect a subpopulation of patients who are less severely ill, and that fluid accumulation reflects the severity of systemic and pulmonary capillary permeability.

This issue was addressed in a prospective, randomized trial in which diuresis and/or fluid restriction was monitored by measuring the extravascular lung water using a double indication technique (46,47). After demonstrating that a treatment strategy based on extravascular lung water was safe and well-tolerated even in hypotensive patients (46), the study was extended to 89 patients who were randomized to be managed either using extravascular lung water measurements or standard management approach including the use of a pulmonary arterial catheter with optimization of the pulmonary arterial wedge pressure (47). Although the initial extravascular lung water was not different, after 24 hours of treatment according to the extravascular lung water protocol, the authors noted a significant decrease in lung water in patients under the lung water protocol (47). With this approach, the patients required a shorter duration of mechanical ventilation and a shorter stay in the intensive care unit (47). However, the survival rate was identical in both groups, and the study population included patients with both hydrostatic and increased-permeability pulmonary edema (see Chap. 4).

Although theory, experimental data, and some clinical studies suggest that clinical strategies designed to reduce pulmonary edema formation through a decrease in pulmonary microvascular pressure may lead to improvement in outcome in early phase of ARDS, these results have to be examined with a greater perspective. A reduction in lung vascular pressure may be associated with a lower cardiac output and tissue perfusion, effects that may translate to more end-organ dysfunction. Thus, a reasonable objective is to maintain the intravascular volume at the lowest level commensurate with reasonable systemic perfusion as measured by metabolic acid/base balance, urine flow, and renal function (30). It may be possible, as discussed in the next section, to maintain a better systemic blood pressure and an adequate cardiac output by using low doses of vasopressor therapy in combination with judicious fluid management.

D. Vasopressors in ARDS

Vasopressors are needed to support systemic blood pressure in patients with septic shock. There is no clear evidence that one particular vasopressor or combination of vasopressors is superior to another. In general, the most prudent guideline is to restore intravascular volume to euvolemic levels (central venous pressure of 4 to 10 mmHg) and then to use dopamine initially to achieve a mean systemic pressure of 55 to 65 mm Hg. However, both the fluid and vasopressor therapy need to be guided by the clinical indices of end-organ perfusion. In particular, the volume of urine flow and the metabolic acidosis, as reflected by arterial pH and base deficit, are most helpful. In some patients, the insertion of a pulmonary arterial catheter can be helpful to optimize fluid and vasopressor therapy by measuring cardiac output, central venous pressure, and pulmonary arterial wedge pressure. Some studies have demonstrated that a significant fraction of patients with ARDS have impaired left ventricular performance so that measurement of cardiac output and the pulmonary arterial wedge pressure may be helpful (Fig. 3) (30). For example, if the patient has left ventricular dysfunction, then dobutamine may be useful to reduce systemic vascular resistance as well as provide a positive inotropic effect for cardiac function. More details regarding use of vasopressors in ARDS are available in detailed reviews (30). The potential effects of dobutamine and dopamine on hemodynamics, fluid balance, and upregulation of alveolar epithelial fluid clearance will be considered in the last section, Future Therapies.

E. Vasodilators in ARDS

In most patients with ARDS, there is evidence of at least mild pulmonary arterial hypertension. In fact, several studies have reported the results of hemodynamic measurements in ARDS patients (Table 3). In some patients, the pulmonary

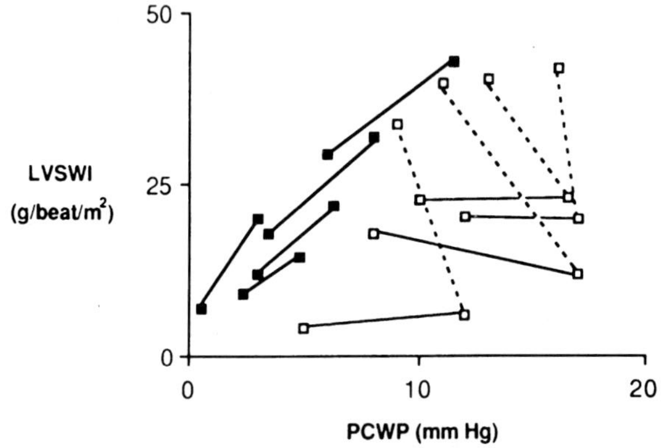

Figure 3 The effect of therapy on left ventricular stroke work index (LVSWI) for the pulmonary capillary wedge pressure (PCWP) in patients with the adult respiratory distress syndrome. Treatment with volume expansion (———) resulted in an improved LVSWI in some patients (n). In other patients volume expansion increased PCWP without an improvement in LVSWI (o). These patients then responded to inotropic therapy (- - - - -). (From Ref. 223.)

Table 3 Initial Systemic and Pulmonary Hemodynamics in Patients with the Acute Respiratory Distress Syndrome with Positive End-Expiratory Pressure of 5 cm H_2O or Less

Study	No. patients	Cardiac index (L/min/m²)	Heart rate (beats/min)	Stroke index (mL/m²)	PCWP (mmHg)	LVSWI (gm-m/m²/beat)	PA (mmHg)	PVR (mmHg/L/min)	BP (mmHg)	SVR (mmHg/L/min)
Normal values[a]	26	3.5 ± 0.7	78 ± 12	46 ± 8	12 ± 2	53 ± 15	17 ± 3	0.9 ± 0.3	91 ± 9	14 ± 3
Jardin et al.	10	4.0 ± 1.0	98 ± 16	41 ± 10	9 ± 2	44			88 ± 20	11
Zimmerman et al.	17	3.8 ± 0.7	118 ± 29	35 ± 10	13 ± 5	37 ± 14	28 ± 9	2.2 ± 1.0	88 ± 16	14 ± 4
Viquerat et al.	11	4.3 ± 1.4	111 ± 20	39 ± 12	18 ± 8	38 ± 12	30 ± 9	1.6 ± 0.8	87 ± 10	10 ± 4
Molloy et al.	11	3.2 ± 1.3	106 ± 22	32 ± 15	11 ± 5	26 ± 11	27 ± 10	4.3 ± 6.7	68 ± 9	13 ± 10
Dhainaut et al.	21	4.5 ± 0.7	109 ± 12	41 ± 3						

[a]Based on Barratt-Boyes et al.

Values equal mean ± standard deviation.

PCWP = pulmonary capillary wedge pressure; LVSWI = left ventricular stroke work index; PA = mean pulmonary artery pressure; PVR = pulmonary vascular resistance; BP = mean systemic blood pressure; SVR = systemic vascular resistance.

Source: Ref. 30.

arterial hypertension leads to cardiac dysfunction due to right ventricular overload (30). Some investigators have tried to lower pulmonary arterial pressure with the goal of reducing right ventricular strain and perhaps to reduce vasoconstriction in the lung.

In the early 1980s, investigators reported that nitroprusside lowered lung water significantly but increased the shunt and lowered the PaO_2. Although nitroprusside decreased pulmonary vascular resistance and increased cardiac output, there was a deterioration of gas exchange. This deterioration in gas exchange was probably secondary to a decrease in hypoxic vasoconstriction (48) as well as an increase in cardiac output to nonventilated regions (49). The use of other vasodilators has also been evaluated. For example, hydralazine seems to be more efficacious in increasing cardiac output than nitroprusside, but it does not increase the shunt (50) because it probably does not influence hypoxic vasoconstriction (51). In an animal model of lung injury (oleic acid), Colley et al. (52) reported that nitroglycerin decreased pulmonary vascular resistance (PVR) by 29% when animals were ventilated with air, but did not influence PVR when breathing oxygen. Nitroglycerin also decreased the arterial blood pressure. These results suggest again that nitrates can modulate the pulmonary circulation, but may be associated with a deterioration in gas exchange and a decrease in blood pressure, which would lead to a decrease in oxygen delivery (53). Prostaglandin E_1 (PGE_1) has also been studied (30). Although some preliminary studies had suggested that continuous infusion of PGE_1 may improve survival (54), a randomized double-blind multicenter study could not confirm these results (55). So, although PGE_1 can improve cardiac output and oxygen delivery while decreasing PVR (56,57), it also induced side effects (56) that offset its potential value as a pulmonary vasodilator. Intravenous prostacyclin has also been evaluated, but its vasodilator effect was also associated with significant changes in systemic hemodynamics (58). The potential role of inhaled nitric oxide will be considered in the last section, Future Therapies. Table 4 summarizes effects of several vasodilators and vasopressors on hemodynamics and oxygenation. In summary, the clinical utility of pulmonary vasodilators in ARDS is limited.

F. Infection Control in ARDS

Patients with ARDS frequently die from uncontrolled infection. The infection may have been the initial cause of the acute lung injury, as in nonpulmonary sepsis from biliary or urosepsis, or severe primary pneumonia with septic shock. In other cases, the cause of the ARDS may be from a noninfectious etiology, such as following major trauma with shock or following drug overdose with aspiration. However, once ARDS is established, there is a high risk of nosocomial pneumonia or other nosocomial infections, such as catheter-related sepsis.

Table 4 Effect of Vasoactive Drugs on Shunt Fraction, Arterial Oxygenation, Cardiac Output, and Systemic Oxygen Delivery in the Setting of Clinical and Experimental Acute Lung Injury

Drug	Shunt fraction	Arterial oxygen tension	Cardiac output	Oxygen delivery	References
Dopamine	No change	Increase or no change	Increase	Increase	30
Dobutamine	Increase	No change	Increase	Increase	30
Isoproterenol	Increase	Decrease	Increase	Increase	30
Nitroprusside	Increase	Decrease	Increase or no change	Increase or decrease	30,49
Hydralazine	No change or increase	No change	Increase	Increase	30,51
Nitroglycerin	Increase	Decrease	Decrease	Decrease	52
Prostaglandin E_1	No change	Increase	Increase	Increase	56,57
Inhaled NO	Slight decrease	Slight increase	No change	No change	144

Uncontrolled infection is, of course, associated with the development of multiple organ dysfunction. Therefore, a major objective of supportive care is to control and prevent infection in ARDS patients.

The diagnosis of nosocomial pneumonia in patients with ARDS is difficult. The usual clinical criteria such as appearance of a new infiltrate, fever, and leukocytosis are common in these patients, even when infection may be absent (59). On the other hand, at autopsy a significant number of patients with ARDS have evidence of undiagnosed pneumonia (60–62). Several attempts have been made to validate the superiority of bronchoscopy with a protected brush to diagnose pneumonia in ARDS patients, but the results have not been reproducible at several medical centers. Currently, clinical judgment is required, recognizing that some patients will be treated with antibiotics who do not have nosocomial pneumonia. It is also important to remember that administration of adequate antibiotics may not always improve outcome (61).

The clinical problem of pneumonia in ARDS has stimulated new approaches to prevent nosocomial pneumonia. Increased colonization of airway epithelium in the critically ill patient and the associated decrease in immunological defenses predisposes to the development of nosocomial pneumonia (62–64). One hypothesis was that the stomach could be the reservoir for gram-negative bacteria. Microorganisms might initially colonize the stomach and subsequently the upper airway, and then could be aspirated into the lung. Gastric colonization might be stimulated by a decrease in gastric acidity as a result of stress ulcer prophylaxis or gastric nutrition (65,66). However, a recent randomized placebo-controlled double-blind study failed to demonstrate differences in incidence of infection, colonization of stomach and respiratory tract, and levels of intragastric acidity between patients receiving either sucralfate or antacids (67). Moreover, sequential analysis of colonization suggested that the stomach might not be the most important source of bacteria in nosocomial pneumonia in these patients. A recent reevaluation of this study confirms that the duration of ventilation and the colonization of the upper respiratory tract are the most important risk factors for nosocomial pneumonia in ventilated patients. Based on these observations, stress ulcer protection should be used according to the recommended criteria (68).

Another alternative that has been considered to control infection in ARDS patients is the use of selective digestive decontamination. With this type of regimen, a combination of topical and intravenous antibiotics is given to modulate the gut flora with the objective of reducing the rate of infection and morbidity and mortality in ICU patients. However, a recent review of this topic (69) has shown that this type of treatment has not been associated with any benefits to the general ICU patient.

G. Nutrition in ARDS

Nutritional supplementation is an important part of supportive therapy for patients with ARDS. Many of the conditions that lead to ARDS, especially sepsis, are associated with hypermetabolism, negative nitrogen balance, and muscle wasting. Although parenteral nutrition had been the preferred approach to administer nutritional support, recent experimental and clinical trials suggest that enteral nutrition may be a superior route for feeding patients. It has been shown in animal models that parenteral nutrition promotes bacterial translocation from the gut (70). Furthermore, in a human study, the response to endotoxin in normal human volunteers who had been fed, either enterally or parenterally, was different. The parenterally fed volunteers had higher levels of systemic and hepatic vein tumor necrosis factor, arterial glucagon, and epinephrine, as well as increased symptomatology and febrile response to endotoxin administration (71). These results suggested that after 1 week of parenteral nutrition, the immunological and hormonal responses to endotoxin were enhanced. If, in fact, enteral nutrition is superior to parenteral nutrition, there should be a decrease in the incidence of multiple organ failure with enteral feeding. Cerra et al. (72) examined the impact of parenteral versus enteral nutrition in 66 septic patients at high risk for organ failure. There was no difference in the incidence of organ failure or mortality in the two groups. So, if enteral nutrition does not provide any changes in the incidence of multiple organ failure, is there any advantage in using this nutritional mode? Several clinical studies have reported that enteral nutrition is associated with a lower incidence of infectious complications than parenteral nutrition (73). Although these results do not clearly differentiate whether enteral feedings decrease the risk of infection or, alternatively, parenteral nutrition increases the risk, they provide enough evidence to support the use of enteral feeding over parenteral nutrition when possible.

IV. Potential New Treatment Strategies for ARDS

There are several promising therapeutic strategies that are currently being explored in a variety of Phase II and III studies. Although no specific new treatment has been proven to reduce morbidity or mortality in clinical acute lung injury, there is reason to be guardedly optimistic that one or more of these new strategies will be successful.

It is important to realize, however, that mortality in clinical acute lung injury relates to several nonpulmonary factors, such as the degree of hepatic insufficiency and the presence and severity of infection (Table 2) (10,11,13,14). Therefore, therapy to reduce mortality in acute lung injury should ideally have some benefit on systemic complications.

This section will briefly review some of the new therapeutic strategies, and when possible refer the reader to other chapters in which these strategies have also been discussed.

A. Surfactant Replacement Therapy for ARDS

The contribution of abnormal surfactant function to the pathophysiology of ARDS was first suggested by Ashbaugh and Petty (23) in their initial description of ARDS. While in the infant respiratory distress syndrome (IRDS) of premature infants, the abnormality of surfactant function is related to a deficiency in the quantity of surfactant, in the adult acute respiratory distress syndrome (ARDS) some of the surfactant is probably inactivated by plasma proteins present in the edema fluid, and there is a change in the lipid composition of the surfactant (74). The abnormalities in surfactant function lead to alveolar instability, a decrease in functional residual capacity, and a decrease in compliance (74). Furthermore, this increase in surface tension in the alveoli may enhance edema formation by creating a more negative hydrostatic force in the alveoli (75). Since surfactant replacement therapy has been shown to improve morbidity and mortality in infant respiratory distress syndrome (76), it was logical to evaluate the potential role of surfactant in the treatment of acute respiratory distress syndrome in adults. Several experimental studies have reported an improvement in pulmonary physiological parameters including compliance, oxygenation, and even survival in different models of lung injury (74).

Although there were some encouraging results from the initial clinical trials with surfactant replacement therapy (77), a recent multicenter randomized placebo-controlled trial involving 725 patients with sepsis-induced ARDS did not demonstrate any impact of an artificial surfactant (Exosurf) on oxygenation, the duration of mechanical ventilation, or the survival of the treated patients (78). There are several possible explanations for the negative results of this trial. First, drug delivery may have been inadequate in this trial. In a study evaluating the delivery of the artificial surfactant (Exosurf), only 4.5% of the dose administered reached the distal air spaces (79). Before concluding that surfactant replacement is not effective in ARDS, surfactant will need to be delivered by a better-aerosolized approach, such as ultrasonic nebulization, or by direct instillation, either by fiberoptic bronchoscopy or with an intratracheal catheter. Also, it is possible that an artificial protein-free surfactant such as Exosurf may not be as efficacious as a natural surfactant preparation or a protein-containing surfactant (74).

Another possible reason for the failure of surfactant therapy is that, despite some similarities, ARDS and neonatal IRDS are fundamentally different. The inflammatory injury in ARDS that often progresses to fibrotic destruction of much of the lung may not be ameliorated by surfactant replacement. Furthermore, as confirmed by the results of the trial by Anzueto et al. (78), most patients with ARDS die from sepsis and multiple organ failure (11,13,60), not from respiratory failure. Surfactant therapy, even if optimally effective, would not be expected to reduce the number of deaths in patients with ARDS that are due to uncontrolled infection and nonpulmonary organ dysfunction.

B. Novel Modes of Mechanical Ventilation and Gas Exchange for ARDS

There have been several major therapeutic efforts to improve outcome in patients with clinical lung injury or ARDS through use of alternative ventilatory strategies. Unfortunately, none have been successful so far. However, it is important to review briefly the major strategies that have been tried and some of the current modalities of new ventilator therapies under study. Table 5 summarizes the major alternative ventilatory strategies that have been evaluated.

ECMO/ECCOR for ARDS

Despite maximal available supportive care, a certain number of patients will have refractory hypoxemia. In the 1970s, multiple investigators suggested that the utilization of extracorporeal membrane oxygenation (ECMO) could be useful as a lifesaving device for these patients. A prospective multicenter randomized trial was then conducted in the mid-1970s to compare ECMO to conventional treatment with continuous positive-pressure ventilation alone (80). ECMO was

Table 5 History of Alternative Ventilator Strategies for the Treatment of the Acute Respiratory Distress Syndrome

Intervention	Year	How studied	Reference
ECMO	1974	Phase III	80
High levels of PEEP	1975	Observational	36
Prophylactic PEEP	1984	Phase III	29
High-frequency ventilation	1983	Phase III	100,101
ECCOR	1994	Phase III	86
Pressure-control inverse-ratio	1993–1998	Observational	112–117
Low tidal volume	1994–1998	Phase II, III	98,99

ECMO = extracorporeal membrane oxygenation: ECCOR = extracorporeal carbon dioxide removal; PEEP = positive end-expiratory airway pressure.

not shown to be superior to conventional therapy, and the mortality rate in both group of patients was 90% (80). Although the high mortality could be related in part to the complications associated with ECMO, it likely also reflects the severity of the disease in that study population.

There have been multiple attempts to improve the technology to decrease complication rates and improve oxygenation. The most noticeable development has been the utilization of extracorporeal carbon dioxide removal ($ECCO_2R$) (81). In true ECMO, oxygenation is the prime objective and the transfer of carbon dioxide occurs as a secondary effect. To achieve effective oxygen transfer, the blood flow rates through the oxygenator need to exceed 50% of the cardiac output. The primary objective of $ECCO_2R$ is to reduce the need for alveolar ventilation, thereby diminishing the potential for ventilator-induced lung injury (see next section). This goal can be achieved with lower blood flow rates, but it provides only 20% to 30% of the total body oxygen requirements (82). Oxygenation is then maintained by providing oxygen by intratracheal insufflation with positive-end expiratory pressure (80).

In 1986, Gattinoni et al. (83) reported a decrease in mortality from 90% to 50% in 47 patients treated with $ECCO_2R$. However, the controls were historical controls based on the entry criteria for the ECMO trials in the 1970s. Brunet et al. (84,85) also reported a survival rate of 50% in their 23 patients treated with $ECCO_2R$. The overall survival rate of the 327 patients treated with $ECCO_2R$ in European countries was 47% in 1992. Although these results were encouraging, the treated patients could not be properly compared with historical controls. Therefore, an NIH-sponsored study was carried out in Salt Lake City at the University of Utah Medical Center to evaluate the efficacy of $ECCO_2R$. There were 40 patients with sufficiently severe ARDS to meet the ECMO entry criteria (86). These patients were randomized to receive either conventional therapy with continuous positive pressure ventilation or pressure-control inverse-ratio ventilation followed by low-frequency positive-pressure ventilation and $ECCO_2R$, as administered by Gattinoni's group in Milan. There was no significant difference in the survival of the patients in the two groups (86). Overall mortality was 62%, much lower than predicted from historical data. Thus, at this time, extracorporeal lung support cannot be recommended as a therapy for ARDS.

Low Tidal Volume/Low Stretch for ARDS

As discussed earlier, one of the clinical hallmarks of ARDS is a decrease in lung compliance (87). It has long been thought that this decrease in compliance was homogeneous through the lung. However, ARDS is not a homogeneous disease (25,27). Instead, the lungs of ARDS patients can be modeled to be composed of three different regions: (1) regions of irreversible damage and alveolar collapse in which no lung volume can be recruited; (2) regions of nearly normal levels of compliance and ventilation; and (3) mixed regions that are infiltrated and consolidated. In these in-between regions, lung volume can be recruited with the application of PEEP (25). In parallel to these observations, some animal experiments have suggested that ventilation of normal lung with large tidal volumes can lead to significant lung injury (see Chap. 13) (88–91). This injury is secondary to an increased permeability of the alveolar capillary membrane (91), which is reversible if the overdistension is not sustained (90). Briefly, Dreyfuss et al. (92) have reported that rats ventilated with large tidal volumes after experimental induction of lung injury had a significant increase in edema compared to injured animals that were ventilated with lower lung volume. However, the major injury occurred with very high tidal volumes in the range of 45 mL/kg, a level that may not occur in the clinical setting of ARDS. Corbridge et al. (93) have also reported that large tidal volumes and low PEEP increase edema accumulation in a canine acid-aspiration model.

All of these new data have led to a serious questioning of the conventional ventilation strategies used in patients with ARDS (94). Although the tidal volumes used to induce injury in the animal model were two or three times greater than the tidal volume used by most clinicians in the intensive care unit, the concern that most of the ventilation is directed to the noninjured portion of the lung has led to the hypothesis that ventilation strategies used in ARDS patients should be reevaluated. In fact, there has been considerable enthusiasm for trials of new ventilator strategies in ARDS. One of the most popular strategies has been the utilization of low-tidal-volume, pressure-limited ventilation associated with permissive hypercapnia. This strategy has been reviewed by many different groups (95–97), but the clinical evidence supporting the benefit of this ventilation strategy has come mainly from two observational studies in which treated patients were compared to their theoretical mortality rate obtained from their Apache II score (98,99). Although these results are encouraging, they are not conclusive. In fact, a recent Phase III trial was carried out primarily in Europe to test the potential value of a low-tidal-volume strategy for reducing mortality in ARDS patients. The trial was stopped after only 107 patients because there was a trend for mortality to be higher in the low-tidal-volume group, although the difference was not significant. The details of this trial have not yet been published, but the results have cast some doubt about the fundamental hypothesis that a reduction in tidal volume and distending airway pressure would have a major favorable impact on outcome in ARDS. The definitive answer should come from an ongoing large, prospective, randomized American trial sponsored by the NIH that is testing the low-tidal-volume strategy. So far, more than 600 patients have been enrolled. The results of the trial are pending. The trial is powered to determine if there is a difference in hospital mortality or the duration of assisted ventilation in patients treated either with 6 mL versus 12 mL/kg tidal volumes with plateau airway pressures of < 30 cm H_2O, or 50 cm H_2O, respectively.

There are other approaches to ventilation of ARDS patients that attempt to combine several strategies. For example, Amato and his colleagues in Brazil have utilized a combination of pressure control, inverse ratio, low tidal volume, and PEEP levels set according to the inflection point on a pressure–volume curve. However, patients must be heavily sedated and paralyzed, and preliminary data from a randomized study at one institution show unusually high mortality rates in control patients (99a). This approach will require further evaluation at other medical centers.

High Frequency and Proportional Assist Ventilation for ARDS

High-frequency ventilation (HFV) was developed in the hope that it could avoid some of the problems associated with conventional ventilation. However, an NIH-sponsored trial in premature infants with respiratory distress syndrome did not demonstrate a significant effect on morbidity or mortality (100). The clinical experience with HFV in ARDS has been disappointing, and the few clinical studies that have been done have reported that mean airway pressures were similar to those used in conventional ventilation if significant improvements in oxygenation were achieved (101). Recently, it has been suggested that ultra-high-frequency ventilation can improve gas exchange and reduce airway pressure for up to 24 hours in severe ARDS patients (102). However, further evaluation of this ventilatory mode is needed before it could become an alternative ventilation strategy in ARDS.

Another recently proposed ventilatory strategy allows the patient to control the extent and timing of lung inflation. This ventilation strategy, called proportional assist ventilation (PAV) (103), adjusts airway pressure in response to patient effort. With this technique, the profile of airway pressure is determined by the subject's inspiratory effort. PAV enables the patient to adjust minute ventilation by allowing complete control of all the elements of any single breath (flow rate, tidal volume, inspiratory time, peak airway pressure, expiratory time). This improves patient comfort and theoretically also minimizes the risk of overdistension. In fact, in one small clinical trial of patients with lung injury, PAV maintained similar minute ventilation to conventional ventilation with a significant decrease in peak airway pressure (104). As with all new approaches, a clinical trial is needed before it can be recommended as a ventilatory strategy in ARDS.

Inverse Ratio Ventilation for ARDS

The major determinant of oxygenation is the mean alveolar pressure because it represents average pressure that is being used to distend the alveoli (105). Although this pressure cannot be measured directly, an estimate of its value can be obtained by measuring the mean airway pressure (MAP). Based on these observations, the level of oxygenation is determined by the MAP (106–109). Since improvement in oxygenation in ARDS occurs primarily because of alveolar recruitment of collapsed regions of the lung, clinicians have tried to use different methods of raising the mean alveolar pressure. PEEP was the first technique used, but it was quite rapidly observed that MAP could be changed independently of PEEP by manipulating the inspiratory time (110). Since the inspiratory time can be set to be longer than the expiratory times, this mode of ventilation has been named inverse-ratio ventilation. This mode of ventilation can be applied either using a pressure-controlled time-cycle ventilation with a long inspiratory time or by using a volume-cycled ventilation applied with either an inspiratory pause or with a slow or decelerating inspiratory flow (105). Several mechanisms have been proposed for the improved oxygenation with inverse-ratio ventilation: there could be an increase in mean airway pressure secondary to the creation of auto-PEEP, or the prolonged inspiratory time with a lower inspiratory flow could enable alveoli with a prolonged time constant to be better ventilated (110).

The application of pressure-controlled inverse-ratio ventilation (PC-IRV) in acute lung injury has some theoretical advantages over conventional techniques. IRV has been shown to improve oxygenation in some ARDS patients (111), and it has also been reported to improve oxygenation when conventional ventilation failed (112). However, there is some evidence that survival of patients treated with this approach is not superior to survival of patients treated with conventional ventilation (113). A more recent study, using a sophisticated computerized protocol, has shown that to achieve similar levels of oxygenation in PC-IRV as conventional volume ventilation requires similar levels of inspired oxygen and PEEP (114). Furthermore, in a recent randomized control study aimed at comparing PC-IRV and $ECCO_2R$ to conventional treatment, the superiority of PC-IRV could not be demonstrated (86). In 21 patients randomized to PC-IRV and $ECCO_2R$, 19 patients had to progress to $ECCO_2R$ since PC-IRV was not effective enough to improve oxygenation in these patients. Furthermore, only one patient of this group improved and survived after PC-IRV alone (86). Another recent study reported no benefit to PC-IRV on oxygenation when there was a careful control of intrinsic PEEP (115).

The utilization of PC-IRV can also be associated with significant adverse effects. If not appropriately monitored, IRV can result in significant air-trapping (intrinsic PEEP), especially when ratios $> 2:1$ are used (105). In fact, one study comparing the efficacy of PC-IRV to PEEP reported a 23% incidence of pneumothoraces with IRV (112). Furthermore, as with the utilization of PEEP, PC-IRV can induce hemodynamic instability (114–117) that seems to be related to a decrease in cardiac output secondary to the increase in MAP and intrinsic PEEP (105). Finally, ventilation with IRV may not be well-tolerated by conscious patients. Some critically ill patients may even require both deep sedation and paralysis to accept this mode of ventilation (105). The prolonged utilization of neuromuscular blocking agents can be associated with either a persistent blockage of the neuromuscular junction or of an acute myopathy (118).

Thus, the superiority of IRV to conventional ventilation and PEEP has not been proven and it could be dangerous to the patient if the proper monitoring is not done. However, its use may be justified in some patients who are refractory to conventional treatment.

Liquivent for ARDS

A recent innovative approach that has been developed for the treatment of hypoxemia secondary to lung injury is liquid ventilation. The development of new organic molecules that are chemically stable, nonbiotransferable, and virtually nontoxic (perfluorocarbon) which dissolve 17 times more O_2 than water (119) stimulated the development of this therapeutic modality. Perfluorocarbon liquids have low surface tension, which allow them to spread easily over the respiratory epithelium. They are minimally absorbed and are eliminated by vaporization through the lungs (119). Liquid ventilation with perfluorocarbon has some possible advantages over conventional ventilation. First, replacing the functional residual capacity of the lung with oxygen-saturated liquid that contains 2.5 times as much O_2 as the same volume of air, could potentially improve gas exchange by increasing alveolar oxygen concentration (119). Furthermore, perflurocarbon has a low surface tension (18 dyne/cm), making it an ideal liquid for lowering surface tension in the injured lung, an effect that might allow adequate ventilation and oxygenation at lower airway pressures. Finally, in comparison to a gas-filled lung, blood flow would be more uniformly distributed in a liquid-filled lung, which should lead to better matching of ventilation and perfusion.

This novel technique of ventilation can be carried out by one of two methods: (1) total liquid ventilation in which the lungs are completely filled with perfluorocarbon and a liquid ventilator assists in the delivery of tidal volumes of perfluorocarbon; or (2) partial liquid ventilation in which the lungs are partially filled with perfluorocarbon to FRC and gas ventilation is continued with a conventional ventilator (119). In different animal models of lung injury, total or partial liquid ventilation improves gas exchange when compared to conventional ventilation (120–124). However, static compliance is significantly increased only by total liquid ventilation (123). The improvement in gas exchange is probably explained by the recruitment and preservation of FRC despite lung injury and inactivation of surfactant. This would prevent alveolar collapse and provide a liquid reservoir of oxygen (120). Furthermore, this improvement in gas exchange is probably secondary to better ventilation/perfusion matching from a redistribution of blood flow to better-ventilated regions of the lung (124). The lack of improvement of gas static compliance with partial liquid ventilation could simply reflect that with a lung partially filled with liquid there is less volume available for distribution of air ventilation.

The use of high-pressure ventilation may still be injurious to pulmonary parenchyma during liquid ventilation as it may be during gas ventilation. In total liquid ventilation, there is also the risk that there could be mechanical interference with venous return (119), although there is minimal hemodynamic instability with partial liquid ventilation administered at around 20 mL/kg (120). Instillation of greater volume of perfluorocarbon may decrease cardiac output in a similar fashion as high PEEP when volumes > 30 mL/kg are instilled (124). Therefore, although there are some clinical reports of the safety and efficacy of partial liquid ventilation in adults (125) and pediatric (126) patients with ARDS, as well as in neonates with IRDS (127), considerable work is needed before this novel technique can be applied in ARDS patients. In fact, a recent unpublished study indicated no major benefits of partial liquid ventilation in a Phase II study of patients with ARDS.

Prone Position for ARDS

Another approach that has been suggested for improving oxygenation is the intermittent prone or lateral positioning of ventilated patients (128,129). Although the exact mechanism explaining this phenomenon is not known, it has been shown that periodic changes in body position will reduce dependent edematous or atelectatic areas present in ARDS patients (130). This may lead to an improvement in the regional ventilation in the dorsal region of the lung, leading to an improvement in the V/Q abnormalities and oxygenation (131). This concept has led to development of a new nursing approach to patients with ARDS named kinetic therapy (132). Patients are nursed in a bed that constantly rotates through 67° each side of horizontal. Although this nursing approach is associated with an improvement in oxygenation and is not usually associated with hemodynamic instability (132), it substantially increases the nursing care of these patients. Unless more data are obtained from randomized controlled trials, positional manipulation should be used in patients only when other therapeutic modalities have failed.

C. Modulation of Pulmonary Vascular Tone (Inhaled Nitric Oxide)

Nitric oxide (NO) is a powerful endogenous vasodilator that is synthesized by NO synthase (133,134). Inhaled as well as endogenous NO leads to the production of cGMP and subsequent relaxation of vascular smooth muscle. The half-life of NO in the body is very short due to oxidation or inactivation by binding to hemoglobin within seconds (134). This rapid inactivation of NO restricts its vasodilatory effects to local blood vessels and to its site of generation or administration. Because its pharmacological action is localized and rapidly terminated, gaseous NO is potentially an ideal agent to affect the pulmonary circulation in ventilated patients. Several experimental studies have been done with inhaled NO in a large number of animal models of acute lung injury (135–139). On balance, some animal studies have reported improvement in the severity of lung injury with inhaled NO while an equal number have reported no benefit, or occasionally a worsening of lung injury.

Encouraging results in some of the animal models (140–142) led to the evaluation of the therapeutic potential of NO in patients with ARDS. Rossaint et al. (143) reported that in 9 of 10 consecutive patients with ARDS, inhaled NO at a concentration of 18 ppm reduced the mean pulmonary artery pressure from 37 to 30 mm Hg and decreased intrapulmonary shunting from 36% to 31%, an effect that led to an average increase of the PaO_2/FiO_2 ratio of 47. No measurements of clinical outcome were made in that study. Recently, an American trial by Dellinger et al. (144) reported the results of a randomized double-blind Phase II study of different doses of inhaled NO (1.25 to 80 ppm) for patients with ARDS. The primary objective was to evaluate safety and the physiologic responses of different doses of inhaled NO with the hope that the results would demonstrate enough benefit to warrant a Phase III trial. Patients were excluded from the trial if they had ARDS from nonpulmonary sepsis and hypotension or if they were immunocompromised. With this design, the investigators hoped to maximize the chance for inhaled NO to show benefit in patients with ARDS and respiratory failure as their primary problem, and to exclude septic patients who have a worse prognosis.

Unfortunately, the results of this Phase II trial were not encouraging (144). Overall, there were no differences among the inhaled NO groups and placebo treatment (provided in a blind fashion) with respect to mortality, the number of days alive and off mechanical ventilation, or the number of days alive after meeting oxygenation criteria for extubation. Even the improvement in oxygenation was modest and not sustained. For example, the fraction of inspired oxygen was significantly lower only on day 1, and the difference compared to the placebo group was trivial (FiO_2 of 0.69 versus 0.71). The PaO_2/FiO_2 was improved only on day 1, and this improvement was not significant on days 2 through 7. Furthermore, only 60% of the patients responded to inhaled NO with an acute improvement (> 4 hours) in arterial oxygenation. In fact, 24% of the placebo group had an acute improvement in oxygenation. Pulmonary arterial pressure was lower only on day 1, and the effect was small (2 mmHg).

The data for the number of days alive and off mechanical ventilation were also not different between placebo and the inhaled NO groups. The authors attempted to find some positive result, so a post hoc analysis was done to examine the percentage of patients alive and off the ventilator at day 28. The 5 ppm inhaled NO group had a slightly higher percent than the placebo group, but this analysis was not significant when a proper statistical analysis for multiple comparisons was done. Since there was no difference in mortality or in days alive and off mechanical ventilation with 5 ppm inhaled NO, this post hoc analysis is neither convincing nor encouraging.

Interestingly, the results of a recent unpublished, prospective, double-blind, randomized French Phase III study of inhaled NO for ARDS in 208 patients also demonstrated no effect on mortality or the duration of mechanical ventilation (personal communication, D. Payen; data presented at Société Française d'Anesthésie Réanimation, September 1997).

Should inhaled NO continue to be tested, possibly for its modest beneficial effects on oxygenation in some ARDS patients? There are other approaches to improving oxygenation, such as a change to the prone position. A change in position may be efficacious in some patients, may be less expensive than inhaled NO, and can probably achieve comparable results in terms of improving oxygenation. It seems unlikely that inhaled NO will become a primary treatment for patients with ARDS. It may have some limited application as a rescue therapy in some ARDS patients with refractory hypoxemia and pulmonary arterial hypertension. Perhaps the major effort now should be directed at determining the contribution of endogenous NO in the pathogenesis of experimental lung injury.

Although the results of the American and French trials diminish enthusiasm for the value of inhaled NO in ARDS patients, it is conceivable that there may be some value in combining inhaled NO in combination with another agent, such as almitrine, for treating severe hypoxemia and moderate to severe pulmonary arterial hypertension in selected ARDS patients (145). Also, there are recent data that inhaled prostacyclin can improve oxygenation and reduce shunt fraction without causing systemic hypotension (146). On balance, however, it seems that these agents will not have a fundamental impact on the morbidity and mortality in patients with ARDS.

D. Augmentation of Systemic Oxygen Delivery for ARDS

Over the years, it has become clear in many patients with ARDS that lung injury is only one of the obvious manifestations of a more generalized process in which multiple organs are involved or are at risk. In fact, most patients with ARDS die with stable though abnormal lung function. The major causes of death appear to be uncontrolled sepsis (11,13,60) and nonpulmonary organ system failure or dysfunction (11,14,60,147,148). Organ system dysfunction may be a complication of a systemic inflammatory response (SIRS) that can be associated with an infectious process (sepsis) (149) and sometimes occurs following severe shock of a noninfectious etiology. One hypothesis is that inadequate tissue oxygen delivery in the early phase of shock predisposes to organ system failure in many critically ill patients, including ARDS patients (150,151).

Although no controlled randomized clinical trials have studied the best approach to correct tissue hypoxia, a recent consensus conference organized by the European Society of Intensive Care Medicine, the Société de Réanimation de Langue Française, and the American Thoracic Society provided guidelines for the optimization of delivery of oxygen to the tissues and for the reduction of oxygen demand (152). To optimize oxygen delivery (DO_2), this group recommends first to proceed with adequate volume resuscitation. If inadequate perfusion persists, vasoactive drugs should be used. Reduction in oxygen demand should be achieved first by giving a proper level of sedation and analgesia, and then by providing mechanical ventilation to the patient in shock since the work of breathing is usually high.

Although timely and adequate intravascular volume resuscitation is essential, is there any benefit in trying to provide the patient with the supranormal level of DO_2? This concept arises from the observation that patients with ARDS may have an abnormal DO_2–VO_2 relationship (153). Under normal conditions, as systemic DO_2 decreases, systemic VO_2 is maintained relatively constant by an increase in tissue oxygen extraction. Below a critical DO_2, VO_2 decreases linearly as DO_2 decreases, a condition called physiological dependence of

VO_2 on DO_2 (153). It has been suggested that in ARDS patients, there is a pathological dependence of VO_2 on DO_2 (153). However, further evaluation of this question has suggested that this linear relationship between VO_2 and DO_2 in ARDS is probably secondary to mathematical coupling of errors in the measurement of shared variables used to calculate VO_2 and DO_2 (154,155). In fact, in a number of clinical studies in which VO_2 is determined independently of DO_2, no pathological dependence of VO_2 on DO_2 could be identified (156).

However, even if the pathological relationship between VO_2 and DO_2 does not really exist, is survival of patients with ARDS who have a supranormal DO_2 better than those with a normal DO_2? At least nine controlled clinical trials investigated this question (Fig. 4). Comparison of these studies is somewhat difficult because they were done with different patient populations and somewhat different goals. In one series of studies, the patient population was mainly a postoperative or posttrauma patient population (157–161). The investigators tried to determine if optimization of DO_2 to a supranormal value could influence the mortality and the development of multiple organ failure in these high-risk patients. In the other groups of studies, investigators evaluated patients with sepsis and/or ARDS to determine if optimization of DO_2 to a supranormal value would decrease mortality (162,163). In the studies of postoperative or post-trauma patients, there was a trend for a decrease in mortality with supranormal oxygen delivery (153–161). However, when sepsis or ARDS was present, there was no apparent benefit of this therapy (162,163). Thus, there are no clinical studies in ARDS patients that support the value of increasing DO_2 to supranormal levels to decrease mortality. Also, since one randomized trial reported an increase in mortality in the treatment group (164), the goal in ARDS should be to normalize hemodynamic parameters without an attempt to provide a supranormal level of oxygen delivery.

E. Anti-Inflammatory Strategies for ARDS

As discussed in several chapters in this book, there are multiple inflammatory mechanisms that mediate acute lung injury with increased permeability pulmonary edema, or what is clinically termed the acute respiratory distress syndrome (ARDS). The inflammatory response is associated with recruitment of large numbers of neutrophils and monocytes to the distal airspaces of the lung. This cellular response is associated with the release of several pro-inflammatory molecules including cytokines, oxygen radicals, and proteases (165). The release of these mediators is associated with injury to the endothelial and epithelial barriers of the lung (166,167). Based on a variety of preclinical experimental studies, several clinical trials have been carried out with the objective of inter-

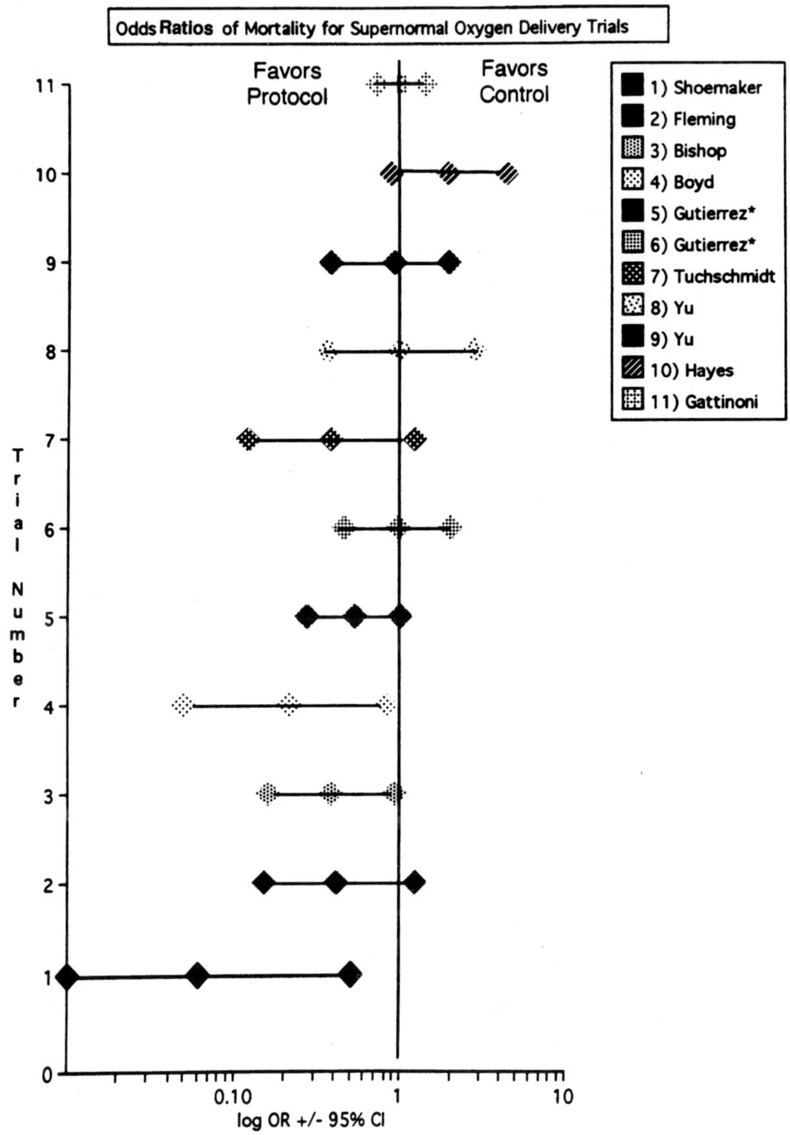

Figure 4 Randomized trials of increased oxygen delivery in critically ill patients. The odds ratio representing the effect on mortality and associated 95% confidence interval is provided. OR = odds ratio; CI = confidence interval. *Gutierrez trial separated into study population with low gastric pH (Trial 6, pHi ≤ 7.35) versus normal or high gastric mucosal pH (Trial 5, pHi > 7.35).

rupting the inflammatory cascade in clinical acute lung injury. Some of the treatments have already been shown to be ineffective in reducing mortality, but a brief review of the negative trials is useful in designing future strategies for more effective treatment.

Therapeutic Strategies to Reduce Sepsis-Induced ARDS

Patients who develop ARDS from sepsis have the highest mortality compared to other causes of ARDS, such as pneumonia without sepsis, aspiration of gastric contents, or shock following major trauma (11,14). Therefore, it seemed logical to treat patients with sepsis either before they developed lung injury or in the early phase of sepsis-induced lung injury. Unfortunately, several clinical trials with a wide variety of anti-inflammatory agents have failed to show clinical benefit in treating septic patients. So far, negative trials have been reported with administration of high doses of glucocorticoids (168–170), antiendotoxin monoclonal antibody therapy, antitumor necrosis factor-α therapy, and anti-interleukin-1 therapy (171). Recently, ibuprofen was also reported to show no major clinical benefit in patients with sepsis (see next section on prostaglandin agonists and inhibitors) (172).

Most of these clinical trials were directed at treating large groups of patients with sepsis, and they provided limited data regarding the incidence of ARDS or the efficacy of treatment in ARDS patients. Two studies have reevaluated the data of some of these trials to address this question. A substudy of the large sepsis trial (173) prospectively evaluated the effects of 24 hours of treatment with methylprednisolone on the development of ARDS in patients with sepsis. There appeared to be a higher mortality in the treated group. In a subgroup analysis of an antiendotoxin trial, there was no effect of the human antiendotoxin on the development or resolution of ARDS (171).

Glucocorticoid Therapy for ARDS

As discussed in the preceding section, high-dose glucocorticoids do not prevent the development of ARDS in patients with sepsis. In addition, controlled clinical studies have shown that there is no benefit to most patients with established ARDS (168–170). Interestingly, in one of these studies, serum complement levels were not lowered in patients with septic-induced ARDS who were treated with high-dose methylprednisolone (169). There have been some recent observational studies suggesting that glucocorticoid therapy may have benefit in some ARDS patients with severe established clinical lung injury (174,175). The studies suggest that some patients with ARDS have ongoing inflammation and release of cytokines in the airspaces of the lung, and that these patients may benefit from high-dose glucocorticoid therapy. It is clear that treatment for several days with high-dose glucocorticoids does increase the risk of nosocomial pneumonia and probably other infections, such as catheter-related infection. In order to test the potential value of high-dose glucocorticoid therapy in established, severe ARDS, the NIH is sponsoring a prospective double-blind randomized trial to test the hypothesis that high-dose methylprednisolone (2 mg/kg q6h for 2 weeks) can reverse the fibroproliferative phase of ARDS. Since this treatment is likely to be associated with a significant increased incidence of infection, it cannot be recommended until a prospective placebo-controlled randomized trial demonstrates efficacy.

Antioxidant Therapy for ARDS

A variety of experimental studies have provided convincing evidence that reactive oxygen species play a major role in mediating injury to the endothelial barrier of the lung in the presence of endotoxin, bacterial sepsis (see Chap. 6), or hyperoxic lung injury (see Chap. 15). Antioxidant therapy has been useful in the prevention and the treatment of acute lung injury in some animal models of clinical lung injury (176). Also, there is evidence that patients with ARDS experience oxidative stress from neutrophil activation, and from treatment with high levels of inspired oxygen. Recent work indicates that patients who do not survive ARDS sustain much greater levels of oxidative molecular damage, suggesting that they are less able to protect themselves against oxidative stress (177).

N-acetylcysteine is a thiol-containing compound that acts as an oxygen free radical scavenger and as a precursor for glutathione, an essential element of the antioxidant defense mechanisms. This compound has been efficacious in some experimental studies (176). In Phase II clinical studies, N-acetylcysteine demonstrated a trend to reduce nonpulmonary organ system dysfunction and the duration of assisted ventilation in patients with ARDS (178); also, there were some trends toward clinical benefit in a Phase II study in septic patients (179). Therefore, a prospective Phase III randomized placebo-controlled American trial began in mid-1997 to test the potential efficacy of Procysteine, an analog of N-acetylcysteine, for the treatment of early ARDS. Treatment with other antioxidants, such as superoxide dismutase, has been limited because of difficulties with delivery of the antioxidant to the site of injury.

Prostaglandin Agonists/Inhibitors for ARDS

Several experimental studies have produced evidence that administration of vasodilating prostaglandins might be beneficial in treating acute lung injury. Prostaglandin E_1 is a vasodilator that can also block platelet aggregation and decrease neutrophil activation. This agent had shown promise in experimental studies of lung injury. One clinical study of 41 surgical patients with ARDS reported improved oxygenation and better mortality with intravenous prostaglandin E_1 (54). However, a larger multicenter study of 100 medical and surgical patients reported no evidence of reduced mortality in ARDS patients treated with intravenous prostaglandin E_1 (55). Recently, prostaglandin E_1 was tried again, but this time it was administered in liposomes with the hypothesis that delivery to the lung and the endothelium would be better. Unfortunately, this Phase III study was stopped recently because there was no benefit even when PGE_1 was given by the improved delivery system.

The synthesis of cyclo-oxygenase products of the prostaglandin pathway, particularly thromboxane, has been linked with abnormalities of airway mechanics, hypoxemia, systemic hypotension, and multiple organ dysfunction in animal models of lung injury, especially from endotoxin and live bacteria. Therefore, a prospective trial was carried out to test the ability of ibuprofen, an inhibitor of the cyclo-oxygenase pathway, to reduce morbidity and mortality in patients with sepsis who were at risk of multiple organ failure including ARDS. Ibuprofen was tested in a double-blind randomized trial of 455 patients with sepsis (172). At baseline, all patients had markedly elevated levels of prostacyclin and thromboxane metabolites; after treatment, the ibuprofen-treated patients had only 11% of the values in the placebo group. However, there was no difference in mortality between the placebo- (40%) and the ibuprofen- (37%) treated groups, and there was no significant effect on the duration of shock or the duration of multiple organ dysfunction (172). For an unexplained reason, there was a trend for lower mortality in patients who presented with hypothermia and in patients who were African-Americans.

Ketoconazole, a potent inhibitor of thromboxane and leukotriene synthesis, was reported in two studies to prevent the development of ARDS in high-risk surgical patients (180). Therefore, this agent was studied in an NIH-sponsored multicenter Phase III randomized placebo-controlled trial to test its efficacy for decreasing mortality and the duration of assisted ventilation in patients who had developed clinical acute lung injury. The drug was administered within 36 hours of meeting criteria for acute lung injury (bilateral pulmonary infiltrates and a $PaO_2/FiO_2 < 300$). A total of 234 patients were studied. Unfortunately, there was no decrease in mortality for ketoconazole treatment (36%) versus the placebo group (37%), and the median number of ventilator-free days was 9 in the placebo group versus 10 in the ketoconazole group. There was a trend for a reduction in urinary thromboxane in the treated group, although the difference did not reach statistical significance.

Thus, attempts to influence outcome in patients at risk for ARDS or with ARDS by inhibiting prostaglandin metabolites or by administering a vasodilating prostaglandin have not been successful in clinical studies. These results are disappointing, particularly in view of the extensive animal data supporting a critical role of prostaglandin metabolites in mediating pulmonary and nonpulmonary injury in patients with ARDS. It is possible, of course, that administration of prostaglandin inhibitors (or an agonist, such as prostaglandin E_2) cannot be given in the clinical setting at a sufficiently early time point to attenuate the inflammatory process. Alternatively, these agents may not have a sufficiently fundamental impact on the pathogenesis of lung injury to be effective clinically.

Lisofylline for ARDS

Pentoxyfylline is a phosphodiesterase inhibitor that inhibits neutrophil chemotaxis and activation in animal models of ARDS (181–183). Although the reported experience in humans so far suggests some benefits, there is not enough information to allow definitive recommendations. Recently, there has been growing interest in lisofylline, an analog of pentoxyfylline. In animal studies, this drug inhibits release of several cytokines including TNF, IL-1, and IL-6 with inhibition of shock-induced lung injury in mice. There are also some experimental data indicating some favorable effect on the course of murine endotoxin shock. Lisofylline was evaluated in a recent Phase II study of 60 patients with hematological malignancies undergoing bone marrow transplant. The results showed fewer infections and less mucositis in the lisofylline-treated patients. Although the exact mechanism of action is unknown, these results are sufficiently encouraging for the drug to now be evaluated in a Phase II/III NIH-sponsored study of early clinical lung injury. The hypothesis is that this agent will protect against endothelial and epithelial injury, hopefully in multiple organs, and thus reduce the severity of lung injury and nonpulmonary organ system dysfunction in ARDS patients.

Anti-Interleukin-8 Therapy and Other Potential Anti-Inflammatory Strategies for ARDS

There are other potential anti-inflammatory strategies that might yet prove to be effective in attenuating ARDS or preventing its development in high-risk patients. One approach is to reduce the number of neutrophils that can migrate into the extravascular space of the lung. This objective theoretically could be accomplished by interfering with neutrophil adhesion to lung endothelium or by reducing the release of chemotactic factors in the extravascular space. Considerable experimental work has been devoted to efforts to reduce integrin- or selectin-mediated neutrophil adhesion in the lung. Although some of the strategies have been successful in preclinical studies, none have yet reached clinical trials. One of the problems with this approach is that the mechanisms for neutrophil adhesion in the lung microcirculation involve mechanical factors that are determined by the pulmonary capillary geometry as well as the size and stiffness of neutrophils. Thus, inhibition of some adhesion molecules, such as CD11,18, will reduce extravascular migration in the systemic circulation, but not necessarily in the pulmonary circulation (184).

There is some compelling support experimentally for a strategy to inhibit the release of interleukin-8 (IL-8), the most important stimulus for migration of neutrophils from an intravascular to an extravascular location. First, experimental data support a role for the efficacy of neutralizing monoclonal antibody therapy to IL-8 to treat and limit acid-induced lung injury in rabbits, even when the anti-IL-8 therapy is given 1 hour after instillation of a pH 1.5 solution (see Chap. 8) (185). This therapy has also been used effectively to limit the extent of pulmonary and systemic injury in an unpublished porcine model of gram-negative sepsis. In addition, several clinical studies indicate that substantial quantities of IL-8 are present in the bronchoalveolar lavage fluid or the pulmonary edema fluid of patients in the early phase of ARDS (186–190). One potential drawback to any anti-neutrophil strategy is that the risk of infection may be increased. However, there is a murine IL-8 receptor knockout mouse model which is not more susceptible to experimental *Pseudomonas* pneumonia. Further preclinical studies are needed, especially relative to the risk of infection. However, clinical trials using anti-IL-8 therapy as prevention in high-risk groups of patients or in early ARDS may now be warranted.

Other potential strategies could include treatments designed to attenuate the effect of platelet-activating factor (PAF), especially in sepsis or severe shock with trauma. PAF is a potent phospholipid mediator that increases cell adhesion and activates endothelial cells by a direct effect or through formation of reactive oxygen species or arachidonic acid metabolites (165). PAF acetylhydrolase (PAF-AH) degrades PAF and related oxidized phospholipids and thus regulates their biological activity. There is some interest in developing a form of PAF-AH that could be given as an anti-inflammatory agent early in ARDS or in septic or trauma patients at high risk for developing ARDS. There is still some interest in the potential role of antiprotease therapy, although BAL studies seem to indicate that the airspaces of the lung in ARDS have an excess of antiprotease activity already, in the form of both endogenous macroglobulin and alpha-1-antitrypsin. As mentioned in the discussion of anti-cytokine trials for sepsis, efforts to neutralize IL-1 or TNF-α have so far been unsuccessful, although it is conceivable that therapy with these agents might still have a role in some patients with ARDS. Therapies to inhibit the coagulation cascade have not reached the level of viable clinical trials in patients at risk of ARDS or patients with established ARDS.

F. Acceleration of Alveolar Epithelial Sodium and Fluid Transport in ARDS

Until recently, most of our attention was focused on the function and dysfunction of the pulmonary endothelium during acute lung injury. However, it is now clear that the structure and function of the alveolar epithelium are also important determinants in lung injury (191,192). The alveolar epithelium is not only an important barrier to alveolar flooding, but is also the site of alveolar fluid reabsorption (192). Reabsorption of alveolar edema is an essential step in the resolution of ARDS, and might have a significant impact on the prognosis of patients with this condition (192). Considerable progress has been made in understanding the mechanisms that regulate alveolar liquid clearance (as discussed in Chaps. 14–18). The evidence indicates that alveolar fluid clearance primarily depends on active sodium transport across the alveolar epithelium. Therefore, the obvious clinical question is whether this process can be upregulated in patients with ARDS. Before attempting to answer this question, the next section will consider the function of the alveolar epithelium in the presence of acute lung injury. A more detailed discussion of these issues is also provided in Chapters 14 through 17.

Transport Properties of the Alveolar Epithelium in the Presence of Acute Lung Injury

The alveolar epithelium is remarkably resistant to injury, particularly compared to the adjacent lung endothelium. Even when mild to moderate alveolar epithelial injury occurs, the capacity of the alveolar epithelium to transport salt and water is often preserved (193–200) (Table 6). In addition, several mechanisms may result in upregulation of the fluid transport capacity of the distal pulmonary epithelium, even after moderate to severe epithelial injury. Even when lung endothelial injury occurs, the alveolar epithelial barrier may remain normally impermeable to protein and retain its normal fluid transport capacity. For example, intravenous endotoxin or bacteria were used to produce lung endothelial injury in sheep and rats (193–195), but permeability to protein across the lung epithelial barrier was not increased. When septic shock was induced in rats, there was a marked increase in plasma epinephrine levels. Even though endothelial injury and mild interstitial pulmonary edema occurred, alveolar epithelial fluid transport was increased by 32% in septic rats. This enhanced liquid clearance was inhibited by instillation of amiloride (10^{-4} M) or propranolol (10^{-4} M) into the distal airspaces, demonstrating that stimulated clearance depended on beta-agonist stimulation of alveolar epithelial sodium transport. When more severe septic shock was produced in sheep, the alveolar epithelial barrier was resistant to injury in the majority of animals, with confinement of edema to the pulmonary interstitium (194). In some sheep, however, more severe systemic and pulmonary endothelial injuries were associated with alveolar flooding, a marked increase in epithelial permeability to protein, and the inability to transport fluid from the airspaces of the lung (195). The inability to remove excess fluid from the airspaces in these sheep may have been related more to a marked increase in paracellular permeability from injury to the epithelial tight junctions than to a loss of salt and water transport capacities of alveolar epithelial cells.

Table 6 Effect of Pathological Conditions on Alveolar Epithelial Fluid Clearance in Several Species

Pathological condition	Species	Severity of lung injury		Alveolar epithelial fluid clearance
		Endothelium	Epithelium	
Endotoxin, intravenous	Sheep	Mild	None	Normal
Endotoxin, alveloar	Sheep	None	None	Normal
	Rat	None	None	Inreased
Exotoxin, alveolar	Rat	None	None	Increased
Bacteria, intravenous[a]	Sheep	Moderate/severe	Mild/severe	Increased/decreased
	Rat	Mild	None	Increased
	Rabbit	Mild	None	Normal
Bacteria, alveolar[a]	Sheep	Mild	Mild	Normal
	Rat	Mild	Moderate/severe	Normal/decreased/increased
	Rabbit	Mild	Moderate/severe	Normal/decreased
Oleic acid, intravenous[b]	Sheep	Moderate	Moderate	Normal
Acid aspiration	Rabbit	Severe	Severe	Decreased
Salt water aspiration	Rabbit	Mild	Mild	Normal
Fresh water aspiration	Sheep	Moderate	Severe	Decreased
Hyperoxia[c]	Rat	Moderate/severe	Mild/moderate	Normal/decreased
Drug-induced (bleomycin, intratracheal)	Rat	Moderate	Mild	Increased
Drug-induced (ANTU, intraperitoneal)	Rat	Moderate	None	Unknown
ARDS	Human	Moderate/severe	Mild/moderate/severe	None/normal/increased

[a]The extent of injury to the epithelial and endothelial barriers is dependent on the dose and virulence of bacteria that are administered.
[b]Initially the injury after intravenous oleic acid is severe, but the alveolar epithelium recovers after 4 hours sufficiently to remove some of the excess edema fluid.
[c]The extent of injury to the epithelial and endothelial barrier depends on the oxygen concentration and duration of exposure of the rats.

Although these studies suggest that active sodium transport can be upregulated during the early phase of acute lung injury, an important issue is whether there is upregulation of active sodium transport during the development of pulmonary edema in vivo. Different groups of investigators have tried to answer this question. Much of the information was obtained in hyperoxic lung injury models (196–200). On balance, the results suggest that there is activation of sodium transport mechanisms during pulmonary edema induced by hyperoxia. However, structural changes may influence interpretation of the data. For example, a proliferative response of alveolar type II cells has been observed in the subacute hyperoxic lung injury model (16). In the acute hyperoxic lung injury model, there is no proliferation of alveolar type II cells, but the number of inflammatory cells in the interstitial space is increased (16).

Because of the potential confounding effect of alveolar cell proliferation, thiourea-induced lung edema was used to study NaK-ATPase activity during recovery from edema because this model is not associated with significant cell proliferation (202). NaK-ATPase activity was measured since NaK-ATPase is the only mechanism for basolateral extrusion of sodium once it is absorbed from the apical membrane (203). Thus, the activity of the enzyme should be a reasonable index of active sodium transport in the lung (204). Lung alveolar type II cell NaK-ATPase activity was increased during recovery from thiourea-induced pulmonary edema. The activity of the enzyme started to increase 4 h after the induction of edema, with maximal activation at 12 h (205). Thus, lung NaK-ATPase can be activated during recovery from experimental pulmonary edema, indicating that active sodium transport mechanisms are upregulated during this process.

Strategies to Increase Removal of Alveolar Edema Fluid

In one study, approximately 40% of patients were able to reabsorb some of the alveolar edema fluid within 12 hours of intubation and acute lung injury (192). These patients recovered more rapidly from respiratory failure and had a lower mortality. In contrast, patients who did not reabsorb any alveolar edema fluid in the first 12 hours after acute lung injury had protracted respiratory failure and a higher mortality (192) (see Fig. 3 in Chap. 6). Additional studies are being carried out in larger numbers of patients at the University of California, San Francisco, to characterize the transport capacity of the alveolar epithelium in the presence of acute lung injury. Preliminary data indicate again that about 40% of ARDS patients have evidence of intact alveolar epithelial fluid transport in the first 12 to 24 hours following clinical lung injury. In contrast, approximately 70% to 80% of patients with severe hydrostatic pulmonary edema have evidence of intact alveolar epithelial fluid transport. Could pharmacological treatment accelerate the resolution of pulmonary edema in patients with intact clearance mechanisms? Secondly, could transport be augmented in patients who have no evidence of net alveolar fluid clearance?

The experimental data provide good evidence that beta-2 adrenergic stimulation can markedly upregulate alveolar fluid clearance in the normal lung, as shown in studies in several species (206). Furthermore, there is good evidence that alveolar epithelial fluid transport can be augmented with beta-2 adrenergic therapy in the ex vivo human lung (207). In most of these studies, the beta-2 agonist was given directly into the airspaces, although there is excellent evidence that intravenous delivery of beta-2 agonist therapy or endogenous release of epinephrine from the adrenal gland into the circulation will also markedly increase the rate of alveolar epithelial sodium and fluid clearance (206).

Recent data indicate that a lipid soluble beta-2 agonist, salmeterol, can maximally upregulate alveolar fluid clearance in the ex vivo human lung at a dose of only 10^{-6} M (Fig. 5). Interestingly, this is exactly the concentration that was achieved in the alveolar compartment in recent sheep studies in which salmeterol was aerosolized in a clinically relevant dose of 5 mg over 1 hour. Thus, there is evidence that a beta-2 agonist can be delivered by nebulization or aerosol in intubated, mechanically ventilated animals and that the required

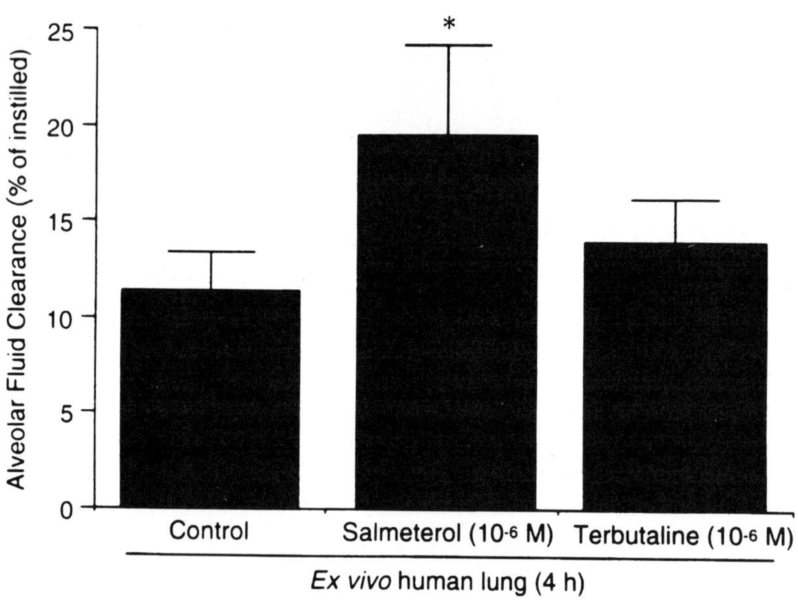

Figure 5 Comparison between the effects of same dose (10^{-6} M) of salmeterol and terbutaline on alveolar fluid clearance in the ex vivo human lung. *$P < .05$ versus rates in the control experiments. (From Ref. 207.)

concentrations can be achieved in the distal airspaces of the lung to accelerate alveolar fluid clearance.

Is there evidence that transport can be stimulated in the presence of lung injury with beta-2 agonists? There are two recent publications in the hyperoxic lung injury model in rats reporting that intra-alveolar terbutaline, a beta-2 agonist, can markedly increase the rate of alveolar fluid clearance, even in the presence of significant lung injury (Figs. 6, 7) (208,209). In both of these studies, the edema was probably confined predominantly to the interstitium. However, the results do establish the principle that exogenous beta-2 agonist therapy can conceivably upregulate alveolar fluid clearance in the injured lung. In addition, as discussed in detail in Chapter 14, alveolar fluid clearance can be markedly upregulated, at least in the short term, by endogenous release of epinephrine in the presence of endotoxemia or bacteremia (206). It is possible, of course, that the epithelium may not respond to beta-2 agonist stimulation, either because of extensive injury and loss of the alveolar type II cells or because the injury itself may downregulate the response to beta-2 agonists. For example, recent work indicates that following prolonged hemorrhagic shock in rats, oxidant mechanisms downregulate the response of the alveolar epithelium to beta-2

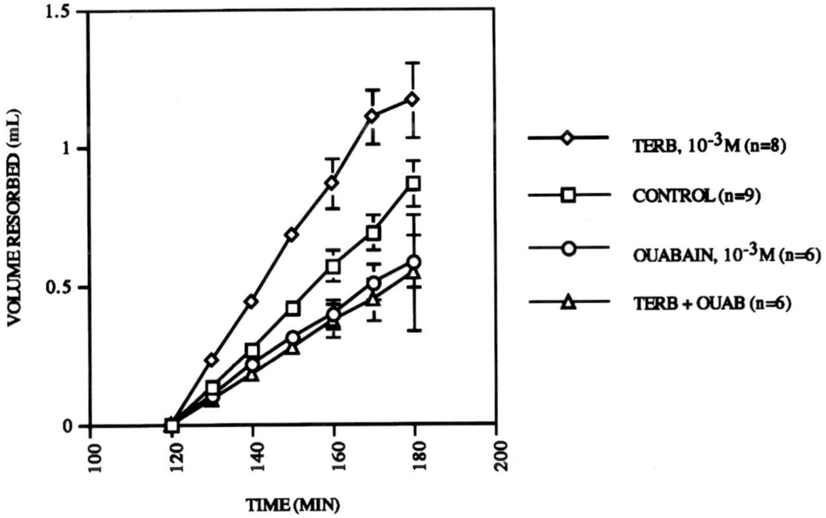

Figure 6 Alveolar fluid resorption from hyperoxic lungs. Values are means ± SE. Where error bars are not shown, range of SE is smaller than symbol. Number of animals for each treatment group is indicated in parentheses. Note that terbutaline increased. (From Ref. 209.)

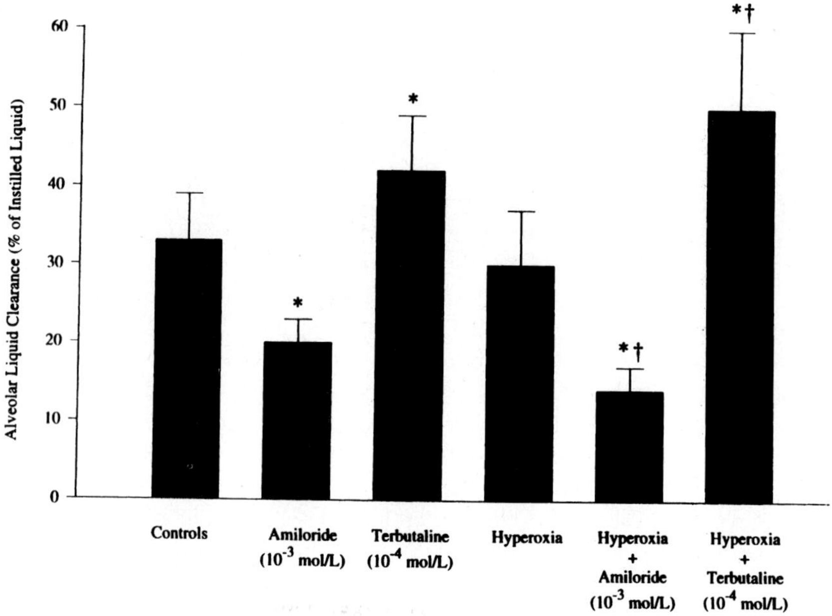

Figure 7 The effects of amiloride and terbutaline on lung liquid clearance in room air-exposed (n=16) and hyperoxic-exposed rats (n=14) are shown. Lung liquid clearance in hyperoxic-exposed rats was similar to room air-exposed rats. Amiloride inhibited lung liquid clearance equally in both oxygen-exposed and room air–exposed rats. Moreover, terbutaline stimulated lung liquid clearance at equal rates in both groups of rats. The effects of amiloride and terbutaline in the hyperoxic rats were similar to the effects in rats exposed to room air alone. $^*P < .05$ vs. control rats; $^\dagger P < .05$ vs. hyperoxia (ANOVA). (From Ref. 208.)

agonist stimulation (see Chap. 9). Controlled clinical trials will be needed to evaluate aerosolized beta-adrenergic agonist therapy in patients with ARDS.

In addition to therapy with aerosolized beta-2 agonists, it is possible that alveolar epithelial fluid clearance could be upregulated with a systemically delivered beta-2 agonist. For example, recent work from our laboratory indicates that dobutamine, a commonly used vasoactive agent in critically ill patients, can markedly upregulate alveolar epithelial fluid clearance when given by an intravenous route in clinically relevant concentrations (Fig. 8) (7). The effect is mediated by stimulation of beta-2 receptors. Another group of investigators has presented evidence that dopamine, another commonly used vasoactive agent, can upregulate alveolar fluid clearance in an isolated perfused rat model, perhaps by increasing the activity of NaK-ATPase (8). Thus, clinically used vasoactive

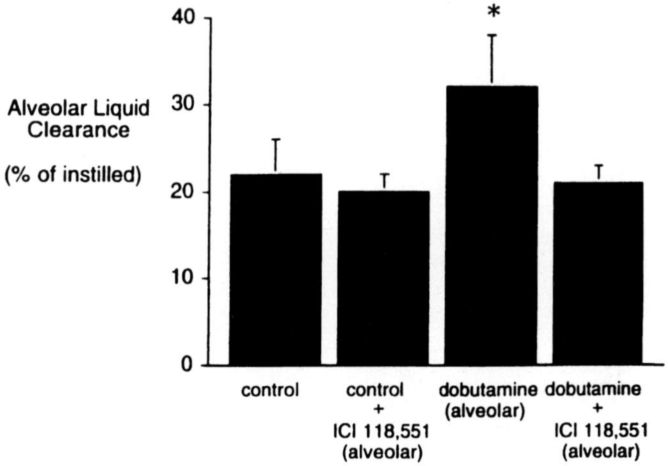

Figure 8 Effects of intra-alveolar ICI 118,551 on alveolar liquid clearance calculated from concentration of ^{125}I-albumin. ICI 118,551 10^{-4} M blocked the dobutamine effect and returned clearance to control levels. Rats given ICI 118,551 10^{-4} M alone also had alveolar liquid clearance rates similar to controls (20% ± 3%). Data shown as mean ± SD. *$P < .05$ versus control, dobutamine + ICI, and control + ICI. (From Ref. 7.)

agents, given at low doses, could be useful in selected patients with hydrostatic or increased permeability pulmonary edema as a pharmacologic treatment to increase the rate of alveolar fluid clearance. Also, dopamine and dobutamine have hemodynamic effects that may directly or indirectly favorably influence lung fluid balance. For example, dopamine can increase cardiac output and augment urine flow, thus facilitating negative fluid balance. Dobutamine lowers left atrial pressure moderately, while increasing cardiac output (Fig. 9).

G. Therapies to Enhance Repair of the Epithelial Barrier in ARDS

As discussed in the previous section, the effective recovery of lung function following acute lung injury will depend on the effective clearance of edema fluid from the lung and the reconstitution of the alveolar structure in the injured areas of the lung. Following the development of severe lung injury, there is disruption of the alveolar epithelium which is due to the death of alveolar type I cell (see Chap. 2). In some patients, the epithelial injury is associated with a fibrosing alveolitis that results in a loss of blood supply to alveoli as well as intra-alveolar fibrosis (210,211). If fibrosis develops, activated myofibroblasts from the interstitium migrate into the alveoli through gaps in the basement membrane and attach to the luminal surface of the damaged membrane.

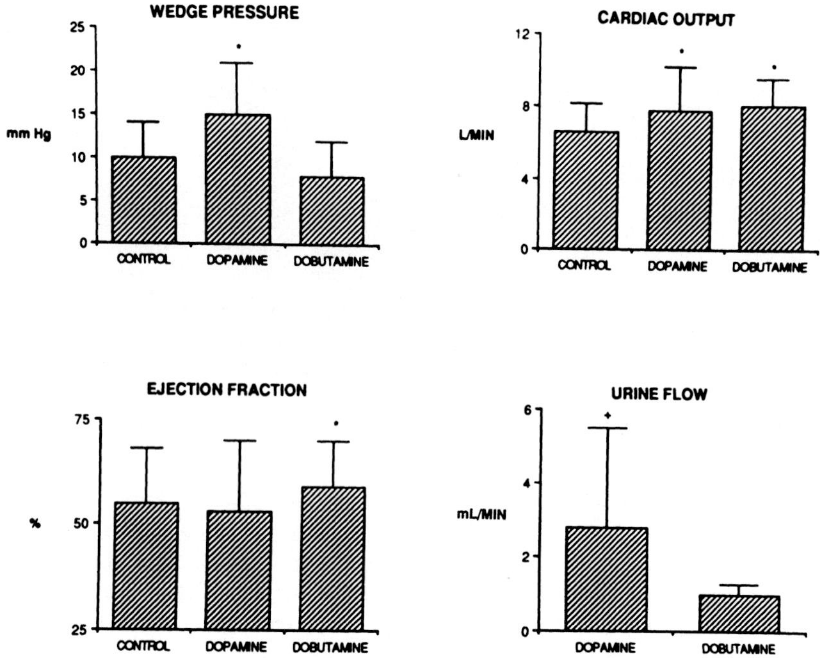

Figure 9 The effect of dobutamine (10 μg/kg/min) and dopamine (13 μg/kg/min) on hemodynamics and end-organ perfusion was studied in eight patients with the acute respiratory distress syndrome. Both dopamine and dobutamine increased cardiac output significantly. However, with dopamine therapy, pulmonary arterial wedge pressure increased by 5 mmHg. Dobutamine decreased the wedge pressure slightly, by 2 mmHg. Dobutamine, however, did not increase urine flow as effectively as dopamine, as illustrated by another study comparing the effects of dopamine and dobutamine on renal function in 12 patients after cardiac surgery. *Significant difference. (From Ref. 30.)

Myofibroblast replication at the air–lung interface eventually obliterates the gas exchange unit. This replication process is under the control of different growth factors, such as platelet-derived growth factor (PDGF) and other peptides (211,212). As part of the repair process, alveolar epithelial type II cells proliferate and provide a provisional new epithelial barrier (213). New experimental work indicates that fibronectin provides a better matrix than collagen in the lung for alveolar epithelial cell haptotaxis (214) and wound healing (215). Ideally, the alveolar epithelial proliferation would occur with a minimal fibrotic response. Interestingly, there is new clinical evidence from our studies of pulmonary edema fluid collected in the early phase of acute lung injury that collagen synthesis occurs in the early phase of ARDS (216). Thus, the patients who are destined to have a fibroproliferative response to lung injury are determined early in the course of lung injury, perhaps because the release of early pro-inflammatory cytokines, such as interleukin-1, may upregulate collagen production in fibroblasts.

The provision of a new epithelial barrier with type II cells may have beneficial effects other than the restoration of air–liquid interface. For example, re-epithelialization of the air–lung interface is associated with a gradual regression of the intra-alveolar granulation tissue, a process that has been called remodeling of the injured lung (211). There is also evidence from experimental work in our laboratory that in the subacute phase following acute lung injury with bleomycin in rats, the rate of alveolar epithelial fluid clearance is upregulated by $> 100\%$ over baseline levels. The primary mechanism for the upregulated alveolar fluid clearance appears to depend on the extensive proliferation of alveolar epithelial type II cells that occurs in the subacute phase following lung injury.

In recent years, considerable work has been devoted to the mechanisms that regulate the repair and remodeling of the injured lung. New information indicates that hepatocyte growth factor (HGF) and keratinocyte growth factor (KGF) are the major mitogens for alveolar epithelial type II cells (217). Recent animal studies indicate that intratracheal pretreatment with KGF (5 m/kg) to rats prior to the induction lung injury from acid, alpha-napthylthiourea, or bleomycin leads to a decrease in the severity of injury (218–221). The mechanism for the protection may occur from increased alveolar fluid transport from the increase in the number of alveolar type II cells or by other mechanisms including potentially a greater release of surface active material or more resistance of the alveolar epithelium to injury. The results of these studies raise the possibility that administration of KGF to patients might accelerate alveolar epithelial repair. Recent work from our clinical studies indicates that levels of KGF in the distal airspaces are < 1 ng/mL early in the course of acute lung injury, indicating that endogenous production of KGF may be low, at least early in acute lung injury. Thus, there may be therapeutic opportunity to administer KGF in the early phase of ARDS (222).

V. Summary

Treatment of ARDS remains mainly supportive since none of the new ventilatory strategies or pharmacologic treatments have been shown to reduce morbidity or mortality in controled clinical trials. However, in recent years, standard supportive therapy seems to have led to a significant decrease in the mortality of ARDS. A further decrease in mortality in ARDS should evolve from a better understanding of the mechanisms of the early inflammatory injury and the process of lung repair and remodeling, as well as from better methods to control infection and nonpulmonary organ dysfunction. There are several reasons to be guardedly optimistic regarding new therapeutic options. For example, improved methods for delivering surfactant to the injured lung in adult patients may prove to be effective in limiting the severity of respiratory failure in ARDS. Some of the new ventilatory strategies may yet prove to be beneficial, although the list of negative trials with different modes of ventilation, including extracorporeal support, is long. New anti-inflammatory strategies, such as anti-interleukin-8 therapy, may attenuate some of the early neutrophil-mediated lung injury without exposing the host to a greater risk of infection. Antioxidant therapy, currently in Phase III clinical trials, may be useful to limit both pulmonary and nonpulmonary organ injury. It may also be possible to administer an epithelial-specific mitogen to the lung, such as KGF, that could accelerate the repair process without increasing fibrosis. Finally, the new insights into the transport function of the alveolar epithelial barrier provide potential therapeutic opportunities to hasten the resolution of alveolar edema in patients with either hydrostatic or increased-permeability edema.

References

1. Osler W. The Principles and Practice of Medicine. New York; D. Appleton and Co., 1927.
2. Parmley WW, Chatterjee MB. Cardiology. Volumes 1 and 2. Philadelphia; J.B. Lippincott & Co., 1988.
3. Jasmer R, Luce JM, Matthay MA. Noninvasive positive pressure ventilation for acute respiratory failure. Chest 1997; 111:1672–1678.
4. Matthay MA, Berthiaume Y, Staub NC. Long-term clearance of liquid and protein from the lungs of unanesthetized sheep. J Appl Physiol 1985; 59:928–934.
5. Woolverton WC, Brigham KL, Staub NC. Effect of positive pressure breathing on lung lymph flow and water content in sheep. Circ Res 1978; 42:550–557.
6. Bhattacharya J, Gropper MA, Shepard JM. Lung expansion and the perialveolar interstitial pressure gradient. J Appl Physiol 1989; 66:2600–2605.
7. Tibayan FA, Chesnutt AN, Folkesson HG, Eandi J, Matthay MA. Dobutamine increases alveolar liquid clearance in ventilated rats by beta-2 receptor stimulation. Am J Respir Crit Care Med 1997; 156:438–444.
8. Barnard ML, Olivera WG, Rutschman DM, Bertorello AM, Sznajder I. Dopamine stimulates sodium transport and liquid clearance in rat lung epithelium. Am J Respir Crit Care Med 1997; 156:709–714.
9. Smith WS, Matthay MA. Evidence for a hydrostatic mechanism in human neurogenic pulmonary edema. Chest 1997; 111:1326–1333.
10. Fowler AA, Hamman RF, Good JT, Benson KN, Baird M, Eberle DJ, Petty TL, Hyers TM. Adult respiratory distress syndrome: risk with common predispositions. Ann Intern Med 1983; 98:593–597.
11. Doyle RL, Szaflarski N, Modin GW, Wiener-Kronish JP, Matthay MA. Identification of patients with acute lung injury: predictors of mortality. Am J Respir Crit Care Med 1995; 152:1818–1824.

12. Milberg JA, Davis DR, Steinberg KP, Hudson LD. Improved survival of patients with acute respiratory distress syndrome: 1983–1993. JAMA 1995; 273:306–309.
13. Montgomery AB, Stager MA, Carrico CJ, Hudson LD. Causes of mortality in patients with the adult respiratory distress syndrome. Am Rev Respir Dis 1985; 132:485–489.
14. Rubin DB, Wiener-Kronish JP, Murray JF, Green DR, Turner J, Luce JM, Montgomery AB, Marks JD, Matthay MA. Elevated von Willebrand factor antigen is an early plasma predictor of acute lung injury in nonpulmonary sepsis syndrome. J Clin Invest 1990; 86:474–480.
15. Falke KJ, Pontoppidan H, Kumar A. Ventilation with end-expiratory pressure in acute lung disease. J Clin Invest 1972; 51:2315–2323.
16. Crapo JD, Barry BE, Foscue HA, Shelburne J. Structural and biochemical changes in rat lungs occurring during exposures to lethal and adaptive doses of oxygen. Am Rev Respir Dis 1980; 122:123–143.
17. Pratt P, Vollmer R, Shelburne J, Crapo J. Pulmonary morphology in a multihospital collaborative extracorporeal membrane oxygenation project. 1. Light microscopy. Am J Pathol 1979; 95:191–214.
18. Barber RE, Lee J, Hamilton WK. Oxygen toxicity in man: a prospective study in patients with irreversible brain damage. N Engl J Med 1970; 283:1478–1484.
19. Clark JM, Lambertson CJ. Pulmonary oxygen toxicity: a review. Pharmacol Rev 1971; 23:37–133.
20. Witschi HR, Haschek WM, Klein-Szanto AJP, Hakkinen PJ. Potentiation of diffuse lung damage by oxygen: determining variables. Am Rev Respir Dis 1981; 123:98–103.
21. Cheney FW, Huang TW, Gronka R. The effects of 50% oxygen on the resolution of pulmonary injury. Am Rev Respir Dis 1980; 122:373–379.
22. Albert RK. Least PEEP: *primum non nocere.* Chest 1985; 87:2–3.
23. Ashbaugh DG, Bigelow DB, Petty TL, Levine BE. Acute respiratory distress in adults. Lancet 1967; 2:319–323.
24. Gattinoni L, Pesenti A, Avalli L. Pressure-volume curve of total respiratory system in acute respiratory failure. Am Rev Respir Dis 1987; 136:730–736.
25. Malo J, Ali J, Wood LDH. How does positive end-expiratory pressure reduce intrapulmonary shunt in canine pulmonary edema? J Appl Physiol 1984; 57:1002–1010.
26. Gattinoni L, Pesenti A, Bombino M. Relationship between lung computed tomographic density, gas exchange, and PEEP in acute respiratory failure. Anesthesiology 1988; 69:824–832.
27. Maunder RJ, Shuman WP, McHugh JW, Marglin SI, Butler J. Preservation of normal lung regions in the adult respiratory distress syndrome: analysis by computed tomography. JAMA 1986; 255:2463–2465.
28. Luce JM, Robertson HT, Huang T. The effects of expiratory positive airway pressure on the resolution of oleic acid-induced lung injury in dogs. Am Rev Respir Dis 1982; 125:716–722.
29. Pepe PE, Hudson LD, Carrico CJ. Early application of positive end-expiratory pressure in patients at risk for the adult respiratory-distress syndrome. N Engl J Med 1984; 311:281–286.

30. Broaddus VC, Berthiaume Y, Biondi JW, Matthay MA. Hemodynamic management of the adult respiratory distress syndrome. J Intens Care Med 1987; 2: 190–213.
31. Jardin F, Farcot J, Boisante L. Influence of positive end-expiratory pressure on left ventricular performance. N Engl J Med 1981; 304:387.
32. Robotham JL, Lixfeld W, Holland L. The effects of positive end-expiratory pressure on right and left ventricular performance. Am Rev Respir Dis 1980; 121: 677–683.
33. Dhainaut JF, Devaux JY, Monsallier JF. Mechanisms of decreased left ventricular preload during continuous positive pressure ventilation in ARDS. Chest 1986; 90: 74–80.
34. Fewell JE, Abendschein DR, Carlson CJ. Mechanism of decreased right and left ventricular end-diastolic volumes during continuous positive-pressure ventilation in dogs. Circ Res 1980; 47:467–472.
35. Weisman IM, Rinaldo JE, Rogers RM. Positive end-expiratory pressure in adult respiratory failure. N Engl J Med 1982; 307:1381–1384.
36. Kirby RR, Downs JB, Civetta JM. High level positive end-expiratory pressure in acute respiratory insufficiency. Chest 1975; 67:156–163.
37. Gattinoni L, D'Andrea L, Pelosi P, Vitale G, Pesenti A, Fumagalli R. Regional effects and mechanism of positive end-expiratory pressure in early adult respiratory distress syndrome. JAMA 1993; 269:2122–2127.
38. Schuster DP. The case for and against fluid restriction and occlusion pressure reduction in adult respiratory distress syndrome. New Horiz 1993; 1:478–488.
39. Prewitt RM, McCarthy J, Wood LDH. Treatment of acute low pressure pulmonary edema in dogs. J Clin Invest 1981; 67:409–418.
40. Ali J, Chernicki W, Wood LDH. Effect of furosemide in canine low-pressure pulmonary edema. J Clin Invest 1979; 64:1494–1504.
41. Huchon GJ, Hopewell PC, Murray JF. Interactions between permeability and hydrostatic pressure in perfused dogs' lungs. J Appl Physiol 1981; 50:905–911.
42. Sznajder JI, Zucker AR, Wood LDH, Long GR. The effects of plasmapheresis and hemofiltration on canine acid aspiration pulmonary edema. Am Rev Respir Dis 1986; 134:222–228.
43. Bone RC. Treatment of adult respiratory distress syndrome with diuretics, dialysis, and positive end-expiratory pressure. Crit Care Med 1978; 6:136–139.
44. Simmons RS, Berdine GG, Seidenfeld JJ, Prihoda T, Harris G, Smith J, Gilbert T, Mota E, and Johanson WG. Fluid balance and the adult respiratory distress syndrome. Am Rev Respir Dis 1987; 135:924–929.
45. Humphrey H, Hall J, Sznajder I, Silverstein M, Wood L. Improved survival in ARDS patients associated with a reduction in pulmonary capillary wedge pressure. Chest 1990; 97:1176–1180.
46. Eisenberg PR, Hansbrough JR, Anderson D, Schuster DP. A prospective study of lung water measurements during patient management in an intensive care unit. Am Rev Respir Dis 1987; 136:662–668.
47. Mitchell JP, Schuller D, Calandrino FS, Schuster DP. Improved outcome based on fluid management in critically ill patients requiring pulmonary artery catheterization. Am Rev Respir Dis 1992; 145:990–998.

48. Colley PS, Cheney FW, Hlastala MP. Ventilation-perfusion and gas exchange effects of sodium nitroprusside in dogs with normal and edematous lungs. Anesthesiology 1979; 50:489–495.
49. Prewitt RM, Wood LDH. Effect of sodium nitroprusside on cardiovascular function and pulmonary shunt in canine oleic acid pulmonary edema. Anesthesiology 1981; 55:537–541.
50. Harrison WD, Raizen M, Ghignone M, Girling L, Slykerman LJ, Prewitt RM. Treatment of canine low pressure pulmonary edema. Am Rev Respir Dis 1983; 128:857–861.
51. Bishop MJ, Kennard S, Artman LD, Cheney FW. Hydralazine does not inhibit canine hypoxic pulmonary vasoconstriction. Am Rev Respir Dis 1983; 128:998–1001.
52. Colley PS, Cheney FW, Alastala MP. Pulmonary gas exchange effects of nitroglycerin in canine edematous lungs. Anesthesiology 1981; 55:114–119.
53. Benoit A, Ducas J, Girling L. Acute cardiopulmonary effects of nitroglycerin in canine oleic acid pulmonary edema. Anesthesiology 1985; 62:754–758.
54. Holcroft JW, Vassar MJ, Weber CJ. Prostaglandin E_1 and survival in patients with the adult repiratory distress syndrome. Ann Surg 1986; 203:371–378.
55. Bone RC, Slotman G, Maunder R, Silverman H, Hyers TM, Kerstein M. Randomized doubled-blind, multicenter study of prostaglandin E_1 in patients with adult respiratory distress syndrome. Chest 1989; 96:114–119.
56. Appel PL, Shoemaker WC. Hemodynamic and oxygen transport effects of prostaglandin E_1 in patients with adult respiratory distress syndrome. Crit Care Med 1984; 12:528–529.
57. Russell JA, Ronco JJ, Dodek PM. Physiologic effects and side effects of prostaglandin E_1 in the adult respiratory distress syndrome. Chest 1990; 97:684–692.
58. Radermacher P, Santak B, Wüst HJ, Tarnow J, Falke KJ. Prostacyclin for treatment of pulmonary hypertension in the adult respiratory distress syndrome: effects on pulmonary capillary pressure and ventilation-perfusion distributions. Anesthesiology 1990; 72:238–244.
59. Meduri GU, Mauldin GL, Wunderink RG, et al. Causes of fever and pulmonary densities in patients with clinical manifestations of ventilator-associated pneumonia. Chest 1994; 106:221–235.
60. Bell RC, Calson JJ, Smith JD, Johanson WG. Multiple organ system failure and infection in adult respiratory distress syndrome. Ann Intern Med 1983; 99:293–298.
61. Seidenfeld JJ, Pohl DF, Bell RC, Harris GD, Johanson WG. Incidence, site, and outcome of infections in patients with adult respiratory distress syndrome. Am Rev Respir Dis 1986; 134:12–16.
62. Rouby J, de Lassale EM, Poete P. Nosocomial bronchopneumonia in the critically ill: histologic and bacteriologic aspects. Am Rev Respir Dis 1992; 146:1059.
63. Estes RJ, Meduri GU. The pathogenesis of ventilator-associated pneumonia. I. Mechanisms of bacterial transcolonization and airway inoculation. Intens Care Med 1995; 21:365–383.
64. Meduri GU, Estes RJ. The pathogenesis of ventilator-associated pneumonia. II. The lower respiratory tract. Intens Care Med 1995; 21:452–460.

65. Pingleton SK, Hinthorn DR, Liu C. Enteral nutrition in patients receiving mechanical ventilation. Am J Med 1986; 80:827–832.
66. Driks MR, Craven DE, Celli BR, et al. Nosocomial pneumonia in intubated patients given sucralfate as compared with antacids or histamine type 2 blockers. N Engl J Med 1987; 317:1376–1382.
67. Bonten MJM, Gaillard CA, van der Geest S, et al. The role of intragastric acidity and stress ulcer prophylaxis on colonization and infection in mechanically ventilated patients: a stratified, randomized, double blind study of sucralfate versus antacids. Am J Respir Crit Care Med 1995; 152:1825–1834.
68. Cook DJ, Fuller HD, Guyatt GH, et al. Risk factors for gastrointestinal bleeding in critically ill patients. N Engl J Med 1994; 330:377–381.
69. Heyland DK, Cook DJ, Jaeschke R, Griffith L, Lee HN, Guyatt GH. Selective decontamination of the digestive tract. Chest 1994; 105:1221–1229.
70. Alverdy JC, Aoys E, Moss GS. TPN promotes bacterial translocation from the gut. Surgery 1988; 104:185–190.
71. Fong Y, Marano MA, Barber A. TPN and bowel rest modify the metabolic response to endotoxins in humans. Ann Surg 1989; 210:449–457.
72. Cerra FB, McPherson JP, Konstantinides FN, Konstantinides KM, Teasley KM. Enteral nutrition does not prevent multiple organ failure syndrome (MOFS) after sepsis. Surgery 1988; 104:727–733.
73. Heyland DK, Cook DJ, Guyatt GH. Enteral nutrition in the critically ill patient: a critical review of the evidence. Intens Care Med 1993; 19:435–442.
74. Lewis JF, Jobe AH. Surfactant and the adult respiratory distress syndrome. Am Rev Respir Dis 1993; 147:218–233.
75. Albert RK, Lakshminarayan S, Hildebrandt J, Kirk W. Increased surface tension favors pulmonary edema formation in anesthetized dog's lungs. J Clin Invest 1979; 63:1015–1018.
76. Long W, Thompson T, Sundell H, et al. Effects of two rescue doses of a synthetic surfactant on mortality rate and survival without bronchopulmonary dysplasia in 700- to 1350-gram infants with respiratory distress syndrome. J Pediatr 1991; 118: 595–605.
77. Spragg RG, Gilliard N, Richman P, et al. Acute effects of a single dose of porcine surfactant on patients with the adult respiratory distress syndrome. Chest 1994; 105:195–202.
78. Anzueto A, Baughman RP, Guntupalli KK, et al. Aerosolized surfactant in adults with sepsis-induced acute respiratory distress syndrome. Exosurf Acute Respiratory Distress Syndrome Sepsis Study Group [see comments]. N Engl J Med 1996; 334:1417–1421.
79. Fulkerson WJ, MacIntyre N, Stamler J, Crapo JD. Pathogenesis and treatment of the adult respiratory distress syndrome. Arch Intern Med 1996; 156:29–38.
80. Zapol WM, Snider MT, Hill JD, et al. Extracorporeal membrane oxygenation in severe acute respiratory failure. JAMA 1979; 242:2193–2196.
81. Gattinoni L, Pesenti A, Bombino M, Pelosi P, Brazzi L. Role of extracorporeal circulation in adult respiratory distress syndrome management. New Horiz 1993; 1:603–612.

82. Evans TW, Keogh BF. Extracorporeal membrane oxygenation: a breath of fresh air or yesterday's treatment? Thorax 1991; 46:692–694.
83. Gattinoni L, Pesenti A, Mascheroni D, Marcolin R, Fumagalli R, Rossi F. Low frequency positive-pressure ventilation with extracorporeal CO_2 removal in severe acute respiratory failure. JAMA 1986; 256:881–886.
84. Brunet F, Mira JP, Belghith M, et al. Extracorporeal carbon dioxide removal technique improves oxygenation without causing overinflation. Am J Respir Crit Care Med 1994; 149:1557–1562.
85. Brunet F, Belghith M, Mira J-P, et al. Extracorporeal carbon dioxide removal and low-frequency positive-pressure ventilation. Chest 1993; 104:889–898.
86. Morris AH, Wallace CJ, Menlove RL, et al. Randomized clinical trial of pressure-controlled inverse ratio ventilation and extracorporeal CO_2 removal for adult respiratory distress syndrome. Am J Respir Crit Care Med 1994; 149:295–305.
87. Lamy M, Fallot RJ, Koeniger E, Dietrich H, Ratliff J, Eberhart R. Pathologic features and mechanisms of hypoxemia in adult respiratory distress syndrome. Am Rev Respir Dis 1976; 114:267–284.
88. Webb HH, Tierney DF. Experimental pulmonary edema due to intermittent positive pressure ventilation with high inflation pressures. Protection by positive end-expiratory pressure. Am Rev Respir Dis 1974; 110:556–565.
89. Kolobow T, Moretti MP, Fumagalli R, et al. Severe impairment in lung function induced by high peak airway pressure during mechanical ventilation. Am Rev Respir Dis 1987; 135:312–325.
90. Dreyfuss D, Soler P, Saumon G. Spontaneous resolution of pulmonary edema caused by short periods of cyclic overinflation. J Appl Physiol 1992; 72:2081–2089.
91. Dreyfuss D, Saumon G. Deleterious effects of mechanical ventilation on the lower lung. Rev Mal Respir 1995; 12:551–557.
92. Dreyfuss D, Soler P, Saumon G. Mechanical ventilation-induced pulmonary edema. Interaction with previous lung alterations. Am J Respir Crit Care Med 1995; 151:1568–1575.
93. Corbridge TC, Wood LDH, Crawford GP, Chudoba MJ, Yanos J, Sznajder JI. Adverse effects of large tidal volume and low PEEP in canine acid aspiration. Am Rev Respir Dis 1990; 142:311–315.
94. Marini JJ, Kelsen SG. Re-targeting ventilatory objectives in adult respiratory distress syndrome. New treatment prospects—persistent question. Am Rev Respir Dis 1992; 146:2–3.
95. Tuxen DV. Permissive hypercapnic ventilation. Am J Respir Crit Care Med 1994; 150:870–874.
96. Bidani A, Tzouanakis AE, Cardenas VJJ, Zwischenberger JB. Permissive hypercapnia in acute respiratory failure. JAMA 1994; 272:957–962.
97. Hickling KG. Permissive hypercapnia in ARDS: current concepts. Intens Care World 1995; 12:121–130.
98. Hickling KG, Henderson SJ, Jackson R. Low mortality associated with low volume pressure limited ventilation with permissive hypercapnia in severe adult respiratory distress syndrome. Intens Care Med 1990; 16:372–377.

99. Hickling KG, Walsh J, Henderson S, Jackson R. Low mortality rate in adult respiratory distress syndrome using low-volume, pressure-limited ventilation with permissive hypercapnia: a prospective study. Crit Care Med 1994; 22:1568–1578.
99a. Amato M, Barbos C, Medeiros D, et al. Effect of a protective ventilation strategy on mortality in the acute respiratory distress syndrome. N Engl J Med 1998; 338: 347–354.
100. Slutsky AS. Nonconventional methods of ventilation. Am Rev Respir Dis 1988; 138:175–183.
101. Standiford TJ, Morganroth ML. High-frequency ventilation—reviews. Chest 1989; 96:1380–1389.
102. Gluck E, Heard S, Patel C, Mohr J, Calkins J. Use of ultrahigh frequency ventilation in patients with ARDS. Chest 1993; 103:1413–1420.
103. Younes M. Proportional assist ventilation, a new approach to ventilatory support. Am Rev Respir Dis 1992; 145:114–120.
104. Younes M, Puddy A, Roberts D, et al. Proportional assist ventilation. Am Rev Respir Dis 1992; 145:121–123.
105. Marcy TW, Marini JJ. Inverse ratio ventilation in ARDS—rationale and implementation. Chest 1991; 100:494–504.
106. Boros S. Variations in inspiratory: expiratory ratio and airway pressure wave form during mechanical ventilation: the significance of mean airway pressure. J Pediatr 1979; 94:114–117.
107. Ciszek T, Modanlou H, Owings D, Nelson P. Mean airway pressure—significance during mechanical ventilation in neonates. J Pediatr 1981; 99:121–126.
108. Gattinoni L, Marcolin R, Caspani M, Fumagalli R, Mascheroni D, Pesenti A. Constant mean airway pressure with different patterns of positive pressure breathing during the adult respiratory distress syndrome. Bull Eur Physiopathol Respir 1985; 21:275–279.
109. Pesenti A, Marcolin R, Prato P, Borelli M, Riboni A, Gattinoni L. Mean airway pressure vs positive end-expiratory pressure during mechanical ventilation. Crit Care Med 1985; 13:34–37.
110. Hinson JR, Marini JJ. Principles of mechanical ventilator use in respiratory failure. Annu Rev Med 1992; 43:341–361.
111. Cole AGH, Weller SF, Sykes MK. Inverse ratio ventilation compared with PEEP in adult respiratory failure. Intens Care Med 1984; 10:227–232.
112. Tharratt RS, Allen RP, Albertson TE. Pressure controlled inverse ratio ventilation in severe adult respiratory failure. Chest 1988; 94:755–762.
113. Lain DC, DiBenedetto R, Morris SL, Nguyem AV, Saulters R, Causey D. Pressure controlled inverse ratio ventilation as a method to reduce peak inspiratory pressure and provide adequate oxygenation and ventilation. Chest 1989; 95:1081–1088.
114. East TD, Böhm SH, Wallace CJ, et al. A successful computerized protocol for clinical management of pressure control inverse ratio ventilation in ARDS patients. Chest 1992; 101:697–710.
115. Lessard MR, Guérot E, Lorino H, Lemaire F, Brochard L. Effects of pressure-controlled with different I:E ratios versus volume-controlled ventilation on respiratory mechanics, gas exchange, and hemodynamics in patients with adult respiratory distress syndrome. Anesthesiology 1994; 80:983–991.

116. Chan K, Abraham E. Effects of inverse ratio ventilation on cardiorespiratory parameters in severe respiratory failure. Chest 1992; 102:1556–1561.
117. Mercat A, Graïni L, Teboul J-L, Lenique F, Richard C. Cardiorespiratory effects of pressure-controlled ventilation with and without inverse ratio in the adult respiratory distress syndrome. Chest 1993; 104:871–875.
118. Hansen-Flaschen J, Cowen J, Raps EC. Neuromuscular blockade in the intensive care unit. Am Rev Respir Dis 1993; 147:234–236.
119. Degraeuwe PL, Vos GD, Blanco CE. Perfluorochemical liquid ventilation: from the animal laboratory to the intensive care unit. Int J Artif Organs 1995; 18: 674–683.
120. Papo MC, Paczan PR, Fuhrman BP, et al. Perfluorocarbon-associated gas exchange improves oxygenation, lung mechanics, and survival in a model of adult respiratory distress syndrome. Crit Care Med 1996; 24:466–474.
121. Tütüncü AS, Faithfull NS, Lachmann B. Intratracheal perfluorocarbon administration combined with mechanical ventilation in experimental respiratory distress syndrome: dose-dependent improvement of gas exchange. Crit Care Med 1993; 21:962–969.
122. Hernan LJ, Fuhrman BP, Kaiser RE, et al. Perfluorocarbon-associated gas exchange in normal and acid-injured large sheep. Crit Care Med 1996; 24:475–481.
123. Hirschl RB, Tooley R, Parent A, Johnson K, Bartlett RH. Evaluation of gas exchange, pulmonary compliance, and lung injury during total and partial liquid ventilation in the acute respiratory distress syndrome. Crit Care Med 1996; 24: 1001–1008.
124. Overbeck MC, Pranikoff T, Yadao CM, Hirschl RB. Efficacy of perfluorocarbon partial liquid ventilation in a large animal model of acute respiratory failure. Crit Care Med 1996; 24:1208–1214.
125. Hirschl RB, Pranikoff T, Wise C, et al. Initial experience with partial liquid ventilation in adult patients with the acute respiratory distress syndrome. JAMA 1996; 275:383–389.
126. Gauger PG, Pranikoff T, Schreiner RJ, Moler FW, Hirschl RB. Initial experience with partial liquid ventilation in pediatric patients with the acute respiratory distress syndrome. Crit Care Med 1996; 24:16–22.
127. Lowe-Leach C, Greenspan JS, Rubenstein SD, et al. Partial liquid ventilation with Perflubron in premature infants with severe respiratory distress syndrome. N Engl J Med 1996; 335:761–767.
128. Douglas WW, Rehder K, Beynen RM, Sessler AD, Marsh HM. Improved oxygenation in patients with acute respiratory failure: the prone position. Am Rev Respir Dis 1977; 115:559–566.
129. Langer M, Mascheroni D, Marcolin R, Gattinoni L. The prone position in ARDS patients. A clinical study. Chest 1988; 94:103–107.
130. Gattioni L, Pelosi P, Vitale G, Pesenti A, D'Andrea L, Mascheroni D. Body positive changes redistribute lung computed-tomography density in patients with acute respiratory failure. Anesthesiology 1991; 74:15–23.
131. Lamm WJ, Graham MM, Albert RK. Mechanism by which the prone position improves oxygenation in acute lung injury. Am J Respir Crit Care Med 1994; 150:184–193.

132. Pape H-C, Regel G, Borgman W, Sturm JA, Tscherne H. The effect of kinetic positioning on lung function and pulmonary haemodynamics in posttraumatic ARDS: a clinical study. Injury 1994; 25:51–57.
133. Rossaint R, Pison U, Gerlach H, Falke KJ. Inhaled nitric oxide: its effects on pulmonary circulation and airway smooth muscle cells. Eur Heart J 1993; 14(suppl 1):133–140.
134. Zapol WM, Hurford WE. Inhaled nitric oxide in the adult respiratory distress syndrome and other lung diseases. New Horiz 1993; 1:638–650.
135. Garat C, Jayr C, Eddahibi S, Laffon M, Meignan M, Adnot S. Effects of inhaled nitric oxide or inhibition of endogenous nitric oxide formation on hyperoxic lung injury. Am J Respir Crit Care Med 1997; 155:1957–1964.
136. McElroy MC, Wiener-Kronish JP, Miyazaki H, Sawa T, Modelska K, Dobbs LG, Pittet JF. Nitric oxide attenuates lung endothelial injury caused by sublethal hyperoxia in rats. Am J Physiol (Lung Cell Mol Physiol) 1997; 272:L631–L638.
137. Kavanagh BP, Mouchawar A, Goldsmith J, Pearl RG. Effects of inhaled NO and inhibition of endogenous NO synthesis in oxidant-induced acute lung injury. J Appl Physiol 1994; 76:1324–1329.
138. Pryor WA, Squadrito GL. The chemistry of peroxynitrite: a product from the reaction of nitric oxide and superoxide. Am J Physiol (Lung Cell Mol Physiol) 1995; 268:L699–L722.
139. Matalon S, De Marco V, Haddad C, et al. Inhaled nitric oxide injures the pulmonary surfactant systems of lamb in vivo. Am J Physiol (Lung Cell Mol Physiol) 1996; 270:L273–L280.
140. Frostell C, Fratacci MD, Wain JC. Inhaled nitric oxide: a selective pulmonary vasodilator reversing hypoxic pulmonary vasoconstriction. Circulation 1991; 83: 2038–2047.
141. Fratacci MD, Frostell C, Chen TY. Inhaled nitric oxide: a selective pulmonary vasodilator of heparin-protamine vasoconstriction in sheep. Anesthesiology 1991; 75:990–999.
142. Shah NS, Nakayama DK, Jacob TD, et al. Efficacy of inhaled nitric oxide in a porcine model of adult respiratory distress syndrome. Arch Surg 1994; 129:158–164.
143. Rossaint R, Falke KJ, Lopez F, Slama K, Pison U, Zapol WM. Inhaled nitric oxide for the adult respiratory distress syndrome. N Engl J Med 1993; 328:399–405.
144. Dellinger RP, Zimmerman JL, Taylor RW, Straube RC, Hauser D, Criner G, Davis K, Hyers TM, and Papadaros P. Effects of inhaled nitric oxide in patients with acute respiratory distress syndrome: results of a randomized phase 2 trial. Crit Care Med 1998; 26:15–23.
145. Wysocki M, Delclaux C, Roupie E, et al. Additive effect on gas exchange of inhaled nitric oxide and intravenous almitrine bismesylate in the adult respiratory distress syndrome. Intens Care Med 1994; 20:254–259.
146. Walmrath D, Schneider T, Schermuly R, Olschewski H, Grimminger F, Seeger W. Direct comparison of inhaled nitric oxide and aerosolized prostacyclin in acute respiratory distress syndrome. Am J Respir Crit Care Med 1996; 153:991–996.
147. Bone RC, Balk R, Slotman G, et al. Adult respiratory distress syndrome—sequence and importance of development of multiple organ failure. Chest 1992; 101:320–326.

148. Suchyta MR, Clemmer TP, Elliott CG, Orme JF Jr, Weaver LK. The adult respiratory distress syndrome. A report of survival and modifying factors. Chest 1992; 101:1074–1079.
149. Bone RC, Balk RA, Cerra FB, Dellinger RP. Definitions for sepsis and organ failure and guidelines for the use of innovative therapies in sepsis. Chest 1992; 101:1644–1655.
150. Cerra FB. Evolving concepts in multiple organ failure syndrome. In: Kinney JM, Tucker HN, eds. Organ Metabolism and Nutrition: Ideas for Future Critical Care. New York: Raven Press Ltd., 1994:457–480.
151. Shoemaker WC, Appel PL, Bishop MH. Temporal patterns of blood volume, hemodynamics, and oxygen transport in pathogenesis and therapy of postoperative adult respiratory distress syndrome. New Horiz 1993; 1:522–537.
152. Consensus conference. Tissue hypoxia. How to detect, how to correct, how to prevent. Am J Respir Crit Care Med 1996; 154:1573–1578.
153. Dantzker DR, Foresman B, Gutierrez G. Pulmonary perspective—oxygen supply and utilization relationships a reealuation. Am Rev Respir Dis 1991; 143:675–679.
154. Hanique G, Dugernier T, Laterre PF, Dougnac A, Roeseler J, Reynaert MS. Significance of pathologic oxygen supply dependency in critically ill patients: comparison between measured and calculated methods. Intens Care Med 1994; 20: 12–18.
155. Phang PT, Cunningham KF, Ronco JJ, Wiggs BR, Russell JA. Mathematical coupling explains dependence of oxygen consumption on oxygen delivery in ARDS. Am J Respir Crit Care Med 1994; 150:318–323.
156. Russell JA, Phang PT. The oxygen delivery/consumption controversy. Am J Respir Crit Care Med 1994; 149:533–537.
157. Schoemaker WC, Appel PL, Kram HB, Waxman K, Lee TS. Prospective trial of supranormal values of survivors as therapeutic goals in high-risk surgical patients. Chest 1988; 94:1176–1186.
158. Boyd O, Grouds M, Bennett ED. A randomized clinical trial of the effect of deliberate perioperative increase of oxygen delivery on mortality in high-risk surgical patients. JAMA 1993; 270:2699–2707.
159. Berlauk JF, Abrams JH, Gilmour IJ, O'Connor SR, Knighton DR, Cerra FB. Preoperative optimization of cardiovascular hemodynamics improves outcome in peripheral vascular surgery. Ann Surg 1991; 214:289–299.
160. Fleming A, Bishop M, Schoemaker WC, et al. Prospective trial of supranormal values as goals of resuscitation in severe trauma. Arch Surg 1992; 127:1175–1181.
161. Bishop MH, Shoemaker WC, Appel PL, et al. Prospective randomized trial of survivor values of cardiac index, oxygen delivery, and oxygen consumption as resuscitation endpoints in severe trauma. J Trauma 1995; 38:780–787.
162. Yu M, Levy MM, Smith P, Takiguchi SA, Miyasaki A. Effect of maximizing oxygen delivery on morbidity and mortality rates in critically ill patients: a propective, randomized, controlled study. Crit Care Med 1993; 21:830–838.
163. Tuchschmidt J, Fried J, Astiz M, Rackow E. Elevation of cardiac output and oxygen delivery improves outcome in septic shock. Chest 1992; 102: 216–220.

164. Hayes MA, Timmins AC, Yau EHS, Palazzo M, Hinds CJ, Watson D. Elevation of systemic oxygen delivery in the treatment of critically ill patients. N Engl J Med 1994; 330:1717–1722.
165. Pittet JF, MacKersie RC, Martin TR, Matthay MA. Biological markers of acute lung injury: prognostic and pathogenetic significance. Am J Respir Crit Care Med 1997; 155:1187–1205.
166. Bachofen H, Bachofen M, Weibel ER. Ultrastructural aspects of pulmonary edema. J Thorac Imag 1988; 3:1–7.
167. Anderson WR, Thielen K. Correlative study of adult respiratory distress syndrome by light, scanning, and transmission electron microscopy. Ultrastruct Pathol 1992; 16:615–628.
168. Sprung CL, Caralis PV, Marcial EH, et al. The effects of high-dose corticosteroids in patients with septic shock. N Engl J Med 1984; 311:1137–1143.
169. Luce JM, Montgomery BA, Marks JD, Turner J, Metz CA, Murray JF. Ineffectiveness of high-dose methylprednisolone in preventing parenchymal lung injury and improving mortality in patients with septic shock. Am Rev Respir Dis 1988; 136:62–68.
170. Bernard GR, Luce JM, Sprung CL, et al. High-dose corticosteroids in patients with the adult repiratory distress syndrome. N Engl J Med 1987; 317:1565–1570.
171. Bernard G. Sepsis trials. Intersection of investigation, regulation, funding and practice. Am J Respir Crit Care Med 1995; 152:4–10.
172. Bernard GR, Wheeler AP, Russell JA, et al. The effects of ibuprofen on the physiology and survival of patients with sepsis. N Engl J Med 1997; 336:912–918.
173. Bone RC, Fisher C, Clemmer TP, Slotman GJ, Metz CA, and the Methylprednisolone Severe Sepsis Study Group. Early methylprednisolone treatment for septic syndrome and the adult respiratory distress syndrome. Chest 1987; 92:1032–1036.
174. Meduri GU, Belenchia JM, Estes RJ, Wunderink RG, El Torky M, Leeper KV Jr. Fibroproliferative phase of ARDS—clinical findings and effects of corticosteroids. Chest 1991; 100:943–952.
175. Meduri GU, Chinn AJ, Leeper KV, et al. Corticosteroid rescue treatment of progressive fibroproliferation in late ARDS. Chest 1994; 105:1516–1527.
176. Bernard GR, Lucht WD, Niedermeyer ME, Snapper JR, Ogletree ML, Brigham KL. Effect of N-acetylcysteine on the pulmonary response to endotoxin in the awake sheep and upon in vitro granulocyte function. J Clin Invest 1984; 73:1772–1784.
177. Quinlan GJ, Lamb NJ, Tilley R, et al. Plasma hypoxanthine levels in ARDS: implications for oxidative stress, morbidity, and mortality. Am J Respir Crit Care Med 1997; 155:479–484.
178. Jepsen S, Herlevsen P, Knudsen P, Bud MI, Klausen N-O. Antioxidant treatment with N-acetylcysteine during adult respiratory distress syndrome: a prospective, randomized, placebo-controlled study. Crit Care Med 1992; 20:918–923.
179. Spies CD, Reinhart K, Witt I, et al. Influence of N-acetylcysteine on indirect indicators of tissue oxygenation in septic shock patients: results from a prospective, randomized, double-blind study. Crit Care Med 1994; 22:1738–1746.

180. Yu M, Tomasa G. A double-blind, prospective, randomized trial of ketoconazole, a thromboxane synthetase inhibitor, in the prophylaxis of the adult respiratory distress syndrome. Crit Care Med 1993; 21:1635–1642.
181. Welsh CH, Lien D, Worthen GS, Weil JV. Pentoxifylline decreases endotoxin-induced pulmonary neutrophil sequestration and extravascular protein accumulation in the dog. Am Rev Respir Dis 1988; 138:1106–1114.
182. Seear MD, Hannam VL, Kaapa P, Raj JU, O'Brodovich HM. Effect of pentoxifylline on hemodynamics, alveolar fluid reabsorption and pulmonary in a model of acute lung injury. Am Rev Respir Dis 1990; 141:1083–1087.
183. Kudoh I, Ohtake M, Nishizawa H, Pittet JF, Wiener-Kronish JP. The effect of pentoxifylline on acid-induced alveolar epithelial injury. Anesthesiology 1995; 82: 531–541.
184. Hogg JC, Doerschuk CM. Leukocyte traffic in the lung. Annu Rev Physiol 1995; 57:97–114.
185. Folkesson HG, Matthay MA, Hébert CA, Broaddus VC. Acid aspiration induced lung injury in rabbits is mediated by interleukin-8 dependent mechanisms. J Clin Invest 1995; 96:107–116.
186. Miller EJ, Cohen AB, Nagao S, Griffith D, Maunder R, Martin TR, Wiener-Kronish JP, Sticherling M, Christophers E, Matthay MA. Elevated levels of NAP-1/interleukin-8 are present in the airspaces of patients with the adult respiratory distress syndrome and are associated with increased mortality. Am Rev Respir Dis 1992; 146:427–432.
187. Chollet-Martin S, Montravers P, Gilbert C, et al. High levels of interleukin-8 in the blood and alveolar spaces of patients with pneumonia and adult respiratory distress syndrome. Infect Immun 1993; 51:4553–4559.
188. Donnelly TJ, Meade P, Jagels M, et al. Cytokine, complement, and endotoxin profiles associated with the development of the adult respiratory distress syndrome after severe injury. Crit Care Med 1994; 22:768–776.
189. Donnelly SC, Strieter RM, Kunkel SL, et al. Interleukin-8 and development of adult respiratory distress syndrome in at-risk patient groups. Lancet 1993; 341: 643–647.
190. Miller EJ, Cohen AB, Matthay MA. Increased interleukin-8 concentrations in the pulmonary edema fluid of patients with acute respiratory distress syndrome from sepsis. Crit Care Med 1996; 24:1448–1454.
191. Montaner JSG, Tsang J, Evans KG, et al. Alveolar epithelial damage. J Clin Invest 1986; 77:1786–1796.
192. Matthay NM, Wiener-Kronish JP. Intact epithelial barrier function is critical for the resolution of alveolar edema in humans. Am Rev Respir Dis 1990; 142:1250–1257.
193. Wiener-Kronish JP, Albertine KH, Matthay MA. Differential responses of the endothelial and epithelial barriers of the lung in sheep to *Escherichia coli* endotoxin. J Clin Invest 1991; 88:864–875.
194. Pittet JF, Wiener-Kronish JP, McElroy MC, Folkesson HG, Matthay MA. Stimulation of lung epithelial liquid clearance by endogenous release of catecholamines in septic shock in anesthetized rats. J Clin Invest 1994; 94:663–671.

195. Pittet JF, Wiener-Kronish JP, Serikov V, Matthay MA. Resistance of the alveolar epithelium to injury from septic shock in sheep. Am J Respir Crit Care Med 1995; 151:1093–1100.
196. Nici L, Dowin R, Gilmore-Hebert M, Jamieson JD, Ingbar DH. Upregulation of rat lung Na-K-ATPase during hyperoxic injury. Am J Physiol (Lung Cell Mol Physiol) 1991; 261:L307–L314.
197. Carter EP, Duvick SE, Wendt CH, Wangensteen D, Ingbar DL. Hyperoxia increases active alveolar Na^+ resorption in vivo and type II cell Na,K,ATPase in vitro. Chest 1994; 105(suppl 3):75S–78S.
198. Olivera WG, Ridge KM, Sznajder JI. Lung liquid clearance and Na,K-ATPase during acute hyperoxia and recovery in rats. Am J Respir Crit Care Med 1995; 152:1229–1234.
199. Sznajder JI, Olivera WG, Ridge KM, Rutschman DH. Mechanisms of lung liquid clearance during hyperoxia in isolated rat lungs. Am J Respir Crit Care Med 1995; 151:1519–1525.
200. Yue G, Russell WJ, Benos DJ, Jackson RM, Olman MA, Matalon S. Increased expression and activity of sodium channels in alveolar type II cells of hyperoxic rats. Proc Natl Acad Sci USA 1995; 92:8418–8422.
201. Olivera W, Ridge K, Wood Ld, Sznajder JI. Active sodium transport and alveolar epithelial Na-K-ATPase increase during subacute hyperoxia in rats. Am J Physiol (Lung Cell Mol Physiol) 1994; 266:L577–L584.
202. Cunningham A, Hurley J. Alpha-napthyl-thiourea induced pulmonary edema in the rat: a topographical and electron-microscope study. J Pathol 1972; 106:25–35.
203. Schultz SG, Hudson RL. How do sodium-absorbing cells do their job and survive? NIPS 1986; 1:185–189.
204. Cheek JM, Kim K-J, Crandall ED. Tight monolayers of rat alveolar epithelial cells: bioelectric properties and active sodium transport. Am J Physiol 1989; 256: C688–C693.
205. Zuege D, Suzuki S, Berthiaume Y. Increase of lung sodium-potassium-ATPase activity during recovery from high-permeability pulmonary edema. Am J Physiol 1997. In press.
206. Matthay MA, Folkesson HG, Verkman AS. Salt and water transport across alveolar and distal airway epithelia in the adult lung. Am J Physiol (Lung Cell Mol Physiol) 1996; 270:L487–L503.
207. Sakuma T, Folkesson HG, Suzuki S, Okanina G, Fujimara S, Matthay MA. Beta-adrenergic agonist stimulated alveolar fluid clearance in *ex vivo* human and rat lungs. Am J Respir Crit Care Med 1997; 155:506–512.
208. Garat C, Meignan M, Matthay MA, Luo DF, Jayr C. Alveolar epithelial fluid clearance mechanisms are intact after moderate hyperoxic lung injury in rats. Chest 1997; 111:1381–1388.
209. Lasnier JM, Wangenstein DD, Schmitz LS, Wangensteen D, Ingbar DL. Terbutaline stimulates alveolar fluid resorption in hyperoxic lung injury. J Appl Physiol 1996; 81:1783–1789.
210. Snyder LS, Hertz MI, Harmon KR, Bitterman PB. Failure of lung repair following acute lung injury—regulation of the fibroproliferative response Part 1. Chest 1990; 96:733–738.

211. Snyder LS, Hertz MI, Peterson MS, Bitterman PB. Acute lung injury: pathogenesis of intraalveolar fibrosis. J Clin Invest 1991; 88:663–673.
212. Kheradmand F, Folkesson HG, Shum L, Derynk R, Pytela R, Matthay MA. Transforming growth factor-a enhances alveolar epithelial cell repair in a new *in vitro* model. Am J Physiol (Lung Cell Mol Physiol) 1994; 267:L728–L738.
213. Adamson IY, Young L. Alveolar type II cell growth on a pulmonary endothelial extracellular matrix. Am J Physiol (Lung Cell Mol Physiol) 1996; 270:L1017–L1022.
214. Kim HJ, Henke CA, Savik SK, Ingbar DH. Integrin mediation of alveolar epithelial cell migration on fibronectin and type I collagen. Am J Physiol (Lung Cell Mol Physiol) 1997; 273:L134–L141.
215. Garat C, Kheradmand F, Albertine KH, Folkesson HG, Matthay MA. Soluble and insoluble fibronectin increases alveolar epithelial wound healing in vitro. Am J Physiol (Lung Cell Mol Physiol) 1996; 271:L844–L853.
216. Chesnutt AN, Matthay MA, Tibayan FA, Clark JG. Early detection of type III procollagen peptide in acute lung injury: pathogenetic and prognostic significance. Am J Respir Crit Care Med 1997; 156:840–845.
217. Ulich T, Yi E, Longmuir K. Keratinocyte growth factor is a growth factor for type II pneumocytes *in vivo.* J Clin Invest 1994; 93:1298–1306.
218. Panos RJ, Bak PM, Simonet WS, Rubin JS, Smith LJ. Intratracheal instillation of keratinocyte growth factor decreases hyperoxia-induced mortality in rats. J Clin Invest 1995; 96:2026–2033.
219. Mason CM, Guery BPH, Summer WR, Nelson S. Keratinocyte growth factor attenuates lung leak induced by alpha-naphthylthiourea in rats. Crit Care Med 1996; 24:925–931.
220. Yano T, Deterding RR, Simonet WJ, Shannon JM, Mason RJ. Keratinocyte growth factor reduces lung damage due to acid instillation in rats. Am J Respir Cell Mol Biol 1996; 15:433–442.
221. Yi ES, Williams ST, Lee H, Malicki DM, Chin EM, Yin S, Tarpley J, Ulich TR. Keratinocyte growth factor ameliorates radiation- and bleomycin-induced lung injury and mortality. Am J Pathol 1996; 149:1963–1970.
222. Matuschak GM, Lechner AJ. Targeting the alveolar epithelium in acute lung injury: keratinocyte growth factor and regulation of the alveolar epithelial barrier [editorial; comment]. Crit Care Med 1996; 24:905–907.

INDEX

A

B

C

D

E

F

G

H

I

R

S